INFECTIOUS DISEASE SECRETS

INFECTIOUS DISEASE SECRETS

ROBERT H. GATES, MD
Associate Clinical Professor of Medicine
Department of Medicine
University of Hawaii at Manoa
John A. Burns School of Medicine
Honolulu, Hawaii

HANLEY & BELFUS, INC./ Philadelphia

Publisher: HANLEY & BELFUS, INC.
Medical Publishers
210 South 13th Street
Philadelphia, PA 19107
(215) 546-7293; 800-962-1892
FAX (215) 790-9330
Web site: http://www.hanleyandbelfus.com

Disclaimer: The opinions or assertions contained in this book are the private views of the authors and are not to be construed as reflecting the views of the Department of the Army, the Department of the Navy, or the Department of Defense.

Library of Congress Cataloging-in-Publication Data

Infectious Disease Secrets / |edited by| Robert H. Gates.
      p.   cm.—(The Secrets Series®)
    Includes bibliographical references and index.
    ISBN 1-56053-266-1 (alk. paper)
    1. Infection—Miscellanea.   2. Communicable diseases—Miscellanea.
  I. Gates, Robert H., 1951–   .   II. Series.
    |DNLM: 1. Communicable Diseases examination questions.
   2. Infection examination questions.   WC 18.2 I43 1998|
RC112.I459 1998
616.9′076—dc21
DNLM/DLC
for Library of Congress   97-42429
                                                      CIP

INFECTIOUS DISEASE SECRETS   ISBN 1-56053-266-1

Last digit is the print number: 9 8 7 6 5 4 3 2 1

CONTENTS

CONTRIBUTORS

David M. Bamberger, M.D.
Professor of Medicine, Section of Infectious Diseases, University of Missouri–Kansas City School of Medicine, Kansas City, Missouri

H. James Beecham III, M.D.
Head, Department of Tropical Medicine, U.S. Navy Environmental and Preventive Medicine Unit No. 6, Pearl Harbor, and Tripler Army Medical Center and University of Hawaii School of Public Health, Honolulu, Hawaii

Benjamin W. Berg, M.D.
Assistant Professor of Medicine, John A. Burns School of Medicine, University of Hawaii, and Chief, Pulmonary and Critical Care Medicine, Tripler Army Medical Center, Honolulu, Hawaii

W. Michael Botkin, M.D.
Chief, Dermatology Service, Department of Medicine, Tripler Army Medical Center, Honolulu, Hawaii

Joel D. Brown, M.D., DTMH, FACP
Professor of Medicine, John A. Burns School of Medicine, University of Hawaii, Associate Director of Medical Education, Queens Medical Center, and Chief, Infectious Diseases Service, Department of Medicine, Tripler Army Medical Center, Honolulu, Hawaii

William J. Burman, M.D.
Assistant Professor, Division of Infectious Diseases, Department of Medicine, University of Colorado School of Medicine and Denver Health Medical Center, Denver, Colorado

Norman Bussell, D.O., Ph.D.
Fellow, Infectious Diseases, Department of Medicine, Walter Reed Army Medical Center, Washington, DC

Paul J. Carson, M.D.
Assistant Professor of Medicine, Division of Infectious Diseases, Department of Internal Medicine, University of North Dakota School of Medicine and Health Sciences and MeritCare Hospital, Fargo, North Dakota

Carmen D. Cetrone, D.O.
Department of Pediatrics, Wilford Hall Air Force Medical Center, San Antonio, Texas

David L. Cohn, M.D.
Professor of Medicine, Division of Infectious Diseases, Department of Medicine, University of Colorado School of Medicine, Denver Public Health, and Denver Health Medical Center, Denver, Colorado

Berjan Collin, M.D.
Infectious Disease Fellow, Division of Infectious Diseases, Department of Internal Medicine, University of Florida School of Medicine, Gainesville, Florida

Eric A. Crawley, M.D.
Division of Pulmonary Medicine, Department of Pulmonary and Critical Care Medicine, Walter Reed Army Medical Center, Washington, DC

Sammi Dali, M.D.
Department of Medicine, William Beaumont Army Medical Center, El Paso, Texas

Jennifer S. Daly, M.D.
Associate Professor of Medicine, University of Massachusetts School of Medicine, and Division of Infectious Diseases and Immunology, Department of Medicine, University of Massachusetts Medical Center, Worcester, Massachusetts

Cecilia I. Del Moral, M.D.
Department of Internal Medicine, William Beaumont Army Medical Center, El Paso, Texas

Denise M. Demers, M.D.
Clinical Assistant Professor, University of Texas–San Antonio School of Medicine, and Chief, Pediatric Infectious Disease Service, Department of Pediatrics, Brooke Army Medical Center, San Antonio, Texas

Chandra Dommaraju, M.D.
Staff Physician, Department of Medicine, Veterans Affairs Medical Center, St. Louis, Missouri

David P. Dooley, M.D.
Chief, Infectious Disease Service, Brooke Army Medical Center, Fort Sam Houston, Texas

James E. Egan, M.D.
Chief, Gastroenterology Service, Department of Medicine, Tripler Army Medical Center, Honolulu, Hawaii

Richard T. Ellison III, M.D.
Professor of Medicine, Molecular Genetics, and Microbiology, University of Massachusetts Medical School, and Clinical Director of Infectious Diseases, Division of Infectious Diseases, University of Massachusetts Medical Center, Worcester, Massachusetts

Lonnie R. Empey, M.D.
Staff Physician, Department of Internal Medicine, Ireland Army Community Hospital, Fort Knox, Kentucky

Joseph C. English III, M.D.
Staff Physician, Dermatology Service, Evans Army Community Hospital, Fort Carson, Colorado

Raymond J. Enzenauer, M.D., FACP
Assistant Chief, Rheumatology Service, Brooke Army Medical Center, Fort Sam Houston, Texas

E. Dale Everett, M.D.
Professor of Medicine, Division of Infectious Diseases, Department of Internal Medicine, University of Missouri–Columbia School of Medicine, Columbia, Missouri

Karen Fagin, M.D.
Infectious Disease Fellow, Section of Infectious Diseases, Department of Medicine, Medical College of Georgia, Augusta, Georgia

Ferric C. Fang, M.D.
Assistant Professor of Medicine, Pathology, and Microbiology, University of Colorado School of Medicine, and Director, Clinical Microbiology Laboratory, University of Colorado Health Sciences Center, Denver, Colorado

Mary Beth Fasano, M.D., M.S.P.H.
Assistant Professor of Medicine and Pediatrics, Section of Infectious Diseases, Department of Internal Medicine, Wake Forest University School of Medicine, Winston-Salem, North Carolina

Tomas M. Ferguson, M.D.
Infectious Disease Service, Department of Internal Medicine, Brooke Army Medical Center, Ft. Sam Houston, Texas

Joel T. Fishbain, M.D.
Infectious Disease Service, Department of Medicine, Tripler Army Medical Center, Honolulu, Hawaii

Susan L. Fraser, M.D.
Infectious Diseases Fellow, Department of Medicine, Brooke Army Medical Center and Wilford Hall Air Force Medical Center, and Instructor in Medicine and Infectious Diseases, University of Texas School of Medicine, San Antonio, Texas; Instructor in Medicine, Uniformed Services University of the Health Sciences, Bethesda, Maryland

Bonnie Cary Freitas, M.D.
Chief Resident, Department of Internal Medicine, Tripler Army Medical Center, Honolulu, Hawaii

Robert H. Gates, M.D.
Associate Clinical Professor of Medicine, Department of Medicine, University of Hawaii John A. Burns School of Medicine, Honolulu, Hawaii; Deputy Commander for Clinical Services, Evans Army Community Hospital, Fort Carson, Colorado

Marie J. George, M.D.
Assistant Professor of Medicine, Division of Infectious Diseases and Immunology, Department of Medicine, University of Massachusetts Medical Center, Worcester, Massachusetts

Kimberly A. Gerstadt, M.D.
Infectious Diseases Fellow, Division of Infectious Diseases and Immunology, Department of Medicine, University of Massachusetts Medical Center, Worcester, Massachusetts

Steve A. Granada, M.D.
Infectious Disease Service, Department of Internal Medicine, William Beaumont Army Medical Center, El Paso, Texas

David R. Haburchak, M.D.
Associate Professor of Medicine, Section of Infectious Diseases, Department of Medicine, Medical College of Georgia, Augusta, Georgia

John H. Hammer, M.D.
Fellow, Division of Infectious Diseases, Department of Medicine, University of Colorado School of Medicine, and Denver Public Health, Denver, Colorado

James Hanley, M.D.
Associate Professor of Medicine and Program Director in Internal Medicine, Department of Internal Medicine, University of North Dakota School of Medicine and Health Sciences, Fargo, North Dakota

Theresa M. Haslett-Essen, Pharm.D., M.S., D.O.
Staff Physician, Department of Internal Medicine, Tripler Army Medical Center, Honolulu, Hawaii

Arthur Herpolsheimer, M.D.
Assistant Professor, Department of Obstetrics and Gynecology, Uniformed Services University of the Health Sciences, Bethesda, Maryland, and Tripler Army Medical Center, Honolulu, Hawaii

Steven C. Johnson, M.D.
Assistant Professor of Medicine, Division of Infectious Diseases, Department of Medicine, University of Colorado School of Medicine, and Practice Director, Infectious Disease Group Practice, University Hospital, Denver, Colorado

Nina J. Karlin, M.D.
Resident, Department of Internal Medicine, William Beaumont Army Medical Center, El Paso, Texas

Kristie J. Lowry, M.D.
Infectious Disease Fellow, Infectious Disease Service, Department of Internal Medicine, Brooke Army Medical Center, Fort Sam Houston, Texas

Nancy E. Madinger, M.D.
Assistant Professor of Medicine and Clinical Laboratory Pathology, Division of Infectious Diseases, Department of Medicine, University of Colorado School of Medicine, Denver, Colorado

Jason D. Maguire, M.D.
Instructor, Department of Internal Medicine, Uniformed Services University of the Health Sciences, and Infectious Diseases Fellow, Division of Infectious Diseases, National Naval Medical Center, Bethesda, Maryland

Stephanie L. Marglin, M.D.
Fellow, Division of Infectious Diseases and Immunology, Department of Medicine, University of Massachusetts Medical School, Worcester, Massachusetts

Mary A. Marovich, M.D.
Clinical Associate, Helminth Immunology Section, Laboratory of Parasitic Diseases, National Institutes of Health, Bethesda, Maryland

C. Kenneth McAllister, M.D.
Consultant to the Surgeon General for Infectious Diseases, Clinical Professor of Medicine, University of Texas–San Antonio School of Medicine, Dean, Military Professional Education, San Antonio Uniformed Services Health Education Consortium, and Infectious Disease Service, Brooke Army Medical Center and Willford Hall Air Force Medical Center, San Antonio, Texas

Cheryl K. McDonald, M.D.
Instructor of Medicine, Division of Infectious Diseases, Department of Medicine, University of Colorado School of Medicine, Denver, Colorado

Colin McDougall, M.D.
Infectious Diseases Fellow, Division of Infectious Diseases, Bowman Gray School of Medicine of Wake Forest University, Winston-Salem, North Carolina

Larry K. Miller, M.D.
Departments of Internal Medicine and Clinical Investigation, Naval Medical Center, San Diego, California

R. Scott Miller, M.D.
Assistant Professor of Medicine, Uniformed Services University of the Health Sciences, Bethesda, Maryland, and Fellow, Infectious Diseases, Department of Medicine, Walter Reed Army Medical Center, Washington, DC

William F. Nauschuetz, Ph.D.
Adjunct Assistant Professor, Department of Microbiology, University of Hawaii–Manoa, and Chief and Medical Director, Section of Microbiology, Department of Pathology and Area Laboratory Services, Tripler Army Medical Center, Honolulu, Hawaii

Christopher Parker, D.O.
Rheumatology Fellow, Department of Rheumatology, Walter Reed Army Medical Center, Washington, DC

Joseph M. Parker, M.D.
Assistant Professor, Uniformed Services University of the Health Sciences, Bethesda, Maryland, and Assistant Chief, Pulmonary and Critical Care Medicine Service, Department of Medicine, Tripler Army Medical Center, Honolulu, Hawaii

P. Samuel Pegram, M.D., FACP
Professor of Medicine, Division of Infectious Diseases, Bowman Gray School of Medicine of Wake Forest University, Winston-Salem, North Carolina

Robert M. Plemmons, M.D.
Infectious Disease Service, Department of Medicine, Brooke Army Medical Center, San Antonio. Texas

Kimberly A. Ratcliffe, M.D.
McDonald Army Community Hospital, Fort Eustis, Virginia

William Roland, M.D.
Division of Infectious Diseases, Department of Internal Medicine, University of Missouri–Columbia School of Medicine, Columbia, Missouri

William Salzer, M.D.
Associate Professor of Clinical Medicine, Division of Infectious Diseases, Department of Internal Medicine, University of Missouri–Columbia School of Medicine, Columbia, Missouri

Donald R. Skillman, M.D., FACP
Assistant Professor of Medicine, Department of Medicine, Uniformed Services University of the Health Sciences, Bethesda, Maryland, and Chief, Infectious Disease Service, Department of Medicine, William Beaumont Army Medical Center, El Paso, Texas

Chun Ho So, M.D.
Infectious Disease Service, Department of Medicine, William Beaumont Army Medical Center, El Paso, Texas

Stephanie Stafford, D.O.
Department of Medicine, William Beaumont Army Medical Center, El Paso, Texas

Robert R. Tight, M.D.
Professor and Chief, Division of Infectious Diseases, Department of Medicine, University of North Dakota School of Medicine and Health Sciences, and Hospital Epidemiologist, MeritCare Medical Group, Fargo, North Dakota

Edmund C. Tramont, M.D.
Professor and Director, Medical Biotechnology Center, University of Maryland Biotechnology Institute, Baltimore, Maryland

T. Keith Vaughan, M.D.
Chief, Dermatology Service, Evans Army Community Hospital, Fort Carson, Colorado

Judy M. Vincent, M.D.
Chief, Pediatric Infectious Disease Service, Department of Pediatrics, Tripler Army Medical Center, Honolulu, Hawaii

Mark R. Wallace, M.D.
Head, Infectious Disease Fellowship Program, Department of Internal Medicine and Clinical Investigation, Naval Medical Center, San Diego, California

Mireya A. Wessolossky, M.D.
Fellow, Infectious Diseases, Division of Infectious Diseases and Immunology, Department of Medicine, University of Massachusetts Medical Center, Worcester, Massachusetts

Wheaton J. Williams, M.D.
Assistant Professor of Medicine, Division of Infectious Diseases, Department of Medicine, University of Colorado School of Medicine, and Attending Physician, University Hospital and Veterans Affairs Medical Center, Denver, Colorado

George R. Winters III, M.D.
Staff Physician, Department of Medicine, Irwin Army Community Hospital, Fort Riley, Kansas

Kelly L. Wirfel, M.D.
Infectious Disease Service, Department of Internal Medicine, William Beaumont Army Medical Center, El Paso, Texas

Edward J. Yang, M.D.
Assistant Clinical Professor of Medicine, Department of Medicine, John A. Burns School of Medicine, University of Hawaii–Manoa, and Allergy Service, Department of Medicine, Tripler Army Medical Center, Honolulu, Hawaii

Robert J. Zabel, D.O.
Infectious Disease Service, Department of Internal Medicine, William Beaumont Army Medical Center, El Paso, Texas

Lisa L. Zacher, M.D., FCCP
Staff Physician, Pulmonary and Critical Care Medicine Service, Department of Medicine, Tripler Army Medical Center, Honolulu, Hawaii

Hasan Syed Zafarul, M.D.
Fellow, Division of Infectious Diseases, Department of Internal Medicine, University of Missouri–Columbia School of Medicine, Columbia, Missouri

Timothy J. Zeien, M.D.
Resident, Infectious Disease Service, Department of Internal Medicine, William Beaumont Army Medical Center, El Paso, Texas

PREFACE

The diagnosis and treatment of infections involve the breadth of medicine—from genetics to microvascular surgery. Infectious diseases span the world and alter history. Infections commonly make the headlines of daily newspapers: "Chicken Flu Erupts," "Hantavirus Linked to Mysterious Four Corner Deaths," "Government Denies Anthrax Kills Sheep," "Ebola Virus Outbreak!," "AIDS Treatment Breakthrough!," "Multiresistant TB Defies Treatment," "Agent of Lyme Disease Discovered," "Flesh-eating Strep Takes Entertainer's Life," and "Chlamydia Infection Linked to Heart Disease." Recognizing that no single volume can do justice to probably the broadest clinical discipline in medicine, this book attempts to cover infections and situations that a physician may reasonably encounter.

No contemporary medical book would be complete without acknowledging Internet sources for timely information. Because the dissemination of information on emerging infections and current outbreaks is a worldwide priority, no field of medicine is better suited to electronic media than infectious diseases. At the risk of being outdated before printing, I recommend the following sites:

For links to many web sites with infectious disease content: http://www.emory.edu/ MED_INF/idsites.html; http://homepages.ihug.co.nz/~jfung/infectious.html; and http://www. idlinks.com. Of particular note is the site of the Centers for Disease Control and Prevention: http://www.cdc.gov (contains links to *Morbidity and Mortality Weekly Report* and the online journal *Emerging Infectious Diseases*). Two other favorites are the sites of the National Institute for Allergy and Infectious Diseases: http://www.niaid.nih.gov and the World Health Organization: http://lynx.who.ch/. Explore but remember that not all sites are created equal with regard to quality and content.

Any student who has stood on rounds and had personal experience with the value of Socratic teaching method can testify to its pleasure, pain, and value. The question-and-answer format of this volume is a convenient way to present the expertise, experience, humanity, and humor from seasoned veterans, as well as perspectives of those still learning the field. Many of the case examples offered are abstracted from true cases. Perhaps this book will help provide the correct answer to a question posed by an attending physician during rounds.

Infectious disease (ID) physicians see and treat some of the most challenging and fascinating illnesses. Ours is one of the few specialties that actually cure patients! It is hoped that the information, scenarios, and examples from our patients and their providers will stimulate the investigative qualities of a Sherlock Holmes or awaken the Salk and Sabin in future medical scholars and clinicians who will discover the hidden "secrets" in the pathogens of today and tomorrow.

I extend my heartfelt thanks and respect to those busy clinicians who gave selflessly of their scarce time to contribute to this volume. Many thanks to Linda Belfus and the expert staff of Hanley & Belfus for their consistently professional efforts, patience, and understanding. Most of all, thanks to my wife, through whose support and encouragement the editing of "Secrets" has become a family tradition.

Robert H. Gates, MD

I. The Approach to Infections

1. CLINICAL USE OF THE MICROBIOLOGY LABORATORY

William F. Nauschuetz, Ph.D.

1. Why should I read this chapter?

Good question with a short answer. One of the basic rules in life is "trash in, trash out." Clinicians require the most rapid diagnosis possible for their patients. But technicians in the microbiology laboratory **must** occasionally reject specimens. If substandard specimens are accepted for processing, the laboratory risks reporting results that do not reflect the patient's condition. Recollection, resubmission, and reprocessing of specimens cost the laboratory extra money and manpower, but that cost is minor compared with the cost to the clinician and patient.

2. Which types of specimens are covered in this chapter?

Clinical microbiology laboratories vary tremendously in size and scope. Some microbiology laboratories provide nothing beyond basic aerobic and anaerobic bacteriology services, offering identification and susceptibility reports on only the most common specimens (urine, throat swabs, sputa, blood, tissues, body fluids, genital exudates and lesions). Other laboratories include services for mycology, mycobacteriology, parasitology, virology, and serology. This chapter discusses topics of specimen submission and processing for the most commonly requested procedures. Every clinical microbiology laboratory is required by the College of American Pathologists to publish and distribute a specimen collection guide for clinicians. One purpose of this chapter is to entice you to examine the specimen collection guide in your hospital more thoroughly.

3. What are the most common causes for rejection of specimens by the microbiology laboratory?

Rejecting a specimen is sometimes the last option, depending on the specimen. Usually the laboratory spends enormous amounts of time correcting common submission errors for surgical specimens, blood cultures, and cerebrospinal fluid (CSF). Clinicians can eliminate many specimen rejections by practicing four simple steps:

1. **Label specimens.** A swab without an indication of the site looks like every other swab in the world. Is it a throat culture? If so, it is set up on one plate. Is it a swab from a surgical site? That requires several more plates, plus a tube of enhancement broth. Furthermore, fluid that comes in a urine cup is not always urine. Think of the difficulty that could arise if shunt fluid were to arrive at the laboratory in a urine cup with no source indicated. Remember that laboratory technicians most likely were not present when the specimen was collected; they probably cannot guess the nature of most unlabeled specimens—nor should they.

2. **Tighten all caps to fluid containers.** If the laboratory receives a leaky cup or tube, the technicians must spray it down with disinfectant and may very well reject it. (If fluid can leak out, some of the disinfectant can leak into the specimen container.)

3. **Put the patient's identification number or name on the specimen.** If the laboratory receives two sets of blood cultures in the same delivery without identification on the bottles, they must be rejected with a request to resubmit new specimens.

4. **Submit the collected specimen to the laboratory as soon as possible.** Culturing specimens, especially swabs, that were submitted a day or two after collection greatly reduces their predictive value. Some laboratories may culture old specimens but often add a disclaimer indicating that the results may not be clinically useful. If it all possible, the laboratory technician should reject the specimen and request another to give clinicians the results that they require.

4. I submit blood cultures daily. What guidelines do I need to follow?

The most common error that we see in the laboratory is failure to collect the recommended number of blood culture bottles from a patient. Submitting the correct number of blood culture bottles has two huge benefits: (1) it increases the total volume of blood screened for bloodstream isolates, and (2) it allows a mechanism for the clinician and the laboratory to predict the relative importance of blood culture isolates. For most patients with suspected bacteremia, the clinical laboratory expects to receive 3 separate sets of blood culture bottles. A set is defined as 2 bottles, 1 aerobe bottle and one anaerobe bottle.

Guidelines for Collection of Specimens for Blood Cultures

	SPECIMEN COLLECTION		
PATIENT PRESENTATION	NO. OF BOTTLES	SCHEDULE	COMMENTS
Acute sepsis	2–3 sets from separate sites	Collect all within 10–15 min	Collect before initiation of antimicrobial therapy
Endocarditis	3 sets from 3 separate sites	Collect over 1–2 hr	Same as above
Subacute bacterial endocarditis	3 samples from separate sites	Collect all within 24 hr; collect sets at least 15 min apart	Repeat on day 2 if laboratory reports no growth after 24 hr
Endocarditis patients on antimicrobial therapy	2 separate sets each day for 3 days	Collect over 1–2 hr on each day	
Other bacteremic patients on antimicrobial therapy	3 sets per day for 2 days	Collect immediately before next dose of antimicrobial	
Patients with fever of unknown origin	Collect 2–3 sets on day 1; collect 2 more sets on day 2	Collect each set at least 1 hr apart	Collect second set before temperature peaks

5. Why is the laboratory so specific when detailing volumes of blood drawn for culture and number of sets collected? How can the number of blood culture bottles help to interpret the significance of blood culture isolates?

Many blood culture bottles are designed to accept 10 ml blood each. Because the concentration of bacteria in bloodstream infections of adults is usually very low, it is essential to obtain the full 10 ml per bottle. Each ml, up to 10 ml, can increase sensitivity of the blood culture by 3%. Therefore, the difference of culturing 5 ml instead of 10 ml can be significant.

The number of sets is also important. Obviously, the more sets submitted, the greater the opportunity to culture bacteria infecting the bloodstream. However, 3 sets per 24 hours is generally considered maximal sensitivity. There is no advantage to submitting a fourth set from a patient within a 24-hour period.

A laboratory may reject blood cultures if only 1 set is received for an adult patient over a 24-hour period. One set lacks the sensitivity to detect bacteremia in many patients and may be a disservice to the physician and patient.

There is another advantage to submitting a total of 4–6 bottles per day. It offers a way to determine the clinical significance of an isolate from a positive bottle. If coagulase-negative

Staphylococcus or *Streptococcus viridans* is isolated from only 1 or 2 of 6 bottles, it is likely to be a contaminant. However, if it is isolated from 3–4 bottles from the set, it then looks more significant in relation to the patient's condition. And, obviously, the same isolate from 5 or 6 bottles is likely to represent an infectious agent in the bloodstream.

Pediatric patients are an exception: only 1 or 2 sets are required. Because bacteremic children usually have high concentrations of bacteria in the bloodstream, the laboratory is likely to recover the pathogen in both bottles of each set, which makes interpreting culture results easier for the clinician.

6. What specimens should I submit to determine whether a septic patient may have a catheter-related bloodstream infection?

If the patient has a catheter-related bloodstream infection, the site of infection is likely to be the insertion point of the catheter or through the lumen of the catheter. Specific laboratory procedures are available to confirm that these sites are involved. Using what has become known as the "Maki semiquantitative method," the catheter is withdrawn from the patient aseptically. The tip and proximal transcutaneous segment are sent to the laboratory in a sterile cup. Once received in the laboratory, the tip is aseptically transferred to a 5% sheep blood agar plate and rolled gently across the surface. A positive culture is said to occur when > 15 colonies of the same bacterium isolated from the patient's blood grow in the culture. The types of bacteria most likely to grow from the tip include coagulase-negative staphylococci, *S. aureus*, enterococci, or *Corynebacterium* spp.

The laboratory can perform specific culturing techniques to determine whether bacteria may have been introduced through a contaminated lumen. Technicians place the catheter segment into a tube of culture broth, tightly cap the tube, and vortex the tube to suspend any bacteria on the segment. The technician then does quantitative cultures of the broth. If the bacterial concentration from the original tubes exceeds 1,000 CFU/ml, and if it is the same organism isolated from the patient's blood culture, the segment lumen was probably the mechanism of infection.

Unfortunately, these procedures require removal of the catheter lines. In some cases, this may be considered a drastic step to determine a possible source of infection. Another method allows the clinician to determine whether a line is involved in a bloodstream infection without removal. This method takes advantage of the Isolator blood culture tube, which can be used to quantitate bacteremia. Peripheral blood is collected into a 1.5-ml pediatric Isolator tube. Blood from the suspected catheter line is collected into a second pediatric Isolator tube. Laboratory technicians process the tube and place 0.5 ml aliquots from each tube onto chocolate agar plates. Cultures are incubated and checked daily for up to 72 hr. Any resulting colonies from the plates are counted. If the blood from the catheter has five times (or more) the number (and type) of colonies resulting from the peripheral blood tube, the results suggest that the catheter is involved in the bloodstream infection. Any other result suggests that the catheter is not a source of infection.

7. A fair number of my urine cultures have been reported as contaminated, with a request to resubmit. Many other reports come back without full identification and susceptibility studies of bacteria grown from culture. Why?

In this world of standardization, clinicians may well find interlaboratory variation in determining what constitutes a "positive urine culture." In the mid 1950s, Kass did his landmark studies that correlated colony counts of bacteria in midstream urine to the clinical condition of patients with upper urinary tract infections (pyelonephritis). He developed the so-called "100,000 rule," suggesting that the cut-off for a "positive" urine culture was 100,000 colony-forming units (CFU) of bacteria/ml. Any number less than 100,000 CFU/ml was thought to represent contamination. The only exceptions were considered to be catheterized urine and urine collected by suprapubic aspirates, from which any growth at all was considered significant, and was worked up for full identification and susceptibility report.

In the early 1980s, Stamm studied the applicability of the "100,000 rule" to women with lower UTI. He found that less than one-half of symptomatic patients with bacterial growth in urine (confirmed by catheterization) would have been diagnosed as having significant UTI using the 100,000 CFU/ml cut-off. In fact, he found that the level of "significant bacteriuria" for some symptomatic women should be as low as 100 CFU/ml. This finding applied to women with acute urethral syndrome (AUS) and to some women with cystitis.

In response to Stamm's data, some laboratories lowered their threshold of "significant bacteriuria" to 100 or 1000 CFU/ml. But other concerns arose immediately. Many patients with < 100,000 CFU/ml in urine one day had fewer, or no, bacteria in the urine on the second day of collection. This finding indicated that colony counts < 100,000 CFU/ml often indicate contamination rather than infection.

In the middle of this controversy, of course, was the clinical bacteriology laboratory. What should be worked up? Many laboratories use a system similar to the system that we use. We define "significant bacteriuria" for most patients as 100,000 CFU/ml. If urine contains that many or more bacteria of a single isolate, we identify and perform a susceptibility study of the isolate. If there are fewer bacteria than 100,000 CFU/ml, we describe and quantitate the isolate (e.g., 10,000 gram-negative bacilli/ml). The plate is held at room temperature for another 72 hours. If low-count bacteriuria is a possibility, the laboratory completes, on request, an identification and antibiotic susceptibility study of the isolate. If the patient is asymptomatic, the physician may well regard the culture as negative. Any growth from catheterized urine and suprapubic aspirates is significant and a full work-up is done. Studies indicate that many cases of low-count bacteriuria are polymicrobial, especially in complicated UTI.

These procedures encourage dialog between physicians and laboratorians, emphasize a team-effort to produce the most timely, significant result, and reduce unnecessary work-ups, thereby reducing cost.

Up to 15% of the urine specimens received for culture may be contaminated. Although they may have become grossly contaminated during collection, it is more likely that they were slightly contaminated during collection and then allowed to sit at room temperature. Many bacteria grow well in urine at room temperature. For this reason, urine should be refrigerated immediately after collection and should remain refrigerated until processed by the laboratory. Refrigeration is a wonderful, inexpensive, low-tech answer to reducing false-positive urine cultures.

8. Some laboratories screen urine to determine whether or not to culture. How do these screens work? Can I use them to screen all urine specimens?

There are many screening techniques for urine. Some, such as the urine Gram stain, have been used for years. In the past decade urine screens have become rapid, inexpensive, easy to interpret, and sensitive. Two of the most common are the LN Dipstick, which has two square matrices for the detection of leukocyte esterase (for pyuria) and nitrite (for bacteriuria), and the UriScreen, which is a semiquantitative catalase test. Both tests are user-friendly and provide excellent turn-around time. Urine samples that are negative for both leukocyte esterase and nitrite can be reported as "urine negative by screening" without the need to culture. If the urine is positive for either test, it is processed for culture. Such methods are sensitive in laboratories that define significant bacteriuria as > 100,000 CFU/ml but should not be used to screen catheterized urine, suprapubic aspirates, or samples from patients with acute urethral syndrome.

9. Some of my lower respiratory specimens were rejected on the basis of a "Q-score." What is a Q-score? How is it used?

Clinical bacteriology is not a matter of identifying all bacteria that grow in all specimens. The laboratory should be able to provide clinicians with clinically relevant answers. The Q-score and its variations are tools for determining the quality of respiratory specimens. Higher specimen quality implies a higher predictive value of results. The microbiology technologist calculates the Q-score by doing a Gram stain of the specimen and comparing the average numbers of polymorphonuclear cells (PMNs) and squamous epithelial cells (SECs) per low-power field. These values are then converted to Q-scores by using the chart below.

Calculation of Q-Scores

	Squamous Epithelial Cells/Field			
	0 (none)	1–9 (few)	10–24 (moderate)	> 25 (many)
Polymorphonculear Cells				
0 (none)	0	–1	–2	–3
1–9 (few)	+1	0	–1	–2
10–24 (moderate)	+2	+1	0	–1
> 25 (many)	+3	+2	+1	0
	Q-Score			

Q-scores are intrepreted as follows:

1, 2, 3   Gram stain is reported with cell types and Q-score. Specimen is accepted for culture.

≤ 0   Gram stain is reported with cell types and Q-score. The report states that the specimen is contaminated and unacceptable for culture. Another specimen is requested. The specimen will be held a few days before it is discarded in case the clinician requests culture of the specimen because of special circumstances.

10. What is the best way to submit sterile body fluids (such as pericardial fluid, ascites, synovial fluid) to the laboratory for culture?

Some laboratories have preferred methods of submission, but there are five basic ways to submit a specimen:

1. **Swabs** are the specimen least encouraged by laboratories for sterile fluids. The reasons are obvious: the amount of fluid on a swab may be inadequate to detect low numbers of bacteria; it is impossible to do a good direct Gram stain; and anaerobic bacteria die quickly during transport.

2. **Syringes** may be the second least encouraged method of submission. A needle and syringe, even if recapped, constitute an infection hazard that requires universal precautions. It is best to inject the specimen into another transport system before sending it to the laboratory.

3. **Sterile tubes or containers**, such as sterile red-top tubes, may be used to transport the specimen. Call the laboratory and ask its preference. Most laboratories request the clinician to use tubes that do not contain anticoagulants.

4. **Blood culture bottles** are a good method for submitting fluids. The physician can even submit specimens for aerobic and anaerobic culture by using appropriate blood culture bottles. But remember to follow the same rule as when filling the tubes with blood. Fill the bottles with 10 ml of specimen, if at all possible. This amount optimizes recovery of low-count pathogens. Because it is impossible for the laboratory to do a direct smear on a specimen submitted in bottles, it is best to submit also a glass slide with a dried smear of the fluid. Thus the laboratory can do a Gram stain and culture.

5. **Biphasic media**, such as the Roche Septi-Chek blood culture bottles, are an alternative method to number 4. They allow the laboratory technician to see isolated colonies as much as 1 day earlier than a broth-only method.

11. In addition to the use of anaerobic blood culture bottles, what other methods of submitting specimens increase the recovery rates of anaerobes?

Before worrying about *how* to submit specimens for anaerobic cultures, it is best to know *what* can and cannot be submitted.

Abbreviated List of Specimens That Can and Cannot Be Cultured for Anaerobic Bacteria

SITE	ACCEPTABLE SPECIMENS	UNACCEPTABLE SPECIMENS
Respiratory tract	Bronchoscopic washing Transtracheal aspirate	Bronchoalveolar washing* Endotracheal aspirate Sputum (induced or expectorated) Nasopharyngeal swab Throat swab
Genitourinary tract	Bartholin's gland Culdocentesis fluid Placenta (by cesarean section) Fallopian tube Intrauterine device Ovary Endometrial aspirate of uterus Urine (suprapubic aspirate)	Cervical swab Endocervical swab (with vaginal secretions) Lochia Perineal swab Urethral swab Prostate fluid Seminal fluid Vaginal swab Urine (voided, catheterized)
Miscellaneous	Blood Bile Bone marrow Surgical specimens (swabs or tissues)	Stool†

* If not submitted in anaerobic transport.
† Except for detection of *Clostridium difficile*.

The best specimens for anaerobic culture are often those collected by a needle and syringe (or catheter). Examples include:

- Abscess material
- Deep-wound drainage
- Ulcers
- Pulmonary aspirates
- Genitourinary tract specimens

Once collected, aspirated materials must be submitted by a system that effectively protects the specimens from oxygen. Fluids can be injected into transport bottles containing an anaerobic environment and prereduced media. This type of product is excellent for the transport of specimens for recovery of anaerobes.

Tissue specimens are also excellent for anaerobic culture. Small tissue chunks can be transported by pushing them into a gel-like material in tubes generally used for anaerobic swabs. Larger tissues can be transported in sealed bags in which catalysts convert free oxygen to moisture or in sterile specimen cups with a small amount of sterile saline to keep the specimen moist.

Several systems are available for the submission of anaerobic swabs. It is best to call the laboratory and find out which transport system is preferred.

12. How can I help the laboratory in ruling out gastrointestinal pathogens in patients with diarrhea?

Stool cultures are one of the most expensive procedures offered by the laboratory. Because of the diverse nature of bacteria, viruses, and parasites commonly associated with diarrhea (see table below), it is clear that the days when the laboratory tried to rule out all pathogens in all stool samples are coming to an end. Clinicians should include patient information with the stool or rectal swab when asking the laboratory to detect stool pathogens. They can provide data that focus the search:

- Did the patient recently return from a trip to an area with inadequate water purification systems?
- Is the patient febrile?
- Has the patient experienced vomiting?
- Has the patient been hospitalized for more than 3 days?
- Is the patient immunocompromised?

Many laboratories reject stool samples for ova and parasite examination if the patient has been in the hospital for more than 3 days. Nosocomial diarrhea in adults is usually caused by toxigenic *Clostridium difficile*; in pediatric patients, it is usually caused by rotavirus or *C. difficile* toxin.

If vomiting is the predominant complaint, the patient may have ingested preformed toxin made by *Staphylococcus aureus* or *Bacillus cereus*. Most clinical laboratories offer little help for such patients. They do not have the capabilities to detect toxin from stool or vomitus, and the patient usually recovers quickly. However, vomiting also may indicate a viral infection. Many laboratories provide rapid detection methods for the human rotavirus, but viruses such as Norwalk and Norwalk-like viruses are best detected by electron microscopy.

A fecal leukocyte smear or the newer lactoferrin test may provide information about likely pathogens. Inflammatory diarrhea may be an indication to focus on invasive organisms (*Salmonella, Shigella,* or *Campylobacter* spp.), toxin-producing *C. difficile* (pseudomembranous colitis), or inflammatory bowel disease.

No universal, standardized guidelines list which pathogens should be ruled out under certain circumstances. It is still basically left to the laboratory and clinicians to determine cost-effective criteria for laboratory-assisted diagnosis of diarrhea.

Stool Pathogens

BACTERIA	VIRUSES	PARASITES
Salmonella spp.*	Rotavirus[∞]	*Giardia lamblia**
Shigella spp.*	Adenovirus[∞]	*Entamoeba histolytica**
Campylobacter spp.*	Human calicivirus[//]	*Cryptosporidium* spp.[†]
Plesiomonas spp.*	Norwalk virus[//]	
*Yersinia enterocolitica**	Norwalk-like virus[//]	
Escherichia coli 0157:H7[†]	Astrovirus[//]	
Clostridium difficile[†]		
Vibrio spp.[†]		
Aeromonas spp.[†]		
Enterotoxigenic *E. coli*[‡]		
Enteroinvasive *E. coli*[‡]		
Bacillus cereus[§]		
Staphylococcus aureus[§]		

* Routine detection.
[†] Usually by special request.
[‡] Usually confirmed by reference laboratory.
[§] Intoxication: not confirmed in most clinical laboratories.
[∞] Enzyme immunoassay.
[//] By electron microscopy only.

13. What specimens and tests optimize my chances for a culture-confirmed diagnosis in patients with aseptic meningitis?

Culture-confirmed diagnosis of aseptic meningitis seems to be one of the solid limitations of routine microbiology; it may be impossible in most patients. Although the culture of enteroviruses, herpes simplex virus (HSV), and mycobacteria involves no inherent difficulty, recovery from cerebrospinal fluid (CSF) is rare. The laboratory should send CSF to a reference laboratory capable of running one of the gene amplification procedures, such as polymerase chain reaction (PCR). This type of technique seems to offer much higher sensitivity than even the best of culture systems.

14. What kind of specimens may be submitted for gene amplification tests? Which bacteria do they detect?

The Food and Drug Administration (FDA) has approved certain gene amplification tests for use in the clinical laboratory. Their most practical application seems to be detection of a bacterium or virus that is difficult to grow in the laboratory or that grows very slowly. The FDA has approved two gene amplification tests for detection of *Mycobacterium tuberculosis* in clinical specimens. One is a PCR test that requires a machine called a thermocycler. A competing product, the transcription assay system (TAS), does not require a thermocycler but is operated in a water bath. Both tests have the same limitations:

- They can be used only on acid-fast bacillus smear-positive respiratory specimens.
- They cannot be used for patients receiving tuberculosis therapy (they cannot be used to detect clearance of the organism).
- They detect all species in the *M. tuberculosis* group, including *M. bovis, M. bovis* BCG, *M. africanum*, and *M. microti* as well as *M. tuberculosis*.
- Both tests give false-positive results with some of the other *Mycobacterium* spp., including *M. celatum* and *M. terrae*-like organisms.

Other gene amplification tests approved by the FDA include direct detection of *Chlamydia trachomatis* in urogenital swabs and urine. The urine test offers a convenient, noninvasive procedure to detect chlamydia in asymptomatic patients who may have been exposed to a *C. trachomatis*-positive sexual partner. All gene amplification tests take about 5 hours. In general, they are expensive but may have overall cost benefits when requested, performed, interpreted, and acted upon appropriately.

BIBLIOGRAPHY

1. Bradley SP, Reed SL, Catanzaro A: Clinical efficacy of the amplified *Mycobacterium tuberculosis* direct test for the diagnosis of pulmonary tuberculosis. Am J Respir Crit Care Med 153:1606–1610, 1996.
2. Isenberg H: Clinical Microbiology Procedures Handbook. Washington, DC, American Society for Microbiology, 1992.
3. Morris AJ, Smith LK, Mirrett S, Reller LB: Cost and time savings following introduction of rejection criteria for clinical specimens. J Clin Microbiol 34:355–357, 1996.
4. Rotbart HA: Enteroviral infections of the central nervous system. Clin Infect Dis 20:971–981, 1995.
5. Sodeman TM: A practical strategy for diagnosis of urinary tract infections. Clin Lab Med 2:233–250, 1995.
6. Yagupsky P, Nolte FS: Quantitative aspects of septicemia. Clin Microbiol Rev 3:269–279, 1990.

2. TAXONOMY FOR THE NOMENCLATURE CHALLENGED

Theresa M. Haslett-Essen, Pharm.D., M.S., D.O.

1. Why is taxonomy important?

A system of classification is needed to provide sense and order to the vast array of organisms that we encounter. A recognized and valid taxonomy functions as a heuristic tool, an interpretive frame, a conceptual paradigm that confers focus and clarity across the spectrum of microorganismal phenomena. Taxonomy strives to bring order to chaos and helps to ensure we are speaking the same language.

2. How are viruses classified?

Taxonomy of viruses may be based on the following:

1. Virion and kingdom of host (use host cell type—e.g., animal viruses, plant viruses, bacterial viruses).

2. Nucleic acid type (ds DNA, ss DNA, ds RNA, ss RNA).

3. Positive or negative polarity of RNA. Positive polarity is able to serve as mRNA. Negative polarity is the complement of positive polarity and must function as a template to make a complimentary strand of positive RNA before translation can occur.

4. Virus coat morphology, i.e., enveloped vs. nonenveloped viruses.

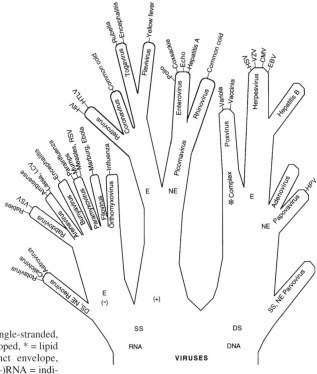

DS = double-stranded, SS = single-stranded, E = enveloped, NE = nonenveloped, * = lipid in outer coat, but no distinct envelope, (+)RNA = direct translation, (–)RNA = indirect translation (after transcription).

Taxonomy of viruses.

3. What is the Baltimore classification of viruses?

The Baltimore classification is named after David Baltimore, who originated the scheme of classifying viruses according to genome types and replication strategies. The various types of virus genomes can be broken down into seven fundamentally different groups that obviously require different basic strategies for their replication.

I   ds DNA viruses

II   ss DNA viruses

III ds RNA viruses

IV ss RNA viruses with (+) sense genomes

V   ss RNA viruses with (–) sense genomes

VI Diploid positive-sense ss RNA viruses that replicate via reverse transcription to and transcription from longer-than-genome-length ds DNA

VII ds DNA viruses that replicate via transcription to and reverse transcription from longer-than-genome-length positive-sense ss RNA

4. What is the universal system of virus taxonomy?

The universal system of virus taxonomy is a scheme developed by the International Committee on Taxonomy of Viruses (ICTV). Virion characteristics are considered and weighted as criteria for making divisions into families and, in some cases, subfamilies and genera. As the species taxon was developed in the 1990s, it became clearer that families and genera may best be defined by a few characteristics, but species are better defined by multiple characteristics.

The ICTV publishes The Classification and Nomenclature of Viruses. The most recent Sixth Report (1995) records a universal taxonomy scheme consisting of one order, 71 families, 9 subfamilies, and 164 genera, including 24 floating genera, and more than 3600 virus species. The system still contains hundreds of unassigned viruses, largely because of lack of data. A major virtue of the universal system of taxonomy is unambiguous virus identification, which is of great value when the editor of a journal requires precise naming of cited viruses.

5. Discuss the importance of databases in taxonomy.

It has been estimated that more than 30,000 viruses, virus strains, and subtypes are being tracked (not to mention bacteria and other microorganisms). It has been estimated that to describe a virus comprehensively, approximately 500–1000 characteristics must be determined. To describe comprehensively all of the known viruses, we must fill in the blanks for 3–21 million data points. The ICTV has laid out a plan to develop the universal virus database over the next 10 years, to manage the scope of data, and to integrate several virus databases currently in operation. Among the many databases are the National Center for Biotechnology Information (NCBI) database, which contains the names of all organisms represented in the genetic databases with at least one nucleotide or protein sequence, and GenBank taxonomy database, which is available for many groups of organisms, including bacteria, protozoa, viruses, and fungi. As of July 1996, there was a total of 18,542 species with sequence data in the genetic databases.

6. How is taxonomy useful in diagnostic virology?

A universal system for taxonomy and nomenclature of viruses is a practical necessity whenever large numbers of distinct isolates are dealt with, as in a reference laboratory. The clinician usually makes a preliminary diagnosis of a viral disease on the basis of four kinds of evidence:

1. Clinical features, which allow recognition with varying certainty in typical cases of many viral diseases (e.g., varicella exanthem, measles exanthem).

2. Epidemic behavior, which in a typical population may allow recognition (e.g., epidemic influenza, arbovirus diseases, enterovirus exanthems).

3. Circumstances of occurrence, which may indicate probable etiology (e.g., respiratory syncytial virus as the primary cause of croup and bronchiolitis in infants; hepatitis C as the likely cause of hepatitis after blood transfusions).

4. Organ involvement, which may suggest a probable etiology (e.g., mumps virus as the cause of parotitis).

Shortcomings in the predictive value of such evidence suggest that the laboratory diagnostician as well as the clinician must appreciate the range of possible etiologic agents in particular disease syndromes. It is often useful to assemble an initial inclusive "long list" of possible etiologic agents so that no candidate agent is overlooked. Usually the list is made informally, and the process is adjusted to the complexity of the case.

The universal system of virus taxonomy may be used as the source of the long list of etiologic candidates. The universal system organizes the list logically, and because the system is comprehensive, it is unlikely that known viruses will be overlooked. The observations that place an etiologic agent in its proper family and genus also should play a role in shortening the list and in most cases should provide etiologic information needed to select immunologic (serologic) identification techniques. For example, the long list of possible etiologies for a slowly progressive central nervous system disease would include many viruses that are difficult or impossible to cultivate. However, the identification of spherical, 45-nm, nonenveloped virions in the nuclei of cells in a brain biopsy from a patient with such a disease shortens the list to the family Papovaviridae, genus *Polyomavirus*, thereby suggesting a diagnosis of JC or SV 40 virus-induced progressive multifocal leukoencephalopathy. In this case, many viruses known to invade the brain and cause slowly progressive neurologic disease would be eliminated from the differential diagnostic list.

7. Why does bacterial nomenclature seem so confusing?

During the past decade, bacterial taxonomy has undergone remarkable changes. Just when one is comfortable with a new genus, it changes names (e.g., *Pseudomonas* changed to *Xanthomonas*, which changed to *Stenotrophomonas*). New categories of information of potential taxonomic value (e.g., chemotaxonomy, DNA base composition, DNA-DNA hybridization) make possible fine distinctions between organisms and reveal dissimilarities not detected before. As Heraclitus said, "You never step in the same river twice." The taxonomic stream is always changing.

8. How are bacteria named?

The naming of bacteria is controlled by the International Code of Nomenclature of Bacteria. The correct name of a bacterial taxon is based on the following factors:
1. Valid publication
2. Legitimacy
3. Priority of publication
4. Effective publication

Since 1 January 1980, priority of bacterial names is based on the Approved Lists of Bacterial Names. Names that were not included in the Approved Lists lost standing in bacterial nomenclature. The Approved Lists contains about 2200 names of genera and species and 123 names of higher taxa.

9. Describe the phenetic system and phylogenetic system used in microbial taxonomy.

The phenetic system groups organisms on the basis of mutual similarity of phenotypic characteristics. This convenient ordering scheme may or may not correctly match evolutionary grouping. For example, flagellated (motile) organisms are put in one group, and nonmotile organisms are put in another group.

The phylogenetic system groups organisms on the basis of shared evolutionary heritage. This ordering scheme displays evolutionary relationships. For example, mycoplasmas (no cell wall) and bacilli (cell wall, gram-positive rods) are not obviously similar and would not be grouped together phenetically. But evolutionarily they are similar, more so than either is to gram-negative organisms.

10. How do phenetic and phylogenetic systems affect bacterial nomenclature?

Phylogeny has attracted increasing attention, and phylogenetic relationships are now an important basis in the classification of bacteria. The integrated use of phenotypic and genotypic characteristics will have great influence not only on classification but also on bacterial nomenclature.

11. What is numerical taxonomy?

Numerical taxonomy uses a variety of characteristics, such as Gram stain, cell shape, motility, size, aerobic/anaerobic capacity, nutritional capabilities, cell wall chemistry, and immunologic characteristics, and relies on similarity coefficients.[10] For example, if organism A and B share 8 characteristics out of 10, the similarity coefficient is 8/10 = 0.8.[10] One can use many such values to establish a similarity matrix. Dendrograms help to display this information clearly.

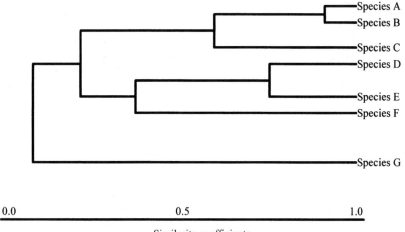

Dendrogram. (Courtesy of T.M. Terry, University of Connecticut.)

A dendrogram is merely a graphic display of similarity coefficients, but one often assumes that these coefficients are representative of a deeper evolutionary relationship.[10] This conclusion may or may not be legitimate, depending on the traits used. The diagram below is a hypothetic evolutionary diagram, similar to a dendrogram but quite different in that it seeks to give an accurate picture of how and when organisms diverged from common ancestors over time.[10] To get accurate phylogeny, one must decide which characteristics give best insight. DNA and RNA sequencing techniques are considered to give the most meaningful phylogenies.

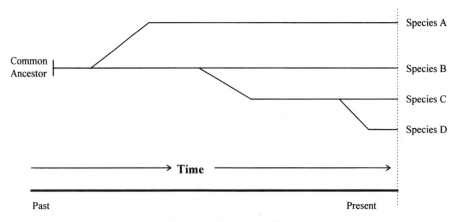

Evolutionary diagram. (Courtesy of T.M. Terry, University of Connecticut.)

12. What is the difference between *classical taxonomy* and *molecular taxonomy*?
Classical taxonomy uses both morphologic and physiologic characteristics. A good example is Bergey's manual, which is a phenetic system. This practical system for clinical laboratory medicine uses successive key features to narrow down an identification. For example, gram-positive or gram-negative? Shape? Motile or not? Eventually only a few organisms match the process of elimination.

Molecular taxonomy attempts to establish a history of evolutionary lineage with the use of 16S RNA sequence homology. 16S RNA is found in a small ribosomal subunit (30S) of procaryotic ribosomes. Since mitochondria and chloroplasts also have these ribosomes, the subunit is found in all three kingdoms. Most ribosomal RNA mutations are deleterious. Therefore, the evolution of 16S RNA is slow. It is a good molecule for comparing organisms that may have diverged as far back as 3 or 4 billion years ago.

13. How has the use of 16S RNA sequence homology helped our understanding of microbial taxonomy?
16S RNA sequence homology has produced remarkable results regarding the bacterial phylogenetic tree. There are three major evolutionary groups, quite different from each other. Archaebacteria must have diverged from Eubacteria as long ago as the origin of Eucaryotes.

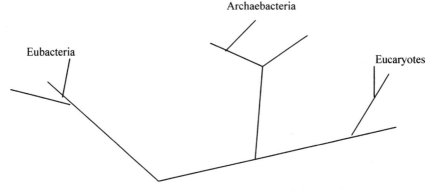

Bacterial phylogenetic tree.

BIBLIOGRAPHY

1. Ax P: The phylogenetic system. The Systematization of Organisms on the Basis of Their Phylogenesis. Chichester, John Wiley, 1987.
2. Bacterial Nomenclature Up-to-date. A database service provided by the DSMZ-Deutsche Sammlung von Mikroorganismen und Zellkulturen GmbH, Braunschweig, Germany, 1996.
3. Gherna R, Pienta P, Cote R: ATCC Catalog of Bacteria and Bacteriophages, 19th ed. Rockville, MD, American Type Culture Collection, 1992.
4. Holt J: Bergey's Manual of Systematic Bacteriology, vol 1–4. Baltimore, Williams & Wilkins, 1989.
5. Minelli A: Biological Systematics. The State of the Art. London, Chapman & Hall, 1993.
6. Moore W, Moore L: Index of the Bacterial and Yeast Nomenclature Changes. Washington, DC, American Society for Microbiology, 1992.
7. Murphy FA: Virus Taxonomy: The Classification and Nomenclature of Viruses. Sixth Report of the International Committee on Taxonomy of Viruses. Vienna, Springer-Verlag, 1995.
8. Sherman V, McGowan V, Sneath P: Approved List of Bacterial Names. Washington, DC, American Society for Microbiology, 1989.
9. Terry TM: Viruses. MCB 229, Virus lecture notes, spring 1996. Available at: http://www.sp.uconn.edu/~terry/spring97/mcb229/viruses.html.
10. Terry TM: Microbial Taxonomy. MCB 229, Microbial Taxonomy lecture notes, spring 1997. Available at: http://www.sp.uconn.edu/~terry/spring97/mcb229/taxonomy.html.

3. THE RIGHT QUESTIONS
THE HISTORY AND INFECTIOUS DISEASES

Kimberly A. Ratcliffe, M.D.

This chapter emphasizes the importance of a detailed history. Often asking one key question can mean the difference between mystery and enlightenment. The chapter is divided into sections based on key parts of a good history. Most of the questions are case scenarios so that you can test yourself and see how good of a medical detective you can be.

EXPOSURE TO ILLNESSES

1. A 33-year-old mother of three children presents with a 3-day history of swollen and painful hands. Her wrists and metacarpophalangeal joints are boggy and inflamed bilaterally. Her 5-year-old son was sent home from school about 3 weeks previously with red cheeks and a blotchy rash on his torso. What does she have?

She has an infection with parvovirus B19, the same agent that caused the childhood exanthem erythema infectiosum or Fifth disease in her son 3 weeks previously, giving him the classic slapped-cheek appearance. Adults typically do not get the facial rash but have arthralgias and arthritis. The distribution of involved joints is similar to that in rheumatoid arthritis: the metacarpophalangeal joints, wrists, knees, and ankles are affected in a symmetric pattern. Onset is typically 3–4 weeks after exposure. Parvovirus B19 is, in general, a self-limited disease lasting 2–3 weeks. A few patients have persistent symptoms. Serologic diagnosis can be made by testing for anti-B19 IgM antibodies, which may remain elevated for up to 2 months after an acute injection. Anti-B19 IgG antibodies are found in up to 77% of adults and are therefore not useful in making the diagnosis.

INGESTIONS

2. A 23-year-old marine stationed in Hawaii develops a severe headache, altered mental status, nuchal rigidity, and paresthesias. A lumbar puncture reveals a leukocyte count of 600/mm^3 with 50% eosinophils. What did he eat?

The marine was dared to eat a raw snail 2 weeks previously. Accidental ingestion of the rat lung worm *Angiostrongylus cantonensis* produced a classic clinical scenario of eosinophilic meningitis. The organism is present in snails and in the slime trail. *A. cantonensis* is typically found in Thailand, Indonesia, Tahiti, Taiwan, and the Hawaiian Islands. Although potentially lethal to children, it is usually a self-limited disease. At present there is no curative treatment.

3. A 38-year-old man in the Northeast presents with diarrhea, periorbital edema, myositis, fever, and eosinophilia. Over the course of a few days he becomes prostrate. Two of his friends complain of diarrhea, fevers, and myalgias. Careful questioning reveals that all three ate barbecued bear meat caught on a recent hunting trip. What do they have?

The men have trichinosis caused by the ingestion of larvae of the roundworms *Trichinella spiralis* found in undercooked meat. Pork is the most common contaminated meat associated with this disease. In the northeastern United States outbreaks have been associated with eating infected raw bear meat.

4. A group of businessmen in Delaware develop hepatitis A. All affected patients were at a local meeting. What ingestions do you ask about?

Ingestion of undercooked shellfish such as oysters and clams has classically been associated with outbreaks of hepatitis A infection. Outbreaks of infection also have been associated with cold milk, salads, lettuce, hamburger, creams, pastries, and strawberries. One of the most recent outbreaks of hepatitis A occurred in April of 1997 after ingestion of fresh strawberries from Mexico that were contaminated with hepatitis A virus. Over 30 children developed hepatitis. Other groups at risk for the development of hepatitis A include patients and staff at long-term care institutions, staff and children in daycare centers, intravenous drug users, travelers from low endemic areas to higher-risk areas, military personnel living in barracks, homosexual men who engage in oral–anal sex, and workers exposed to sewage.

PETS AND ANIMALS

5. A 4-year-old boy presents with 1 day of loose stools, fevers, abdominal cramping, headache, and myalgia. He has no blood in his stool and tells you that he wants to go back home to play with his new pet Tommy the turtle. What is the cause of his diarrhea?
This is a classic scenario for *Salmonella* spp. gastroenteritis or enterocolitis. Patients with achlorhydria or alterations in gastric acidity, sickle cell disease, or defects in cellular and humoral immunity and children younger than 5 years of age have a more severe course and increased incidence of *Salmonella* infections. After the Food and Drug Administration banned the interstate shipment of pet turtles in 1975, the frequency of turtle-associated salmonellosis decreased dramatically.

6. A 37-year-old woman complains of headache, backache, and a dry hacking cough productive of scant sputum. She has fevers as high as 40° C. Her respiratory rate is 32 breaths per minute, and she has a pale macular rash on her trunk. Lung exam reveals fine, crepitant rales in the lower lung fields and a pleural rub. Abdominal exam reveals nontender splenomegaly. What type of pet does she have at home?
She recently purchased a pet parakeet and now is suffering from psittacosis. Psittacosis is caused by *Chlamydia psittaci*, an obligate intracellular parasite. Any species of bird can host the organism. Pet shop employees, pigeon handlers, and poultry workers are the largest groups at risk today.

7. What is the name of the macular rash associated with psittacosis?
Horder's spots.

8. A 13-year-old girl has painful adenopathy in her left axilla. She has scratches on her left arm with a papule at the proximal site of one scratch. What pets do you ask about?
You should ask if she has a kitten. The patient has the classic symptoms of cat scratch disease (CSD) caused by the bacillus *Bartonella henselae* (formerly *Rochalimaea henselae*). CSD is a self-limited disease with onset of symptoms 3–10 days after an inoculating scratch. The organism can be isolated from kittens, typically less than 1 year of age. A history of a new kitten in the house and the papule at the site of a scratch with regional painful adenopathy define the classic scenario for CSD.

OCCUPATIONS AND HOBBIES

9. A 28-year-old veterinarian presents with a 1-month history of malaise, chills, drenching sweats, fatigue, and weakness. He has anorexia and has lost 15 pounds. He has intermittent fevers as high as 103° F. He complains of visual blurring. Physical exam reveals mild lymphadenopathy, petechiae, and a new murmur or aortic insufficiency. Several weeks previously he helped to deliver an aborting calf fetus. What does he have?
He has brucellosis endocarditis, caused by *Brucella abortus*, which is found in cattle. The organism was first isolated in Baltimore in 1922 and typically causes a mild disease. However, *Brucella* sp. can infect the cardiovascular system and cause a localized infection. *B. abortus* is the most common species of *Brucella* to cause endocarditis (80% of cases). The aortic valve has been most commonly involved, followed by the mitral valve and then both valves together. Up to 43% of patients with endocarditis have underlying valvular disease.

10. What is Malta fever?
Malta fever, also known as Mediterranean remittent fever, is a form of brucellosis caused by *Brucella melitensis*. The organism was first isolated in British soldiers dying of Malta fever in 1886. Later it was found that unpasteurized goat milk was the source of the infection.

11. A 55-year-old butcher presents with a purplish-red, swollen, painful area surrounding a cut on his right hand. No suppuration or pitting surrounds the site. The initial lesion shows central fading and the development of new purplish-red areas at the periphery. He has a sense of burning, throbbing, and itching on his hand. What does he have?
Erysipelothrix rhusiopathiae is a pleomorphic gram-negative rod that causes a localized skin infection. Erysipelothrix is considered an occupational disease of fisherman, fish handlers, butchers, meat-processing workers, poultry workers, farmers, veterinarians, abattoir workers, and housewives. The infection usually spreads from a scratch or abrasion 1–4 days after trauma. Rarely it spreads to the heart valves and causes endocarditis. Treatment is with penicillin.

12. An amateur florist presents with painless, violaceous nodules spreading proximally along her arm. What does she have?
She has lymphocutaneous sporotrichosis caused by the fungus *Sporothrix schenckii*. The organism is most often found in soil, plants, straw, hay, and thorns of plants (such as rose bushes). Infection causes formation of subcutaneous granuloma. Secondary lesions develop superficially along the lymphatic chain.

13. A weekend spelunker complains of fever, headache, malaise, and nonproductive cough. He has no coryza or sore throat. What should you suspect as the cause?
Acute pulmonary histoplasmosis caused by *Histoplasma capsulatum* is an inhalation-acquired mycosis. *H. capsulatum* is found in soil that tends to be moist and acidic. Although birds do not become infected with the organism, bats may become infected and excrete *H. capsulatum* in their droppings. Spelunkers who disturb the dust and dirt on cave floors are at risk for acute pulmonary histoplasmosis. The severity of the disease is proportional to the amount of organisms inhaled. Up to 90% of primary pulmonary infections are asymptomatic.

14. A 32-year-old man from Arkansas presents with fevers, nonproductive cough, and myalgias for several days. His pulse is 70 beats per minute, and his temperature is 101° F. He has painful right inguinal adenopathy and a tender ulcer with raised borders on his right calf. He was rabbit hunting every day of the previous week and had a tick bite. What is the most likely cause of his illness?
Francisella tularensis, which causes tularemia, is the most likely culprit. Fifty percent of cases have been reported in Missouri, Arkansas, and Oklahoma. Infection can be transmitted by tick bites or by handling of animals such as rabbits, squirrels, beavers, and muskrats.

15. A 19-year-old college student on a summer archeology dig in California complains of fevers, cough, night sweats, and anorexia. Physical exam reveals erythema nodosum. What does he have?
He has primary coccidioidomycosis caused by *Coccidioides immitis*. Miniepidemics have been reported in archeology students digging for Native American artifacts.

NATIONALITY AND GEOGRAPHIC LOCATION

16. Why is it important to inquire about the nationality of the patient with coccidioidomycosis?
Disseminated disease occurs most often in certain dark-skinned races such as Filipinos, Mexicans, and Africans.

17. A 29-year-old Navajo Indian presents to the hospital in New Mexico with complaints of fever, myalgias, and cough for 4 days. On exam he is tachypneic and uses accessory muscles

to breathe. **Shortly after admission, he is intubated and diagnosed with adult respiratory distress syndrome. What infection must you consider?**

Hantavirus pulmonary syndrome, first noted in an outbreak in 1993, consists of fever, myalgia, and rapid development of respiratory failure leading to death. The initial cases were mostly in young Navajo Indians. The syndrome has been documented in many states and Canada but is most frequent in New Mexico, Colorado, Utah, and Arizona. Diagnosis is possible by enzyme-linked immunosorbent assay for IgM and IgG antibodies to hantavirus.

18. A 30-year-old man from Mississippi is treated for a chronic draining leg ulcer. He has received multiple courses of antibiotics without improvement. He has a well-circumscribed osteolytic lesion on plain film. A wet preparation of the pus reveals broad-based, budding yeast. What does he have?

He has skeletal blastomycosis caused by the dimorphic fungus *Blastomyces dermatitidis*. After skin, the skeletal system is the second most frequent extrapulmonary site. Any bone may be involved, although long bones are most common. The well-circumscribed osteolytic lesion and visualized budding yeast confirm the diagnosis. Immunocompetent patients are treated with itraconazole.

COMORBID ILLNESSES

19. A 72-year-old woman with diabetes presents with ear pain and drainage of pus. She has swelling and tenderness over the mastoid bone. What should you be concerned about?

Invasive malignant otitis externa is a severe necrotizing infection of the external canal, usually with *Pseudomonas aeruginosa*. Infection may spread to the mastoid bone, temporal bone, sigmoid sinus, base of the skull, meninges, and even brain. Patients at increased risk include the elderly, diabetics, and immunocompromised hosts.

20. What is the most common etiologic agent of osteomyelitis in sickle cell disease?

Salmonella species cause up to 80% of cases of osteomyelitis in sickle cell patients.

21. What diseases should you suspect in patients with *Streptococcus bovis* bacteremia?

Every patient with *S. bovis* bacteremia should undergo gastrointestinal and cardiac evaluation. In one study up to 50% of patients with *S. bovis* bacteremia had a colonic malignancy. In another study, 25–50% of cases of *S. bovis* bacteremia were associated with endocarditis, especially in patients with preexisting valvular lesions.

22. A 65-year-old man with a history of bullous emphysema complains of hemoptysis for 3 weeks. What do you suspect?

Aspergilloma. In addition to *Aspergillus* spp. infections, atypical mycobacteria such as *M. chelonei* must be considered in superinfection in patients with bullous lung disease.

23. A 13-year-old girl undergoing chemotherapy for acute lymphocytic leukemia is neutropenic. She presents with a fever, right lower quadrant pain and guarding, and guaiac positive stools. What do you suspect?

Typhlitis. The setting of neutropenia with abdominal findings and evidence of bowel involvement strongly suggests the diagnosis. Blood cultures may be positive despite appropriate antibiotic therapy because of the high-grade bacteremia and compromised host defenses.

BIBLIOGRAPHY

1. Bryan CS: Fever, famine, and war: William Osler as an infectious diseases specialist. Clin Infect Dis 23:1139–1149, 1996.
2. Nathanson N, Alexander ER: Infectious disease epidemiology. Am J Epidemiol 144(Suppl 8):S34–S38, 1996.
3. Regnery R, Tappero J: Unraveling mysteries associated with cat-scratch disease, bacillary angiomatosis, and related syndromes. Emerg Infect Dis 1:16–21, 1995.
4. Satcher D: Emerging infections: getting ahead of the curve. Emerg Infect Dis 1:1–6, 1995.
5. Wilson ME: Travel and the emergence of infectious diseases. Emerg Infect Dis 1:39–46, 1995.

4. CLUES FROM THE PHYSICAL EXAMINATION

William J. Burman, M.D.

1. A 46-year-old man is admitted to the hospital with pneumonia. He had acute onset of fevers, severe myalgias, headache, and nonproductive cough 3 days previously. His vital signs on admission are temperature of 40° C, pulse of 92 beats/min, and blood pressure of 126/86 mmHg. The remainder of the physical examination is notable for crackles in both lower lung fields posteriorly. What is notable about the vital signs? What does this suggest about the etiology of the pneumonia?

The patient has a markedly elevated temperature, and a normal pulse—a pattern termed **pulse–temperature dissociation**. Because acute bacterial infections, such as pneumococcal pneumonia, typically cause an elevation of both temperature and pulse, pulse-temperature dissociation suggests that the pneumonia is not due to an acute bacterial infection. On the other hand, viral infections often cause fever without tachycardia. Other intracellular pathogens, such as *Salmonella*, *Chlamydia*, and *Mycoplasma* species, also have been associated with pulse-temperature dissociation. The patient's chest radiograph showed diffuse infiltrates, and his white blood cell count was normal—further evidence against acute bacterial pneumonia. A nasopharyngeal culture was positive for influenza A. His symptoms improved rapidly with amantadine.

2. Fever is often considered the hallmark of infection. Give examples of situations in which infections are not associated with fever.

Fever is a host response (as are many other clinical manifestations of infections), not a direct effect of the infecting organism. Therefore, specific host factors may result in afebrile infections. Corticosteroids, particularly in high doses, can completely ablate the febrile response, despite the presence of life-threatening bacterial infection. Acetaminophen and nonsteroidal antiinflammatory drugs certainly affect fever but rarely ablate the febrile response. Because the febrile response is impaired in very young and very old patients, fever is not a consistent feature of infections in either population.

A number of chronic infections rarely cause fever. For example, although febrile illnesses are common complications of AIDS, HIV infection itself rarely causes fever (apart from the acute retroviral syndrome during initial seroconversion). A specific source should be sought for febrile illnesses in patients with AIDS. Similarly, uncomplicated viral hepatitis rarely causes fever. Fever is not a consistent feature of chronic fungal and mycobacterial infections; a surprising percentage of patients with active tuberculosis, particularly of the genitourinary tract, are consistently afebrile.

3. A patient with advanced AIDS (CD4 cell count = 23/ml) is admitted for treatment of bacterial pneumonia. On review of systems, he complains of several painful oral ulcers, which now make it difficult for him to eat. Examination reveals two ulcers, one under the tongue and one on the right tonsillar pillar. Both ulcers are approximately 1.5 cm in diameter. What causes painful oral ulcers in people with AIDS?

Painful oral ulcers are a common problem for patients with advanced AIDS and may be a source of considerable morbidity due to the pain itself and the inability to eat and resultant weight loss. The common causes are herpesvirus infections and apthous (idiopathic) ulcers. Of the herpesviruses, herpes simplex (HSV) is the most common cause of oral ulcers. HSV typically causes multiple small painful ulcers on the lips or hard palate; involvement of the tongue and tonsillar pillars, as in this case, is unusual. Herpes zoster may cause intraoral "shingles," multiple small ulcers on one side of the palate (due to infection of the maxillary division of the trigeminal nerve). Large apthous ulcers are common in advanced AIDS and may be particularly severe when they occur in the esophagus. The cause is unknown; apthous ulcers are not thought to be caused by an opportunistic infection. Apthous ulcers tend to occur on the gingiva, pharynx (and tonsillar pillars), and on or under the tongue. Apthous ulcers are usually few in number (1–3), though a variant called herpetiform apthous ulcers may present with multiple small ulcers. If untreated, apthous ulcers can become large (> 1.5 cm). Less common but important causes of oral ulcers include fungal infections (such as histoplasmosis or cryptococcosis), syphilis, medications (such as zalcitabine), and tumors (such as non-Hodgkin's lymphoma). Effective treatments are available for most causes of oral ulcers. Initial treatment (acyclovir for HSV, topical corticosteroids for apthous ulcers) is often based on clinical appearance; ulcers with an atypical appearance and ulcers that do not respond to an initial course of therapy should be biopsied.

4. Cutaneous and mucous membrane problems are common throughout the course of HIV disease. What are cutaneous and mucous membrane signs of early HIV disease?

Several cutaneous and mucous membrane problems can be valuable signs of early HIV disease. During the initial infection with HIV, approximately one-third of patients have symptomatic HIV seroconversion illness, which most often is a mononucleosis-like illness with fever and sore throat. Up to 50% of patients with seroconversion illness also have a maculopapular rash. This symptom complex in a person with risk factors for exposure to HIV should prompt specific testing for seroconversion illness (p24 antigen or reverse transcriptase polymerase chain reaction [PCR] for HIV RNA). Herpes zoster certainly occurs in immunocompetent individuals, but it is quite uncommon in persons younger than 40 years. However, persons with asymptomatic HIV infection have a 10-fold increased risk of zoster; thus, shingles in a young person should raise the question of HIV infection. Seborrheic dermatitis is a common dermatologic condition, but it is particularly common and unusually severe in persons with HIV infection. Oral hairy leukoplakia is aptly named—patches of the mucosa of the sides of the tongue become hyperplastic and appear "hairy." This finding is due to poorly controlled Epstein-Barr infection and is highly suggestive of HIV infection. Oral thrush is rare in adults and should suggest the possibility of HIV infection (other causes of thrush in adults are poorly controlled diabetes mellitus and severe immunosuppression, such as from aggressive cytotoxic chemotherapy). Vaginal candidiasis is common in reproductive-age women, but candidiasis that is refractory to therapy should suggest HIV infection (the other common cause of recurrent or refractory vaginal candidiasis is poorly controlled diabetes mellitus).

5. An injection drug user is admitted with fever without an apparent focus of infection. A serious cause of this syndrome is endocarditis. What cutaneous signs of endocarditis should be sought?

Most cutaneous lesions in endocarditis represent embolization of infected material to subcutaneous arterioles. As such, cutaneous lesions strongly suggest left-sided endocarditis (because emboli from right-sided endocarditis go to the pulmonary circulation and cause septic pulmonary emboli) and are most commonly seen in acute, destructive forms, such as *Staphylococcus aureus* endocarditis. Perhaps the most common cutaneous manifestation of endocarditis are petechiae, usually seen on the palate and conjunctiva. The counterparts in the eye are known as Roth spots—small petechiae with a pale (infarcted) center. The examination then should focus on the hands and feet. Splinter hemorrhages—linear hemorrhages running the length of the nail bed—occur in endocarditis. Larger emboli cause Osler nodes—painful, nodular, violaceous lesions on the pads of the fingers and toes. Janeway lesions are larger, macular, ecchymotic lesions on the palms and soles. Occasionally Janeway lesions are so large and prominent as to suggest the purpura fulminans of disseminated meningococcemia.

6. A 33-year-old man presents with fevers and chills for 2 days. His medical history is notable for a splenectomy 2 years ago, and the physical examination is notable for scattered petechiae on the arms and legs. What is the differential diagnosis of fever and petechiae?

The presence of petechiae signifies abnormal bleeding from small arterioles. One of the pathophysiologic mechanisms of petechiae is the occurrence of severe thrombocytopenia. A number of viral infections, particularly HIV, can trigger immune thrombocytopenia. Intestinal infection with certain strains of *Escherichia coli* (0H157) cause vasculitis and thrombocytopenia—the hemolytic-uremic syndrome—probably due to an overly vigorous immune response to the initial infection. Petechiae may also be due to inflammation of the blood vessel (i.e., vasculitis). Infectious agents are common causes of vasculitis. Acute bacterial sepsis, most notably *Neisseria meningitidis* sepsis, may cause a severe febrile illness with petechiae. Asplenic patients are at markedly increased risk of this syndrome, most commonly due to *Streptococcus pneumoniae* and occasionally *Haemophilus influenzae*. Because *Rickettsia* species directly infect endothelial cells, petechiae are a common manifestation of rickettsial infection. In the United States, the most common rickettsial infection is Rocky Mountain spotted fever (*Rickettsia rickettsiae*), which typically causes petechiae that initially appear on the extremities and subsequently spread to involve the torso. Microemboli also may cause petechiae; thus, petechiae are a common cutaneous manifestation of endocarditis. Finally, severe malaria, due to *Plasmodium falciparum*, may cause severe thrombocytopenia and high fevers.

The patient was emergently started on intravenous ceftriaxone and promptly improved. Blood cultures from admission grew *S. pneumoniae*.

7. A 53-year-old woman presents with lesions on the right arm for 1 month. The first lesion began near the wrist and was raised and painful. Similar lesions then appeared proximal to the initial lesion, progressing up the right arm. What is this syndrome called? What infections should be suspected?

The presentation of multiple nodular lesions along an extremity suggests infection of the lymphatics. This syndrome is called **nodular lymphangitis** or **sporotrichoid lymphangitis** because the classic cause is infection by *Sporothrix schenckii*, an environmental fungus. Other causes include environmental mycobacteria, such as *Mycobacterium marinum*, and *Nocardia brasiliensis*. In a patient with a history of travel to Central or South America, cutaneous leishmaniasis should be considered. Finally, although lymphangitis due to pyogenic bacteria such as *Streptococcus pyogenes* or *S. aureus* is usually an acute, rapidly evolving illness, occasionally these organisms cause a more indolent form of lymphangitis, which may have a sporotrichoid appearance. A biopsy from one of the patient's lesions showed noncaseating granulomata, and the culture grew *Sporothrix schenckii*.

8. A 58-year-old woman presents with fevers and progressively severe abdominal pain for the past 2 days. Her history is notable for non–insulin-dependent diabetes mellitus. On examination her temperature is 38.5° C, and a large area of erythema extends from the vulva onto the anterior abdominal wall. In the center of this area, the patient has no pinprick sensation. What is the differential diagnosis? How can the physical examination help to distinguish between the major possibilities?

Fever and cutaneous erythema are most commonly due to infection of the dermis, termed cellulitis. However, infection of deeper structures—subcutaneous fascia and muscle—also may result in fever and cutaneous erythema. The distinction between cellulitis and infections of deeper structures is crucial because the therapy is radically different: cellulitis generally responds well to antibiotic therapy, but necrotizing fasciitis or myositis requires aggressive debridement in addition to systemic antibiotics. The distinction between cellulitis and necrotizing fasciitis or myositis is made almost entirely on the basis of the physical examination. Infection of the subcutaneous tissue often causes infarction of the blood vessels serving the skin and related structures; this is the basis of many of the physical findings in necrotizing fasciitis, including severe pain, local anesthesia (infarction of cutaneous nerves), and skin necrosis. Diabetes mellitus is a major risk factor for necrotizing fasciitis of the abdominal wall. The patient's presentation warrants emergent surgical consultation as well as broad-spectrum intravenous antibiotics.

Comparison of the Clinical Features of Cellulitis and Necrotizing Fasciitis/Myositis

	CELLULITIS	NECROTIZING FASCIITIS/MYOSITIS
Frequency	Common	Uncommon
Systemic toxicity	Uncommon	Common
Pain	Mild to moderate	Often severe
Skin color	Erythema	Erythema progressing to blue-black discoloration
Local anesthesia	Absent	Sometimes present
Crepitance	Absent	Sometimes present
Bullae	Usually absent	Sometimes present

9. What organisms cause necrotizing fasciitis?

The anatomic location of necrotizing fasciitis is an important clue to its microbiologic etiology. Necrotizing fasciitis of the extremities is often monomicrobial; the common pathogens are *S. pyogenes* (group A beta-hemolytic streptococci) or clostridial species. Involvement of the trunk is more often due to a mixed infection of enteric organisms (aerobic gram-negative bacilli and anaerobes such as *Bacteroides* and/or *Fusobacterium* species).

10. A 21-year-old man was diagnosed with acute myelogenous leukemia 10 days previously. He received chemotherapy and quickly became pancytopenic. He developed fevers to 38.5° C 3 days ago and was started on ceftazidime and gentamicin. However, the fevers have continued, and he has now developed diffuse pustular skin lesions. What causes skin lesions in the setting of neutropenia?

Skin lesions are a valuable clue in the evaluation of febrile immunosuppressed patients. Bacterial sepsis, particularly due to *Pseudomonas aeruginosa* and *S. aureus*, is a relatively common cause of skin lesions in febrile neutropenic patients. Candidal septicemia is a major consideration in the neutropenic patient with pustular lesions, especially when the lesions appear during treatment with broad-spectrum antibacterial agents. Other fungi, including molds, also may cause this syndrome, particularly in the setting of prolonged granulocytopenia (> 21 days). Disseminated herpesvirus infections (varicella zoster virus, herpes simplex virus) usually cause diffuse vesicular lesions. Finally, drug reactions are a common cause of rash and fever and are not easily differentiated from infection on clinical grounds. However, skin biopsy helps to distinguish between infectious and noninfectious causes of skin lesions.

11. A 28-year-old man with AIDS presents with fevers for 3 weeks. On examination he has diffuse 0.5-mm nodular skin lesions. What causes nodular skin lesions in the setting of AIDS?

Patients with AIDS have a profound deficiency in cell-mediated immunity, but usually granulocytic function is relatively preserved. Therefore, the spectrum of infections with cutaneous manifestations is different in AIDS than in neutropenic patients. In contrast to neutropenic patients, bacterial infections and candidal septicemia seldom are causes of skin lesions in febrile patients with AIDS. Instead the differential diagnosis of skin lesions in febrile patients with AIDS primarily involves fungal and viral infections. Dimorphic fungal infections, such as histoplasmosis, coccidioidomycosis, or cryptococcosis (or disseminated *Penicillium marneffei* in patients from southeast Asia) commonly present with nodular or ulcerative skin lesions. Given the rapidly progressive, severe nature of fungal infections in AIDS and the difficulties in diagnosis (due to the need for specialized media and slow growth of organisms in culture), skin biopsy can be a valuable tool and should be considered early in the evaluation of such patients. Mycobacterial infections, such as tuberculosis or disseminated *Mycobacterium avium* complex, are common in patients with AIDS and occasionally present with skin lesions. Viral infections that commonly present as skin lesions include herpesviruses (most commonly presenting as vesicles, but occasionally causing nodules) and molluscum contagiosum (a common cause of nodular lesions). Finally, an unusual bacterial infection may present with nodular skin lesions in patients with AIDS. Infection with several *Bartonella* species causes bacillary angiomatosis, characterized by multiple violaceous skin lesions similar in clinical appearance to the cutaneous lesions of Kaposi's sarcoma. The first test in the evaluation of the patient was a skin biopsy, which showed many small yeast forms with morphologic characteristics suggestive of *Histoplasma capsulatum* (eventually confirmed by culture).

12. A 24-year-old man presents with a week-long history of an ulcer on the penis. What features on physical examination help to distinguish the common causes of a genital ulcer?

The common causes of genital ulcer are herpes simplex virus (HSV), syphilis, chancroid, and trauma. No single feature is diagnostic, but characteristic features of these etiologies are listed in the table below.

Feature	HSV	Syphilis	Chancroid	Trauma
Pain	Prominent	Usually absent	Prominent	Variable
Number of ulcers	Multiple	Usually single	Usually single	Usually single
Size of ulcers	Small	Moderate	Moderate	Variable
Appearance of ulcers	Not indurated, tender	Clean base, indurated edge	Friable base, tender	Variable
Associated adenopathy	Bilateral during primary HSV, absent during recurrences	Unilateral, nontender	Unilateral, sometimes fluctuant	Usually absent

13. Infections that are introduced through the skin may result in a lesion at the site of initial inoculation followed by dissemination to the rest of the body. The lesion at the site of initial inoculation is called a chancre. What infections cause chancres?

Syphilis is the classic infection that presents with a chancre. Lyme disease, also caused by a spirochete, frequently causes an expanding skin lesion (erythema migrans) at the site of initial inoculation. Chancres are common in several rickettsial diseases (boutonneuse fever in the Mediterranean and scrub typhus in the South Pacific). Finally, a chancre is characteristic of African trypanosomiasis.

14. A 32-year-old man presents with diffuse nontender adenopathy. What infections should be included in the differential diagnosis?

A number of viral infections may cause diffuse adenopathy (e.g., measles, mononucleosis). In a person with risk factors for exposure, HIV infection is probably one of the most common causes of diffuse adenopathy. Disseminated bacterial infections, usually due to intracellular pathogens, also may cause diffuse adenopathy; examples include secondary syphilis, leptospirosis, and typhoid fever. Of the parasitic infections, toxoplasmosis is the common cause of diffuse lymphadenopathy in the United States. Given an appropriate exposure history, leishmaniasis, trypanosomiasis, and filariasis are considerations.

15. Polyarticular arthritis has many causes. What infections should be considered? How can physical examination help in the differential diagnosis?

Arthritis related to infection can be due either to direct infection of the joints or to an immune reaction to an infection. Symmetric polyarticular arthritis is a relatively common manifestation of a number of viral infections in immunocompetent adults, most likely due to an immune response to viremia. Hepatitis B and parvovirus B19 are common causes of acute, nondestructive polyarthritis (prior to high rates of vaccination, rubella and mumps were the common viral causes of this syndrome).

Immune reactions to bacterial infections also may cause arthritis; examples include the arthritis of rheumatic fever and the reactive arthritis following urethral or gastrointestinal infections

(Reiter's syndrome). The reactive arthritides related to bacterial infections most commonly result in asymmetric, oligoarticular arthritis involving large joints. Direct bacterial infection usually presents as monoarthritis but may cause polyarthritis, especially in patients with pre-existing polyarticular arthritis (such as rheumatoid arthritis). Polyarticular arthritis is also relatively common in gonococcal arthritis and Lyme disease. However, the involvement of multiple joints from direct infection is generally limited to a few joints and is seldom symmetric. Finally polyarticular arthritis can be a manifestation of lepromatous leprosy.

BIBLIOGRAPHY

1. Brook I: Clinical and microbiological features of necrotizing fasciitis. J Clin Microbiol 33:2382–2387, 1995.
2. Cohen PR, Bank DE, Silvers DN, Grossman ME: Cutaneous lesions of disseminated histoplasmosis in human immunodeficiency virus-infected patients. J Am Acad Dermatol 23:422–428, 1990.
3. Holmberg SD, Buchbinder SP, Conley LJ, et al: The spectrum of medical conditions and symptoms before acquired immunodeficiency syndrome in homosexual and bisexual men infected with the human immunodeficiency virus. Am J Epidemiol 141:395–406, 1995.
4. Itin PH, Lautenschlager S, Fluckiger R, Rufli T: Oral manifestations in HIV-infected patients: Diagnosis and management. J Am Acad Dermatol 29:749–760, 1993.
5. Kingston ME, Mackey D: Skin clues in the diagnosis of life-threatening infections. Rev Infect Dis 8:1–11, 1986.
6. Kostman JR, DiNubile MJ: Nodular lymphangitis: A distinctive but often unrecognized syndrome. Ann Intern Med 118:883–888, 1993.

II. Major Syndromes

5. FEVER AND FEVER OF UNKNOWN ORIGIN: THE "WHO DUNNIT" OF INFECTIOUS DISEASE

Kelly L. Wirfel, M.D., and Donald R. Skillman, M.D., FACP

There is only one way to be born and a thousand ways to die.

Serbian Proverb

1. How is fever defined?

Fever is a controlled elevation of body temperature above normal range as a result of a shift in the hypothalamic set point. Fever is distinguished from other forms of hyperthermia by a response to pyrogens in the central nervous system thermoregulatory functions. It is the only form of hyperthermia that responds to aspirin and aspirin-like compounds and functions by upregulation of the body temperature set point. Heat stroke, in contrast, is a result of excessive heat storage and faulty heat dissipation.

2. How was a "normal" body temperature decided?

The normal temperature for healthy adults was determined in the nineteenth century by Carl Reinhold August Wunderlich, who took nearly 1 million **axillary** temperatures from approximately 25,000 adults. The mean temperature of 37.0° C (98.6° F) was identified with a range of 36.2–37.5° C (97.2–99.5° F). Temperatures were recorded with the nadir at 6 AM and the zenith between 4–6 PM. Axillary temperatures are uniformly unreliable, as are oral temperatures taken after hot or cold drinks or smoking or in a mouth-breathing patient. Rectal temperatures are typically 0.6° C (1° F) higher than oral temperatures.

3. What is the pathogenesis of fever?

The fundamental step in raising the hypothalamic set point involves the ability of pyrogenic (derived from the Greek word *pyr*, meaning fire) molecules to increase the production of hypothalamic arachidonate metabolites. Pyrogens can be either endogenous or exogenous. Cytokine interleukin-1 (IL-1) is an example of an endogenous pyrogen, whereas lipopolysaccharides from bacteria may be exogenous pyrogens. In addition to upregulating the hypothalamic thermostat, the peripheral mechanisms regulating heat loss and/or production must be intact for the production of fever.

4. What does fever do for us?

The purpose of fever is to enhance the inflammatory response, inhibit bacterial growth, and create an undesirable physiologic environment for the infection or other disease process.

5. What is the significance of relative bradycardia in the presence of fever?

The magnitude of fever and the associated pulse rate sometimes give a clue to the cause of fever. Most infectious diseases produce temperatures between 37.0–41.0° C. Temperatures greater than 41.0° C are usually not infectious and result from drug fevers, malignant hyperthermia, heat stroke, and central nervous system fevers.

6. How can I know if relative bradycardia is present in a patient with fever?

Relative bradycardia is identified by calculating the appropriate pulse rate for a given temperature deviation above 102° F. Subtract 1 from the last digit of the Fahrenheit temperature, multiply by 10, and then add that number to 100. For example:

$$103° F = 3 - 1 = 2; 2 \times 10 = 20; 20 + 100 = 120 \text{ beats/minute.}$$

Any pulse less than 120 is considered relative bradycardia.

7. Give examples of fevers with relative bradycardia and relative tachycardia.

Relative bradycardia	Relative tachycardia
Dengue fever	Diphtheria
Central nervous system fever	Clostridial sepsis
Drug fever	Hyperthyroidism
Epidemic typhus	Pulmonary embolism
Legionnaires' disease	Cardiac arrhythmias
Malaria	
Lymphoma	
Typhoid/yellow fever	
Factitious fever	

8. Fever curves, although not diagnostic, sometimes suggest the underlying cause of fever. What are the confusing and sometimes ridiculous names of the characteristic fever curves seen with adult-onset Still's disease (juvenile rheumatoid arthritis), *Plasmodium malariae*, *P. vivax* or *P. ovale*, and cyclic neutropenia?

Adult-onset Still's disease is characterized by a double quotidian fever curve consisting of two fever spikes within a 24-hour period. *P. malariae* may present with a quartan fever curve with fevers and suppuration occurring every third day. In contrast, *P. vivax* or *P. ovale* may have tertian fevers occurring on alternate days. Cyclic neutropenia manifests as fever and associated neutropenia every 21 days.

Malaria is derived from the Latin *malus aer* (bad air). Quartan must pertain to the fourth; paroxysms of fever recur every fourth day, counting the day of the previous temperature spike as day number one. Tertian refers to the recurrence of fever every third day.

9. What is the likely cause of fever in a diabetic patient who presents with leukocytosis, pleuritic left upper quadrant pain, a new heart murmur, left pleural effusion, and constitutional symptoms?

The likely cause is bacterial endocarditis with septic emboli to the spleen resulting in a splenic abscess. Splenic abscesses develop most frequently with endocarditis, sickle cell anemia, splenic trauma, and immunocompromised states, including AIDS, chemotherapy-induced immunosuppression, chronic steroid use, and diabetes mellitus. Common organisms are *Escherichia coli*, *Streptococcus* spp., *Staphylococcus aureus*, and *Salmonella* spp.

10. What disease process is commonly associated with fever and an evanescent salmon-colored rash?

Adult-onset Still's disease or juvenile rheumatoid arthritis is a systemic inflammatory disorder of unknown etiology and pathogenesis. A double quotidian fever curve (see question 8), arthralgias and/or arthritis, polyserositis, and leukocytosis characterize Still's disease. The transient macular-papular, salmon-colored rash is noted with fever spikes. Elevation of serum ferritin is suggestive and correlates with disease activity. Still's disease is the most common rheumatologic disorder causing fever of unknown origin (FUO).

11. When is it appropriate to treat fever?

It is common practice to treat temperature elevations with antipyretics despite some evidence that fever may enhance host defense mechanisms. Several animal studies, but few human studies, suggest benefits of fever. In vitro data reveal enhanced B- and T-cell activity and increased immunoglobulin synthesis in response to fevers greater than 39° C. In vitro growth of some microbes (e.g., *Plasmodium* spp.) is suppressed at elevated temperatures. At least two notorious infectious disease doctors (Jeff Lennox and Don Skillman) live by the motto that "fever is our friend."

Obviously children at risk for febrile seizures and patients with extremely high temperatures or underlying cardiac or pulmonary disease should be treated with acetaminophen or other nonsteroidal antiinflammatory drugs (NSAIDs). Aspirin and NSAIDs should be used with caution in children because of the increased risk of Reye's syndrome. Fever increases oxygen demand. For every 1° C over 37° C, oxygen consumption increases by 13%.

12. What is the definition of fever of unknown origin (FUO)?

The original criteria by Petersdorf and Beeson described an illness with temperatures greater than 38.0° C, evolving during at least a 3-week period with no diagnosis reached after 1 week of inpatient investigation. Most causes of FUO are not so much obscure diseases as unusual presentations of common diseases. The UO is part of FUO because the illnesses are sufficiently atypical to fool technology as well as the clinician.

13. In the era of cost-containment, has the definition of FUO changed?

If the patient's condition allows, a substantial portion of the evaluation should be done in the outpatient setting. Under Medicare, the federally allotted stay in the hospital is substantially less than the time required to arrive at a diagnosis. Petersdorf recently suggested that the third criterion be modified to no diagnosis despite 1 week of intensive evaluation. Wherever you do it, there is no substitute for observing, repeatedly talking to, and thinking about the patient.

14. Name three usual suspects (categories of disease) that give rise to FUO.

Infections, neoplasms, and connective tissue diseases are the major categories. Infections still represent the majority of cases of FUO, followed closely by connective tissue diseases. Tumors have become a less important cause of FUO, presumably related to improvements in diagnostic modalities.

In addition to these classic categories, other authors have suggested a further breakdown of categories to include nosocomially acquired infections, neutropenic fevers, and HIV-associated infections. Important considerations in nosocomial infections are *Clostridium difficile* colitis, sinusitis, drug fever, and septic thrombophlebitis. Perianal and fungal infections should be considered in neutropenic patients refractory to antibiotic treatment. The myriad opportunistic infections should be high on the differential diagnosis in patients with HIV infection as well as drug fever, lymphoma, and tuberculosis.

15. Give several examples of the more common infections and neoplasms that cause FUO in the United States.

Infections	Neoplasms
Endocarditis	Leukemia
Osteomyelitis	Lymphoma
Vascular catheter infections	Malignant histiocytosis
Hepatitis	Pancreatic cancer
Prostatic abscess	Myelodysplastic syndromes
Sinusitis	Sarcoma
Tuberculosis	Benign atrial myxoma
Intraabdominal abscess	Renal cell carcinoma
HIV	Hepatoma

16. Give several examples of connective tissue diseases and miscellaneous conditions that cause FUO in the United States.

Connective tissue disease	Miscellaneous conditions
Adult-onset Still's disease	Drug fever
Temporal arteritis	Factitious fever
Polymyalgia rheumatica	Familial Mediterranean fever
Sarcoidosis	Hyperthyroidism
Systemic lupus erythematosus	Adrenal insufficiency
Sjögren's syndrome	Pulmonary emboli
Wegener's granulomatosis	Cyclic neutropenia
Erythema nodosum	Postmyocardial infarction
Behçet's syndrome	Crohn's disease

17. What is the most common neoplastic disease responsible for FUO?

Lymphoma, including both Hodgkin's and non-Hodgkin's disease. Patients commonly have a daily temperature spike. The Pel-Ebstein fever, characterized by a relapsing fever that disappears and reappears at an interval of 3–10 days, rarely occurs but is classic for Hodgkin's lymphoma.

18. Name the most common solid tumor causing FUO.

Renal cell carcinoma. Fever occurs in approximately 20% of cases, and may be the only symptom in rare patients. Patients occasionally present with liver function abnormalities or coagulopathy suggesting a primary liver disorder.

19. What is the most common systemic bacterial infection causing FUO?

Tuberculosis. Not infrequently, patients have disseminated (miliary) disease, often associated with a negative tuberculin skin test. Chest roentgenogram is normal in approximately 50% of extrapulmonary tuberculosis. Characteristic small opacities (2-mm diameter) on chest roentgenogram may go unseen until several weeks into the course of the illness.

Infectious agents still remain the most common source of FUO since the original description of FUO in 1961 (despite advances in antibiotic therapy). Other systemic bacterial illnesses to consider include salmonellosis, brucellosis, syphilis, chronic meningococcemia, tularemia, borreliosis, leptospirosis, and Lyme disease, among many others.

20. What is the most common viral cause of FUO?

Cytomegalovirus commonly produces atypical lymphocytosis, with elevated transaminases and alkaline phosphatase enzymes on presentation and often with a fever of more than 3 weeks' duration. Other common symptoms include general malaise, myalgias, splenomegaly, sore throat, and, on rare occasions, cervical lymphadenopathy. HIV and infectious mononucleosis also should be considered. HIV rarely produces isolated fever, but fever may be an indication of other underlying infections.

21. How do you figure out when your patient has a drug fever?

Patients may present with high spiking fevers (above 40.0° C [104° F]) associated with rigors, hypotension, and leukocytosis. Other patients present with a characteristic rash or eosinophilia. Patients may appear clinically well or ill. Relative bradycardia, as noted above, may be seen. Virtually any medication can be the culprit, including those administered for long periods or those previously administered without difficulty. Fever typically abates within 24–72 hours after discontinuation of the suspect drug, and reinstitution of the drug elicits fever within several hours. Withdrawal of all drugs should be considered in the early evaluation of FUO when the diagnosis is unclear.

22. What is factitious fever?

Factitious fever is a rare entity seen most commonly in young women with paramedical experience. Such patients commonly manipulate thermometers, inject infectious agents, and fabricate extensive historical information to simulate disease. Clues to this entity include a healthy-appearing female in the face of extremely high temperatures, which may lack diurnal variation, and associated tachycardia or diaphoresis. Also consider this diagnosis when sequential blood cultures are positive for multiple organisms. Take temperatures with a nurse in the room, check simultaneous rectal and oral temperatures, and search the room for needles, syringes, preset thermometers, vaccines, and toxins to evaluate for this condition. The electric thermometers make it hard for people to "fake" a fever.

23. What is Sutton's law? Petersdorf's law?

Petersdorf and Beeson's original article popularized Sutton's law in 1961 to emphasize the importance of targeting diagnostic tests toward the historical and physical findings rather than conducting random tests. The law has been ascribed to the thief Willie Sutton, who, when asked why he robbed banks, replied "Why, that's where the money is." Willie later denied making this famous statement.

The cause of fever remains unknown in approximately 5–15% of cases of FUO. Often FUOs resolve without emergence of serious disease. It is important to consider repeat history and physical exams when the cause remains obscure. New observers often add important data to the differential diagnosis that may not have been previously acquired. After a reasonable work-up, observation may be as beneficial as further diagnostic tests in a stable patient.

In 1982, Petersdorf's law is as follows: "When the diagnosis is obscure, look at the surgical scar for sure." In my experience getting a surgeon to consider seriously that the patient's recent operation may be the cause of FUO is like getting a turtle to jump through a flaming hoop.

BIBLIOGRAPHY

1. Hirschmann JV: Fever of unknown origin in adults. Clin Infect Dis 24:291–302, 1997.
2. Cunha BA: Clinical implications of fever. Postgrad Med 85:188–200, 1989.
3. Cunha BA: Fever of unknown origin. Infect Dis Clin North Am 10:111–127, 1996.
4. Knockaert DC, Vanneste LJ, Vanneste SB, et al: Fever of unknown origin in the 1980's: An update of the diagnostic spectrum. Arch Intern Med 152:51–55, 1992.
5. Mandell GL, Bennet JE, Dolin R (eds): Principles and Practice of Infectious Disease, 4th ed. New York, Churchill Livingstone, 1995.
6. Petersdorf RG, Beeson PB: Fever of unexplained origin: Report of 100 cases. Medicine 40:1–30, 1961.

6. SEPSIS IN ADULTS

Syed Hasan, M.D., and William Roland, M.D.

1. Define infection and bacteremia.

Infection: the presence of microorganisms at a normally sterile site with an inflammatory response.

Bacteremia: presence of bacteria in the blood (may be transient) detected by culture.

2. Define sepsis, severe sepsis, septic shock, and refractory septic shock.

Sepsis: infection accompanied by systemic host response in two or more of the following ways: (1) temperature > 38°C or < 36°C, (2) heart rate > 90 beats/min, (3) respiration > 20 breaths/min or $PaCO_2$ < 32 mmHg, and (4) white blood cell count > 12,000 cell/mm^3 or < 4,000 cell/mm^3 or > 10% bands.

Severe sepsis: sepsis associated with altered organ perfusion or dysfunction or hypotension often manifested by one of the following: (1) elevated lactic acid, (2) acute oliguria, or (3) altered mental status.

Septic shock: sepsis-induced hypotension with systolic blood pressure < 90 mmHg or drop of 40 mmHg from baseline despite adequate fluid challenge (500 ml saline).

Refractory septic shock: septic shock that does not respond to fluid or pharmacologic resuscitation for 1 hour.

3. Define systemic inflammatory response and multiorgan dysfunction.

Systemic inflammatory response (SIRS): a systemic response like sepsis with or without documented infection. It also may be secondary to noninfectious etiology (e.g., burns or pancreatitis).

Multiorgan dysfunction (MODS): presence of two or more organ system dysfunctions in the clinical setting of sepsis. It is a hyperdynamic, hypermetabolic state with a 60% mortality rate.

4. How common are sepsis and its associated conditions? What is the prognosis?

The CDC estimates 71,000–140,000 cases of sepsis per year (1.3% of hospital discharges) and 550–900 episodes of SIRS per 1000 patient days. The mortality rate is about 6% for sepsis, 7% for SIRS, 20% for severe sepsis, and 46% for septic shock.

5. Name the risk factors for higher mortality rates in sepsis.

For **early death:** severe acidosis, shock, and failure of two or more organ systems.

For **late death:** preexisting heart or liver disease, hypothermia, thrombocytopenia, and multiple sources of infection.

6. What are the common signs and symptoms of sepsis?

Signs and symptoms may be nonspecific. Fevers, chills, hyperventilation, hypothermia, skin lesions (e.g., meningococcemia, pseudomonal sepsis), and mental status changes are common.

7. Name the major complications of sepsis.

Hypotension, leukopenia, thrombocytopenia, bleeding from disseminated intravascular coagulation (DIC), adult respiratory distress syndrome (ARDS), renal failure, and multiple organ failure.

8. What is the proposed pathogenetic sequence in sepsis?

Endotoxin and other bacterial products, such as lipoteichoic acid, act on responsive immune effector cells (macrophages, neutrophils, endothelial cells, and lymphocytes). These cells release secondary inflammatory mediators such as cytokines, prostanoids, leukotrienes, platelet-activating factor, and kinins. These mediators produce hypotension through vasodilation and myocardial depression, along with tissue damage through hypoperfusion, neutrophil accumulation, reactive oxygen metabolites, and proteolytic enzymes.

9. Name the most important mediators of sepsis.

Tumor necrosis factor alpha (TNF-α); interleukins (IL) 1, 2, 6, and 8; complement components (C5a, kinins); myocardial depressant factor; and nitric oxide (NO).

10. What are the effects of tumor necrosis factors?

Inflammation: fever, margination of polymorphonuclear neutrophils, activation of antimicrobial activity of phagocytes.

Wound effect: increased vascular proliferation, osteoclastic activity, collagen synthesis.

Cardiovascular effects: tachycardia, hypotension, myocardial depression, capillary leak.

Central nervous system: anorexia, fever, headache.

Metabolic effects: acidosis, bone resorption, gluconeogenesis, increased production of pituitary and adrenal hormone.

Hematologic effects: decreased hematopoiesis.

Renal effects: oliguria, cortical necrosis.

11. How is production of NO regulated?

Nitric oxide is produced in endothelial cells and macrophages by the action of inducible nitric oxide synthetases on arginine. Activators include interferon (IFN)-γ, lipopolysaccharide (LPS), TNF-α, IL-1, and IFN-α.

12. What are the beneficial effects of NO?

NO dilates microvessels to maintain perfusion, blocks platelet aggregation, inhibits leukocyte adhesion to protect endothelium, and scavenges oxygen radicals. NO also is partially responsible for the microbicidal activity of macrophages.

13. Name the deleterious effect of NO.

NO dilates vessels, leading to hypotension from loss of autoregulation in capillary beds and myocardial depression. It also causes free radical damage and direct tissue damage.

14. What is the role of platelet-activating factor (PAF)?

PAF is a phospholipid mediator produced in response to endotoxin and cytokines. It increases vascular permeability, aggregates platelets and leukocytes, promotes arachidonic acid release, and has a negative inotropic effect on the heart.

15. What organisms are commonly involved in community-acquired sepsis?

The common organisms are streptococci and *Staphylococcus aureus*. Among the gram-negative organisms, *Escherichia coli* is the most common.

16. What are the common organisms for nosocomial sepsis?

Gram-negative bacilli (*Pseudomonas* sp., *Proteus* sp., *Klebsiella* sp., *E. coli*) and gram-positive organisms (*S. aureus*, and enterococci).

17. What are the three key features of sepsis management?

1. **Recognition** of sepsis through a high index of suspicion
2. **Prompt diagnosis and treatment** of the nidus of infection and broad spectrum of antibiotic coverage
3. **Adjunctive therapy** with fluids, inotropic support, and electrolyte management

18. What is the role of nonantibiotic therapies such as steroids, anticoagulants, naloxone, morphine, prostaglandin inhibitors, and antiserum to TNF in the management of sepsis?

To date no benefit has been proved for any of the above agents.

19. What should be the order of inotropic agent use?

Dopamine usually is the first inotropic agent used. It causes vasodilation of renal, coronary, and cerebral vessels as well as an increase in systolic blood pressure and heart rate and an effective reduction in blood flow to skeletal muscle. Dobutamine is the next choice. Its inotropic effects are greater than its chronotropic effects. Isoproterenol is the third choice; it increases cardiac index but has little effect on mean arterial pressure. Norepinephrine, which is an alpha agonist, should be reserved only for patients in whom it is not possible to support systemic blood pressure and vascular perfusion with dopamine or isoproterenol. Norepinephrine has intense peripheral vasoconstricting activity that can compromise perfusion of vital organs and increase myocardial irritability.

20. What is the appropriate empiric treatment for community-acquired sepsis in a non-neutropenic host with the urinary tract suspected as the source?

If the urinary tract is the suspected source, consider a third-generation cephalosporin, antipseudomonal penicillin or a quinolone with or without an aminoglycoside. These agents provide broad-spectrum gram-negative bacterial coverage along with some gram-positive coverage.

21. If the urinary tract is not the source, what antibiotics should you use?

A third-generation cephalosporin and metronidazole or any of the following: (1) ticarcillin/clavulanate, (2) piperacillin/tazobactam, or (3) ampicillin/sulbactam with or without an aminoglycoside. These combinations provide broad-spectrum gram-negative and anaerobic coverage along with some gram-positive coverage. Choice is guided by the clinical setting of the sepsis and the suspected source of infection.

22. What is an appropriate empiric choice of antibiotics for nosocomial sepsis?

An antipseudomonal cephalosporin or antipseudomonal penicillin with a beta-lactamase inhibitor or imipenem with or without an aminoglycoside. These combinations provide broad gram-negative, gram-positive, and anaerobic coverage. The choice should be guided by the clinical setting (i.e., problematic bacteria in the ICU if the infection is acquired there and antibiotic susceptibility patterns for organisms in your hospital). Being familiar with the results of the antibiogram in a particular institution greatly assists in the selection of the appropriate antibiotic(s) for empiric therapy.

23. When should you add vancomycin?

When methicillin-resistant *Staphyloccus aureus* (MRSA) or multidrug resistant pneumococci are suspected. Knowing the relative importance of MRSA in your institution is useful in making this decision.

24. What are the drugs of choice in patients with thermal injury to at least 20% of the body surface area?

A third-generation cephalosporin, aminoglycoside, and vancomycin or antipseudomonal penicillin, vancomycin, and aminoglycoside provide broad-spectrum staphylococcal, pseudomonal, and gram-negative coverage.

BIBLIOGRAPHY

1. Bone RC, Balk RA, Cerra FB, et al: Definition for sepsis and organ failure and guidelines for the use of innovative therapies in sepsis. Chest 107:1644–1655, 1992.
2. Bone RC, Grodzin CJ, Balk RA: Sepsis: A new hypothesis for pathogenesis of disease process. Chest 112:235–243, 1997.

pyogenic abscesses more likely, but overlap is considerable. Serologic studies detecting the presence of antibodies are 90% sensitive in patients with amebic liver abscesses. Aspiration revealing organisms by Gram stain and/or culture is diagnostic of pyogenic abscesses. Aspiration of amebic abscesses usually produces a material akin to anchovy paste. Organisms, however, may not be seen in material from the center of an amebic abscess. Hydatid cysts may show internal septations on computed tomographic (CT) scans. Serologic studies are 60–85% sensitive, but aspiration may be dangerous due to leakage of the fluid. Hepatosplenic candidiasis is usually seen during or after an episode of neutropenia. The CT scan typically reveals multiple bull's-eye lesions.

6. List the clinical clues that should make one suspect an anaerobic lung abscess.
 • History of altered consciousness
 • Esophageal disease
 • Periodontal disease or gingivitis
 • Cavitary involvement of the posterior segments of the upper lobes (right more common than left)
 • Fever and cough for more than 2 weeks
 • Foul smelling sputum
 • Presence of mixed bacterial flora on Gram stain of sputum

7. Describe the different types of renal abscesses.
 Renal cortical abscesses (renal carbuncle) are usually due to hematogenous spread of *Staphylococcus aureus*. Urinalysis may be normal. Antibiotic therapy without drainage is often successful.
 Because renal corticomedullary abscesses usually are secondary to an underlying urinary tract infection, the usual pathogens are enteric gram-negative rods. Urinalysis typically reveals pyuria and bacteria. Percutaneous drainage and antibiotics are the usual treatment.
 Most perinephric abscesses are secondary to extension from urinary tract infections; enteric gram-negative organisms are the usual pathogens. Perinephric abscesses less commonly result from hematogenous seeding. Typically patients have a urinary tract obstruction, kidney stone, or diabetes. These abscesses require drainage and antimicrobial therapy.

8. What anatomic spaces are involved when head and neck abscesses result in life-threatening complications?
 Maxillary abscesses may extend into the orbit and result in cavernous sinus thrombosis. Bilateral submandibular and sublingual space involvement (Ludwig's angina) may result in asphyxia from obstruction by the tongue. Infections involving the submandibular space or masticator spaces may extend into the lateral pharyngeal space and then the retropharyngeal space. From the lateral pharyngeal space, extension into the jugular vein may cause thrombosis or carotid artery erosion. Infections of the retropharyngeal space may cause respiratory distress due to forward displacement of the pharyngeal wall or extend into the mediastinum.

9. When should one suspect involvement by anaerobic bacteria in patients with cellulitis?
 • Human bites
 • Facial infections after ear, nose, and throat infections
 • After intraabdominal infections
 • Decubitus ulcers
 • Foot infections in diabetics
 • Trauma

10. Which antimicrobial agents are consistently active against almost all anaerobic bacteria?
 Metronidazole, combination beta-lactam and beta-lactamase inhibitors (ampicillin + sulbactam, ticarcillin + clavulanate, piperacillin + tazobactam), carbapenems (imipenem and meropenem), and chloramphenicol are active against almost all *Bacteroides* spp., *Fusobacterium*

spp., and *Clostridium perfringens.* Clindamycin, cefoxitin, cefotetan, and piperacillin are active against most anaerobes, but 5–15% of *Bacteroides* spp. are resistant. Metronidazole has no activity against microaerophilic streptococci, *Actinomyces* sp., and *Propionibacterium acnes.*

11. A previously healthy 23-year-old man develops a sore throat, then becomes progressively more ill with a high fever, hypotension, cough, and pleuritic chest pain. The laboratory states that a slender gram-negative rod is growing in the blood. What is the patient's diagnosis? How should the patient be treated?

Postanginal sepsis (Lemiere's syndrome) is usually seen in adolescents and young adults. It is characterized by septic phlebitis of the jugular vein and widespread metastatic involvement, often involving the lung. The microbiologic cause is usually *Fusobacterium necrophorum.* The organism is susceptible to penicillin G.

12. What are the clinical clues of early gas gangrene?

Clostridial myonecrosis usually follows a traumatic or penetrating wound, intraabdominal or pelvic surgery, septic abortion or delivery, soft tissue infection with vascular insufficiency, or neutropenic enterocolitis. Occasional cases may arise spontaneously. The earliest symptoms are intense pain, followed by edema. The wound may appear normal early in the course. Soft tissue gas may be noted but may not be impressive. As the course progresses, the wound may develop a bronze discoloration that leads to a hemorrhagic bulla. Gram stains of the thin brownish discharge may reveal gram-positive rods. Systemic findings include tachycardia, diaphoresis, and fever.

13. What are the three main types of infections due to actinomycosis?

1. Cervicofacial, often after a dental infection, usually involving the paramandibular or submandibular spaces.

2. Thoracic, involving the lungs, pleura, mediastinum, and chest wall.

3. Abdominal or pelvic, most commonly after surgery. Pelvic actinomycosis is associated with use of intrauterine devices.

Less commonly, actinomycosis involves the central nervous system.

14. What are the most common pathogens in clenched fist injuries of the hand?

Viridans streptococci, *S. aureus*, *Bacteroides* sp., *Fusobacterium* sp., peptostreptococci and *Eikenella corrodens* (notice the striking resemblance to normal oral flora).

15. What are the indications for the use of tetanus immune globulin (TIG)?

TIG should be given as prophylaxis to a patient who presents with a tetanus-prone wound and has not completed a series of three vaccinations with absorbed tetanus toxoid. Tetanus-prone wounds include wounds that are contaminated with dirt, feces, or saliva; puncture wounds; avulsions; and wounds resulting from missiles, crushing, burns, or frostbite. TIG is also used in the therapy of clinical tetanus as soon as possible after the disease is recognized.

BIBLIOGRAPHY

1. Bamberger DM: Outcome of medical treatment of bacterial abscess without therapeutic drainage: Review of cases reported in the literature. Clin Infect Dis 23:592–603, 1996.
2. Blomquist IK, Bayer AS: Life-threatening deep fascial space infections of the head and neck. Infect Dis Clin North Am 2:237–264, 1988.
3. Joiner KA, Lowe BR, Dzink JL, Bartlett JG: Antibiotic levels in infected and sterile subcutaneous abscesses in mice. J Infect Dis 143:487–494, 1981.
4. Seidenfeld SM, Sutker WL, Luby JP: *Fusobacterium necrophorum* septicemia following oropharyngeal infection. JAMA 248:1348, 1982.

8. ULCEROGLANDULAR INFECTIONS

Tomas Ferguson, M.D., and Donald R. Skillman, M.D., FACP

1. Briefly describe the history of ulceroglandular infections and its relevance to tularemia.

Infections consistent with ulceroglandular fever have been described worldwide, dating back to reports in the 19th century by Homma Soken in Japan. Hachiro Ohara worked to identify a pathogen that seemed to spread by contact with a hare. In an attempt to identify the causative agent he infected his wife, with her permission, by rubbing organs from dead hares all over her body. He then isolated the organism from her excised lymph nodes. The infection was dubbed Ohara-Haga disease. In 1911 McCoy described a plaguelike illness common to the California ground squirrel, and in 1912 Chapin successfully cultured the causative agent. They named it *Bacterium tularense* because they were working in Tulare County. Tule is a variety of bullrush, a large reed once common in the extensive marshy areas of Tulare County. The work of Edward Francis prompted a name change to *Francisella tularensis*. Other synonyms for this infection are rabbit fever, deerfly fever, market men's disease, yato-byo, and water-rat trapper's disease.

2. Just exactly what kind of germ is *F. tularensis*?

F. tularensis is a pleomorphic gram-negative coccobacillus. It is aerobic and catalase-positive. *F. tularensis* is often separated into Jellison A and B groups based on subspeciation and distinct variations in the organism's biochemistry. Jellison A *F. tularensis* is specific for North America and is the more virulent of the Jellison classes. *F. tularensis* possesses a lipopolysaccharide capsule and is capable of causing endotoxin-mediated sepsis.

3. What are the natural reservoirs and vectors of *F. tularensis*?

Natural reservoirs and vectors are legion. Insect-parasitized mammals that may harbor the organism include rabbits, hares, squirrels, cats, dogs, opossum, raccoon, sheep, voles, muskrats, and beavers. Blood-feeding arthropods and flies are the most important vectors, but the disease is mainly tick-borne in the central and Rocky Mountain states. Although some 13 species of tick have been reported to be naturally infected with *F. tularensis*, the dog tick (*Dermacentor variabilis*), wood tick (*D. andersoni*), and Lone Star tick (*Amblyomma americanum*) are common vectors in North America. The germ may be found in tick saliva or feces, and transmission may be through direct or indirect inoculation into the bite wound. Biting flies are the predominant vectors in California, Nevada, and Utah. Mosquitoes are the most frequent insect vector in Sweden, Finland, and the former Soviet Union. Organisms have been isolated from water, mud, grain, and bird and vole feces. There are anecdotal reports of spread from indirect contact with most of the above.

4. Is *F. tularensis* endemic anywhere?

The organism is widely reported in the northern hemisphere: Japan, Europe, Russia, southwestern Asia, and North America. The only American state that has not reported a case of infection is Hawaii. States reporting the highest incidences are in the South and Midwest; Arkansas, Missouri, Texas, Virginia, Illinois, and Tennessee top the list. The infection has not been found in the United Kingdom, Africa, South America, or Australia.

5. How do humans acquire tularemia?

The most common manner of acquisition is from handling rabbits and hares. Skinning, dressing, or eating infected animals occasionally leads to large outbreaks in hunters. Arthropods are the next most common fashion. The organism gains a portal of entry through injection, breaks in normally intact barriers, or inhalation. The mode of entry determines the type of infection.

Injections via arthropods most often produce an ulceroglandular infection. Tick-borne infection and entry through broken barriers and inhalation may produce both the typhoidal and the ulceroglandular forms of infection. The disease is rarely spread to spouses in the name of science (see question 1). Carnivores may transiently carry *F. tularensis* in their mouth or on their claws after killing or feeding on an infected animal. Domestic cats occasionally transmit tularemia in this manner.

6. What is an ulceroglandular infection?

Ulceroglandular tularemia is the most common manifestation of the disease, appearing in up to 87% of cases. It most often starts as enlarged, tender lymphadenopathy in the anatomic distribution of the inoculation with a skin lesion at the site of inoculation. A papule then forms, eventually drains into the involved lymph nodes, and becomes an ulcer. The ulcer may take weeks to heal and may leave a scar. Inoculation via animal handling usually leads to hand and forearm involvement. Tick inoculation most often involves the lower extremities, but may involve any area to which a tick can gain access. Consider resigning your membership at the nudist camp.

7. Describe the other forms of infection with *F. tularensis*.

1. **Glandular infection** is similar to ulceroglandular infection without the cutaneous manifestations.

2. **Oculoglandular infection** occurs when the organism gains entry to the host through the conjunctiva, most often by inoculation from the host or aerosolized bacteria. Oculoglandular infection is manifested by lacrimation, photophobia, conjunctivitis, soft tissue edema, and ulceration. The lymphatic drainage of these areas also may become involved.

3. **Pharyngitis** results from invasion in the oropharynx. Inoculation is thought to be secondary to ingestion of infected materials or aerosolized pathogens. Symptoms include sore throat and lymphadenopathy in the involved area. Erythema and exudates are often seen, and pseudomembranes have been described.

4. **Pneumonic infection** is manifested by cough productive of sputum, pleuritic chest pain, shortness of breath, and hemoptysis. Chest radiographs may confirm infiltrate, adenopathy, effusion, or nothing at all.

5. **Typhoidal disease** is a nonspecific clinical syndrome starting with fever, chills, prostration, nausea, vomiting, abdominal pain, malaise, anorexia, and diarrhea. The patient may have meningismus, but meningitis rarely has been attributable to *F. tularensis*. It is important to note that typhoidal tularemia is not associated with lymphadenopathy, and a high clinical suspicion may be all that leads to the correct diagnosis.

8. Does tularemia cause a skin rash?

Dermatologic manifestations include erythema nodosum, diffuse maculopapular and vesiculopapular rashes, erythema multiforme, erythema nodosum, acneiform lesions, and nonspecific urticaria. Secondary skin rashes usually appear within the first 2 weeks of symptoms and may be found in up to 35 % of cases. A rash is more common in women. Any type of secondary rash may be seen in any form of tularemia, but erythema nodosum most commonly occurs with pneumonic tularemia.

9. Which type of tularemia has the highest mortality rate?

The typhoidal form of the disease has the highest mortality rate, especially when accompanied by a pneumonic process. Because it is hard to diagnose and mimics other deadly diseases, the clinician easily can be misled and fail to deliver the proper therapy.

10. Without antibiotics, what is the natural course of *F. tularensis* infection?

F. tularensis usually manifests as one the above syndromes in 3–6 days after exposure to the pathogen. Before treatment the rule of thumb had been "31 days of fever, 31 days in bed, and total duration of $3\frac{1}{2}$ months." Ulceroglandular infection usually responds appropriately to therapy, but all forms, as noted above, may progress to gram-negative–related sepsis, and each has been associated with an adult respiratory distress syndrome, especially the pneumonic variant and Jellison A organism.

11. Can *F. tularensis* be diagnosed by Gram stain and culture?

Yes, but you have to work at it. The diagnosis is made by smart people with a high clinical suspicion. The organism is difficult to visualize with Gram stain or in tissues, even when the bacterial load is high. The germ requires selective media to grow in the laboratory; glucose cysteine with thiamine agar, cysteine blood agar, thioglycolate broth, modified Thayer-Martin medium, and charcoal-yeast agar are suitable. *F. tularensis* may be isolated from suspected sites using the above means. Care must be used in the attempt to diagnose tularemia because laboratory workers may become infected inadvertently while working with the organism.

12. What are the newer, more sophisticated ways to diagnose tularemia?

Indirect methods such as enzyme-linked immunosorbent assay (ELISA), microagglutination, hemagglutination, and tube agglutination are the most commonly used diagnostic tests. Agglutinins may be detectable by 10–14 days after infection and are maximally elevated within 42 days. Acute and convalescent titers also may be used; a titer of 1:160 is considered consistent with exposure.

Newer methods to confirm the organism's presence include polymerase chain reaction, RNA hybridization with a probe directed at the 16S protein, direct fluorescent antibody staining, and urine antigen detection. Animal or spouse inoculation is rarely used because it requires a specific lab set-up (or a willing spouse—see question 1).

13. How is tularemia treated?

The gold standard is streptomycin. Streptomycin is not widely available because of its toxic side effects (vestibulotoxicity) and the availability of other suitable agents. Gentamicin is a good alternative. Tetracycline and chloramphenicol may be used with the caveats that they are bacteriostatic for the organism, the full course must be completed, and the host must have an intact immune system. Chloramphenicol should be added to streptomycin or gentamicin if meningeal infection is suspected. Reports are favorable for the use of fluoroquinolones. Other antibacterial therapies thought to be active against *F. tularensis* are erythromycin, rifampin, cefoxitin, ceftazidime, cefotaxime, imipenem/cilastin, and the other aminoglycosides. Erythromycin resistance has been reported.

14. Is tularemia fatal?

With the advent of antibiotics the mortality rate for all comers with tularemia has declined from 33% to about 5%. The typhoidal form of the disease has a higher mortality rate, especially when accompanied by significant pleuropneumonic disease. Other risk factors associated with a worse prognosis include increasing age, serious coexisting medical conditions, presence of symptoms for a month or longer before treatment, renal failure, delay in diagnosis, and inappropriate antibiotic therapy. Some patients with tularemia may experience months of debility, often associated with late lymph node suppuration and/or persistent fatigue.

15. What kind of complications may occur with tularemia?

The most common complication currently is suppuration of involved lymph nodes, which may occur after effective antibiotic therapy. Patients with severe disease may manifest disseminated intravascular coagulation, renal failure, rhabdomyolysis, jaundice, and hepatitis. Meningitis, encephalitis, pericarditis, peritonitis, osteomyelitis, splenic rupture, and thrombophlebitis have become rare since the availability of antibiotic therapy. The cerebrospinal fluid in meningitis almost always shows a mononuclear cell pleocytosis, with high protein and hypoglycorrhachia.

16. How can tularemia be prevented?

People who fall into high-risk groups for developing the disease should receive the vaccine, which is a live attenuated form of the bacteria. High-risk groups include trappers and others working in this field. Forms of passive immunity are available after exposure, and high-risk exposures may warrant antibiotic prophylaxis as well. When tularemia is suspected, it is important to let the laboratory know so that infected samples may be held for longer intervals; notification also facilitates isolation of the organism and promotes personal protection. Do not allow the infected organs of suspected carriers to be rubbed on your body.

17. What kind of isolation is advocated for patients with tularemia?

Because person-to-person spread does not occur, hospitalized patients do not need special isolation. Standard universal precautions for contaminated secretions are adequate in handling drainage from wounds or eyes.

18. Can you get tularemia twice?

Protective immunity for life seems to be the rule after recovery from tularemia. However, a few recurrent infections have been documented. Most recurrences were clinically mild ulceroglandular disease; systemic symptoms were uncommon. Consequently, vaccination or preemptive antibiotic therapy after a known exposure is not necessary for people with a history of tularemia.

19. Tularemia is not the only cause of ulceroglandular infection. What should you know about rat-bite fever?

Two germs can cause rat-bite fever: *Spirillum minus* and *Streptobacillus moniliformis*. Both are denizens of the oral cavity of rats, and rat bite is the most common form of transmission. *S. minus*, a gram-negative, flagellated spiral rod, is found only in Asia. *S. moniliformis* a gram-negative nonmotile rod, also has been transmitted by turkey, milk, or water contaminated with rat excrement (Haverhill fever).

After inoculation an incubation period, usually less than 10 days, is followed by systemic complaints of fever, malaise, headache, and myalgia/arthralgias. Because the rat bite often occurs at night, is unrecognized, and has healed completely by the time that symptoms begin, it takes a clever doctor to suspect the diagnosis.

A significant leukocyte count is often present, and a false-positive syphilis serology is found in about 25%. *S. minus* is most often described as the mimicker of tularemia, causing regional lymphadenitis and chancre formation as well as an eschar at the site of inoculation. Both entities cause a skin rash (nonpruritic maculopapular, morbilliform, or petechial rash) over the palms, soles, and extremities. Skin lesions may become purpuric or confluent and eventually may desquamate. Asymmetric polyarthritis or true septic arthritis develops in approximately 50% of cases concurrently with the rash or shortly thereafter. Fevers last 3–5 days, with gradual resolution of symptoms over the next 2 weeks, but the patient may relapse over weeks and months.

S. moniliformis is diagnosed by history and direct visualization of the organism. *S. minus* is diagnosed on clinical suspicion and visualization of spiral organisms on dark field examination. Both germs may be cultured on enriched media. The agents of rat-bite fever are susceptible to penicillin; tetracycline is the recommended alternative for penicillin-allergic patients.

20. Describe the forms of infection with *Bacillus anthracis*.

Anthrax is caused by a spore-forming gram-positive rod. It is rare in the United States but is endemic in Southwest Asia and is a good candidate to use as a biologic weapon. There are three types of infection with *B. anthracis:* cutaneous inoculation, gastrointestinal infection, and inhalation anthrax. Inhalational infection (woolsorter's disease) causes an abrupt and usually fatal hemorrhagic mediastinal lymphadenitis. Cutaneous inoculation, which is seen in 95% of anthrax cases, is characterized by toxin-induced edema and necrosis. It is common to find a black eschar with surrounding vesicular or bullous edema (the so-called ring of pearls). Regional lymphadenopathy is often present. The cutaneous form is rarely fatal when treated but kills about

20% of victims if not treated. Gastrointestinal anthrax also usually kills its victims; hemorrhagic abdominal lymphadenitis is a prominent finding.

21. What is cat scratch fever? Why is it included here?

Cat scratch fever is a cool name for a good rock-n-roll tune popularized by the legendary Ted Nugent. Cat scratch disease is an infectious syndrome caused by *Bartonella henselae* or *Afipia felis*. Regional lymphadenopathy is associated with an erythematous papule at a cat scratch or bite distal to the involved node(s). Stellate caseating granulomas, microabscesses, and hyperplasia are seen in affected lymph nodes. *B. henselae* is implicated in most cases; *A. felis* rarely causes the syndrome. The patient's history is often positive for inoculation by a cat, either through a bite or scratch to skin or eye. Symptoms begin 7–10 days after exposure. Systemic sequelae are rare but sometimes quite severe.

Diagnosis is made by visualization of the organisms on a Warthin-Starry stain, confirmed by serology. Culture can be difficult. The natural history of cat scratch disease is resolution within 1–2 months. Treatment with trimethoprim-sulfamethoxazole, gentamicin, erythromycin, ciprofloxacin, or rifampin has been tried for severe manifestations, but it is debatable whether antibiotics affect the resolution of milder cases.

22. Like polio, plague has been eliminated from the United States. True or false?

Unfortunately the statement is false. Squirrels and prairie dogs in the Southwest United States are the reservoirs for the causative agent, *Yersinia pestis*. Fleas found on these rodents are the vectors.

BIBLIOGRAPHY

1. Evans ME, Gregory DW, Schaffner W, McGee ZA: Tularemia: A 30 year experience with 88 cases. Medicine 64:251–269, 1985.
2. Laforce FM: Anthrax. Clin Infect Dis 19:1009–1013, 1994.
3. Mandell GL, Bennett J, Dolin R: Principles and Practice of Infectious Diseases, 4th ed. New York, Churchill Livingstone, 1995.
4. Sanders CV, Hahn R: Analysis of 106 cases of tularemia. J La State Med Soc 120:391–403, 1968.
5. Schwartzman W: Bartonella infections: Beyond cat scratch. Ann Rev Med 47:355–364, 1996.
6. Spach DH, Liles WC, Campbell GL, Quick RE: Tick-borne diseases in the United States. N Eng J Med 330:936–947, 1993.

9. TICK-BORNE DISEASES

Joel T. Fishbain, M.D.

1. What are the diagnostic criteria for Lyme disease?

Lyme disease is diagnosed by finding a lesion consistent with erythema migrans. The lesion must be 5 cm or greater in diameter. Patients usually reside in an area known to be endemic for Lyme disease, but exposure history and history of a tick bite are variable. Patients with late-stage Lyme disease must have a compatible clinical syndrome and a reasonable history for exposure in an endemic area.

2. What tests are available for serologic testing of Lyme disease?

Two categories of serologic testing are currently available: an enzyme-linked immunosorbent assay (ELISA) and an immunoblot assay (also known as Western blot assay). The ELISA screening system uses sonicated whole organism as the target in some kits. In patients with borderline (indeterminate) values and positive values, the results are confirmed with the Western blot. The organism's main proteins are separated on a gel and transferred to a membrane. The patient's antibody reaction to specific proteins is then examined. A positive test is based on the number of visible "bands." A cut-off point is chosen that limits false-negative and false-positive results. The level of positivity chosen for the Western blot may make it a more sensitive test, but the specificity may decrease. Follow-up studies in patients with suspected Lyme disease show increasing numbers of positive bands on Western blot. For suspected cases, follow-up testing is warranted. Specific bands that appear early may be highly suggestive of Lyme disease, yet the total number of bands may be less than the number required for diagnosis. It is important to be aware of the method used by each laboratory and also to know which bands are present in patients who are reportedly negative but have a clinical syndrome suggestive of Lyme disease. The second point must be kept in mind for patients with symptoms highly suggestive of Lyme disease and negative ELISA tests. Western blot testing of such patients may still be used, and early bands on Western blotting are suggestive of Lyme disease. Thus early disease will not be missed.

3. When do false-negative and false-positive Lyme serologies occur?

Unfortunately, only 30–40% of patients with erythema migrans have positive serologic tests. Therefore, the diagnosis is clinical, and therapy should not be based on serologic testing in early Lyme disease. In addition, serologic testing in patients with erythema migrans is a waste of money. Patients who reside or have lived in endemic areas may have asymptomatic infection, which occurs in roughly 5–10% of patients. Random screening of patients with clinical syndromes not compatible with Lyme disease may be given a false diagnosis based merely on a positive serologic test. Serologic testing should be used selectively and the results viewed with a careful clinical eye.

4. What findings would you expect from spinal fluid testing in a patient with erythema migrans, fever, headache, and stiff neck?

The most common spinal fluid findings in patients with early Lyme disease and meningeal signs are normal protein, normal glucose, and normal numbers of cells. Lyme meningitis is a late or at least not an early finding, and one can expect the spinal fluid to be normal in patients with early Lyme disease. Systemic symptoms are common in early disease. Fever, headache, and paraspinal myalgias may suggest meningitis, but the diagnosis may turn out to be false.

5. A 40-year-old woman from New York state presents with a right facial palsy and meningeal signs. Spinal fluid analysis reveals a mild lymphocytic pleocytosis and elevated protein. Routine spinal fluid studies are negative, and an ELISA and Western blot are positive for Lyme disease. What test(s) may assist with your diagnosis of neuroborreliosis?

Sending the patient's cerebrospinal fluid (CSF) and serum for Lyme testing may reveal intrathecal antibody production strongly suggestive of neuroborreliosis. The tests must be run by an identical method and should be run together. A CSF/serum ratio > 1 is suggestive of intrathecal antibody production. Other tests, such as culture and polymerase chain reaction, are either too insensitive or too experimental to be helpful.

6. What are the major clinical characteristics of tick-borne borreliosis?

Tick-borne borreliosis, also known as tick-borne relapsing fever, is caused by *Borrelia* spp., but not by *B. burgdorferi*. The particular *Borrelia* species is given the same species name as its tick vector (*Borrelia hermsii* takes its name from the tick *Ornithodoros hermsii*). Patients rarely report a tick bite since the vectors, *Ornithodoros* spp., are soft-body ticks that feed at night. Patients may note a small papule or eschar at the site of inoculation but more commonly report only fever, chills, headache, myalgias, arthralgias, and malaise. The classic pattern in patients who do not receive therapy is recurrent fever with associated symptoms after approximately 1 week. Subsequent relapses are usually of a less severe nature and shorter duration. Without therapy relapses range in number from 3–5.

7. You suspect that a patient has tick-borne relapsing fever. What is the quickest and most specific method of diagnosis? What are the therapeutic options? What precautions should be taken once therapy is instituted?

Tick-borne relapsing fever is best diagnosed by examining a blood smear (stained by Wright or Giemsa) from the patient during a febrile period. The spirochete can be visualized in the extracellular portion of the smear. Treatment with a tetracycline-like doxycycline is recommended, but erythromycin also may be effective. Failures have been reported with penicillin. Patients may develop the Jarisch-Herxheimer reaction when therapy is instituted. If this occurs, supportive therapy with intravenous fluids for hypotension is all that is necessary.

8. What seasonal variations are associated with tularemia? What epidemiologic factors are responsible for these variations?

Tularemia has two yearly peaks, summer and winter. These peaks correspond to the primary modes of transmission. The summer peak occurs when ticks are most active, and the clinical syndromes appropriate to tick bites occur. The winter peak occurs as a result of rabbit hunting. Be sure to take a careful history in any patient with a febrile illness of unclear etiology. Environmental exposures are frequently clues to the underlying illness and should be meticulously sought.

9. Name at least four of the six clinical syndromes associated with *Francisella tularensis* infection (tularemia).

1. **Ulceroglandular.** This is the most common form of tularemia and consists of an ulcerative lesion at the site of inoculation with associated regional adenopathy. Systemic symptoms frequently occur and are of a nonspecific infectious nature.

2. **Glandular.** Adenopathy is noted with no associated ulcer at the site of inoculation.

3. **Typhoidal.** This is the most severe and dreaded form of tularemia. Fortunately it is not common. Patients present with severe signs and symptoms of systemic illness with no immediately identifiable source. An abnormal chest radiograph may be noted. The nonspecific nature of the symptoms makes diagnosis difficult, and the appropriate epidemiologic history must be obtained to increase the index of suspicion.

4. **Oculoglandular.** This syndrome of painful conjunctivitis, usually unilateral, with associated preauricular adenopathy, is initiated by direct conjunctival inoculation with the organism.

5. **Primary pneumonic.** Patients present with signs and symptoms of community-acquired pneumonia, but the organism stains poorly by Gram stain, requires special culture media, and is dangerous to culture for laboratory personnel. The appropriate epidemiologic history may provide a clue.

6. **Oropharyngeal.** This rare form of tularemia occurs after ingestion of contaminated meat. An exudative pharyngitis with associated adenopathy is noted. Obviously tularemia is difficult to distinguish from other far more common etiologies.

10. What are the most important diagnostic and therapeutic issues in all forms of tularemia?

Physicians rarely make a definitive diagnosis of tularemia before institution of appropriate therapy. The clinician must know the epidemiology of the disease and ask all the important questions. Once it is determined that the patient has a clinical syndrome compatible with tularemia, therapy should be initiated. Acute and convalescent sera should be obtained and sent for diagnostic study at the same time. If culture is attempted, the laboratory should be notified, and in many cases the risks of culture are inappropriate. Early therapy consists of streptomycin or gentamicin before the diagnosis is confirmed by serology. Tetracycline and chloramphenicol are alternative agents. Therapy for 14 days is required to avoid relapse.

11. Bonus question: What is the difference between a rabbit and a hare?

Hares have longer ears and larger feet with strong legs for jumping.

12. What four states had the highest incidence of Rocky Mountain spotted fever in 1990?

The disease is most prevalent in south Atlantic, western, and south central states. North Carolina, South Carolina, Oklahoma, and Tennessee had the highest reported incidence in 1990.

13. Name the classic triad associated with Rocky Mountain spotted fever. What percent of patients report this triad?

The classic triad of fever, rash, and history of a tick bite is noted in only 60–70% of patients. This obviously creates a significant diagnostic dilemma. Delay in diagnosis and appropriate therapy is responsible for increased mortality rates.

14. A 14-year-old boy presents to the emergency department at a local hospital in North Carolina in July with fevers, headache, myalgias, and malaise. He has no rash. You suspect Rocky Mountain spotted fever. What other clinical symptoms may be found? What do you think about the lack of a rash?

Rocky Mountain spotted fever has been associated with significant gastrointestinal manifestations, including nausea, vomiting, abdominal pain, and diarrhea. These symptoms have led physicians down the wrong pathway and are frequently forgotten as associated symptoms in Rocky Mountain spotted fever. In addition, aseptic meningitis has been reported in patients who underwent spinal fluid sampling and analysis. You should not be surprised by the lack of a rash. The classic rash appears anywhere from 1–15 days after onset of fever, and in 10–15% of patients no rash is reported. Darker-skinned people often have a difficult-to-identify rash, thus confusing the issue and making a clinical diagnosis difficult.

15. You have elected to treat the patient in question 14 for Rocky Mountian spotted fever. What agents would you consider for therapy?

Tetracycline agents are recommended for therapy in nonpregnant adults and children over the age of 8. Therapy is given for 5–7 days and should be continued for a minimum of 48 hours after resolution of fever. Chloramphenicol is an alternative agent for patients in whom tetracyclines are relatively contraindicated, but its risks must be taken into consideration. Given the brief duration of therapy necessary with tetracyclines, they could be considered viable options in patients younger than 8 years for a single course of therapy.

16. A 25-year-old hiker from New York state presents with complaints of fever, headache, myalgias, arthralgias, and a history of a tick bite 2 weeks previously. The patient has no rash, and laboratory findings reveal a white blood cell count of 2500, a platelet count of 68,000, an alanine aminotransferase level of 210, and an aspartate aminotransferase level of 230. What is the major diagnostic consideration?

Ehrlichiosis must be included on the list of diagnostic considerations. This disease presents with various manifestations, but most are of the nonspecific infectious type. Clues to the diagnosis include leukopenia and/or thrombocytopenia. Liver enzyme elevations are extremely common.

17. Name the two forms of human ehrlichiosis. How do they differ from pathogenetic and epidemiologic points of view?

Monocytic ehrlichiosis was the first described human form in the United States. The causative organism was named *Ehrlichia chaffeensis* because it was first identified in a soldier who had returned from Ft. Chaffee, Arkansas. *E. chaffeensis* infects human monocytes and is closely related to canine ehrlichia. Infection occurs primarily in the distribution of the ticks *Dermacentor variabilis* (dog tick) and *Amblyomma americanum* (lone star tick). Most cases are reported in the southern Atlantic and south central states.

Recently, a second species was identified. The organism has only recently been cultivated and has no species name to date; therefore, the term *human granulocytic ehrlichiosis* (HGE) is used. As the name suggests, this organism primarily infects cells of granulocyte origin. It appears to be most prominent in the northeastern states and Wisconsin and Minnesota. The vector may be *Ixodes scapularis*, but data are limited.

18. Describe the clinical manifestations of ehrlichiosis.

Clinical Manifestations of Ehrlichiosis

SYMPTOM	% PATIENTS	SYMPTOM	% PATIENTS
Fever	100	Chills	73
Headache	63	Nausea	50
Myalgias	43	Arthralgias	33
Fatigue or malaise	30	Vomiting	27
Back pain	20	Diarrhea	10
Rash	20	Cough	< 10
Testicular pain	< 10	Abdominal pain	< 10

Modified from Everett ED, Evans KA, Henry RB, et al: Human ehrlichiosis in adults after tick exposure. Ann Intern Med 120:730–735, 1994.

19. You suspect that one of your patients has ehrlichiosis. How do you diagnose and treat the illness?

The only way to diagnose ehrlichiosis immediately is to identify intracellular inclusions in monocytes or granulocytes. These inclusions, known as morula (meaning mulberry), are located in the cytoplasm and consist of a vacuole containing many organisms. Despite valiant efforts, however, attempts to identify morula are more often than not unsuccessful. The reader is referred to appropriate references for excellent photographs.[1,3]

The identification of morula in a peripheral smear is not at all sensitive. Wright or Giemsa staining of buffy coat smears is easy to do, but the longer the duration of illness, the less likely the identification of morula. Bone marrow aspirate and biopsy may be better for this purpose. Serologic tests for both *E. chaffeensis* and HGE are available from various laboratories and the Centers for Disease Control and Prevention in Atlanta. The polymerase chain reaction has also been used at some laboratories in buffy coat specimens. The best therapeutic agent appears to be doxycycline; other agents, such as erythromycin, have failed to produce consistent results.

20. A 23-year-old man reports a tick bite 3 weeks before presentation and now complains of fevers, chills, headache, myalgias, weakness, abdominal pain, vomiting, and anorexia. He has a history of posttraumatic splenectomy 3 years earlier. His white blood cell count is 4500, and his platelet count is 90,000. What particular organism should you be concerned about?

Babesia microti is a well-described source of tick-borne illness in the United States. It primarily affects patients who are asplenic, have other underlying diseases, or are of advanced age. Normal host-related infections are also reported. Infections with *Babesia* spp. and *Babesia*-like organisms result in a spectrum of illness. Patients may be asymptomatic, mildly symptomatic, or develop life-threatening illness with hemolytic anemia, renal failure, and hypotension. Transfusion-related infections also have been reported. A newly described organism, known as WA-1, has been identified in a patient from the Pacific Northwest, and three patients from northern California had reactive serologic tests.

21. What is the epidemiology of babesiosis? How is it diagnosed and treated?

At present, babesiosis appears to be located primarily in areas of *Ixodes scapularis* and *Ixodes pacificus* habitat in the United States, including the Northeast, Midwest (Wisconsin and Minnesota), and Pacific Northwest. Diagnosis of babesia or piroplasm species is made with Giemsa-stained blood smears. The organisms are intraerythrocytic parasites similar to malaria. The tetrad form of the organisms within a red cell resembling a Maltese cross is diagnostic, but pairs, singles, and ring forms are more common. Quinine and clindamycin appear to offer effective therapy for babesiosis.

22. Describe the condition known as tick paralysis.

Tick paralysis is defined by the presence of a tick, usually within the scalp (thus escaping detection), in association with symmetric neurologic symptoms. Symptoms are typically described as progressive weakness of the lower extremities with sensory sparing. Isolated ataxia without muscle weakness also has been reported. Careful inspection for an embedded tick is critical for diagnosis, and prompt removal with resolution of symptoms is both diagnostic and therapeutic. The pathogenesis appears to be related to the presence of a neurotoxin in tick saliva.

BIBLIOGRAPHY

1. Eagle K: Images in clinical medicine: Ehrlichiosis. N Engl J Med 332(21):1417, 1993.
2. Everett ED, Evans KA, Henry RB, et al: Human ehrlichiosis in adults after tick exposure. Ann Intern Med 120:730–735, 1994.
3. Goodman JL, Nelson C, et al: Direct cultivation of the causative agent of human granulocytic ehrlichiosis. N Engl J Med 334:209–215, 1996.
4. Mandell GL, Bennett JE, Dolin R (eds): Principles and Practice of Infectious Diseases. New York, Churchill Livingstone, 1995.
5. Persing DH, Herwaldt BL, Glaser C, et al: Infection with a *Babesia*-like organism in northern California. N Engl J Med 332:298–303, 1993.
6. Spach DH, Liles WC, Campbell GL: Tick-borne diseases in the United States. N Engl J Med 329:936–947, 1993.

10. BITE WOUND INFECTIONS

Robert M. Plemmons, M.D.

1. How common are bite wounds? What species are most often responsible?

As many as 2 million people may sustain bite wounds each year in the United States. Most of these injuries are fairly trivial and are not brought to medical attention. Other cases may involve infectious complications ranging from simple cellulitis to severe sepsis and death. Dogs account for most bite wounds in the U.S., and cat bites are the next most common. Human bite wounds, most of which are related to physical assault, appear to be the third most common form.

2. What are the major risk factors for infection of a bite wound?

The risk of infection following a bite wound depends on the immune status of the person bitten, the nature of the wound, and the location of the wound. Elderly people and people with systemic immune deficits (including asplenia, diabetes mellitus, and alcoholism) are obviously at increased risk for infection, but patients with local immune defects such as chronic edema or vascular insufficiency in an extremity are also at increased risk if an affected extremity is bitten. Puncture wounds and wounds with extensive crush injury are more likely to become infected than tears or scratches. Wounds of the hands and feet are at increased risk because of the many tissue planes and compartments that facilitate persistence and spread of infection,

3. What are the major bacterial pathogens causing dog-bite wound infections?

The bacteria most frequently isolated from dog-bite wounds are alpha-hemolytic streptococci, but the vast majority of bite wound infections are mixed. *Staphylococcus aureus*, beta-hemolytic streptococci, *Pasteurella multocida*, and *Capnocytophaga canimorsus* are among other important aerobic pathogens isolated from dog-bite wounds. Various anaerobic bacteria (including *Actinomyces* sp., *Bacteroides* sp., and fusobacteria) are also commonly recovered. In contrast to the anaerobes isolated from human bite wounds (which are often beta-lactamase producers), the anaerobes recovered from animal bite wounds have been almost uniformly susceptible to penicillin.

4. What is *C. canimorsus*? What types of patients are at greatest risk for severe infections?

C. canimorsus (formerly designated CDC group DF-2) is an aerobic, gram-negative rod that comprises part of the normal oral flora of dogs and cats. This organism has been shown to cause bacteremia and fatal sepsis in immunocompromised patients after dog bites. Cat bites occasionally result in fulminant illness, but the syndrome is more strongly associated with dog bites. Asplenic patients seem to be at particularly high risk for sepsis due to *C. canimorsus*, but patients with various other predisposing conditions (including corticosteroid use, malignancy, and liver disease) have been reported. Roughly 20% of patients who develop infection after a dog bite have no obvious predisposing condition, but fatal infections have occurred even in this group. *C. canimorsus* is susceptible to penicillin, cefoxitin, cefotaxime, erythromycin, tetracycline, ciprofloxacin, and clindamycin.

5. How do cat bites differ from dog bites in terms of likelihood of infection?

Cat bites become infected more than twice as often as dog bites. This finding may be partly due to the fact that a cat bite tends to produce deep small-caliber puncture wounds that may be difficult to irrigate adequately. Another factor may be the higher oropharyngeal carriage rate of *P. multocida* in cats compared with dogs. Cat bites are also more likely than dog bites to result in septic arthritis and osteomyelitis, a finding that has been attributed to the sharpness of a cat's teeth and their ability to penetrate joint capsules and bones.

6. What are the major bacterial pathogens causing cat-bite wound infections?

P. multocida is the pathogen most frequently isolated from infected cat-bite wounds. Like all other bite wound infections, however, cat-bite wounds tend to result in mixed infections. Aside from the increased presence of *P. multocida* with cat-bite wound infections, the common pathogens causing cat-bite and dog-bite wounds are similar (i.e., *S. aureus*, streptococci, occasional aerobic gram-negative organisms, and various anaerobes). Cat scratch disease, a lymphadenitis syndrome most often caused by *Bartonella henselae*, can also follow a cat bite (see chapter 64).

7. What is *P. multocida*? What is the typical clinical course of infection?

P. multocida is an oxidase-positive, aerobic, gram-negative coccobacillus that is part of the normal oral flora of cats and dogs. Bite wound infections involving *P. multocida* tend to become symptomatic quickly. Onset of pain, erythema, and edema at the wound site within 24 hours of injury is frequent. Up to 40% of patients with bite wound infections due to *P. multocida* may develop tenosynovitis, septic arthritis, abscess, or osteomyelitis. *P. multocida* bacteremia with metastatic infection also has been reported, along with cases of fatal sepsis.

8. What animals other than cats and dogs may have *P. multocida* as a component of their normal oral flora?

P. multocida infections have been reported after bite wounds caused by various animals, including lions, panthers, pigs, opossums, rabbits, wolves, and rats. There is even one reported case of *P. multocida* infection after a Tasmanian devil bite. Nasopharyngeal colonization with *P. multocida* also been described in humans, and cases of sinusitis and pneumonia due to this organism in humans are thought to have resulted from such colonization.

9. What antibiotics are most useful for treating infections due to *P. multocida*?

P. multocida is characteristically susceptible to penicillins (with the notable exception of antistaphylococcal penicillins such as oxacillin and dicloxacillin), second- and third-generation cephalosporins (cefuroxime, cefoxitin, cefotaxime), doxycycline, trimethoprim-sulfamethoxazole, and fluoroquinolones. *P. multocida* is usually resistant to erythromycin and first-generation cephalosporins.

10. What type of human bite wound is most likely to have serious infectious complications?

The clenched-fist injury, in which a combatant's fist strikes the tooth of an opponent resulting in a wound to the assailant's hand (often at the third metacarpophalangeal joint), is one of the most dangerous bite wounds. Because of the hand's many tendon sheaths, fascial planes, and compartments, along with the tendency of such wounds to involve penetration of joint capsule or bone, complications such as tenosynovitis, abscess, septic arthritis, and osteomyelitis are more frequent than with other types of bite wounds. An orthopedic surgeon specializing in the hand should be consulted early in the management of clenched fist injuries.

11. What is *Eikenella corrodens*? What is its significance in human bite wound infections?

E. corrodens, an aerobic gram-negative rod, is a normal component of human oral flora and is associated with clenched-fist wound infections. Because most clenched-fist wound infections also involve anaerobes, empiric therapy must take into account both *E. corrodens* (which has an antibiotic susceptibility profile similar to *P. multocida*) and beta lactamase-producing oral anaerobes.

12. When should prophylactic antibiotics be given after a bite injury?

Most authorities recommend a 3–5 day course of antibiotics for anything more than a trivial bite wound when the wound is seen early (< 8 hours after injury). A significant bite wound in an immunocompromised host or involving a high-risk site (bone, joint, hand) should always be treated. All patients presenting with cat bites should be given prophylactic antibiotics.

13. What antibiotic regimens are most appropriate for prophylaxis and empiric therapy of bite wound infections?

Appropriate prophylactic/empiric treatment for a bite wound must take into account the unique oral flora of the biting species (e.g., *P. multocida* in animals, *E. corrodens* in humans) along with streptococci and beta lactamase-producers such as *S. aureus* and certain anaerobes. Amoxicillin-clavulanate (or a parenteral beta-lactam/beta-lactamase inhibitor combination, if indicated) is uniquely suited for this application. Patients with serious penicillin allergy may be treated with doxycycline or a combination regimen (e.g., fluoroquinolone/clindamycin or trimethoprim-sulfamethoxazole/clindamycin). Wound cultures should be obtained before starting therapy, with any subsequent modifications based on culture results.

14. What other prophylactic agents should be considered in the management of a bite wound?

Rabies immunization (both with vaccine and human rabies immunoglobulin) should be considered in patients with bite wounds, depending on the species that inflicted the wound and the circumstances of the biting. Most patients with wild animal bites require rabies prophylaxis. Local health authorities should be contacted to determine the risk of rabies in a given species. A tetanus booster is usually given after a bite wound if more than 5 years have passed since the last tetanus immunization, although the risk of contracting tetanus from a bite wound appears to be low.

15. What adjunctive measure has been shown to make the difference between clinical success and failure in some cases of bite wound infection?

Control of edema at the site of the wound (accomplished by elevating the injured extremity) appears to be an important factor in elimination of infection. Bite wound infections have failed to resolve, even with appropriate antibiotic therapy, when edema was not addressed through appropriate elevation. Other cornerstones of bite wound management include adequate debridement and liberal irrigation at the time of presentation.

16. Should patients receive antibiotic prophylaxis after snake-bite wounds?

In general, snake-bite wounds are not at high risk for infection. Rattlesnake venom actually has some antibacterial properties. Nevertheless, a snake's oral flora include the fecal flora of its prey (primarily rodents), and antibiotic prophylaxis is recommended for wounds with bullae or tissue necrosis and when manipulation of the wound in the field may have introduced contaminants.

BIBLIOGRAPHY

1. Brook I: Human and animal bite infections. J Fam Pract 28:713–718, 1989.
2. Goldstein EJC: Bite wounds and infections. Clin Infect Dis 14:633–640, 1992.
3. Griego RD, Rosen T, Orengo IF, et al: Dog, cat, and human bites: A review. J Am Acad Dermatol 33:1019–1029, 1995.
4. Kalb R, Kaplan MH, Tenenbaum MJ: Cutaneous infection at dog bite wounds associated with fulminant DF-2 septicemia. Am J Med 78:687–690, 1985.
5. Lewis KT, Stiles M: Management of cat and dog bites. Am Fam Physician 52:479–485, 1995.

11. NOSOCOMIAL INFECTIONS

Robert J. Zabel, D.O.

1. What is the National Nosocomial Infections Surveillance (NNIS) System?

In 1970 the Centers for Disease Control (CDC) created a national database to track nosocomial infections, noting the associated pathogens and their antimicrobial susceptibility. The database uses a standard definition of a nosocomial infection to monitor groups of patients in the hospital. Participation by hospitals is voluntary, and the identity of the institutions is protected by public law. This national tracking system not only has yielded valuable information about specific trends in infection, but also has helped to define rational strategies for monitoring nosocomial infections within individual hospitals.

2. Which nosocomial infection is associated with the highest mortality?

Although nosocomial pneumonia accounts for only 15% of all nosocomial infections, it is associated with the highest mortality rate, 20–50%. It is the second most common hospital-acquired infection overall and the most common in intensive care units. There is a 7–20-fold increased incidence in mechanically ventilated patients.

3. Which pathogens are most often reported to cause nosocomial pneumonia?

The most common pathogens, in decreasing order of frequency, are *Pseudomonas aeruginosa, Staphylococcus aureus, Enterobacteriaceae* sp., *Klebsiella* sp., *Escherichia coli, Haemophilus influenzae*, and *Serratia marcescens*. In reported surveys, *P. aeruginosa* and *S. aureus* ranked first or second in frequency. Approximately 60% of all nosocomial pneumonias are caused by aerobic gram-negative bacilli.

4. What is the risk of a health care worker acquiring hepatitis B virus (HBV) infection from a single needlestick from a patient infected with hepatitis B?

In general, the risk of acquiring any infection from a needlestick injury is related to how contagious the infection is and the degree to which the health care worker is exposed to the infected blood (i.e., the deeper stick and the more blood inoculated, the greater the risk). In the specific case of HBV, the presence of the hepatitis e antigen (HBeAg) imparts a much greater risk of infection for the health care worker. Without HBeAg the risk of infection from a single needlestick to a susceptible health care worker has been estimated at 6%. When HBeAg is present in the blood, the risk to the health care worker of HBV infection from a single needlestick increases to 30%.

5. Can hepatitis C (HCV) be transmitted by needlestick or percutaneous exposure?

Yes. From seroconversion studies of the needlestick victims, the risk of acquisition of infection from a single exposure has been estimated to range from as low as 0% to as high as 10%.

6. Which organism is most often responsible for infecting percutaneous intravascular devices?

Coagulase-negative staphylococci, usually *S. epidermidis*. As a genus, staphylococci are responsible for one-half to two-thirds of all infected percutaneous intravascular devices.

7. What are the main ways in which a percutaneous intravascular device becomes infected?

Migration down the insertion tract by microorganisms colonizing the skin is the most common method of infection. A less common method is through contamination of the catheter hub-infusion tubing junction. A third way is hematogenous seeding of the device. Lastly, the device may become infected by a contaminated infusate.

8. Does the absence of inflammation surrounding a percutaneous intravascular device rule out infection?

Signs of local inflammation are present in only approximately one-half of cases and should not be relied on for diagnosis of infection. However, local inflammation, especially purulent drainage, is correlated highly with infection. Blood cultures and intravascular device cultures also help with the diagnosis of infection.

9. Infectious diarrheas acquired in the hospital are caused by what?

When an etiologic agent is found, the most common pathogen in children is rotavirus, followed by adenovirus. In adults the most common pathogen is *Clostridium difficile*, which accounts for 21–52% of cases. Other causes in adults include *Salmonella*, *Shigella*, and *Campylobacter* spp., but they are rare causes of nosocomial diarrhea. Some medical centers do not even routinely process stools for the latter pathogens if the patient has been in the hospital for 3 or more days. Diarrhea from parasites (e.g., *Giardia* spp.) is for practical purposes never acquired nosocomially.

10. What factors predispose hospitalized patients to infection with *C. difficile*?

The normal microbial flora of the gastrointestinal tract are protective against clinically evident infection with *C. difficile*. Predisposing factors for infection are therefore associated with the disruption of normal microbial flora. Examples include antibiotic use, older age, increasing length of stay in the hospital, nasogastric tube feeding, severe illness, some chemotherapy regimens, and enemas.

11. How is *C. difficile* most commonly transmitted?

Indirect transmission of *C. difficile* accounts for over 50% of cases. Indirect methods include contaminated bedrails, commodes, bed pans, and other sites that become contaminated by spores, which may remain viable for up to 6 months. Direct person-to-person transmission between other patients or hospital personnel is reported in about 25% of cases. No source of transmission can be found for another 25%. Transmission can be reduced through good hand-washing, glove use, enteric precautions, and private rooms or cohorting for infected patients.

12. What is the most common nosocomial infection?

Urinary tract infections (UTIs) are clearly the most common infections acquired in the hospital, accounting for approximately 40%. About 80% of nosocomial UTIs are catheter-associated. Another 5–10% occur after genitourinary manipulation. The remainder most likely were present but asymptomatic before hospitalization.

13. What pathogens most frequently cause nosocomial UTIs?

Escherichia coli is the most frequently isolated pathogen. Other common pathogens include *P. aeruginosa*, *Klebsiella pneumoniae*, *Proteus mirabilis*, *S. epidermidis*, enterococci, and (when antibiotics have been used) yeast. With long-term catheterization, defined as 30 days or more, 95% of infections are polymicrobial.

14. What measures can be taken to reduce the incidence of nosocomial UTIs?

The most important measure is to avoid urinary catheters. When avoidance is not possible, keep the catheter system closed to prolong the onset of bacteriuria and remove the catheter as soon as possible. Alternatives to urinary catheters include condom catheters for males and suprapubic catheters.

15. What are the risk factors for vancomycin-resistant enterococci (VRE) infection or colonization?

Risk factors include critically ill patients, immunosuppression, intraabdominal or cardiothoracic surgeries, indwelling urinary or central venous catheters, prolonged hospital stay, and multiantimicrobial or vancomycin therapy. This list seems to include just about everybody in your hospital, doesn't it?

16. What is the major source for VRE infections?

Enterococci are part of the normal flora of the gastrointestinal tract and female genital tract. These endogenous sources are responsible for most infections. However, VRE can be transmitted by direct patient-to-patient contact, hospital personnel contact, or contaminated environmental surfaces.

17. What steps can control and limit the spread of VRE? Why should you care?

Prudent use of vancomycin (especially oral administration), educating hospital staff about VRE, early reporting of VRE by the hospital lab, and immediate use of vigorous infection control measures hopefully will reduce the spread of VRE. Control of spread is important for many reasons:

1. The isolation requirements are expensive and complicate access to VRE-infected patients by members of the health care team.

2. Some VREs are also resistant to every other antibiotic available (a factor that significantly impairs effective therapy).

3. High-level vancomycin resistance can be readily transferred from *Enterococcus faecalis* to *S. aureus* in both in vitro and in vivo models. In the words of Edmond, Wenzel, and Pasculle, "The emergence of vancomycin-resistant *S. aureus* would represent the most important issue in antibiotic resistance since the dawn of the antibiotic era. A common, virulent, and transmissible bacterial agent with no known effective therapy would set infectious diseases back 60 years." Yes—reports are beginning to appear of vancomycin-resistant *S. aureus*.

18. If the hospital lab reports a positive VRE culture for your patient, what isolation precautions should you implement?

Notify the infection control team immediately. Place the VRE-infected patient in a private room. Gloves should be worn by anyone entering the room; a protective gown also should be worn if contact with the patient or any environmental surface is anticipated. Gloves and gown should be removed before leaving the room and placed in regulated medical waste containers. Most importantly, wash your hands immediately after removing personal protective equipment. Dedicate the use of a stethoscope, sphygmomanometer, and rectal thermometer to the infected patient alone, and leave them in the room. Place a sign on the patient's door informing all who come near that contact isolation precautions are needed. Place a similar sign on the patient's chart.

19. What are the common modes of transmission of methicillin-resistant *S. aureus* (MRSA)?

MRSA is most commonly transmitted via the transiently colonized hands of evil hospital personnel. They acquire the organism from direct contact with a source patient or contaminated environmental surface and stupidly fail to wash their hands properly. Airborne transmission may be an important mode for patients with tracheostomies, extensive burns, and dermatitis. Transmission via hospital personnel who are chronic carriers appears to be uncommon. However, a physician who carried MRSA in the nose has been documented to become a "cloud adult," with a 40-fold increase in airborne dispersal of MRSA when he (or she) developed a rhinovirus infection.

20. How do you rule out infection or colonization with MRSA?

When infection is suspected, cultures should be obtained from sites of presumed infection, based on clinical evaluation. To detect colonization, cultures should be obtained from the nose, throat, perineum, sites of abnormal skin lesions, or wounds, insertion sites of intravascular lines, catheter urine samples, sputum, and tracheostomy site (if present).

21. What precautions should you take to prevent the spread of MRSA from one patient to others?

Contact isolation is the rule, including a private room (or cohorting if absolutely necessary), gloves, and gowns for direct patient contact, strict hand washing after removal of gloves, and masks if aerosolization or splashing of infected secretions is expected.

22. What is the most common nosocomial fungal infection?

Candida species are responsible for approximately 70% of nosocomial fungal infections. In the 1980s, the rate of nosocomial candidemia increased by 200–500%, depending on the institution. This trend has continued throughout the 1990s. During this same period, *Candida* species were the sixth most common hospital acquired pathogen overall and the fourth most common bloodstream infection. *Candida albicans* is responsible for 50–70% of candidal infections.

23. What are risk factors for invasive candidal infections?

Intravascular catheters, antibiotic and steroid exposure, mucosal colonization, severe burns, major surgery, and neutropenia have been identified as major risk factors for candidal infections.

24. Your patient is about to receive a blood transfusion and asks what infections can be transmitted with this procedure. How do you respond?

Over 25 different pathogens have been transmitted through the use of blood products. The more common ones include hepatitis B virus, hepatitis C virus, and HIV virus. The frequency of acquiring hepatitis B is 0.002% per person transfused. For hepatitis C the frequency is 3 per 10,000 units transfused and for HIV 6.5–28 per 1,000,000 units transfused.

BIBLIOGRAPHY

1. Edmond MB, Wenzel RP, Pasculle AW: Vancomycin-resistant *Staphylococcus aureus:* Perspectives on measures needed for control. Ann Intern Med 124:329–334, 1996.
2. George DL: Epidemiology of nosocomial pneumonia in intensive care unit patients. Clin Chest Med 16:29–40, 1995.
3. Hospital Infection Control Practices Advisory Committee: Recommendations for preventing the spread of vancomycin resistance: Recommendations of the Hospital Infection Control Practices Advisory Committee (HICPAC). Am J Infect Control 23:87–94, 1995.
4. McFarland LV: Epidemiology of infectious and iatrogenic nosocomial diarrhea in a cohort of general medicine patients. Am J Infect Control 23:295–305, 1995.
5. Mulligan ME, Murray-Leisure KA, Ribner BS, et al: Methicillin-resistant *Staphylococcus aureus:* A consensus review of the microbiology, pathogenesis, and epidemiology with implications for prevention and management. Am J Med 94:313–325, 1993.
6. Pfaller MA: Epidemiology of fungal infections: Current perspectives and future directions. Clin Infect Dis 20:1525–1530, 1995.
7. Sheretz RJ, Reagan DR, Hampton KD, et al: A cloud adult: The *Staphylococcus aureus*–virus interaction revisited. Ann Intern Med 124:539–547, 1996.

12. DOES AGE MAKE A DIFFERENCE? INFECTIONS AND THE ELDERLY

Berjan Collin, M.D., and James Hanley, M.D.

1. What predisposes the elderly to infectious diseases?
1. Aging and alteration of the immune system
2. Poor nutrition
3. Functional impairment, such as incontinence, weakness, and being bedridden
4. Comorbid conditions such as chronic obstructive pulmonary disease, atherosclerotic heart disease, diabetes mellitus, renal insufficiency, cerebrovascular disease
5. Environmental conditions, such as residing in a nursing home
6. Indwelling devices

2. How do you define fever in the elderly?
Although the definition is somewhat controversial, a lower threshold should be used, particularly in the frail elderly. Guidelines include:
- Temperature > 100° F or
- Change in body temperature > 2.4° over baseline ("the old tend to be cold")

3. What are the best ways to measure temperature?
Be careful in measuring temperature in the elderly. The standard method of measurement is the oral thermometer, but the rectal thermometer is most accurate. The omnipresent tympanic thermometer has an ill-defined track record. In at least one observational study the tympanic thermometer missed 60% of low-grade fevers in the elderly. The reason is not clear; possibilities include changes in aging anatomy, presence of cerumen, or changes in blood flow and associated temperature gradients.

4. What is the significance of fever in the elderly?
Fever is always a red flag, but it is especially important in the elderly. In one recent emergency department study, 76% of elderly patients who had a temperature > 100° F had a serious illness. In many of these patients, no other clinical feature associated with serious illness was identifiable. Be aggressive in your evaluation, and consider hospitalization of elderly patients with fever.

5. What are the atypical (often typical) presentations of infection in the elderly?
The key to appreciating the atypical presentation of infection in the elderly is loss of function. Cognitive changes—delirium, in particular—are good indicators of homeostatic imbalances seen with infections. Other changes in functional state that may indicate an infection include:

1. New onset of incontinence   4. Weight loss
2. Weakness   5. Loss of appetite
3. Falls

These maladaptive responses to infections occur more commonly in the fragile elderly.

6. What are the differences in presentation of community-acquired pneumonia in the elderly?
1. Less pain   6. More tachypnea
2. Less cough   7. More confusion
3. Less fever and chills   8. More complications, such as bacteremia,
4. Less leukocytosis   empyema, and meningitis
5. Less sputum

7. What factors are prognostic for poor outcomes in elderly patients with community-acquired pneumonia?

The mortality rate attributable to pneumonia is > 20%. The following factors have been associated with a poor outcome:

1. A bedridden patient
2. Temperature < 98.6° F on admission
3. Swallowing disorder
4. Respiratory rate > 30 breaths/min
5. Shock
6. Elevated creatinine (> 1.4 mg/dl)
7. Involvement of > 3 lobes on chest radiograph

8. Should you screen for bacteriuria in elderly patients?

No. Asymptomatic bacteriuria is common in the elderly and increases with both age and decline in functional status. It is more common in women than in men. At the age of 80, up to 50% of women and 20% of men have bacteriuria. Surprisingly, the presence of asymptomatic bacteriuria in ambulatory women is not associated with any change in mortality.

9. What is the best way to treat asymptomatic bacteriuria in ambulatory elderly women?

Not with antibiotics—you may try cranberry juice. A recent controlled clinical trial demonstrated that the elderly women who were treated with antibiotics for asymptomatic bacteriuria, although less likely to have another positive culture, were more likely to have symptomatic urinary tract infection than a control group who were culture-positive and not treated with antibiotics.

10. If you do not treat asymptomatic elderly patients with bacteriuria, which elderly patients do you treat?

Patients with symptoms. Most elderly patients have the classic symptoms of urinary tract infection:

1. Fever
2. Urgency
3. Frequency
4. Dysuria
5. Increasing nocturia

However, a small subset have atypical symptoms:

1. New urinary incontinence
2. Delirium
3. Functional decline in the activities of daily living
4. Changes in appetite or nausea

11. Is cellulitis more frequent in the elderly? If so, why?

Cellulitis is clearly a more common problem in the elderly. Predisposing factors include (1) peripheral vascular disease, (2) chronic venous stasis, (3) edema, and (4) trauma. The most common bacterial organisms are still beta-hemolytic streptococci and *Staphylococcus aureus*. The dilemma is when to hospitalize such patients. Again one must be aware of atypical symptoms.

12. Should topical antibiotics be used to treat local infection in patients with pressure ulcers?

Probably not. Outcome studies to date have demonstrated no improvement in healing in patients with pressure ulcers treated with topical antibiotics.

13. Do antibiotics have any role in treatment of patients with pressure ulcers?

Clearly antibiotics are required in patients with surrounding cellulitis, underlying osteomyelitis, or sepsis. Sepsis is usually associated only with a stage 3 (full-thickness skin loss) or stage 4 (full-thickness skin loss with extensive destruction) pressure ulcer. The presence of bacteremia and pressure ulcers is associated with a high mortality rate.

14. What is the best way to treat herpes zoster in an immunocompetent elderly patient?

A recent trial demonstrated that a course of acyclovir (800 mg 5 times/day for 21 days) and prednisone (60 mg/day for the first 7 days; 30 mg/day for days 8–14 and 15 mg/day for days 15–21) was superior to matched controls in terms of (1) accelerated time to cessation of acute neuritis, (2) time to return to uninterrupted sleep, (3) return to usual activities, and (4) time to cessation of analgesic.

15. What is the most common parasitic infection in nursing homes?

Scabies outbreaks are a major problem in hospitals and nursing homes where patients require hands-on nursing care, which leads to transmission of disease between patients and nursing personnel. The major symptom of scabies is severe pruritus with crusted papular or nodular skin lesions, usually within folds of the skin.

16. Why must one be vigilant about tuberculosis in the nursing home?

Twenty-six percent of all cases of tuberculosis and 60% of deaths due to tuberculosis occur in patients older than 65 years. The annual incidence of tuberculosis in nursing home patients is 2–4 times that of community-dwelling elders. Although transmission is not uncommon within the nursing home, most active cases are caused from reactivation of old disease.

17. How should you screen for tuberculosis in patients entering a nursing home?

1. All new patients should receive a two-step tuberculin test. The first step is the standard tuberculin skin test. All patients with a negative test (< 10 mm) should have the tuberculin skin test repeated in 1–2 weeks. An anergy panel may be included with the tuberculin test.

2. All patients with positive skin test should have a chest radiograph to evaluate for pulmonary involvement.

3. An abnormal chest radiograph requires further evaluation, including sputum for *Mycobacterium tuberculosis*.

18. How should you monitor the tuberculin reactors?

Tuberculin reactors represent an ongoing risk for active tuberculosis. The results of the skin test must be recorded so that the staff is aware of the potential problem. In addition, sputum specimens should be obtained in every patient who has symptoms consistent with tuberculosis. Examples include unexplained weight loss, prolonged fever, cough for longer than 3 weeks, or functional decline.

19. What is the most common bacterial cause of diarrhea in nursing home patients?

Diarrhea due to *Clostridium difficile* is endemic in most nursing homes and has on average a colonization rate of 7–10%. Unfortunately, the high incidence no doubt results from overutilization of antibiotics in nursing home patients.

20. What vaccinations are recommended in the elderly?

Pneumococcal vaccine. In patients over 65 the incidence of pneumonia is 50/100,000. In patients with bacteremia, the case fatality rate remains high. Older people have lower antibody titers to certain pneumococcal serotypes before and after immunization than do the young; nonetheless, the mean antibody level will rise at least 10-fold. Case-control studies show that the aggregate efficacy of vaccination is 55–75%.

Influenza vaccine. Elderly patients account for 80–90% of all influenza-associated deaths. Protection correlates with antibody titers of 1:40 or more. Some elderly patients have a reduced antibody titer compared with young patients. Uncontrolled studies in patients with a protective antibody response show a protection rate of 70–100% against death by influenza as well as reduced rate of hospitalization. Estimated vaccination effectiveness is about 40%.

Tetanus toxoid vaccine. More than 50% of cases of tetanus are in patients older than 65 years. Forty percent of elderly people have inadequate levels of antitoxin antibody.

21. What is the magnitude of methicillin-resistant *Staphylococcus aureus* (MRSA) as a problem in nursing homes?

The prevalence of MRSA colonization in nursing homes is 10–25%; however, only 3–4% are clinically infected. Eradication is not indicated. Transmission of MRSA from roommate to roommate is rare.

Contact isolation is advised—wear gloves when caring for affected patients. MRSA carriers may remain in the same room as patients who are at low risk. Another option is to have MRSA carriers share a room.

BIBLIOGRAPHY

1. Abrutyn E, Berlin J, Mosey J, et al: Does treatment of asymptomatic bacteriuria in older ambulatory women reduce subsequent symptoms of urinary tract infection? J Am Geriatr Soc 44:293–295, l996.
2. Abrutyn E, Mosey J, Berlin JA, et al: Does asymptomatic bacteriuria predict mortality and does antimicrobial treatment reduce mortality in elderly ambulatory women? Ann Intern Med 120:827–833, 1994.
3. Dutt AK, Stead WW: Tuberculosis. Clin Geriatr Med 8:761–775, 1992.
4. Marco CA, Schoenfeld CN, Hansen KN, et al: Fever in geriatric emergency patients: Clinical features associated with serious illness. Ann Emerg Med 26:18–24, 1995.
5. Riquelme R, Torres A, El-Ebiary M, et al: Community-acquired pneumonia in the elderly: A multivariate analysis of risk and prognostic factors. Am J Respir Crit Care Med 154:1450–1455, 1996.
6. Smith DM: Pressure ulcers. In Besdine RW, Rubenstein LZ, Snyder L (eds): Medical Care of the Nursing Home Resident: What Physicians Need to Know. Philadelphia, American College of Physicians, 1996, pp 61–74.
7. Walker KJ, Gilliland SS, Vance-Bryan K, et al: *Clostridium difficile* colonization in residents of long-term care facilities: Prevalence and risk factors. J Am Geriatr Soc 41:940–946, 1993.
8. Whitley RJ, Weiss H, Gnann JW Jr, et al: Acyclovir with and without prednisone for the treatment of herpes zoster. A randomized placebo-controlled trial. The National Institute of Allergy and Infectious Disease Collaborative Antiviral Study Group. Ann Intern Med 125:376–383, 1996.
9. Yoshikawa TT, Norman DC: Fever and infection. In Besdine RW, Rubenstein LZ, Snyder L (eds): Medical Care of the Nursing Home Resident: What Physicians Need to Know. Philadelphia, American College of Physicians, l996, p 47–59.

III. Clinical Considerations of Infections in the Immunocompromised

13. PRIMARY IMMUNODEFICIENCIES

Mary Beth Fasano, M.D., M.S.P.H.

1. What is the overall incidence and relative distribution of primary immunodeficiencies (excluding asymptomatic IgA deficiency)?

Recent studies suggest that the overall incidence of primary immunodeficiencies (excluding asymptomatic selective IgA deficiency) is 1:10,000, with about 400 new cases annually of primary immunodeficiency in children born in the United States and 5,000–10,000 total cases.

The immune system is commonly divided into distinct categories: antibodies, T cells, phagocytes, and complement. The relative distribution of deficiencies in each is illustrated in the diagram below.

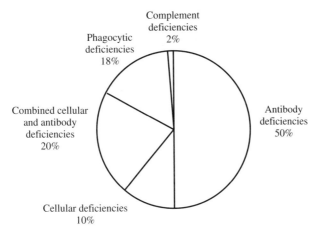

Relative distribution of primary immunodeficiencies. (Data from Stiehm ER (ed): Immunologic Disorders in Infants and Children, 4th ed. Philadelphia, W.B. Saunders, 1996.)

2. Under what circumstances should you suspect the diagnosis of a primary immunodeficiency?

- Recurrent or chronic infections
- Infection caused by opportunistic or unusual pathogens
- Failure to respond as expected to standard treatments for an infectious process
- Unusual complications to a usual infection
- A constellation of findings associated with an identified primary immunodeficiency (e.g., eczema and bleeding = Wiskott-Aldrich syndrome; hypocalcemic tetany and congenital heart disease = DiGeorge anomaly; partial oculocutaneous albinism and giant cytoplasmic granules in circulating leukocytes = Chédiak-Higashi syndrome)
- Family history of an identified primary immunodeficiency

3. What is the most common non-HIV immunodeficiency?

Selective IgA deficiency is the most common primary immunodeficiency with a reported incidence of 1:500.

4. What types of infections might you expect to see with deficiencies in different arms of the immune system?

Infections Associated with Immunodeficiencies

SPECIFIC DEFICIENCY	TYPES OF INFECTIONS
T-cell deficiencies	Pneumonia: bacterial, opportunistic viral, fungal, mycobacterial, *Pneumocystis carinii* Gastrointestinal: viruses Skin/mucous membranes: fungal
Antibody deficiencies	Sinopulmonary: bacterial, particularly gram-positive organisms Gastrointestinal: enteroviruses, giardiasis
Phagocytic cell deficiencies	Skin/soft tissue: staphylococcal, gram-negative, fungal, mycobacteria
Complement deficiencies	Sepsis/blood-borne: *Neisseria* spp., pneumococci, streptococci

5. What initial screening tests should you consider in evaluating a patient for a possible primary immunodeficiency?

A screening complete blood count (CBC) with differential and platelet count and quantitative immunoglobulins (IgG, IgA, IgM) should be performed in all patients suspected of having a primary immunodeficiency. Other initial tests depend on which arm or arms of the immune system are suspected of deficiency. In addition, one wants to exclude secondary causes of immune deficiency such as HIV infection or drug-induced immunosuppression.

Screening Tests for Immunodeficiencies

SUSPECTED ABNORMALITY	DIAGNOSTIC SCREENING TEST
Antibody deficiency	Quantitative immunoglobulins (IgG, IgA, IgM) Antibody response to immunizations (tetanus, diphtheria, rubella)
T-cell deficiency	Total lymphocyte count Delayed-type hypersensitivity tests T-lymphocyte subset analysis (CD4$^+$, CD8$^+$)
Complement deficiency	CH$_{50}$
Phagocytic deficiency	Neutrophil count and morphology Nitroblue tetrazolium (NBT) dye test IgE level

6. Give examples of primary immunodeficiencies that are inherited in an X-linked (XL) fashion.

- XL chronic granulomatous disease (gp91-phox)
- Properdin deficiency
- Wiskott-Aldrich syndrome
- XL severe combined immunodeficiency (SCID) (γ_c defect)
- XL agammaglobulinemia (Bruton's agammaglobulinemia)
- XL hyper-IgM
- XL lymphoproliferative syndrome

7. Give examples of primary immunodeficiencies that are inherited in an autosomal recessive (AR) fashion.

- AR chronic granulomatous disease (p22-phox, p47-phox, p67-phox)
- Adenosine deaminase (ADA) deficiency; ADA-SCID

• Purine nucleoside phosphorylase (PNP) deficiency; PNP-SCID
• Ataxia-telangiectasia
• Leukocyte adhesion deficiency type 1 (LAD1)
• Major histocompatibility complex (MHC) class II deficiency (Bare lymphocyte syndrome)

8. Define selective IgA deficiency. What are the common manifestations of this primary immunodeficiency?

Selective IgA deficiency is defined as a serum IgA level ≤ 5 mg/dl, normal levels of serum IgG and IgM, and normal cell-mediated immunity. Many patients with IgA deficiency are completely asymptomatic. Others present with an increased incidence of allergies, asthma, or recurrent sinopulmonary infections. Gastrointestinal diseases have been reported in association with IgA deficiency, including giardiasis, pernicious anemia, malabsorption, celiac disease, and nodular lymphoid hyperplasia. Several autoimmune diseases are associated with selective IgA deficiency; the most frequent are rheumatoid arthritis and systemic lupus erythematosus.

9. What is the cause of selective IgA deficiency?

The underlying pathogenesis is unknown, although a T-cell defect has long been suspected. Studies have shown that IgA deficiency is associated with certain MHC haplotypes, suggesting that the inheritance of a certain gene in the MHC region of chromosome 6 confers susceptibility to IgA deficiency. Acquired IgA deficiency has been reported after certain infections (congenital rubella, Epstein-Barr virus, toxoplasmosis) and with the use of certain drugs (e.g. penicillamine, sulfasalazine, gold, phenytoin, valproic acid, captopril). Drug-induced IgA deficiency is usually transient; the mechanism is unknown.

10. Discuss the management of patients with selective IgA deficiency.

Selective IgA deficiency has been reported in association with IgG subclass deficiency and/or functional antibody deficiency. Therefore, once IgA deficiency is diagnosed, it is important to assess for additional immunologic deficits. There is no specific treatment for IgA deficiency. Intermittent or continuous antibiotics may be helpful in patients with recurrent infections. Associated diseases are treated with standard therapies. In patients with associated IgG subclass deficiency or impaired functional antibody responses, immunoglobulin replacement with IgA-depleted intravenous immunoglobulin (IVIG) preparations (Gammagard S/D or Polygam S/D) may be warranted. In general, IVIG is contraindicated in patients with selective IgA deficiency for two reasons: (1) currently available immunoglobulin preparations contain little IgA, and (2) transfusions with blood or blood products containing IgA (e.g., IVIG) may sensitize patients, resulting in the formation of IgG or IgE anti-IgA antibodies and thus placing them at risk for systemic reactions with subsequent blood or blood product transfusions. Therefore, patients with IgA deficiency who require blood products should be given blood from an IgA-deficient donor, autologous preparations, or saline-washed products. IgA deficient patients with anti-IgA antibodies should wear a Medic-Alert bracelet.

11. How do immunoglobulin levels change with age?

At birth, the full-term infant's IgG is equal to or slightly higher than the mother's serum IgG as a result of active transport of IgG across the placenta. Preterm infants may have diminished IgG because the bulk of placental transfer of immunoglobulin is thought to occur during the third trimester. After birth, IgG levels fall rapidly (half-life = ~ 21 days), reaching a nadir at about 3–4 months of life. Thereafter the infant's endogenous IgG production becomes evident and reaches adult levels by about 8–12 years of age. Because IgM and IgA do not cross the placenta, serum concentrations at birth are very low. IgM concentrations rise rapidly after birth and reach approximately 60% of adult levels by 1 year of age. IgA concentrations increase more slowly and do not reach adult levels until close to adolescence. It is therefore extremely important to interpret serum immunoglobulin levels with respect to age.

12. What are the best screening tests for suspected deficiencies in the classic, terminal, and alternative complement pathways?

The CH_{50} represents the best screening test for classic and terminal complement component deficiencies. The AH_{50} is the best screening test for alternative complement component deficiencies.

13. What is the best screening test for chronic granulomatous disease?

The NBT dye reduction test represents the best screening test for chronic granulomatous disease.

14. What chromosomal abnormality may be found in DiGeorge anomaly?

DiGeorge syndrome is usually a sporadic event but may be inherited. Most familial cases are associated with microdeletions on the long arm of chromosome 22 (22q11.2). Special chromosome analysis using fluorescence in situ hybridization (FISH) with specific probes should be ordered in evaluating an infant for suspected DiGeorge syndrome.

15. What embryonic defects are seen with DiGeorge syndrome?

DiGeorge anomaly is defined as a deficiency of the derivatives of the third and fourth branchial pouches, which results in aplastic thymus (T-cell deficiency), aplastic parathyroids (hypocalcemia), and abnormal development of the aortopulmonary and conotruncal septa. The most common cardiac malformations are interrupted aortic arch type B, truncus arteriosus, right aortic arch, and tetralogy of Fallot. Craniofacial anomalies include hypertelorism, small ears with notched pinnae, micrognathia, and short philtrum of the lip.

16. What is severe combined immunodeficiency syndrome (SCID)?

SCID is a heterogenous group of disorders characterized by gross functional impairment of both T and B cells. Patients usually die of overwhelming infection within the first year or two of life unless immunologic reconstitution can be achieved. Early features include persistent thrush, chronic diarrhea, failure to thrive, and pneumonia (*Pneumocystis carinii*, bacterial, viral, mycobacterial). The average age of diagnosis is $6\frac{1}{2}$ months. SCID may result from diverse pathogenic mechanisms with different inheritance patterns that lead to defects at different levels of cellular differentiation. The frequency of SCID is 1:100,000 to 1:500,000.

17. List the most common genetic forms of SCID.
- Reticular dysgenesis (generalized hematopoietic hypoplasia)
- Adenosine deaminase deficiency
- Purine nucleoside phosphorylase deficiency
- Janus-associated kinase (JAK)-3 deficiency
- XL defect in common gamma chain (γ_c)
- Bare lymphocyte syndrome—MHC class II deficiency
- Cartilage hair hypoplasia
- Recombinase activating gene (RAG)-1 or RAG-2 mutations
- Abnormal T-cell receptor (TCR)/CD3

18. What is the molecular defect for X-linked SCID?

The molecular basis for XSCID is a mutation of the gene encoding the common γ chain (γ_c) of the interleukin (IL)-2 receptor and several other cytokine receptors (IL-4, IL-5, IL-7, IL-15).

19. What is the classic clinical triad for Wiskott-Aldrich syndrome?

Eczema, thrombocytopenia (small platelets), and recurrent infections.

20. Describe the molecular defect responsible for X-linked agammaglobulinemia (XLA)?

The primary defect in XLA is failure in maturation from pre-B to B cell. The defective gene in XLA, named *Btk* (Bruton's tyrosine kinase), encodes a cytoplasmic tyrosine kinase. It was identified in 1993 as the target of mutations responsible for XLA. Tyrosine kinases are important in the signaling pathways regulating B-cell development. Btk is preferentially expressed in the B lymphoid and myelomonocytic lineages and is undetectable in T lymphoid cells. Btk is a member of a unique tyrosine kinase subfamily and is essential for normal B-cell maturation and for responsiveness to a subset of T-cell–independent antigens. Much remains to be learned about the regulation and function of Btk.

21. What is ataxia-telangiectasia?

Ataxia-telangiectasia (AT) is an autosomal recessive disorder characterized by (1) telangiectasias primarily around the bulbar conjunctivae and ears; (2) progressive cerebellar ataxia; (3) extreme sensitivity to ionizing radiation and abnormality in DNA repair mechanisms; (4) increased incidence of cancer; (5) combined immunodeficiency usually consisting of IgA and IgG_2 deficiency, cutaneous anergy, and depressed in vitro lymphocyte responsiveness; (6) premature aging; (7) endocrine disorders; and (8) recurrent sinopulmonary infections. Diagnosis is made in the presence of the classic cutaneous and neurologic findings (which generally develop between 2–6 years of age), an elevated serum α-fetoprotein and carcinoembryonic antigen, and excessive chromosomal breakage. Family members are at increased risk for the development of malignancy, especially breast cancer in heterozygote females.

22. IgA deficiency may be seen with what other immunodeficiencies?

Ataxia-telangiectasia, IgG subclass deficiency, functional antibody deficiencies.

23. Describe the metabolic abnormality in chronic granulomatous disease (CGD).

Although phagocytes from patients with chronic granulomatous disease ingest microorganisms normally, killing is deficient because the capacity of the phagocytes to produce superoxide and related microbicidal oxygen intermediates is impaired by deficiency of reduced nicotinamide adenine dinucleotide phosphate (NADPH) oxidase. NAPDH oxidase is a multicomponent complex that includes a unique membrane-bound cytochrome b and several cytosolic components. The cytochrome b is a heterodimer consisting of a 91-kd glycosylated heavy chain and a 22-kd light chain, termed gp91-phox (phagocyte oxidase) and p22-phox, respectively. The gene for the heavy chain is the site of mutations responsible for X-linked CGD. Deficiency of p47 phox, a 47-kd cytosolic protein required for oxidase activity, accounts for most autosomal recessive forms of CGD. Two rare subgroups of autosomal recessive CGD are due to defects in the gene for the light chain of the cytochrome b (p22-phox) or a defect in the product of the gene encoding p67-phox, a 67-kd cytosolic protein.

24. What are the most common organisms causing infection in patients with chronic granulomatous disease?

Staphylococcus aureus, *Aspergillus* spp., *Serratia* sp., *Escherichia* sp., *Pseudomonas* spp., *Proteus* spp., *Salmonella* spp., and *Candida* spp. Aspergillus lung infections are associated with a high mortality rate.

25. Describe the clinical presentation of CGD.

Classically, patients with CGD present in the first years of life with recurrent infections involving the skin, lymph nodes, liver, lungs, bones, and gastrointestinal tract. Disseminated visceral granulomatous lesions result. Other features include eczematous dermatitis, ulcerative stomatitis, and abscesses of the liver, spleen, lungs, bones, and perianal area. Infections are most frequently caused by the organisms listed in question 24.

26. What is the hyper-IgE syndrome (HIE)?

Hyper-IgE (Job's) syndrome is a rare, complex immunoregulatory disorder characterized by recurrent staphylococcal abscesses and markedly elevated serum IgE levels. Patients have a lifelong history of severe and recurrent staphylococcal abscesses involving the skin, lungs, joints, and other sites. In addition, patients have a unique tendency to form persistent pneumatoceles after staphylococcal pneumonias. IgE levels range from 2,150–90,000 IU/ml with a mean of > 20,000 IU/ml. IgD levels may be elevated; however, levels of IgG, IgA, and IgM are normal. Diminished T-cell function has been reported in some patients as well as poor functional antibody responses to immunization. High levels of anti-*S. aureus* IgE help to confirm the diagnosis. Mild-to-moderate eosinophilia in blood and sputum may be seen. Associated allergies and asthma are rare.

27. What primary immunodeficiency is associated with delayed separation of the umbilical cord?

Leukocyte adhesion deficiency (LAD) type 1 is an autosomal recessive disorder of neutrophils characterized by recurrent, life-threatening bacterial infections, and impaired pus formation and wound healing. During the neonatal period, septicemia and omphalitis may occur and separation of the umbilical cord may be delayed for 21 days or longer. Absent or deficient expression of the adhesion molecules CD11 and CD18 on the surface of neutrophils and other leukocytes results in defective cellular adherence. The hallmark of LAD-1 is absence of granulocytes at sites of infection in the presence of marked peripheral blood leukocytosis. This finding is secondary to defective neutrophil and monocyte adhesion to vascular endothelium.

28. What is the CD40 ligand? What immunodeficiency is caused by defects in the CD40 ligand gene?

CD40 ligand is a T-cell activation protein. Its receptor, CD40, is expressed by antigen-presenting cells, including B cells. CD40 plays a major role in B-cell proliferation and differentiation. The interaction of CD40 and its ligand induces the formation of memory B cells and the switch from IgM to other immunoglobulin isotypes. A defect in expression of CD40 ligand on the surface of T cells is the basis for the X-linked form of hyper-IgM syndrome. This defect results in the laboratory findings of low serum levels of IgG, IgA, and IgE, with normal or increased IgM.

29. The first clinical use of gene therapy in humans involved which primary immunodeficiency?

Treatment of SCID syndrome secondary to ADA deficiency represents the first clinical use of gene therapy. In 1990 Blaese et al. at the National Institutes of Health started a clinical trial with retroviral-mediated transfer of the ADA gene into the T cells of two children with ADA-SCID.

30. List the current uses for intravenous immunoglobulin approved by the Food and Drug Administration.

- Primary immunodeficiency states (e.g., XL agammaglobulinemia, common variable immunodeficiency, Wiskott-Aldrich syndrome, XL hyper-IgM, SCIDs)
- Idiopathic thrombocytopenic purpura
- Chronic lymphocytic leukemia
- Kawasaki syndrome
- Bone marrow transplantation
- Pediatric AIDS

31. List the major potential risks of treatment with IVIG.

Adverse reactions occur in approximately 5% of infusions of IVIG. These reactions are generally mild and may include fever, chills, headache, myalgia, nausea, vomiting, chest tightness, wheezing, flushing, urticaria, or alterations in blood pressure. Most reactions are associated with rapid infusion of IVIG and subside with temporary discontinuation or reduction in the infusion rate. Rare anaphylaxis to IVIG has been reported. Less common are delayed reactions, including aseptic meningitis, pulmonary toxicity, renal toxicity, transient neutropenia and hemolysis, and disseminated intravascular coagulation. Finally, the risk of transmission of infectious agents accompanies the use of this blood-derived product. The manufacturing process, as well as the recent addition of extra viral inactivation steps, makes the transmission of an infectious agent extremely low.

32. Why is IVIG usually administered at 3–4 week intervals in the treatment of primary immunodeficiencies?

The half-life of IgG is approximately 23 days. For this reason a 3–4 week dosing interval is usually selected.

33. What is common variable immunodeficiency?

Common variable immunodeficiency (CVID) is a heterogenous disorder characterized by hypogammaglobulinemia, absence of functional antibody, normal or decreased numbers of circulating B cells, and recurrent bacterial infections, primarily involving the sinopulmonary tract. CVID can present in children or adults; the average age of diagnosis is 29–30 years. Associated T-cell dysfunction may develop in up to 50% of patients over time. Treatment is with regular infusions of IVIG. The molecular basis for CVID has yet to be defined but most likely involves a number of gene defects and/or environmental factors.

34. Other than recurrent infections, what conditions might you see in association with CVID?

Although recurrent sinopulmonary infections are the most common presenting complaint in patients with CVID, other disorders are frequently seen. Autoimmune disease occurs in about 26% of patients and may even be the presenting symptom. Examples of autoimmune disorders seen in CVID include autoimmune hemolytic anemia, idiopathic thrombocytopenic purpura, and rheumatoid arthritis. Gastrointestinal disease occurs in 17% of patients, and Crohn's disease and ulcerative colitis are relatively common. Chronic giardiasis and nodular lymphoid hyperplasia also may occur. Granulomatous lesions may be seen, often in association with autoimmune hemolytic anemia or autoimmune thrombocytopenia. Finally, malignancies, especially lymphomas and carcinoma of the stomach, are found with increased frequency in CVID.

35. How does a late complement component deficiency (LCCD) classically present?

The hallmark of persons with LCCD (C5, C6, C7, C8, C9) is meningococcal disease, which occurs in 50–60% of patients. Typically the initial infection presents at a median age of 17 years as meningitis caused by an uncommon serogroup of meningococci. Recurrent meningococcal disease is classic in LCCD as is relapse of infection within 1 month of treatment. Of interest, the mortality rate from meningococcal disease in LCCD patients is 5–10 fold lower than in a normal host.

Late Complement Component Deficiency and Meningococcal Infections

PARAMETER	NORMAL	LCCD
Frequency of infection (%)	0.0072	57
Male-to-female ratio	1.3:1	2.2:1
Median age (yr) of first episode	3	17
Recurrence rate (%)	0.34	41
Relapse rate (%)	0.6	7.6
Mortality/100 episodes (%)	19	1.5
Infecting serogroup		
No. of isolates	3,184	67
% B	50	19.4
% Y	4.4	32.8

Adapted from Figueroa JR, Densen P: Infectious diseases associated with complement deficiencies. Clin Microbiol Rev 4:359–395, 1991.

36. Which primary immunodeficiency is frequently associated with polyendocrinopathies?

Polyendocrinopathies are seen in one subgroup of patients with chronic mucocutaneous candidiasis. Chronic mucocutaneous candidiasis is characterized by persistent or recurrent infections of the skin, nails, and mucous membranes with *Candida* species (almost always *C. albicans*).

The six clinical subgroups are defined by the extent and location of infections, genetic factors, and associated disorders, such as polyendocrinopathy, thymomas, autoimmune disorders, and interstitial keratitis. The candidiasis-polyendocrinopathy syndrome most frequently presents during infancy with thrush and extensive cutaneous candidiasis. Endocrinopathies may develop at any time from childhood through adulthood. The parathyroids, adrenals, and thyroid are most commonly involved. Most studies of pedigrees with the candidiasis-polyendocrinopathy syndrome are suggestive of an autosomal recessive mode of inheritance.

BIBLIOGRAPHY

1. Blaese RM, Culver KW, Miller AD, et al: T lymphocyte-directed gene therapy for ADA-SCID: Initial trial results after 4 years. Science 270:475–480, 1995.
2. Buckley RH, Schiff RI, Schiff SE, et al: Human severe combined immunodeficiency: Genetic, phenotypic, and functional diversity in one hundred eight infants. J Pediatr 130:378–387, 1997.
3. Figueroa JE, Densen P: Infectious diseases associated with complement deficiencies. Clin Microbiol Rev 4:359–395, 1991.
4. Primary immunodeficiency diseases: Report of a WHO Scientific Group. Clin Exp Immunol 99(Suppl 1):1–24, 1995.
5. Sneller MC, Strober W, Eisenstein E, et al: New insights into common variable immunodeficiency. Ann Intern Med 118:720–730, 1993.
6. Stiehm ER (ed): Immunologic Disorders in Infants and Children, 4th ed. Philadelphia, W.B. Saunders, 1996.

14. NATURAL HISTORY OF HIV INFECTION, ANTIRETROVIRAL THERAPY, AND PREVENTIVE CARE

Wheaton J. Williams, M.D., and Steven C. Johnson, M.D.

1. Which laboratory test is the best surrogate marker of HIV-1 disease progression?

At present, the level of HIV-1 RNA in plasma (viral load) is the most useful laboratory test for estimating the risk for progression to AIDS or death. The quantity of HIV-1 RNA in plasma is determined by assays such as branched-chain DNA (bDNA) and reverse transcription polymerase chain reaction (RT-PCR). Most HIV-1 replication occurs within lymphoid tissues, with spillover of virus into the bloodstream. HIV-1 in plasma has a half-life of only about 6 hours. Therefore, the quantity of HIV-1 in plasma serves as an indirect measure of the total HIV-1 viral load and provides important information about the current level of HIV-1 replication.

In a study of 180 HIV-infected persons for whom the duration of infection was unknown, Mellors et al. found that a single baseline determination of HIV-1 RNA level was highly predictive of the risk of progression to AIDS or death. Patients with a 3-fold higher baseline level of HIV-1 RNA had a 1.5-fold greater risk of death within 10 years. The prognostic significance of the viral load was independent of the baseline CD4 cell count. Fifty percent of persons with a CD4 count $\geq$ 500 cells/μl and a plasma viral load > 10,900 copies/ml died within 6 years of study entry compared with only 5% of persons with a CD4 count $\geq$ 500 cells/μl and a plasma viral load < 10,900 copies/ml.

2. How should viral load measurements be used in clinical practice?

Reasonable recommendations for use of viral load measurements in clinical practice include:

1. Obtain baseline viral load (consider two separate viral load determinations 4 weeks apart to serve as a baseline).

2. Obtain viral load measurements routinely every 3–4 months to detect elevations in viral load that indicate the need to initiate or change antiretroviral therapy.

3. Obtain a viral load measurement 4 weeks after starting or changing antiretroviral therapy to assess virologic response to therapy.

4. Viral load measurements should not be obtained within 4 weeks of immunization or acute infection.

5. Viral load measurements should be delayed if the patient has been noncompliant with antiretroviral therapy.

Most experts agree that HIV-infected persons with a viral load of > 30,000 copies/ml should initiate or change antiretroviral therapy, and antiretroviral therapy should be considered for patients with a viral load > 5,000 copies/ml.

3. Describe indications for starting or changing antiretroviral therapy.
Indications for initiation of antiretroviral therapy

1. Primary HIV infection (acute retroviral syndrome) - all patients
2. Established HIV infection if:
   - CD4 < 500, *or*
   - Viral load > 5,000–10,000 copies/ml
3. Vertical transmission prophylaxis (maternal-fetal transmission)
4. Postexposure prophylaxis
5. HIV-related immune thrombocytopenic purpura (ITP)
6. AIDS-related dementia

Indications for changing antiretroviral therapy
1. Treatment failure
   - Increase in viral burden ≥ 0.5 log ($\geq$ 3-fold)
   - Decrease in CD4 cell count
   - Clinical progression (fever, wasting, opportunistic infection)
2. Drug toxicity or intolerance
3. Current use of a suboptimal treatment regimen: monotherapy with zidovudine (AZT), zalcitabine (ddC), or lamivudine (3TC)

4. What are the advantages of combination antiretroviral therapy compared with monotherapy?

In general, combination antiretroviral therapy results in greater and more sustained decreases in viral load and increases in CD4 cell count than monotherapy. For example, in antiretroviral naive patients, superior virologic and immunologic responses have been demonstrated with combinations of zidovudine (AZT) + didanosine (DDI), AZT + zalcitabine (ddC), and AZT + lamivudine (3TC) compared with AZT monotherapy. The most impressive reductions in viral load and increases in CD4 cell counts have occurred in patients receiving a three-drug regimen, including a protease inhibitor. Examples include AZT + 3TC + indinavir (IDV) or AZT + 3TC + ritonavir (RTV). These three-drug combinations have resulted in up to 100- to 1000-fold reductions in viral load and increases of up to 150 CD4 cells/μl.

Combination therapy also slows the progression of HIV disease and improves survival. Compared with AZT monotherapy, the combination of AZT + DDI, AZT + ddC, or AZT + 3TC delays disease progression in antiretroviral naive patients. When used as the initial antiretroviral therapy, combination therapy with AZT + DDI or AZT + ddC results in improved survival compared with AZT monotherapy. Multidrug regimens, including a protease inhibitor, have been shown to prolong survival in antiretroviral-experienced patients with CD4 cell counts < 100/μl and are likely to prolong life in patients with higher CD4 cell counts.

Finally, combination therapy delays the emergence of drug-resistant HIV-1 isolates. For instance, after 12 weeks of therapy, only 9% of patients taking AZT + 3TC have HIV-1 isolates with genotypic resistance to AZT compared with 44% of patients on AZT monotherapy.

5. Describe reasonable options for initial antiretroviral therapy.

The decision to initiate or change therapy and the selection of an antiretroviral regimen are complex issues that require consideration of factors such as viral load, CD4 cell count, history of prior antiretroviral therapy, potential drug interactions, concurrent medical problems, cost, compliance, and the patient's willingness to take multiple medications. Currently, most experts favor the use of three-drug combinations (see question 4):
1. Any of the following + protease inhibitor (indinavir, nelfinavir, or ritonavir)
2. Any of the following + nonnucleoside reverse transcriptase inhibitor (nevirapine or delavirdine)
   - Zidovudine + lamivudine (AZT + 3TC)
   - Zidovudine + didanosine (AZT + DDI)
   - Zidovudine + zalcitabine (AZT + ddC)
   - Stavudine + lamivudine (D4T + 3TC)
   - Didanosine + stavudine (DDI + D4T)

6. Do treatment-induced reductions in plasma HIV-1 RNA levels reduce the risk of HIV disease progression?

Treatment-induced reductions in plasma viremia are associated with a reduced risk of HIV-1 disease progression. The degree of clinical benefit is related to both the magnitude and duration of the reduction in plasma HIV-1 RNA levels. For instance, in a study comparing the efficacy of AZT vs. DDI vs. AZT + DDI vs. AZT + DDC, a decrease of 1.0 log in the level of HIV RNA from baseline to week 8 of the study was associated with a 65% reduction in the risk of AIDS or death. Furthermore, if the 1.0 log reduction in viral load persisted to week 56 of the study, there was a 90% reduction in disease progression.

7. Describe the most common adverse reactions associated with each of the currently available antiretroviral agents.

Generic Name	Brand Name	Adverse Reactions
Reverse transcriptase inhibitors		
Zidovudine (AZT)	Retrovir	Fatigue, headache, GI upset, myopathy, anemia, leukopenia
Didanosine (DDI)	Videx	Peripheral neuropathy, pancreatitis, hepatitis, unpalatable tablets
Zalcitabine (ddC)	Hivid	Peripheral neuropathy, oral ulcers
Stavudine (D4T)	Zerit	Peripheral neuropathy
Lamivudine (3TC)	Epivir	Rarely nausea, headache
Nevirapine	Viramune	Rash (potentially severe), fever, nausea, headache
Delavirdine	Rescriptor	Rash, nausea, elevated liver enzymes
Protease inhibitors		
Saquinavir	Invirase	Nausea, diarrhea, abdominal pain
Ritonavir	Norvir	Nausea, vomiting, diarrhea, circumoral paresthesias, drug interactions
Indinavir	Crixivan	Asymptomatic bilirubin elevation, nausea, kidney stones, drug interactions
Nelfinavir	Viracept	Diarrhea, nausea, headache, drug interactions

8. What are the clinical manifestations of primary HIV infection? Which tests are needed for diagnosis?

About one-half of all patients with primary HIV infection experience an acute symptomatic illness within 2–6 weeks of last exposure to HIV. Patients typically present with a mononucleosis-like illness with significant constitutional symptoms and lymphadenopathy. The most common signs and symptoms are summarized in the table below. Dermatologic findings are common and include an erythematous maculopapular eruption, primarily involving the face and trunk, and oral aphthous ulcers. Hematologic abnormalities include leukopenia and thrombocytopenia. Neurologic manifestations may be prominent features of the illness; examples include aseptic meningitis, encephalitis, and peripheral neuropathy.

Signs and Symptoms of Primary HIV Infection (n=139)

SIGN OR SYMPTOM	FREQUENCY (%)
Fever	97
Adenopathy	77
Pharyngitis	73
Rash	70
Myalgia or arthralgia	58
Thrombocytopenia	51
Leukopenia	38
Diarrhea	33
Headache	30
Elevated serum aspartate aminotransferase or alanine aminotransferase	23
Nausea or vomiting	20
Hepatosplenomegaly	17
Oral thrush	10
Encephalopathy	8
Neuropathy	8

From Clark SJ, Saag MS, Decker WD, et al: High titers of cytopathic virus in plasma of patients with symptomatic primary HIV-1 infection. N Engl J Med 324:954–960, 1991, with permission.

Because symptomatic primary HIV infection precedes or accompanies the development of HIV-1-specific antibody response, diagnostic tests such as the enzyme-linked immunosorbent assay (ELISA) and Western blot, which detect the presence of viral antibodies, are not helpful in this setting. Instead, it is necessary to demonstrate the presence of the HIV virus by detection of p24 antigen, HIV RNA, or HIV DNA.

9. What is the estimated period between infection with HIV-1 and development of an AIDS-defining illness?

HIV infection is a chronic illness that after many years results in profound immunodeficiency manifested by opportunistic disease. Within 10 years of estimated seroconversion, 51% of a cohort of homosexual and bisexual men from San Francisco developed AIDS.

Effective antiretroviral or prophylactic therapies alter the natural history of HIV infection by delaying the development of opportunistic disease and changing the frequency with which certain opportunistic diseases develop. Prophylaxis against *Pneumocystis carinii* pneumonia (PCP) has been shown to delay the first AIDS-defining illness for 6–12 months and to decrease the frequency of PCP. Patients receiving PCP prophylaxis often present with other AIDS-defining illnesses such as wasting syndrome, disseminated *Mycobacterium avium* complex disease, cytomegalovirus disease, and esophageal candidiasis. It is anticipated that the widespread use of combination antiretroviral therapy and MAC prophylaxis will also change the clinical manifestations of AIDS.

10. What clinical findings predict disease progression in HIV-infected patients?

Thrush, oral hairy leukoplakia, unexplained fever and diarrhea, and involuntary weight loss have been associated with subsequent progression to AIDS. Generalized lymphadenopathy is a common finding in patients with HIV infection but is not associated with progression to AIDS.

11. Which laboratory tests should be performed during the initial evaluation of a patient with HIV infection?

The initial laboratory studies are obtained to stage HIV infection and to identify HIV-related complications and risk-behavior–related complications.

Laboratory study	Clinical relevance
Complete blood count	Leukopenia, anemia, immune thrombocytopenic purpura
Chemistries, liver function tests	Nephropathy, hepatitis
CD4 count and percent	Assess immunologic status, risk for opportunistic infection
Plasma HIV-1 RNA	Assess amount of viral replication, risk for disease progression
Purified protein derivative test	Screen for tuberculosis
Rapid plasma reagin test	Identify coinfection
Hepatitis B serologies	Nonimmune patients receive immunization
Hepatitis C serologies	Identify coinfection
Toxoplasma serology	Identify patients at risk for toxoplasma encephalitis
Cervical Papanicolaou smear	Screen for cervical cancer
Chest x-ray	Identify pulmonary pathology, baseline for comparison

12. Which immunizations are recommended for patients with HIV infection? Which are contraindicated?

Whenever possible, HIV-infected patients should receive immunizations early in the course of infection (CD4 > 500), because patients with symptomatic HIV infection (CD4 < 200) are likely to have suboptimal immunologic responses to vaccines. In general, live vaccines are contraindicated in persons with HIV infection. However, the measles, mumps, and rubella vaccine (MMR) is recommended for HIV-infected patients with CD4 > 200 who would otherwise be eligible for the MMR vaccine. The following table summarizes the recommendations of the Advisory Committee on Immunization Practices for the use of immunizations for persons with HIV infection:

Immunizations for HIV-infected Patients

VACCINES TO CONSIDER FOR ALL HIV-INFECTED-PATIENTS	VACCINES THAT ARE SAFE IF BOOSTER IS NEEDED	VACCINES THAT ARE SAFE IF INDICATED	VACCINES THAT ARE CONTRAINDICATED
Pneumococcal	Tetanus toxoid	Hepatitis A	Bacille Calmette-Guérin
Influneza	MMR (CD ≥ 200)	Rabies	Oral polio[†]
Hepatitis B*	Inactivated polio	Inactivated typhoid	Oral typhoid
Hemophilus B		Cholera	Yellow fever
		Meningococcal	MMR (CD4 < 200)

MMR = measles, mumps, and rubella vaccine.
* Consider for patients who are nonimmune and at risk for acquiring hepatitis B.
† Oral polio vaccine should not be administered to healthy household contacts of HIV-infected persons because of the risk of transmission of vaccine-strain polio.

Some studies suggest that immunization with viral or bacterial vaccines may result in transient increases in plasma viral load measurements. However, it is not clear that the transient increase in viral replication results in accelerated progression of HIV infection. Therefore, most experts favor immunization of HIV-infected patients when indicated.

13. Describe the indications for primary prophylaxis and the preferred preventive regimens for infection with *Pneumocystis carinii*, *Toxoplasma gondii*, *Mycobacterium avium* complex, and *Mycobacterium tuberculosis*.

Infection	Indication	Preferred Agent	Alternative Agent
Pneumocystis carinii	CD4 < 200 CD4 < 14% Thrush, other opportunistic infection	Trimethoprim-sulfamethoxazole	Dapsone Pentamidine
Toxoplasma gondii	CD4 < 100 and IgG antibody to *Toxoplasma*	Trimethoprim-sulfamethoxazole	Dapsone + pyrimethamine
Mycobacterium avium complex	CD4 < 75	Clarithromycin or azithromycin	Rifabutin
Mycobacterium tuberculosis	Purified protein derivative (PPD) ≥ 5 mm History of positive PPD without treatment, contact with case of active tuberculosis	Isoniazid	Rifampin

Primary prophylaxis refers to prevention of the first episode of an infection. It is not routinely recommended for infection with *Candida* species, *Cryptococcus neoformans, Histoplasma capsulatum, Coccidioides immitis,* herpes simplex, and cytomegalovirus.

14. What are the benefits of prophylaxis against *Pneumocystis carinii*, *Toxoplasma gondii*, and *Mycobacterium avium*?
Prophylaxis reduces the risk of developing these common opportunistic infections and delays the development of an AIDS-defining illness until later in the course of HIV infection, when CD4 cell counts are lower. HIV-infected patients who have access to comprehensive care, including prophylaxis against opportunistic infections, generally develop opportunistic infections at CD4 cell counts < 50. The use of broad-spectrum antimicrobial agents such as trimethoprim-sulfamethoxazole, clarithromycin, and azithromycin also reduces the risk of developing common bacterial infections such as sinusitis. Finally, prophylaxis against PCP and *Mycobacterium avium* complex improves survival.

15. What is the relationship between HIV infection and cervical neoplasia?

Cervical neoplasia is associated with infection with one of several oncogenic serotypes of human papillomavirus (HPV serotypes 16, 18, and 31). The cell-mediated immunodeficiency resulting from HIV infection presumably impairs control of both HPV viral replication and development of neoplasia.

Immunodeficiency due to HIV infection is associated with an increased risk of cervical intraepithelial neoplasia (CIN), the precancerous lesion of the cervical squamous epithelium. Women with HIV infection tend to have more severe and extensive CIN and suffer from higher recurrence rates of CIN after standard ablative therapy. Although CIN is more common in HIV-infected women, it is not clear that invasive cervical cancer develops more rapidly or more frequently in this population if adequate screening programs are available. However, cervical cancer in HIV-infected women seems to be more aggressive and less responsive to treatment. In 1992, the Centers for Disease Control and Prevention added invasive cervical cancer in an HIV-infected woman to the list of conditions diagnostic of AIDS.

The optimal method of screening for CIN in HIV-infected women is controversial. At a minimum, HIV-infected women should receive an annual Papanicolaou smear. Consider performing smears every 6 months if the patient has (1) a previous smear with a squamous intraepithelial lesion, (2) a history of HPV infection, (3) a CD4 cell count < 200, or (4) a history of multiple male sexual partners. Women should be referred for colposcopic examination if a screening Papanicolaou smear reveals squamous cell carcinoma or a high-grade squamous intraepithelial lesion. If the smear reveals a low-grade squamous intraepithelial, consider a repeat smear in 3 months, and refer for colposcopy if the squamous intraepithelial lesion persists.

Some experts recommend routine use of colposcopy in HIV-infected women because it seems to be a more sensitive test for the detection of cervical neoplasia.

16. What should health care providers advise HIV-infected patients about the risks of pet ownership?

Persons infected with HIV are at increased risk of acquiring a number of animal-associated infections, including *Toxoplasma gondii, Bartonella henselae, Cryptosporidium* sp., *Salmonella* sp., *Campylobacter* sp., *Giardia* sp., *Listeria* sp., *Mycobacterium marinum,* and *Cryptococcus neoformans.* However, most of these infections are usually acquired from sources other than exposure to pet animals. Because the risk of acquiring infections from pets is low and the psychological benefits of pet ownership may be significant, health care providers should not prohibit HIV-infected individuals from owning pets. Instead, they should educate patients about the potential risks and the means to reduce the likelihood of acquiring pet-related infections.

Cats. Potential risks include *T. gondii, B. henselae,* and enteric infections. To minimize the risk of transmission of *T. gondii* and enteric infections, HIV-infected cat owners should avoid cleaning litter boxes or should wear gloves when cleaning litter boxes and wash hands thoroughly immediately afterward. Flea control and avoidance of cat scratches and bites may decrease the risk of *B. henselae* transmission.

Dogs. Potential source of enteric pathogens. HIV-infected dog owners should avoid contact with dog feces and thoroughly wash hands after exposure to feces. Dogs with prolonged diarrheal illness should be examined by a veterinarian. Puppies are more likely to carry infections than adult dogs.

Birds. Potential source of *C. neoformans* and *M. avium.* Pet birds seem to be a low risk for patients with HIV infection. Avoid contact with bird droppings. Ill birds should be examined by a veterinarian.

Reptiles. Reptiles have a high carriage rate of *Salmonella* sp. HIV-infected patients should avoid contact with reptiles or wear gloves when handling reptiles or cleaning their cages.

Fish. Potential source of *M. marinum.* HIV-infected patients should wear gloves when handling fish or cleaning aquariums.

17. What should health care providers advise HIV-infected patients about the risks of travel to foreign countries?

Travelers to foreign countries, especially to countries with a tropical climate or a poor standard of living, are at risk of exposure to pathogens that are not present in the country in which they reside. HIV-infected travelers are more likely to develop severe illness if they acquire infection with pathogens such as *Salmonella* sp., *Cryptosporidium* sp., *Leishmania* sp., and *M. tuberculosis*. In addition, HIV-infected persons should not receive the live vaccines, such as oral polio, oral typhoid, and yellow fever, that are commonly given to travelers. Despite these concerns, HIV infection should not prohibit travel abroad. However, travelers with HIV infection should receive accurate advice and preventive strategies to reduce the risk of exposure to infectious diseases. Travel advice should include the following components: (1) measures to reduce transmission of food- and water-borne pathogens, (2) ways to reduce transmission of arthropod-borne infections, (3) management of traveler's diarrhea, (4) chemoprophylaxis for malaria, if indicated, and (5) recommendations for immunizations. If possible, patients should consult with an expert in travel medicine.

BIBLIOGRAPHY

1. Centers for Disease Control: Recommendations of the Advisory Committee on Immunization Practices (ACIP): Use of vaccines and immune globulins for persons with altered immunocompetence. MMWR 42(RR-4):1–12, 1993.
2. Carpenter CJ, Fischl MA, Hammer SM, et al: Antiretroviral therapy for HIV infection in 1997. Recommendations of an international panel. JAMA 277:1962–1969, 1997.
3. Chaisson RE, Volberding PA: Clinical manifestations of HIV infection. In Mandell GL, Bennett JE, Dolin R (eds): Principles and Practice of Infectious Diseases. New York, Churchill Livingstone, 1995, pp 1217–1252.
4. Clark SJ, Saag MS, Decker WD, et al: High titers of cytopathic virus in plasma of patients with symptomatic primary HIV-1 infection. N Engl J Med 324:954–960, 1991.
5. Glaser CA, Angulo FJ, Rooney JA: Animal-associated opportunistic infections among persons infected with the human immunodeficiency virus. Clin Infect Dis 18:14–24, 1995.
6. Hammer SM, Katzenstein DA, Hughes MD, et al: A trial comparing nucleoside monotherapy with combination therapy in HIV-infected adults with CD4 cell counts from 200 to 500 per cubic millimeter. N Engl J Med 335:1081–1090, 1996.
7. Katzenstein DA, Hammer SM, Hughes MD, et al: The relation of virologic and immunologic markers to clinical outcomes after nucleoside therapy in HIV-infected adults with 200 to 500 CD4 cells per cubic millimeter. N Engl J Med 335:1091–1098, 1996.
8. Mellors JW, Rinaldo CR Jr, Gupta P, et al: Prognosis in HIV-1 infection predicted by the quantity of virus in plasma. Science 272:1167–1170, 1996.
9. Moore RD, Chaisson RE: Natural history of opportunistic disease in an HIV-infected urban clinical cohort. Ann Intern Med 124:633–642, 1996.
10. Sande MA, Volberding PA (eds): The Medical Management of AIDS, 5th ed. Philadelphia, W.B. Saunders, 1997.
11. USPHS/IDSA Prevention of Opportunistic Infections Working Group: 1997 USPHS/IDSA Guidelines for the prevention of opportunistic infections in persons infected with human immunodeficiency virus. MMWR 46(RR-12):1–47, 1997.
12. Wilson ME, von Reyn F, Fineberg HV: Infections in HIV-related travelers: Risks and prevention. Ann Intern Med 114:582–592, 1991.

15. DIAGNOSIS AND TREATMENT OF COMMON HIV-RELATED COMPLICATIONS

Steven C. Johnson, M.D., and Wheaton J. Williams, M.D.

This chapter outlines important general considerations, common clinical syndromes, and diagnosis and management of the most common opportunistic infections in HIV-infected persons. Because the standard of care for AIDS is a rapidly moving target, there should be a low threshold to seek advice from experts in the field. References 2 and 8 in the bibliography are well-written, relatively concise handbooks on many aspects of HIV infection and AIDS; they are good resources for additional information about diseases and treatments, including specific doses and adverse drug reactions for medications discussed in this chapter.

1. What are the important general considerations in the approach to acutely ill patients?

1. **Understand the types of diseases for which HIV-infected patients are at risk.** Despite a seemingly endless number of diagnostic possibilities, the specific types of diseases to consider in HIV-infected patients include the classic opportunistic infections (e.g. *Pneumocystis carinii* pneumonia [PCP], cryptococcosis, central nervous system toxoplasmosis, cytomegalovirus retinitis), certain bacterial infections (e.g., pneumonia, sinusitis, line-related infections, enteric bacterial infections), and certain malignant conditions (especially non-Hodgkin's lymphoma and Kaposi sarcoma). In addition, patients may have illnesses related to underlying risk behavior (e.g. endocarditis in an injection drug user or secondary syphilis related to sexual activity). Finally, HIV-infected patients also develop diseases common to the general population (e.g., viral gastroenteritis, influenza).

2. **Review recent CD4 lymphocyte counts when interpreting signs and symptoms.** Certain opportunistic illnesses are likely only when significant immunodeficiency is present. For example, headache in a patient with a CD4 lymphocyte count of 600 cells/mm^3 is much more likely to be benign (e.g. migraine or tension headache) than due to cryptococcal meningitis. Conversely, a new headache in a patient with a CD4 lymphocyte count of 60 cells/mm^3 requires a more aggressive diagnostic approach to exclude opportunistic processes such as cryptococcal meningitis, central nervous system (CNS) toxoplasmosis, or CNS lymphoma.

3. **Recognize the common causes of a given clinical syndrome.** Although there may be over 100 different causes of pulmonary symptoms in HIV-infected patients, the vast majority of respiratory syndromes are due to PCP, bacterial pneumonia, tuberculosis, and viral respiratory infections. Knowing what is common helps to guide the initial diagnostic work-up and empiric therapy.

4. **Consider first illnesses that may be life-threatening.** This list includes extensive pneumonia (bacterial, fungal, mycobacterial, or PCP), space-occupying CNS lesions, bacterial sepsis, and meningitis (fungal, tuberculous, and bacterial). Hospitalization or close outpatient monitoring may be necessary prior to exclusion of these diagnoses.

2. What findings help to distinguish PCP from other pulmonary infections?

Even in the era of prophylaxis, PCP remains one of the most common opportunistic infections in patients with advanced HIV disease (CD4 lymphocyte count < 200 cells/mm^3). The clinical symptoms of fever, cough, shortness of breath, and dyspnea on exertion are clearly nonspecific, and other diagnoses, such as bacterial pneumonia, tuberculosis, and other opportunistic infections, must be considered. Differentiating PCP from bacterial pneumonia is particularly important. Abrupt onset of symptoms, high fever, purulent sputum, and focal infiltrate are more common with bacterial pneumonia. The classic radiographic appearance of PCP is bilateral reticular infiltrates. However, a less common radiographic appearance of PCP may be more likely than typical manifestations of many less common diseases. Focal infiltrates, apical infiltrates, pneumatoceles, and pneumothorax may be seen with PCP. In addition, approximately 10% of cases of PCP are associated with a normal chest x-ray. Pleural effusion, hilar adenopathy, and lobar consolidation are unlikely to be due to PCP and should prompt a search for other causes. An increased serum level of lactate dehydrogenase (LDH) is often listed as a helpful sign, but it is highly nonspecific. Specific microbiologic confirmation is the only way to be sure of the diagnosis.

3. Should all cases of PCP be microbiologically confirmed?

Although PCP is common and may have a characteristic clinical presentation, it is important to confirm the diagnosis in most, if not all, cases. Examination of an induced sputum sample for *P. carinii* should be the initial diagnostic step in most patients. This is an excellent, noninvasive test but lacks sensitivity (approximately 75%). If the test is positive, the patient can be treated without additional diagnostic testing. If the test is negative, bronchoalveolar lavage should be performed. Rarely, transbronchial biopsy or open lung biopsy may be required. The only situation in which empiric treatment of PCP is defensible is an extremely mild case (A–a gradient < 20, mildly abnormal chest x-ray, induced sputum for *P. carinii* negative). However, it is good practice to confirm all cases, especially in patients who develop pneumonia while on PCP prophylaxis (which makes other causes more likely).

4. What is the best antibiotic treatment for PCP?

Trimethoprim-sulfamethoxazole remains the treatment of choice for PCP of all degrees of severity. Adverse reactions such as fever, rash, and hepatitis may limit its use in selected cases. Suitable alternatives for severe disease include intravenous pentamidine or intravenous trimetrexate with folinic acid. Suitable alternatives for milder forms of PCP include trimethoprim-dapsone, atovaquone, or clindamycin-primaquine. Adjunctive therapy may include intravenous fluids, supplemental oxygen, mechanical ventilation, or corticosteroids.

5. When should corticosteroids be used in PCP?

Several studies have clearly shown improved survival in patients with severe PCP who are treated with concomitant corticosteroids. The established criteria are based on a $pO_2 < 70$ mmHg or an A–a gradient > 35. Because these criteria are arbitrary and arterial blood gas measurements have some laboratory variability, moderate cases of PCP that do not meet these criteria are still reasonable candidates for corticosteroids. Given some risk for adverse events, patients with mild cases of PCP should not receive steroids.

6. When should an HIV-infected patient be hospitalized for PCP?

Many cases of PCP are diagnosed and treated in the outpatient setting. However, PCP can be serious and still has a mortality rate of approximately 10%. Inpatient care should be considered if any one of the following criteria is present:
- Severe pneumonia (A–a gradient > 35, extensive radiographic involvement, respiratory distress)
- Pneumothorax
- Significant volume depletion that does not correct easily
- Inability to take oral medications
- Unreliable patient or difficult social situation

7. What are the clinical syndromes caused by cytomegalovirus (CMV) in patients with HIV infection?

CMV disease is a complication of advanced HIV infection; most cases occur when the CD4 lymphocyte count is below 50 cells/mm^3. CMV retinitis is by far the most common clinical syndrome, and diagnosis is typically based on ophthalmologic appearance alone. Other sites of CMV disease require microbiologic confirmation, which often involves culture or immunostaining from a biopsy specimen. Other important syndromes due to CMV are colitis, pneumonitis, esophagitis, encephalitis, and radiculopathy.

8. What is the treatment of choice for CMV retinitis?

The number of treatment options for CMV retinitis is growing. However, intravenous ganciclovir or intravenous foscarnet are still the treatments of choice and are similar in efficacy. In general, ganciclovir is more commonly used because of ease of administration and predictable, treatable toxicities (leukopenia, anemia, thrombocytopenia). Cidofovir, a new agent with remarkable pharmacokinetics, allows infrequent dosing (once per week for induction, every 2 weeks for maintenance), but its proper role has not been determined. The ganciclovir ocular implant is also an option in selected patients. The clinical course for most patients involves the use of several different agents over time, given the predilection for relapse.

Treatment Option	Advantages	Disadvantages
Intravenous ganciclovir	Easy to administer Protects other parts of body Easily managed cytopenias	Need for venous access and daily infusions Relapse common
Ganciclovir intra-ocular implant	Excellent protection of affected eye Removes need for chronic indwelling catheter in some cases	Surgical implantation risk of endoph-thalmitis and retinal detachment Does not protect sites outside eye
Intravenous foscarnet	Highly effective Protects other parts of body Initial studies suggested survival advantage over ganciclovir	Side effects, including nephrotoxicity, low calcium and magnesium, nausea
Intravenous cidofovir	Pharmacokinetics (1 dose/wk for induction and 1 dose per 2 wk for maintenance) No need for chronic indwelling catheter	Nephrotoxicity Requires concomitant probenecid (may cause rash) and intravenous fluids Complete efficacy data lacking

Oral ganciclovir is available for the treatment of CMV disease and offers the advantage of a non-parenteral regimen. However, it is not as effective as any of the parenteral therapies and it should not be used alone as induction therapy for CMV disease. It clearly has a role for secondary prophylaxis of individuals with stable disease including CMV retinitis if the retinitis is not close to the macula. Oral ganciclovir is also reasonable in conjunction with the ganciclovir intraocular implant to protect the other eye and other tissues from CMV. The clear advantage of oral ganciclovir over parenteral therapies is the lack of venous access and its attendant complications of thrombosis and infection.

9. What are the most common manifestations of disseminated *Mycobacterium avium* complex (DMAC) disease?

DMAC is a complication of advanced HIV disease; nearly all cases occur in patients with a CD4 lymphocyte count < 75–100 cells/mm^3. Usual symptoms of DMAC include fever, chills, sweats, anorexia, weight loss, abdominal pain, and diarrhea. It is one of the leading diseases to consider in HIV-infected patients who present with fever of unknown origin (FUO) or wasting syndrome. Clinical findings include anemia, other cytopenias, increased liver enzymes (especially alkaline phosphatase), hepatosplenomegaly, and lymphadenopathy. Occasionally, patients present with acute localized lymphadenitis. Anecdotally, acute localized lymphadenitis has been seen soon after the initiation of potent antiretroviral therapy, perhaps indicating an augmented immune response against MAC.

10. How is DMAC disease diagnosed?

DMAC is commonly associated with mycobacteremia, and most cases are diagnosed by a blood culture processed for acid-fast bacilli (AFB). Blood cultures are often positive within 1–2 weeks. This lag in diagnosis is often not clinically significant because DMAC is typically a slowly progressive illness. Bone marrow biopsy with AFB staining and culture may allow an earlier diagnosis. In cases with localized, accessible lymphadenopathy, biopsy is a useful method of diagnosis. Empiric treatment for presumed DMAC is generally hazardous and not recommended.

11. What is the treatment of choice for DMAC disease?

The new macrolides (clarithromycin, azithromycin) represent a clear advance in the management of DMAC disease. Of the two, clarithromycin appears to be slightly more effective. All cases of DMAC disease are treated with multidrug chemotherapy, as in the management of tuberculosis. The combination of clarithromycin, ethambutol, and rifabutin is a well-tolerated, highly effective regimen. The duration of therapy is lifelong.

12. What is the role of lumbar puncture in the diagnosis and management of cryptococcosis in HIV infection?

Cryptococcosis is an opportunistic fungal infection most common in patients with a CD4 lymphocyte count < 100 cells/mm³. Although pneumonia or systemic infections without CNS involvement may occur, most cases present with meningitis. Thus, lumbar puncture (LP) is part of the diagnostic approach. The cryptococcal antigen test of cerebrospinal fluid (CSF) has a sensitivity greater than 90%, but some cases can be diagnosed only by culture. The serum cryptococcal antigen has an even greater sensitivity and is a useful diagnostic test in patients who refuse lumbar puncture. Although serial LPs have been used to document improvement, patients who respond well to treatment do not need follow-up LPs.

13. What is the preferred treatment for cryptococcosis in HIV infection?

The four effective regimens that have been studied for the initial treatment of cryptococcosis are amphotericin B alone, amphotericin B plus flucytosine, fluconazole alone, and fluconazole plus flucytosine. Of these, an amphotericin B-containing regimen continues to be the treatment of choice. The most potent regimen, amphotericin B plus flucytosine, is particularly useful in patients who present with severe disease (mental status changes, positive India Ink, increased intracranial pressure). For milder cases, all of the approaches are probably acceptable. However, use of fluconazole alone should probably not be considered until additional trials (especially those using higher doses) are completed. Fluconazole alone is the treatment of choice for lifelong secondary prophylaxis.

14. What is the most common presentation of tuberculosis in HIV infection?

Extrapulmonary presentations of tuberculosis (TB) have been reported frequently in persons with HIV infection, including lymphadenitis, pericarditis, peritonitis, visceral abscesses, and meningitis. These presentations are certainly more common in HIV-infected patients than in the general population. However, pulmonary TB remains the most common presentation in HIV-infected persons. TB is an illness that may occur early in the course of HIV infection with normal or mildly reduced CD4 lymphocyte counts. When it occurs early in HIV infection, it appears similar to the classic disease in HIV-seronegative persons. When TB occurs late in HIV infection, miliary disease or extrapulmonary presentations are more common.

15. How does the management of syphilis differ in HIV infection?

The epidemiology of syphilis and HIV infection overlaps significantly, and coinfection is common. Over the past 10 years, a series of case reports and case series have raised concerns that persons with HIV infection may be more likely to fail standard syphilis treatment. Some of these failures have been dramatic, including rapid development of neurosyphilis, relapses of secondary syphilis despite appropriate treatment, and development of uncommon complications such as ocular syphilis. For this reason, the proper approach to coinfected patients is unclear. Standard regimens appropriate to the stage of syphilis (e.g., benzathine penicillin, 2.4 million units intramuscularly for primary and secondary syphilis) are currently recommended in the 1993 CDC STD treatment guidelines. However, some experts favor more aggressive therapy, such as that used for neurosyphilis (e.g., intravenous penicillin), for all stages of disease. Regardless of the treatment used, close follow-up with serial serologic testing to assess the clinical and serologic response to therapy is strongly recommended. There should also be a low threshold to perform lumbar puncture to clarify the extent of CNS involvement.

16. What are the diagnostic considerations in HIV-infected patients who present with dysphagia and odynophagia?

Dysphagia and odynophagia suggest inflammation in the hypopharynx, esophagus, or stomach. Of these anatomic areas, the esophagus is the most common site of pathology. The major causes of esophagitis are *Candida albicans*, herpes simplex, and cytomegalovirus. Other causes to consider are aphthous esophageal ulcers, pill-induced esophagitis, and acid-induced disease (reflux esophagitis). In most situations, an empiric trial of fluconazole is a reasonable approach to patients with dysphagia or odynophagia because candidal esophagitis is a common explanation. If improvement is noted, a presumptive diagnosis of candidal esophagitis is made. If there is no improvement, upper endoscopy should be performed to determine the cause.

17. What are the common causes of fever of unknown origin (FUO) in HIV-infected patients?

The classic definition of FUO requires fever > 101° F on several occasions, illness of at least 3 weeks' duration, and absence of a diagnosis despite 1 week of intensive study. FUO is a common syndrome in HIV infection, although the causes are somewhat different from those in classic studies. Over 10 studies of FUO in HIV infection have been reported. Mycobacterial infections (MAC and MTB), lymphoma, PCP, toxoplasmosis, and drug fever are particularly common causes of FUO in HIV infection. Although the diagnostic approach varies from case to case, mycobacterial blood culture, bone marrow biopsy, lymph node biopsy, and computed tomography of the abdomen and pelvis are often helpful. Fever should not be ascribed to HIV itself until other causes are excluded.

18. What are the appropriate diagnostic tests for acute diarrhea in HIV infection?

Alterations in bowel habits (diarrhea, loose stools, and hyperdefecation) are common complaints in patients with HIV infection. Chronic, mild complaints may have no discernible etiology. In addition, the side effects of many medications include diarrhea. However, the acute onset of diarrhea usually implies an infection. The table below lists some of the etiologic agents and the appropriate tests relative to the level of immunodeficiency.

Level of Immunodeficiency	Diagnostic Considerations	Diagnostic Tests
CD4 lymphocyte count ≥ 200 cells/mm^3	Viral gastroenteritis Enteric bacterial infections Antibiotic-associated colitis Food poisoning Giardiasis	Stool culture, including studies for *Clostridium difficile* Stool exam for ova and parasites (O&P)
CD4 lymphocyte count 100–199 cells/mm^3	All of the above plus crypto-sporidiosis and isosporiasis	Stool culture Stool O&P with acid-fast bacillus (AFB) stain
CD4 lymphocyte count < 100 cells/mm^3	All of the above plus MAC, CMV colitis, and micro-sporidiosis	Stool culture Stool O&P Stool exam for microsporidium AFB blood culture Colonic biopsy

19. What clinical findings and diagnostic tests are helpful in distinguishing the cause of CNS mass lesions in the absence of or prior to brain biopsy?

The three most common causes of mass lesions in the brain of patients with HIV/AIDS are toxoplasmosis, lymphoma, and progressive multifocal leukoencephalopathy (PML). Brain abscess, tuberculosis, cryptococcosis, nocardiosis, and many other infections are occasional causes of mass lesions. Although brain biopsy is definitive for many of these conditions, certain clinical findings may lead to a relatively secure diagnosis without brain biopsy.

Diagnosis	Supportive Findings
CNS toxoplasmosis	Ring-enhancing lesions on MRI or CT scan Positive *Toxoplasma* serology CD4 lymphocyte count < 100 cells/mm^3 Response to empiric antitoxoplasmosis therapy
CNS lymphoma	Enhancement on thallium 201 SPECT scan Ring-enhancing lesions on MRI or CT scan with negative *Toxoplasma* serology Positive cerebrospinal fluid (CSF) cytology Positive CSF Epstein-Barr virus polymerase chain reaction
Progressive multifocal leukoencephalopathy	White matter involvement with lack of enhancement on MRI or CT scan Positive CSF JC virus polymerase chain reaction
Cryptococcoma, tuberculoma, metastatic cancer, nocardiosis, brain abscess, many other causes	These diseases are uncommon and seldom diagnosed without brain biopsy. However, CSF examination and systemic findings of these diseases (e.g., bacteremia with brain abscess) may be helpful in diagnosis.

20. What complications of HIV infection lead to hospitalization?

In 1996, we prospectively measured the reasons for 137 consecutive hospitalizations in our clinic cohort of 456 HIV-infected patients (58% with AIDS).[10] The reasons for hospitalization were diverse with over 50 different diagnoses. Common categories of illness included opportunistic infections (28%), bacterial infections (23%), malignancy-related complications (11%), need for surgical or diagnostic procedure (9%), and adverse drug reactions (7%). Specific diagnoses that were common reasons for admission included PCP, DMAC disease, non-Hodgkin's lymphoma, bacterial pneumonia, cellulitis, sepsis (line-related and other types), pancreatitis, and fever with volume depletion. Uncertainty of the correct diagnosis and concern for life-threatening illnesses were common reasons for admission. Ninety percent of all admissions involved persons with AIDS (CD4 lymphocyte count < 200 cells/mm^3), and 70% of all admissions involved patients with a CD4 lymphocyte count < 50 cells/mm^3. Potent combination antiretroviral therapy, prophylactic medications and vaccines, and early diagnosis and treatment of opportunistic diseases significantly reduce the frequency of hospitalization.

BIBLIOGRAPHY

1. Barnes PF, Bloch AB, Davidson PT, Snider DE Jr: Tuberculosis in patients with human immunodeficiency virus infection. N Engl J Med 324:1644–1650, 1991.
2. Bartlett JG. Medical Management of HIV Infection, 1996 ed. Glenview, IL, Physicians & Scientists Publishing, 1996.
3. Chuck SL, Sande MA: Infections with *Cryptococcus neoformans* in the acquired immunodeficiency syndrome. N Engl J Med 321:794–799, 1989.
4. Luft BJ, Hafner R, Korzun AH, et al: Toxoplasmic encephalitis in patients with the acquired immunodeficiency syndrome. N Engl J Med 329:995–1000, 1993.
5. Musher DM, Hamill RJ, Baughn RE: Effect of human immunodeficiency virus (HIV) infection on the course of syphilis and on the response to treatment. Ann Intern Med 113:872–881, 1990.
6. National Institutes of Health–University of California Expert Panel for Corticosteroids as Adjunctive Therapy for Pneumocystis Pneumonia: Consensus statement on the use of corticosteroids as adjunctive therapy for pneumocystis pneumonia in the acquired immunodeficiency syndrome. N Engl J Med 323:1500–1504, 1990.
7. Polis MA, Masur H: Promising new treatments for cytomegalovirus retinitis. JAMA 273:1457–1459, 1995.
8. Sande MA, Volberding PA (eds): The Medical Management of AIDS, 5th ed. Philadelphia, W.B. Saunders, 1997.
9. Shafran SD, Singer J, Zarowny DP, et al: The Canadian Randomized Open-Label Trial of Combination Therapy for MAC Bacteremia. N Engl J Med 335:377–383, 1996.
10. Williams W, Hageman A, Calhoon B, Johnson S: Factors associated with hospitalization and inpatient length of stay (LOS) in a university-based HIV clinical program [abstract 662]. Fourth Conference on Retroviruses and Opportunistic Infections, Washington, DC, January 22–26, 1997.

16. RHEUMATIC SYNDROMES ASSOCIATED WITH HIV INFECTION

Raymond J. Enzenauer, M.D., FACP

1. What is the only rheumatic syndrome *not* routinely associated with HIV infection?

Although systemic lupus erythematosus, a Sjögren's-like syndrome, systemic vasculitis, seronegative spondyloarthropathies (particularly psoriatic arthritis and Reiter's syndrome), inflammatory myositis, infectious arthritis, and pyomyositis have been reported in association with HIV, rheumatoid arthritis (RA) is *rarely* seen in association with HIV infection. RA is believed to be primarily mediated by CD4-positive lymphocytes; thus, the profound CD4 lymphopenia in HIV infection may protect the patient from RA. There have been isolated case reports of patients with RA who have gone into clinical remission when they acquired HIV infection.

2. How is the Reiter's syndrome in HIV disease different from non–HIV-related Reiter's syndrome?

Reiter's syndrome was the first rheumatic syndrome recognized in association with HIV infection. The incomplete form is more commonly seen in HIV disease than the classic triad. Patients with HIV-associated Reiter's syndrome have much less axial involvement or sacroiliitis compared with non–HIV-related Reiter's syndrome. Most cases of HIV-associated Reiter's syndrome are venereally acquired. HLA-B27 positivity is similar in the two groups. Some authors suggest that HIV-associated Reiter's syndrome is a more aggressive disease and is less responsive to treatment. Clearly some patients with HIV-associated Reiter's have progressed to AIDS with immunosuppressive treatment. Most authors recommend concomitant antiviral therapy in all patients with HIV-associated Reiter's syndrome who are being considered for immunosuppressive therapy.

3. How is psoriatic arthritis different in HIV-infected and non–HIV-infected patients?

It is estimated that 5–7% of non–HIV-infected persons with psoriasis develop psoriatic arthritis, whereas 32% of HIV-infected psoriatics develop arthritis. Like HIV-associated Reiter's syndrome, HIV-associated psoriatic arthritis rarely affects the spine. Most studies suggest a more aggressive skin and joint disease in HIV-affected psoriatics compared with non–HIV-infected psoriatics.

4. List the autoimmune phenomena associated with HIV infection.

1. Polyclonal gammopathy
2. Circulating immune complexes
3. Autoantibodies
   - Rheumatoid factor
   - Antinuclear antibodies
   - Anticardiolipin antibodies
4. Anticellular antibodies
   - Antiplatelet antibodies
   - Anti-red blood cell antibodies
   - Antilymphocyte antibodies
   - Antibrain antibodies
   - Anti-parietal cell antibodies

5. What is diffuse infiltrative lymphocytic syndrome (DILS)? How does it differ from non–HIV-associated Sjögren's syndrome?

Like primary Sjögren's syndrome, DILS is associated with keratoconjunctivitis sicca. Minor salivary biopsy in DILS reveals a CD8-predominant lymphocytic infiltrate, whereas primary Sjögren's syndrome has a CD4-predominant cellular infiltrate. Treatment is primarily symptomatic, and HIV-infected patients with DILS have a longer survival than HIV-infected patients with other rheumatic manifestations, such as psoriasis.

Comparison of Diffuse Infiltrative Lymphocytic Syndrome (DILS) and Sjögren's Syndrome

	DILS	SJÖGREN'S SYNDROME
Sex: Male	+++	+
Female	+	+++
Sicca symptoms	+++	+++
Lymphadenopathy	+++	+
Hypergammaglobulinemia	+++	+++
SS-A	0	++
SS-B	0	++
HIV antibody	+++	0
HLA	DR5	B8/DR3
Minor salivary gland biopsy	CD8-predominant	CD4-predominant

6. What is the "painful articular syndrome" associated with HIV infection?

Painful articular syndrome is characterized by severe articular pain of 2–24 hours' duration. It is often incapacitating, unresponsive to oral nonsteroidal and analgesic (including narcotic) medications, and requires emergency care with intravenous narcotic medication. Patients have no evidence of local inflammation, and results of all tests are normal. The etiopathogenesis remains to be elucidated.

7. Describe the "arthralgias" associated with HIV infection.

Arthralgias are seen in as many as one-third of patients with HIV infection. The pain involves two or more joints, it is of moderate intensity and frequently intermittent.

8. Describe HIV-associated arthropathy.

HIV-associated arthropathy is a distinct seronegative arthropathy associated with inflammatory arthritis and no recognizable rheumatic disease or syndrome. Most patients have oligo- or monoarticular arthritis that persists for 1–24 weeks. HIV-associated arthropathy is not associated with HLA-B27, and none of the patients develop extraarticular symptoms.

9. Describe the various forms of myopathy associated with HIV infection.

Generalized myalgias are frequent in patients with HIV infection. They tend to recur and respond readily to analgesic compounds. Muscle wasting has been reported and is usually related to the underlying presence of neurologic, nutritional, and/or infectious disorders. Several cases of inflammatory myositis have been reported in HIV infection. The clinical picture is indistinguishable from idiopathic polymyositis (PM). Some patients respond to immunosuppressive therapy with prednisone; again, concomitant antiviral treatment is usually recommended.

Zidovudine (AZT) therapy also may cause a myopathy clinically similar to idiopathic PM. Most authors recommend discontinuation of AZT in such patients. If muscle symptoms persist for 2 weeks after discontinuation of AZT, muscle biopsy is recommended to evaluate the patient for inflammatory myositis.

10. Describe the septic arthritis of HIV infection.

Systemic opportunistic infections are highly prevalent during the course of HIV infection. Septic joint involvement, however, is rare, despite the often profound state of immunodeficiency. HIV-infected hemophiliac patients are considered to be at high risk for development of septic arthritis because of their propensity for intraarticular bleeding.

11. What are the pathogenic considerations in HIV-related rheumatic diseases?

1. Direct effect of HIV infection
2. Indirect effect of HIV infection

- Role of cytokines
- Proliferative effects of HIV-derived growth factors

3. Reactive immune mechanisms
- Autoimmunity
  Circulating immune complexes
  Anticardiolipin antibodies
- Opportunistic infection
  Arthrogenic organisms
  HLA-B27-related
- HIV antigens

12. Name the various forms of vasculitis reported in HIV infection.

Although vasculitis is rare in HIV infection (0.4% of cases), various types have been described, including medium-vessel vasculitis (similar to periarteritis nodosa), CNS vasculitis, lymphomatoid granulomatosis, mononeuritis multiplex, leukocytoclastic vasculitis, and eosinophilic vasculitis. Pathogenesis is believed to be either direct viral invasion of the vessel wall or immune-mediated vascular damage. Treatment consists of high-dose corticosteroids, again usually in combination with antiretroviral therapy.

13. What is the association of fibromyalgia with HIV infection? How does it differ from non–HIV-related fibromyalgia?

Fibromyalgia is seen in 11–29% of HIV-infected patients and represents over 40% of all rheumatic complaints in HIV infection. Unlike non–HIV-related fibromyalgia, fibromyalgia in HIV is more common in men than women, and the incidence of associated depression may be higher in HIV-related fibromyalgia.

14. How does pediatric HIV differ from adult HIV with respect to rheumatic complaints?

HIV-infected children do not display the serious rheumatic manifestations seen in HIV-infected adults. Arthritis, vasculitis, and Reiter's syndrome are never seen in pediatric HIV infection. Arthralgias are seen in 20% and myalgias in 8% of pediatric HIV infections, although little evidence indicates that they are immune-mediated. Possible reasons for the difference include immaturity of the pediatric immune system, different modes of HIV acquisition, shorter duration of HIV infection, and lack of exposure to other sexually transmitted diseases.

BIBLIOGRAPHY

1. Calabrese LH: The rheumatic manifestations of infection with the human immunodeficiency virus. Semin Arthritis Rheum 18:225–239, 1989.
2. Espinoza LR, Aguilar JL, Berman A, et al: Rheumatic manifestations associated with human immunodeficiency virus infection. Arthritis Rheum 32:1615–1622, 1989.

17. INFECTIONS AFTER CHEMOTHERAPY

Robert H. Gates, MD

1. Are infections an important cause of mortality in patients with cancer?

Yes. Infections are the major cause of mortality in many types of cancers. Infection has replaced bleeding as the major cause of mortality in leukemia. Data about causes of death from cancer centers vary; however, about 75% of patients with acute leukemia and 50% with lymphoma die as a result of infection.

2. What factors place patients with cancer at risk for infection?

Multiple factors place patients with cancer at risk for infection. They range from factors associated with the cancer itself to factors associated with therapy for cancer and previous antibiotic therapy.

Factors Predisposing to Infection in Patients with Cancer

FACTOR PROMOTING INFECTION	EXAMPLES OF ASSOCIATED ORGANISMS	EXAMPLES OF DISEASE STATES
Diminished antibody response	Encapsulated organisms: Pneumococci *Haemophilus influenzae* *Neisseria* species Staphylococci Streptococci	Multiple myeloma Poor nutrition B-cell lymphomas Post-splenectomy (Hodgkin's disease) Myelophthisis
Poor white blood cell function or number	Aerobic gram-positive organisms Staphylococci Enterococci Aerobic gram-negative organisms *Pseudomonas aeruginosa* *Enterobacter* species Fungi *Candida* species *Aspergillus* species	Leukemias Lymphomas Myelophthisis processes Chemotherapy
Poor cellular immunity	Listeria Herpes Mycobacteria Cryptococci *Legionella* species *Pneumocystis* species	Hodgkin's disease Non-Hodgkin's lymphoma Poor nutrition Chronic leukemias Chemotherapy, especially fludarabine Steroids
Skin and mucosal defects	Staphylococci *Candida* species Herpes Aerobic gram-negative organisms	Chemotherapy Radiation therapy Vascular access devices
Environmental problems Construction Poor airflow	*Aspergillus* species Tuberculosis *Legionella* species	Organ transplants Neutropenia
Contaminated water supply, raw foods	Aerobic gram-negative organisms	Organ transplants Neutropenia

Table continued on following page.

Factors Predisposing to Infection in Patients with Cancer (Continued)

FACTOR PROMOTING INFECTION	EXAMPLES OF ASSOCIATED ORGANISMS	EXAMPLES OF DISEASE STATES
Anatomic mechanical problems	Anaerobes Staphylococci Aerobic gram-negative organisms	Lung cancer causing airway blockage Skin or mucosal disruption from primary or metastatic cancer Bowel obstruction from primary or metastatic cancer Urinary tract obstruction from renal or cervical cancer
Prior infection with organism that has propensity to recur	*Aspergillus* species *Candida* species Herpes group virus	Not disease-specific

3. What is the most significant predisposing factor for infection in patients with cancer?

Neutropenia is the single most important factor in determining whether a patient with cancer will become infected. The absolute neutrophil count (ANC) is calculated by multiplying the granulocyte percent (neutrophils or segments + bands) by the total white blood cell (WBC) count. The risk of infection rises as the WBC count falls; the risk is greatest with neutrophil counts less than 500/mm^3. Most serious infections occur with neutrophil counts below 100/mm^3. In addition to presence and degree, duration of neutropenia is also important. As the duration increases, the risk of infection increases, ultimately reaching 100%. A duration of 3–7 days poses much less of a risk than a duration beyond 14 days. Currently, about one-third of neutropenic patients with fever have a microbiologically proven infection (positive cultures), whereas about one-fifth have clinically apparent infection with negative cultures.

4. What are neutropenic precautions?

The following precautions are initiated to protect the neutropenic patient from other people:

1. Strict handwashing is the most important precaution.

2. Routinely, it is not necessary for health care providers to wear masks. Healthcare providers with a transmissible respiratory disease should not care for the patient. The practice of requiring the patient to wear a mask when leaving the room varies by institution.

3. Ideally, the airflow in the patient's room should be positive compared with the hall. The intent is to avoid exposure to airborne pathogens such as *Aspergillus* spp.

4. The patient's room should not be cleaned in a manner that will cause dust to be shed (e.g., from drapes) because of transient but significant increases in *Aspergillus* spore counts.

5. Sources of gram-negative organisms should be avoided (e.g., live flowers in water, raw food, fresh fruits and vegetables).

5. What else can be done to prevent infections in neutropenic patients?

1. High-efficiency particulate air (HEPA) filtration is used by many centers for patients who undergo organ transplantation or are expected to have prolonged neutropenia from therapy. The intent is to remove airborne pathogens such as *Aspergillus* spp.

2. Generally, immunizations should be up to date, including pneumococcal and *Haemophilus* vaccines. Special consideration should be given to patients about to undergo elective splenectomy. Such patients should receive the above vaccines and meningococcal vaccine.

3. The use of prophylactic antibiotics is often determined according to institutional practice. Experience with the use of prophylactic agents has been a mixed bag, ranging from spectacular success with acyclovir and ganciclovir in bone marrow transplant recipients to failure with nystatin. The major problems of prophylactic agents are that they promote resistant bacteria and are partially responsible for the emergence of *Staphylococcus epidermidis* and enterococci as significant

pathogens in neutropenic patients. To prevent or delay infection in patients with cancer undergoing chemotherapy, several different prophylactic agents have been used:

- **Antibiotics:** quinolones, trimethoprim-sulfamethoxazole, oral aminoglycosides, and oral amphotericin B for selective bowel decontamination. Selective antibiotic suppression appears to be most appropriate for patients anticipated to have prolonged or severe neutropenia. Note that the agents used do not affect the anaerobic flora of the bowel. The use of trimethoprim-sulfamethoxazole is well established in bone marrow transplant recipients to prevent the development of *Pneumocystis carinii* infection.
- **Antifungal agents:** nystatin, clotrimazole, and the imidazoles.
- **Antiviral agents:** acyclovir and ganciclovir. Acyclovir may be effective for patients with recurrent Herpes simplex infections by helping to prevent relapses during periods of neutropenia; it has the added benefit of maintaining mucosal integrity, thereby lessening the risk of mucosal colonization and invasion by fungi and bacteria.
- **Isoniazid (INH):** to prevent reactivation of tuberculosis in patients with a positive tuberculosis skin test, particularly in patients with lymphoreticular cancer.

6. What is the source of most bacteria that infect a neutropenic patient?

Although some infections are acquired from the environment, about 50% of infections in neutropenic patients with cancer come from bacteria that make up the patient's own endogenous flora, such as *Escherichia coli*, *Enterobacter* spp., *Klebsiella* spp., other gram-negative bacteria, yeast, and anaerobes. Even *Staphylococcus epidermidis* isolated from blood is likely to have originated from the bowel. A patient's flora may change rapidly on admission to the hospital. In immunosuppressed patients, the bacterial flora can change in a matter of hours, quickly resembling the bacteria found in the hospital setting.

7. When is fever in neutropenic patients significant?

Fever in the presence of neutropenia is always significant and should be treated as a medical emergency. A patient can die literally within hours if prompt and effective therapy is not begun. Fever is usually regarded and treated in neutropenic patients as indicating the presence of bacteria in the blood (bacteremia).

Despite the lack of universal agreement, most authorities define significant fever in neutropenic patients as a single oral temperature greater than 38.3° C (101° F) in the absence of a clear cause (e.g., the administration of blood products) or a temperature greater than 38° C (100.4° F) for 1 hour or more. In certain situations the febrile response may be greatly blunted, absent, or less than expected. Steroid therapy is the most common culprit. Nonsteroidal antiinflammatory drugs, old age, renal failure, and overwhelming infection also can blunt the normal fever response. Unfortunately, the absence of fever does *not* mean that the patient does *not* have a potentially serious infection.

8. Are all fevers due to infections?

No. Fevers in patients with cancer are commonly related to drug-induced fevers or to cancer itself (e.g., leukemias, lymphomas, renal cell cancer, liver cancer). A cause for a significant number of fevers is not found; undetermined fevers are termed FUOs (fever of unknown origin) or PUOs (pyrexia of unknown origin).

9. What is drug-induced fever?

Drug-induced fever is caused by the drug itself. Drugs that may induce fevers include antibiotics, antifungals (e.g., amphotericin B), and allopurinol. The usual mechanism is antibody-mediated with either a type II (cytotoxic with a drug such as hapten) or type III (immune complex-mediated) reaction. The diagnosis of drug fever may be relatively easy or obscure and challenging. Clues to the presence of drug-induced fever include the following:

1. Timing of the fever. If the fever occurs with each administration of the drug or after 10–14 days of a treatment course (a typical time frame for the immune system to develop antibodies to

the drug), drug-induced fever is likely. The time to development of drug-induced fever may be accelerated if the patient has received the drug before and already made antibodies.

2. Appearance of the patient. The patient often appears well. The pulse may not be elevated in proportion to the fever. Patients also may appear quite ill with shaking chills, as seen in reactions to quinidine.

3. Rash (not due to infection) and/or other evidence of drug-induced end-organ dysfunction such as interstitial nephritis or hepatitis.

4. No other reason for fever after thorough investigation.

10. What should be done when a neutropenic patient becomes febrile?

After appropriate cultures are obtained, antibiotic therapy should be promptly ordered and administered, ideally within 1 hour of recognizing the fever. The assessment and evaluation should proceed without delay. Obtain cultures of blood, urine (even in patients with no signs or symptoms), throat (in patients with abnormal findings), stool (in patients with diarrhea; order *Clostridium difficile* toxin assay in patients currently or recently on antibiotics), and IV sites (in patients with evidence of inflammation). For new skin findings, consider immediate evaluation with biopsy and culture. A baseline chest radiograph must be obtained in the presence of signs or symptoms attributable to the lungs. A question of sinus disease should prompt an early computed tomography (CT) scan of the sinuses; plain radiographs are often not sensitive enough to pick up early evidence of infection.

Brilliant diagnoses are usually made by ordinary people in a dull and methodical manner. Without neutrophils many of the expected signs and symptoms of inflammation may be minimal or absent. Remember to take the vital signs and look for the early signs and symptoms of serious infection:

- Decrease in mentation
- Decrease in urine output
- Decrease in platelet count
- Increase in glucose
- Increase in heart rate or respiration
- Decrease or increase in temperature

In the physical assessment pay particular attention to the following areas:

1. Skin
   - Check all current and previous IV sites.
   - New rashes—consider drug reaction, blood-borne spread of bacteria or fungi.
   - Perianal pain or inflammation—consider infected hemorrhoids, fissure, phlegmon.
2. Head, ears, eyes, nose, and throat
   - Headache, sinus, or jaw pain—consider sinusitis.
   - Nasal ulcers or mucosal necrosis—consider fungal involvement.
   - Cotton-wool spots in front of retina—consider candidal infection.
   - Oral mucosal white patches that rub off and bleed—consider candidal infection.
   - Oral ulcers—consider herpes, gram-negative bacteria, chemotherapy.
   - Odynophagia (pain when swallowing): with oral ulcers—consider herpes; with thrush—consider candidal esophagitis.
3. Lungs: Findings on exam may be minimal or may precede x-ray abnormalities
4. Abdomen: Rebound tenderness, especially involving the right lower quadrant—consider typhlitis.

11. How many blood cultures? How much blood per culture? How far apart should the blood cultures be done? Should blood cultures be obtained from venous access devices (VADs)?

Two pairs of aerobic and anaerobic blood cultures are usually enough to obtain a positive result. More than two contribute little to the statistical likelihood of a positive culture but may help to make the patient anemic. It is important to obtain the amount of blood required by the hospital laboratory. Many culture systems are optimized for a given amount of blood; indeed, the blood itself may help to provide the nutrients that the bacteria need to grow. Too little blood may decrease the yield from the culture. The interval between cultures need be only as long as it takes to prepare the second site after the first culture is obtained. Delaying therapy so that a second blood culture can be done in 30 or 60 minutes places the patient at needless risk. Whether to draw blood through a VAD is controversial, but it is usually done. The advantage is that a positive culture from the VAD may suggest the catheter as the source of infection. The bad news is that it may be a contaminant from the hardware of the VAD. If the laboratory can do quantitative cultures, comparing the yield from the VAD and from the peripheral culture may suggest whether the VAD was the source. Unfortunately, this service is not available in most microbiology labs.

12. What empirical antibiotics should be prescribed to neutropenic febrile patients?
  In the absence of findings that might direct therapy (e.g., pus from a VAD exit site and a Gram stain showing gram-positive cocci in clusters suggest a *Staphylococcus* species), all broad-spectrum regimens (containing antibiotics effective against the commonly found gram-negative bacteria) appear to work well. Initial clinical responses vary from 60–80%. Varying response rates are explained by differences in study design, patient populations, antibiotic use, and antibiotic susceptibility (according to the institution). Broad-spectrum combination antibiotic regimens may include an extended-spectrum penicillin (e.g., ticarcillin or piperacillin) plus an aminoglycoside (e.g., gentamicin or amikacin) or a third-generation cephalosporin (e.g., ceftazidime).
  The following factors should be considered in choosing an antibiotic regimen:

- Patient drug allergies
- Route of administration
- Concomitant drugs
- Suspected organism
- Antibiotic resistance patterns
- Previous antibiotic therapy
- Previous infecting organisms
- Duration of neutropenia
- Patient exposure to pathogens

Most authorities believe that two antibiotics with activity against *Pseudomonas aeruginosa* should be given initially. Clinical trials and experience also support the use of broad-spectrum monotherapy with agents that have anti-pseudomonal activity (e.g., ceftazidime, imipenem-cilastatin, or a quinolone). Some physicians prefer two antibiotics when the patient has had prolonged, severe neutropenia or shows altered vital signs due to infection. The decision is usually determined by the institution's antibiotic susceptibilities. For example, if a patient is on a medical or surgical ward with infection problems from a resistant *Enterobacter* sp., initial therapy should cover the possibility that the patient may be infected with that organism. Coverage for staphylococci is not initially given unless there is a reason to suspect a source for staphylococci. Other agents may be added as necessary for special circumstances (e.g., to cover anaerobes in the case of suspected typhlitis).

Commonly Used Antibiotics

ANTIBIOTIC CLASS	EXAMPLES	SPECTRUM/ACTIVITY	CAUTIONS
Penicillins	Ticarcillin Piperacillin	Streptococci Gram-negative anaerobes	Allergic reactions Potassium loss (especially with amphotericin B) Rash with allopurinol Drug-induced neutropenia
Carbapenems	Imipenem-cilastatin Meropenem	Gram-negative Gram-positive anaerobes	Fungal superinfection
Cephalosporins	Ceftazidime Cefepime	Streptococci Gram-negative	Allergic reactions Drug-induced neutropenia Enterococcal superinfections
Quinolones	Ciprofloxacin Ofloxacin	Gram-negative *Legionella* sp.	Aluminum, magnesium, iron, zinc, and sucralfate interfere with GI absorption

Table continued on following page.

Commonly Used Antibiotics (Continued)

ANTIBIOTIC CLASS	EXAMPLES	SPECTRUM/ACTIVITY	CAUTIONS
Aminoglycosides	Gentamicin Tobramycin Amikacin	Gram-negative	Avoid with cisplatin Avoid with cyclosporine Ototoxicity Nephrotoxicity Avoid with amphotericin B
Sulfonamides	Sulfamethoxazole (with trimethoprim)	Gram-negative *Pneumocystis* sp.	Allergic reactions Marrow suppression
Vancomycin	Vancomycin Teicoplanin	Gram-positive	Red neck, red man Drug-induced neutropenia
Imidazoles	Ketoconazole Fluconazole Itraconazole	*Candida* sp. *Aspergillus* sp. (itraconazole)	Antacids decrease GI absorption

13. Why is it necessary to review the patient's previous antibiotic regimens?

Prior antibiotics can greatly affect the likely organisms currently infecting a neutropenic patient. If an antibiotic that kills or suppresses one kind of bacteria is given, other bacteria or fungi that are resistant to the antibiotic will try to replace the killed bacteria. In treating a patient with a quinolone antibiotic, beware of anaerobic bacteria and yeast. Vancomycin therapy leaves gram-negative organisms without the usual competition from gram-positive organisms. Broad-spectrum antibiotics permit the fungi a free hand. Even the imidazole class of antifungal agents (ketoconazole, fluconazole, itraconazole) may permit or allow resistant fungi to grow.

14. How long should antibiotics be continued?

In general, antibiotics are continued for the duration of the neutropenia. The following guidelines may help:

1. **No fever and ≥ 500 neutrophils**
   - No source of infection—stop antibiotics.
   - Known source of infection—give course appropriate for source.
2. **No fever and < 500 neutrophils**—continue antibiotics for up to 14 days.
3. **Fever and ≥ 500 neutrophils**—consider changing or stopping therapy after evaluation for:
   - Hidden site of infection
   - Abscess, catheter-related
   - Resistant bacteria, fungi, virus
   - Drug fever
   - Tumor fever
4. **Fever and < 500 neutrophils**—continue antibiotics and consider:
   - Fungal superinfection
   - Inadequate antibiotic dosing
   - Resistant bacteria
   - Viral infection
   - Abscess or catheter-related infection

The suggested duration for antibiotic therapy depends on many variables. A case in point is the recent report from Chile of children with a variety of cancers treated with chemotherapeutic agents. Neutropenic patients with new fever were assessed with C-reactive protein determinations on day 1 and day 2. If the C-reactive proteins were normal (suggesting a nonbacterial cause of fever) and cultures were negative, antibiotics were stopped on day 3 with good outcomes, whether or not the patient was afebrile.

15. What is antibiotic lock therapy?

Antibiotic lock therapy is a relatively new approach to the management of an infected catheter line. A small volume of a concentrated antibiotic solution is placed in the lumen of the catheter and allowed to remain for hours. The approach is said to work poorly for candidal infections.

Another exciting approach intended to prevent infection in indwelling lines is to impregnate the lines with a combination of (1) silver and chlorhexidine, (2) tetracycline and rifampin, or (3) tetracycline and ethylenediamine tetraacetic acid (EDTA).

16. What about colony-stimulating factors?

Colony-stimulating factors are glycopeptides that stimulate the bone marrow to speed the production and maturation of neutrophils. Granulocyte colony-stimulating factor (G-CSF) and granulocyte/macrophage colony-stimulating factor (GM-CSF) have been shown to shorten the duration of chemotherapy-induced neutropenia and may enhance the function of neutrophils. They are expensive and may cause symptoms such as myalgias. The cost-benefit ratio works best for patients with an expected prolonged duration of neutropenia (> 7–10 days), in whom the risk of infection with agents such as *Aspergillus* spp. is high. G-CSF is started after chemotherapy and continued until the neutrophil count recovers.

17. Amphotericin B has a bad reputation for side effects during administration and for causing problems with kidney and bone marrow function. Is the reputation deserved? If so, what can be done to lessen the problems?

Considerable folklore has arisen around the administration of amphotericin B ("ampho-terrible"). Signs and symptoms commonly seen include chills and fever, phlebitis, and nausea and vomiting. Renal problems include tubular dysfunction, which leads to loss of electrolytes (particularly potassium and bicarbonate), and suppression of erythropoietin production. Common myths include the following:

1. Heparin in the amphotericin B solution decreases the risk of phlebitis.

Fact: Heparin is unproven to prevent phlebitis. It is not needed when amphotericin B is given through a central line. Indeed, the use of heparin even in small amounts may lead to immune-mediated platelet destruction.

2. A test dose of amphotericin B is required to avoid anaphylaxis.

Fact: The test dose came about as a result of side effects seen with the administration of the early, relatively impure preparations of amphotericin B. In patients who have never received amphotericin B before, the test dose may be safely omitted.

3. Steroids should be added to the amphotericin B infusion to decrease the occurrence of febrile reactions.

Fact: Although steroids are often used, there is little scientific evidence of their efficacy. Some authorities argue against the routine use of steroids because of the theoretical concern of increasing the patient's immune suppression. If steroids are used, they should be the shortest-lived preparations available (e.g., hydrocortisone succinate). Methylprednisolone should *not* be used.

4. Amphotericin B is better tolerated if the infusion is given over at least 4–6 hours.

Fact: Although bolus therapy is dangerous, amphotericin B is tolerated by most patients when given over 1–2 hours.

18. What should be done to assist in the administration of amphotericin B?

- Individualize the symptomatic medications to the patient's needs.
- Reassure the patient that tolerance increases with time.
- Use meperidine, 25–50 mg intravenously, to terminate chills and fever. Rare intractable chills and fever may be treated with dantrolene.
- To help avoid renal toxicity, maintain an adequate volume status. Saline boluses given with the infusions are often used for this purpose.
- Consider using the newer preparations of amphotericin B. Lipid-complexed and liposomal preparations *may* be better tolerated and have less renal and bone marrow toxicity; thus, larger doses may be given.

19. A patient who is receiving vancomycin and experiences flushing, wheezing, and hypotension is most likely allergic to vancomycin. True or false?

False. The so-called red neck or red man syndrome (from the flushed appearance of the face, neck, and upper torso) is not, strictly speaking, an allergy. Classic allergic reactions are defined by the presence of an antibody that reacts with the patient's immune system to produce the allergic response. Vancomycin interacts with mast cells (no antibody role) and directly causes release of histamine. The histamine causes the vasodilation, flushing, and wheezing. As histamine release from mast cells is also important in anaphylactic reactions (an IgE-mediated mast cell degranulation), it is not difficult to understand how the patient may appear clinically to have an allergic reaction. The patient is *not* allergic to vancomycin in this setting.

Tolerance to vancomycin infusions tends to improve with time. Do not infuse the drug rapidly; infusion over 60–90 minutes is recommended.

20. What is typhlitis?

Typhlitis or neutropenic enterocolitis is a necrotizing infection of the bowel secondary to a combination of factors causing mucosal damage and allowing bacterial invasion. The infection, usually involving the large bowel (especially the cecum), results in bowel wall edema, thinning, and perforation. Patients may present with symptoms suggestive of appendicitis, such as abdominal pain, nausea and vomiting, and fever. The condition is particularly common in children. Blood cultures may be positive despite the fact that the patient is receiving effective antibiotic therapy. The diagnosis may be made by CT scan, which shows a thickened bowel wall, in the proper clinical setting. Peritoneal lavage with a positive culture for the same organisms found in the blood cultures is confirmatory. Medical therapy includes antibiotics to cover the gram-negative organisms, *Candida* spp., and anaerobic organisms. Laxatives and enemas should be avoided. Surgical intervention may be indicated. Unfortunately, surgery is usually a difficult undertaking because patients are critically ill and poor surgical risks.

21. What is ecthyma gangrenosum?

Ecthyma gangrenosum is a skin manifestation of the vascular spread of bacteria, usually gram-negative bacteria. *Pseudomonas aeruginosa* is the most commonly involved organism. Other responsible organisms include staphylococci and fungi such as *Aspergillus* spp. and *Alternaria* sp. Blood cultures are often positive for the causative bacteria. The lesions begin as nodular papules that quickly progress to central blebs, then ulcerate with underlying induration and central necrosis. The lesions are usually erythematous, often with a violaceous hue; not unlike petechiae, they may be somewhat hidden in the skin folds, buttocks, and perineum.

22. What is bacterial translocation?

Bacterial translocation is the movement of living bacteria from the gastrointestinal tract to the mesenteric lymph nodes and blood stream and thus to other organs. Every moment of our lives, the bowel flora are prevented from translocating or quickly cleared when they try to move across the bowel wall. In the presence of neutropenia and other immunosuppression, life-threatening infections may result from mucosal disruption of the bowel wall caused by chemotherapy, invading organisms, or antibiotic suppression of normal bowel anaerobic bacteria (the predominant normal bowel flora that help to prevent translocation). Gram-negative organisms most likely to translocate include *E. coli*, *Klebsiella* species, and *Pseudomonas aeruginosa*. Nutritional counseling may be important. Many authorities believe that fiber ingestion assists in mucosal preservation, thus decreasing the rate at which bacterial translocation occurs.

23. What is low-risk neutropenia?

Low-risk neutropenia is a relative term used to describe neutrophil counts < 500/mm^3 but > 100/mm^3, with an expected neutropenia duration of < 7–10 days. Low-risk neutropenia is often seen during chemotherapy for solid tumors, whereas neutropenia after therapy for leukemias or bone marrow transplant is usually more severe. Patients with low-risk neutropenia usually respond well to initial antibiotic therapy.

Some centers have begun the practice of outpatient therapy for low-risk neutropenia after an initial inpatient treatment with good response. Outpatient management should be done only by clinicians experienced in the management of neutropenic fevers. Candidates for outpatient therapy should have no comorbid conditions (e.g., no heart or kidney failure), responsive tumor, good outpatient support systems, and easy access for follow-up and readmission.

24. What are the indications to remove an infected VAD?

- No response to appropriate antibiotic therapy
- Persistent positive blood cultures
- Deteriorating status
- Line malfunction

25. What strategies are used to guide therapy for infected VADs?

Therapy is guided by the infecting organism and location of infection:

1. *Staphylococcus epidermidis*
   - Exit site—medical therapy.
   - Tunnel infection—consider removal.
   - Port—remove Huber needle and give antibiotic at remote IV site.
2. *Staphylococcus aureus*
   - Exit site—medical therapy.
   - Line or tunnel—remove line.
   - Port—consider removal.
3. *Candida* species
   - Exit site—remove line.
   - Tunnel infection—remove line.
   - Port—remove line.
4. Gram-negative organisms
   - Exit site—try medical therapy.
   - Line—remove line.
   - Tunnel—50% failure rate with medical therapy.

Still another factor to consider is the type of VAD. A recent report suggested that in hemodialysis catheters gram-negative infections were salvaged better by antibiotics alone than were gram-positive infections.

26. Why should a dental consultation be performed prior to chemotherapy?

Before administering myelosuppressive chemotherapy, it is good practice to take care of sites that are actively infected and to consider preventive care for potential sources of infection. A minor dental problem in a normal host may become a life-threatening source of infection in a neutropenic patient.

27. Does it matter what type of dressing is placed on the exit site of a central VAD?

After reviewing the data from clinical trials, noting the good results from institutions with catheter care teams, and discussing the advantages and disadvantages of various dressings with nurses and physicians, my recommendation is to pay meticulous attention to institutional protocol in caring for central VAD exit sites. The kind of dressing is not as important as the attention given by the provider and patient to the care of the line. A reasonable strategy is to use a gauze dressing immediately after line placement and while drainage continues. After the site is healed or drainage has stopped, a transparent, semipermeable occlusive dressing may be used alone or with gauze. It is also appropriate to use no dressing for tunneled catheters.

DISCLAIMER

The views and opinions in this chapter are solely the author's and do not reflect the views or the policies of Evans Army Community Hospital, the Department of Defense, or the United States government.

BIBLIOGRAPHY

1. Chanock SJ, Pizzo PA: Fever in the neutropenic patient. Infect Dis Clin North Am 10:777–796, 1996.
2. Giamarellou H: Empiric therapy for infections in the febrile, neutropenic, compromised host. Med Clin North Am 79:559–580, 1995.
3. Hathorn JW, Lyke K: Empirical treatment of febrile neutropenia: Evolution of current therapeutic approaches. Clin Infect Dis 24(Suppl 2):S256–S265, 1997.
4. Hoeprich PD: Clinical use of amphotericin B and derivatives: Lore, mystique, and fact. Clin Infect Dis 14(Suppl 1):S114–S119, 1992.
5. Hughes WT, Armstrong D, Bodey GP, et al: Guidelines for the use of antimicrobial agents in neutropenic patients with unexplained fever. J Infect Dis 161:381–396, 1990.
6. Malik IA, Khan WA, Karim M, et al: Feasibility of outpatient management of fever in cancer patients with low-risk neutropenia: Results of a prospective randomized trial [see comments]. Am J Med 98:224–231, 1995.
7. Schimpff SC, Scott DA, Wade JC: Infections in cancer patients: Some controversial issues [see comments]. Support Care Cancer 2:94–104, 1994.

18. POSTTRANSPLANT INFECTIONS

Kimberly A. Gerstadt, M.D., and Marie J. George, M.D.

1. What type of immunodeficiencies occur in bone marrow transplant (BMT) recipients? What are the most prevalent associated infections?

The time at risk for infection in bone marrow transplant recipients can be roughly divided into three phases:

1. During the first 30 days after transplant, recipients follow a bone marrow eradicating regimen of irradiation and chemotherapy. Immunosuppressive medication such as cyclosporine is also used. Profound, prolonged neutropenia is present with the possibility of gram-negative and gram-positive infections. Antibiotic treatment promotes *Candida* spp. as pathogens. A striking concern is the risk for herpes simplex virus (HSV) in patients already seropositive for herpes virus before transplant.

2. After this 30-day period the initial engraftment of the transplanted marrow begins. Cytomegalovirus (CMV) replaces HSV as the major viral concern, with the potential for severe involvement of multiple organ systems. *Aspergillus* spp. replace *Candida* spp. as major fungal pathogens.

3. After 90–100 days, the bone marrow engraftment is completed. Unfortunately, the immune system does not completely recover for up to 1–2 years. The recipient remains at increased risk for infections with organisms that affect patients with poor immunoglobulin function, particularly the pneumococci. Varicella zoster virus (VZV) replaces CMV as the principal viral pathogen. Another major problem is graft vs. host disease, which may begin during the time of bone marrow engraftment. Graft vs. host disease may require immunosuppressive therapy, further increasing the risk of infection.

Bone Marrow Transplant-associated Infections

IMMUNODEFICIENCY	TIME POST-TRANSPLANT	TYPE OF INFECTION
Mucositis (oral, GI)	1–3 wk	Bacterial, HSV
Granulocytopenia	0–4 wk	Bacterial, *Candida* spp., *Aspergillus* spp.
T-cell deficiencies	1–3 mo*	EBV, respiratory viruses, CMV, HSV, PCP, *Aspergillus* spp., other fungi
Humoral	4–8 mo*	Encapsulated bacteria, PCP, VZV, *Staphylococcus* spp., *Aspergillus* spp.

* Time extended with graft vs. host disease.
HSV = herpes simplex virus; EBV = Epstein-Barr virus; respiratory viruses = adenovirus, respiratory syncytial virus, rhinovirus, influenza, parainfluenza; CMV = cytomegalovirus; PCP = *Pneumocystis carinii* pneumonia; VZV = varicella zoster virus.

2. What are the common causes of bacteremia after BMT?

Bacteremias account for one-third of all infections in the early posttransplant period. Gram-positive cocci, especially *Staphylococcus aureus* and coagulase-negative staphylococci, are the most common isolates. Indwelling intravascular catheters, mucositis, and use of prophylactic antibiotics such as the quinolones have been associated with a rise in the number of gram-positive infections. More recently, other gram-positive organisms such as viridans streptococci, *Enterococcus* spp., and *Streptococcus pneumoniae* have become important causes of bacteremias. Gram-negative organisms such as *Escherichia coli* and *Klebsiella* spp. are isolated in 30–40% of posttransplant bacteremias.

3. List the risk factors for invasive fungal infection after BMT.

- Duration and intensity of neutropenia (absolute neutrophil count < 500 cells/mm^3)
- Broad-spectrum antimicrobial agents
- Corticosteroids
- Acute leukemia in relapse
- Acute and chronic graft vs. host disease
- Older age
- Donor-recipient mismatch
- Cytotoxic chemotherapy
- Indwelling central venous catheter

4. Which findings on physical exam suggest fungemia in BMT recipients?

Fungemia may be difficult to diagnose by physical exam, but certain findings strongly suggest the diagnosis. The recognition of these findings is extremely important because blood cultures may be persistently negative. Careful physical exam may reveal pathognomonic fluffy retinal exudates or single or grouped macronodular skin lesions.

5. Which organisms cause fungemia in BMT recipients? How is it treated?

Historically, *Candida albicans* caused most infections. More recently, other *Candida* species, such as *C. lusitaniae*, *C. glabrata*, *C. krusei*, and *C. parapsilosis*, have increased in incidence after BMT. Mucositis, which may involve the entire gastrointestinal tract, and indwelling intravascular catheters are the usual sources of fungemia. Removal of the catheter alone is not adequate treatment. Systemic antifungal therapy for presumed deep-seated infection must be instituted.

6. What is chronic hematogenously disseminated candidiasis in BMT recipients?

It is a chronic infection of the liver, kidney, spleen, lungs, and eye that usually is recognized as neutrophil counts begin to recover. Suspect this type of infection when fever persists despite broad-spectrum antibiotics and adequate circulating neutrophils. About 40–60% of patients may have negative blood cultures. CT scan of the abdomen shows diffuse small abscesses in affected organs.

7. What is the most common site for *Aspergillus* infection in BMT recipients?

BMT recipients acquire pulmonary aspergillosis via exogenous airborne exposure. Neutropenia is the most important risk factor. A nodular cavitary lesion on chest radiograph or a zone of low attenuation around a mass (halo sign) on chest CT suggests *Aspergillus* involvement. Diagnosis usually requires tissue biopsy because blood cultures are routinely negative. Aspergillosis also may present as invasive sinusitis or central nervous system abscesses or infarction.

8. How may HSV present in BMT recipients?

HSV may cause limited or disseminated skin infections, oral herpes, genital herpes, esophagitis, keratitis, pneumonia, hepatitis, or encephalitis. Such infections are most likely due to reactivation of latent HSV. All herpesviruses lie dormant after initial infection and may cause recurrent disease at times of cellular immunodeficiency.

9. When does CMV infection occur after BMT? What are the manifestations?

Without prophylaxis, CMV infections usually occur between 30 and 100 days after transplant. Interstitial pneumonitis is the most common manifestation and is associated with high morbidity and mortality rates. Gastroenteritis, retinitis, and CMV syndrome, manifested as fever, fatigue, hepatitis, and leukopenia, also occur.

10. Is the BMT recipient still immunosuppressed after engraftment?

Cell-mediated immunity, humoral immunity, and phagocytic defenses may remain suppressed for months after engraftment. These defects include decreased number and function of natural killer cells, T cells, CD4 cells, and CD8 cells; decreased levels of IgG and IgM; and decreased chemotaxis.

11. What are the drug interactions between antimicrobial agents and commonly used immunosuppressants?

Cyclosporine and tacrolimus (FK506) are metabolized by cytochrome P450 in the liver. Antimicrobials that induce or inhibit cytochrome P450 affect the metabolism of these immunosuppressants. Rifampin and rifabutin upregulate cytochrome P450, increasing cyclosporine metabolism and resulting in low serum levels. Erythromycin, azithromycin, clarithromycin, ketoconazole, itraconazole, and fluconazole downregulate cytochrome P450, decreasing cyclosporine metabolism and resulting in high serum levels. In addition, cyclosporine may potentiate aminoglycoside nephrotoxicity.

12. Name the major community-acquired infections that can reactivate after transplant to cause significant disease in solid organ recipients.

- *Mycobacterium tuberculosis*
- Hepatitis B and C
- *Strongyloides stercoralis*
- Human immunodeficiency virus (HIV)
- CMV
- EBV
- Blastomycosis
- Histoplasmosis
- Coccidioidomycosis
- HSV
- VZV

13. What type of infections occur in the first month after solid organ transplant?

Most infections are bacterial, such as pneumonia, line-related bloodstream infections, wound infections, and infections related to technical problems (e.g., infection of a vascular suture line causing rupture). Liver and lung transplants carry the highest incidence of technical problems. In most cases, patients have not taken immunosuppressive agents long enough to allow opportunistic infections.

14. What type of infections occur 2–6 months after solid organ transplant?

1. **Viruses.** Newly acquired or reactivated CMV is the single most important cause of morbidity and mortality in solid organ recipients. Patients are also at risk for EBV and recurrent hepatitis B and C.

2. **Opportunistic infections**, such as PCP, *Listeria* sp., and *Aspergillus* spp.

15. What type of infections occur more than 6 months after solid organ transplant?

Most patients (70–80%) have good allograft function and are on maintenance doses of immunosuppressants. They remain at risk for the usual community-acquired infections such as urinary tract infection, influenza, respiratory syncytial virus, and pneumococcal pneumonia. Ten percent of patients have chronic viral infection such as hepatitis B or C (after liver transplant), CMV chorioretinitis, or EBV-induced lymphoproliferative disorders. Another 10% have chronic rejection and therefore require higher than normal doses of immunosuppressive drugs for longer periods. This leaves them at risk for opportunistic infections, especially PCP, cryptococcosis, listeriosis, and nocardiosis.

16. Which solid organ transplant recipients have the highest rates of infection?

Heart-lung recipients have the largest number of episodes per patient (3.19) and the largest number of deaths from infection (45%). The most common infection is bacterial pneumonia. Patients also have high rates of mediastinitis, invasive fungal infections, PCP, and cytomegalovirus pneumonia. The reason for the increased rate of infection is multifactorial: immunosuppression, allograft reactions, anastomotic leak, rejection, and ablation of the cough reflex below the tracheal anastomosis.

17. What are the three patterns of CMV transmission in recipients of solid organ transplants?

1. **Primary CMV infection** occurs when a CMV-negative patient receives a CMV-positive organ. Rarely (< 10% of cases) infection occurs via CMV-infected leukocytes in blood transfusions.

2. **Reactivation CMV infection** occurs when a CMV-positive patient reactivates latent virus. Patients receiving antilymphocyte antibody therapy (OKT3) for treatment of rejection are more likely to become ill.

3. **Superinfection with CMV** occurs in CMV-positive patients who receive CMV-positive organs. The virus causing infection can be shown by DNA restriction enzyme analysis to be of donor origin.

18. Which organ is most at risk for CMV disease in solid organ recipients?

The transplanted organ is far more vulnerable to infection than native organs. CMV hepatitis is an important problem in liver transplants, CMV myocarditis in heart transplants, and CMV pancreatitis in pancreas transplants. The reason is not completely clear. One theory is that cytotoxic T cells are unable to eliminate HLA complex-mismatched cells infected with CMV in the allograft.

19. What other complications may occur in solid organ recipients after they become infected with CMV?

CMV pneumonitis causes macrophage dysfunction, leading to opportunistic superinfection with *Pneumocystis carinii* and *Aspergillus fumigatus*. CMV also facilitates the colonization of the upper respiratory tract with gram-negative bacilli, increasing the risk of gram-negative pneumonia. Patients with severe CMV disease are at risk for sepsis with *Listeria monocytogenes*, *Candida* spp., and gram-negative bacteria.

CONTROVERSIES

20. Does CMV cause allograft injury in solid organ recipients?

For: Some believe that CMV may cause a specific glomerular lesion in kidney transplants, specific hepatic lesions and the vanishing bile duct syndrome in liver transplants, accelerated coronary atherosclerosis in heart transplants, and bronchiolitis obliterans in lung transplants.

Against: Although CMV infection and the organ-specific lesions listed above may occur at the same time, a causal relationship has not been established. These lesions are also found in patients without viral infection.

21. Should antimicrobial agents be used for prophylaxis in BMT patients?

For: Antibiotics such as the quinolones reduce the incidence of serious gram-negative bacteremia.

Against: Prophylactic antibiotics are associated with an increase in infections due to resistant organisms. For example, quinolones used for bacterial prophylaxis are associated with increased incidence of streptococcal and staphylococcal infection in some transplant centers.

BIBLIOGRAPHY

1. Bennett JV, Brachman PS (eds): Hospital Infections, 4th ed. Philadelphia, Lippincott-Raven, 1998.
2. Kucers A, Croew SM, Grayson ML, Hoy JF: The Use of Antibiotics. A Clinical Review of Antibacterial, Antifungal, and Antiviral Drugs, 5th ed. Oxford, Butterworth-Heinemann, 1997.
3. Mandell GL, Bennett JE, Dolin R (eds): Principles and Practice of Infectious Disease, 4th ed. New York, Churchill Livingstone, 1995.
4. Mormin F, Chandrasekar PH: Antimicrobial prophylaxis in bone marrow transplantation. Ann Intern Med 123:205–215, 1995.
5. Rubin R, Moellering RC (eds): Infection in Transplantation. Philadelphia, W.B. Saunders, 1995.
6. Sable CA, Donowitz GR: Infections in bone marrow transplant recipients. Clin Infect Dis 18:273–281, 1994.

IV. Antibiotics

19. CHOICE OF ANTIBIOTICS FOR PROPHYLAXIS AND THERAPY

Mark R. Wallace, MD

1. Empiric treatment of dog, cat, and human bites should be directed against which pathogens?
- Staphylococci (dogs, cats, humans)
- Streptococci (dogs, cats, humans)
- *Pasteurella multocida* (dogs and cats)
- Anaerobes (dogs, cats, humans)
- *Capnocytophaga canimorsus* (dogs)
- *Eikenella corrodens* (humans)

2. Antimicrobial prophylaxis of significant dog, cat, and human bites should be initiated as soon as possible after the injury is identified. Which oral antibiotic regimens offer broad coverage of the likely pathogens?
- Amoxicillin-clavulanate (preferred)
- Penicillin plus dicloxacillin or an oral first-generation cephalosporin
- An oral quinolone plus clindamycin

3. A patient is admitted to the ICU with fulminant bilateral pneumonia. You include legionnaires' disease in the differential diagnosis and want to provide coverage for this possibility until diagnostic studies are complete. List three appropriate antibiotic regimens.
- Macrolides (erythromycin, azithromycin, clarithromycin)
- Quinolones (ofloxacin, ciprofloxacin, levofloxacin)
- Tetracyclines
- Rifampin may reasonably be combined with any of the above regimens, but rifampin cannot be used alone because of the rapid development of resistance.

4. Treatment of necrotizing streptococcal soft tissue infections ("flesh-eaters") involves which agents and modalities?

1. Aggressive surgical intervention (debridement, fasciotomy, amputation if needed) must be performed immediately upon suspicion of the diagnosis.

2. An intravenous beta-lactam agent effective against group A beta-hemolytic streptococci (a penicillin or cephalosporin) *plus* clindamycin should be started as soon as blood and wound cultures have been obtained. Clindamycin is needed to compensate for a possible lack of beta-lactam activity in high inoculum streptococcal infections ("Eagle effect") and to limit exotoxin production.

3. Intravenous immunoglobulin also may be used, but it is controversial.

5. Slow-growing, fastidious gram-negative bacteria of the HACEK group cause about 5–10% of all native valve endocarditis. Name the HACEK organisms. What is the antibiotic of choice for treatment of infections?

H = *Haemophilus aphrophilus* and *H. parainfluenzae*
A = *Actinobacillus actinomycetemcomitans*
C = *Cardiobacterium hominis*
E = *Eikenella corrodens*
K = *Kingella kingae*
Ceftriaxone (or another parenteral third-generation cephalosporin) is the preferred therapy.

6. Multiple reasonable oral antibiotic regimens can be used for outpatient therapy of sinusitis. List common oral antibiotic approaches and the benefits and drawbacks of each.

- Amoxicillin: inexpensive and usually effective, but not active against beta-lactamase-producing *Haemophilus influenzae, Moraxella catarrhalis*, and anaerobes.
- Amoxicillin–clavulanate: covers common bacterial pathogens, but diarrhea can be problematic; more expensive than amoxicillin.
- Second-generation oral cephalosporins (cefuroxime axetil, cefprozil): good coverage but also more expensive than amoxicillin.
- Azithromycin and clarithromycin: dosing regimens promote compliance, but not dependable against anaerobes or resistant pneumococci.
- Some highly penicillin-resistant pneumococci (MIC > 2.0) may not respond to any of the above agents and may require vancomycin therapy for a severe, refractory infection.

7. Which antibiotics may induce hemolytic anemia in G6PD-deficient people?

Nalidixic acid, nitrofurantoin, primaquine, sulfamethoxazole (although trimethoprim is safe), and dapsone.

8. Describe the appropriate empiric antibiotic coverage for acute bacterial meningitis in adults.

A third-generation cephalosporin (cefotaxime or ceftriaxone) provides coverage for cephalosporin-sensitive *Streptococcus pneumoniae* as well as all *Neisseria meningitidis* and *H. influenzae*. Vancomycin should be added to provide coverage for possible cephalosporin-resistant pneumococci until cultures yield a susceptible organism or are negative at least 2–3 days. Ampicillin should be added as a third empiric drug to cover *Listeria monocytogenes* in patients over 50 years old and immunocompromised hosts. Ceftazidime is not an acceptable substitution for the other third-generation cephalosporins because of its relatively poor activity against *S. pneumoniae*.

9. *Clostridium difficile* is an emerging nosocomial pathogen. Which oral agent is preferred for initial therapy? Why?

Metronidazole and vancomycin are the traditional oral drugs of choice. There is no reliable intravenous therapy. Although both oral agents are comparable in response rates, relapses, and toxicity, metronidazole is favored because of its lower cost and the tendency of oral vancomycin to select for vancomycin-resistant enterococci (VRE).

10. Pelvic inflammatory disease (PID) is usually treated according to guidelines published by the CDC. This is done because cultures are usually not obtained and therapy is (of necessity) empiric. All PID regimens must provide coverage for which four pathogens?

Neisseria gonorrhoeae, Chlamydia trachomatis, aerobic gram-negative rods, and anaerobes.

11. List the likely organisms involved in diabetic foot infections. What are the best oral and intravenous antibiotic approaches?

Organisms

Aerobic gram-negative bacteria (enterics and *Pseudomonas aeruginosa*)

Anaerobes

Staphylococcus aureus

Most diabetic foot infections are polymicrobial

Antibiotic regimens

Intravenous beta-lactam/beta-lactamase inhibitor combination drugs (ticarcillin-clavulanate, piperacillin-tazobactam, ampicillin-sulbactam)

Intravenous second-generation cephalosporins with anaerobic activity (cefotetan or cefoxitin)

An oral fluoroquinolone plus either clindamycin or amoxicillin-clavulanate

12. What is the optimal duration of therapy for uncomplicated cystitis in a nonpregnant young woman? Which agents are preferred?

Three-day therapy with either trimethoprim-sulfamethoxazole or a quinolone has a cure rate of about 95%. Single-dose regimens have an unacceptably high rate of failure and relapse, whereas longer (7–14 days) regimens increase toxicity and cost without a corresponding increase in efficacy.

13. Name the common bacterial causes of febrile, invasive diarrhea. Which antibiotic agents are most dependably effective against these organisms?

- *Shigella* spp.
- *Campylobacter jejuni*
- *Salmonella* spp.
- *Yersinia enterocolitis*

Quinolones are the most effective agents currently available, but resistance is emerging, especially among *C. jejuni* isolates.

14. In a patient with a history of bacterial endocarditis, which of the following procedures carry a significant risk of bacteremia and require antibiotic prophylaxis?

- Teeth cleaning (scaling)
- Sclerotherapy for esophageal varices
- Dental fillings above the gumline
- Gastrointestinal surgery
- Urinary tract and/or prostate surgery
- Bronchoscopy (flexible)

Answer: All but fillings above the gumline and flexible bronchoscopy require prophylaxis.

15. List appropriate empiric antibiotic regimens for the treatment of febrile neutropenic patients.

1. An antipseudomonal beta-lactam agent (ceftazidime, piperacillin, or ticarcillin) plus an aminoglycoside with or without vancomycin

2. A carbapenem (imipenem or meropenem) plus an aminoglycoside with or without vancomycin

3. Vancomycin should be considered in febrile neutropenics when an indwelling intravascular device is present and when penicillin-resistant streptococci and methicillin-resistant *S. aureus* are possible pathogens.

4. Imipenem or ceftazidime monotherapy has been advocated by some authorities but should be avoided in severely ill patients and patients with an absolute neutrophil count (ANC) < 100.

CONTROVERSIES

16. Should fluoroquinolone antibiotics be used as prophylaxis for bacterial infections in neutropenic patients?

For: Multiple studies have shown a reduction in gram-negative bacteremias in neutropenic patients receiving quinolone prophylaxis.

Against: No major study has demonstrated a favorable effect on outcome. The use of quinolone prophylaxis adds both expense and potential toxicities to the management of neutropenic patients.

17. Should sputum Gram stains be used to guide therapy in acute pneumonia?

For: If a sputum Gram stain has more polymorphonuclear neutrophils (PMNs) than epithelial cells and a predominant organism is noted, antibiotic therapy can be narrowly targeted at the probable pathogen.

Against: Many patients with pneumonia have a nonproductive cough or produce poor quality sputum. Sputum Gram stains are occasionally falsely positive, demonstrating a predominant organism, while simultaneous cultures of a sterile site (blood of pleural fluid) later yield the (unsuspected) causative agent.

18. Prophylactic fluconazole in patients receiving intensive chemotherapy—useful or not?

For: 5–20% of intensive chemotherapy courses are complicated by fungal infections. Antifungal prophylaxis with fluconazole has been shown to reduce morbidity and mortality due to fungal infections after bone marrow transplantation.

Against: Antifungal prophylaxis with fluconazole has not been shown to favorably affect *overall* mortality or prognosis in patients undergoing bone marrow transplantation or any intensive chemotherapy. It offers no protection against molds (such as *Aspergillus*) and may select for resistant *Candida* species.

19. How long should antibiotic prophylaxis be continued after cardiac surgery?

Single doses of an antistaphylococcal antibiotic (perhaps repeated once during a long case) are adequate, but many surgeons administer antibiotics for 2–5 days. No data support this approach.

20. Should a CT scan be performed before a lumbar puncture in the evaluation of possible bacterial meningitis in an immunocompetent patient with a nonfocal neurologic examination?

For: Intracranial mass lesions can exist in patients without focal findings or papilledema. Empiric antibiotics can be given without affecting cerebrospinal fluid culture results for 1 hour or more. This time can be used to evaluate the patient with a noncontrast CT scan of the head before lumbar puncture, eliminating any risk of herniation from an unsuspected mass lesion.

Against: In normal hosts presenting with the clinical picture of meningitis and a nonfocal neurologic examination, the risk of herniation is extremely remote. The CT scan adds considerable cost, delays the lumbar puncture, and rarely contributes any relevant information.

ACKNOWLEDGMENT

The Chief, Bureau of Medicine and Surgery, Navy Department, Washington, DC, Clinical Investigation Program, sponsored this report, no. 84-16-1968-646, as required by HSETCINST 6000.41A. The views expressed in this article are those of the author and do not reflect the official policy or position of the Department of the Navy, Department of Defense, or the United States Government.

BIBLIOGRAPHY

1. Beutler E: Glucose-6-phosphate dehydrogenase deficiency. N Engl J Med 324:169–174, 1991.
2. Bow EJ, Mandell LA, Louie TJ, et al: Quinolone-based antibacterial chemoprophylaxis in neutropenic patients: Effect of augmented gram-positive activity on infectious morbidity. Ann Intern Med 125: 183–190, 1996.
3. Cruciani M, Rampazzo R, Malena M, et al: Prophylaxis with fluoroquinolones for bacterial infections in neutropenic patients: A meta-analysis. Clin Infect Dis 23:795–805, 1996.
4. Durack DT: Prevention of infective endocarditis. N Engl J Med 332:38–44, 1995.
5. Edelstein PH: Antimicrobial chemotherapy for legionnaires' disease: A review. Clin Infect Dis 21(Suppl 3): S265–S276, 1995.
6. Evans RS, Pestotnik SL, Classen DC, et al: A computer-assisted management program for antibiotics and other antiinfective agents. N Engl J Med 338:232–238, 1998.
7. Gold HS, Moellering RC: Antimicrobial-drug resistance. N Engl J Med 335:1445–1454, 1996.
8. Goldstein EJ: Bite wounds and infection. Clin Infect Dis 14:633–640, 1992.
9. Gwaltney JM: Acute community-acquired sinusitis. Clin Infect Dis 23:1209–1225, 1996.
10. Haas DW, McAndrew MP: Bacterial osteomyelitis in adults: Evolving considerations in diagnosis and treatment. Am J Med 101:550–561, 1996.
11. McCormack WM: Pelvic inflammatory disease. N Engl J Med 330:115–120, 1994.
12. Schaffher A, Schafflier M: Effect of prophylactic fluconazole on the frequency of fungal infections, amphotericin B use, and health care costs in patients undergoing intensive chemotherapy for hematologic neoplasias. J Infect Dis 172:1035–1041, 1995.
13. Stamm WE, Hooton TM: Management of urinary tract infections in adults. N Engl J Med 329: 1328–1334, 1993.
14. Stevens DL: Invasive group A streptococcus infections. Clin Infect Dis 14:2–13, 1992.
15. Talan DA: Infectious disease issues in the emergency department. Clin Infect Dis 23:1–14, 1996.
16. Quagliarello VJ, Scheld WM: Treatment of bacterial meningitis. N Engl J Med 336:708–716, 1997.
17. Wenisch C, Parschalk B, Hasenhundl M, Hirschl AM: Comparison of vancomycin, teicoplanin, metronidazole, and fusidic acid for the treatment of *Clostridium difficile*-associated diarrhea. Clin Infect Dis 22:813–818, 1996.
18. Wilson WR, Karchiner AW, Dajani AS, et al: Antibiotic treatment of adults with infective endocarditis due to streptococci, enterococci, staphylococci, and HACEK microorganisms. JAMA 274:1706–713, 1995.

20. ANTIINFECTIVE THERAPY

P. Samuel Pegram, M.D., and Colin McDougall, M.D.

ANTIBACTERIAL AGENTS

1. How do antibiotics kill or inhibit microorganisms?

1. **Inhibition or disruption of cell wall growth** (beta-lactams, vancomycin, bacitracin).

2. **Inhibition of protein synthesis.** Erythromycin/macrolides, clindamycin, and chloramphenicol bind to the 50S ribosomal subunit; aminoglycosides and tetracyclines, to the 30S subunit.

3. **Interference with DNA or RNA synthesis.** Quinolones interfere with DNA gyrase; rifamycins inhibit DNA-dependent RNA polymerase; and trimethoprim/sulfamethoxazole sequentially blocks the formation of tetrahydrofolic acid needed for nucleic acid synthesis.

4. **Inhibition of cell membrane function** (mostly antifungal agents such as amphotericin B, azoles, nystatin).

2. Which antibiotics are bactericidal? Which are bacteriostatic?

Bactericidal	**Bacteriostatic**
Beta-lactams (e.g., penicillins, cephalosporins, carbapenems, monobactams)	Tetracyclines
	Erythromycin/macrolides
Aminoglycosides	Chloramphenicol
Quinolones	Clindamycin
Glycopeptides (vancomycin, teicoplanin)	Sulfonamides
Rifamycins (rifampin)	
Metronidazole	

This list is highly generalized; several agents are bactericidal against some organisms and bacteriostatic against others.

3. Name the settings in which bactericidal antibiotics are preferred.

Bactericidal agents are preferable if the host is compromised (especially neutropenic) or if the host defense mechanisms do not operate well (e.g., patients with bacterial endocarditis or meningitis).

4. Describe time-dependent vs. concentration-dependent bactericidal effects.

Concentration-dependent effects: increased bactericidal effect correlates with increased drug concentration.

Time-dependent effects: bacterial killing has little relationship to concentration; as long as the antibiotic level at the site of infection is above the minimal inhibitory concentration (MIC), the drug is effective.

5. Which antibiotics are time-dependent? Which are concentration-dependent?

Time-dependent	**Concentration-dependent**
Beta-lactams	Aminoglycosides
Vancomycin	Quinolones
	Chloramphenicol

6. What are the implications of time- vs. concentration-dependent bactericidal effect for the dosing of antibiotics?

Antibiotics that are time-dependent should be dosed so that the levels achieved are as low as possible (to reduce toxicities) but remain as long as possible above the MIC. This goal may be achieved best by a continuous slow infusion, but the traditional method has been moderate doses

99

at short intervals. Concentration-dependent antibiotics should be given as large, infrequent doses to achieve the desirable high levels. Infrequent dosing decreases exposure to the drug and limits toxicities (e.g., once-daily aminoglycoside dosing).

7. What is the postantibiotic effect?

The postantibiotic effect was first described in vitro in the 1940s. It was noted that after short exposure to an antibiotic, an affected organism was unable to grow for a certain period after the antibiotic was removed. Although the exact mechanism is not known, residual drug binding to target proteins, delayed recovery of metabolism, and prolonged bacterial morphologic alterations are thought to play a role. In vivo experiments also have shown this effect, although the results are not necessarily compatible with in vitro outcomes. This difference is thought to result from factors that are not modeled in vitro, such as increased susceptibility to phagocytosis after exposure to antibiotics. Aminoglycosides, carbapenems (imipenem, meropenem), quinolones, and vancomycin show significant postantibiotic effect.

8. What is the rationale behind once-daily aminoglycoside dosing?

1. Aminoglycosides are concentration-dependent; higher levels show faster bactericidal effect.

2. Aminoglycosides have an extended postantibiotic effect (often lasting 2–3 times longer than the half-life of the drug); even after levels have dropped, bacteria are still killed.

3. Aminoglycosides exhibit first-exposure effect; exposed bacteria (in particular *Pseudomonas* spp.) show decreased uptake of the drug for several hours. Dosing at longer intervals has been shown to decrease this effect.

4. Toxicities of aminoglycosides may be time-dependent.

5. Uptake into renal tubular cells and into the inner ear is saturable and greater with constant, low serum levels.

Comparative trials have shown that once-daily dosing is effective and may have fewer clinical failures. Most studies have shown either no difference or significantly less nephrotoxicity with once-daily dosing, especially in patients under 65 years of age. Time to onset of nephrotoxicity was significantly longer with once-daily dosing. No significant difference in inner ear toxicity has been shown, although this finding may be due to the relatively infrequent occurrence of clinically significant ototoxicity or vestibulotoxicity with commonly used aminoglycosides and the small number of patients enrolled in the studies.

9. List the antibiotics that are active against intracellular organisms.

Tetracyclines	Erythromycin/macrolides
Chloramphenicol	Clindamycin
Trimethoprim/sulfamethoxazole	Rifamycins
Quinolones	

To be active intracellularly, an agent must enter the cell at adequate levels, penetrate into the microenvironment that contains the bacteria (e.g., phagosome), and be stable to the conditions in the microenvironment in the cell (e.g., low pH, lytic enzymes). Agents that rely on rapid cell growth for their antibacterial effect (e.g., beta-lactams) may not be as active against bacteria already inhibited to some degree by intracellular defenses.

10. List common indications for using antibiotic combinations.

1. Empirical treatment of the febrile, neutropenic patient to cover an array of potential deadly pathogens (gram-negative and gram-positive organisms).

2. Treatment of polymicrobial infections to cover organisms with dissimilar antimicrobial sensitivities (e.g., intraabdominal infections).

3. Synergism to enhance bacterial killing in serious or difficult-to-treat infections (e.g., penicillin and gentamicin against many enterococcal infections).

4. Historically prevention of the emergence of resistance has applied primarily to the treatment of tuberculosis.

11. **List antibiotics primarily excreted by the liver and kidney.**

Liver as major pathway of excretion	Kidney as major pathway of excretion
Cefoperazone	Aminoglycosides
Chloramphenicol	Aztreonam
Clindamycin	Cephalosporins (other than cefoperazone)
Doxycycline	Imipenem
Erythromycin	Quinolones
Metronidazole	Penicillins
Nafcillin	Trimethoprim
Rifampin	Tetracyclines (other than doxycycline)
Sulfamethoxazole	Vancomycin

Drugs primarily excreted by the kidney need dosage reductions with renal insufficiency; drugs excreted or detoxified by the liver need dose adjustments with hepatic insufficiency.

12. **Which antibiotics penetrate the central nervous system (CNS) and are most useful for CNS infections?**

Penicillins, third-generation cephalosporins, chloramphenicol, rifampin, and trimethoprim/sulfamethoxazole generally penetrate the CNS well and have been clinically useful in bacterial meningitis caused by different pathogens. The early-generation cephalosporins, clindamycin, and especially the aminoglycosides do not penetrate the CNS well.

13. **What are the Food and Drug Administration (FDA) ratings for use of antibiotics in pregnancy?**

A = Controlled studies show no risk: adequate, well-controlled studies in pregnant women have failed to demonstrate risk to the fetus.

B = No evidence of risk in humans: either animal findings show risk but human findings do not, or, if no adequate human studies have been done, animal findings are negative.

C = Risk cannot be ruled out: human studies are lacking, and animal studies are either positive for fetal risk or lacking; however, potential benefits may justify the potential risk.

D = Positive evidence of risk: investigational or postmarketing data show risk to the fetus; nevertheless, potential benefits may outweigh the potential risk.

X = Contraindicated in pregnancy: studies in animals or humans or investigational or postmarketing reports have shown fetal risk that clearly outweighs any possible benefit to the patient.

14. **Describe the two general categories of antibiotic resistance.**

Antibiotic resistance may be **intrinsic** (an inherent property present in virtually all isolates of the species) or **acquired** (a change in the genetic material of a previously susceptible organism, either by mutation or acquisition of new DNA).

15. **List the general mechanisms of resistance to antibiotics with examples.**

• Diminished intracellular drug concentration: tetracycline (increased efflux) and beta-lactams (decreased outer membrane permeability).

• Drug inactivation: beta-lactams (beta-lactamases), aminoglycosides (modifying enzymes), and chloramphenicol (inactivation by acetyltransferase).

• Target modification: beta-lactams (decreased affinity for penicillin-binding proteins), quinolones (DNA gyrase modification), and macrolides (rRNA methylation).

• Target bypass: glycopeptides and trimethoprim (thymine-deficient strains).

16. **What is the spectrum of action of natural penicillins?**

Penicillin V and G are active against many gram-positive and anaerobic organisms. Despite the wide production of penicillinase (staphylococci acquired resistance soon after penicillin was introduced), natural penicillins are the agent of choice for syphilis and can be used in meningococcal infections (rare resistance) and *Pasteurella multocida* infection.

17. Which bacteria do the aminopenicillins cover that natural penicillins do not?

The aminopenicillins (ampicillin, amoxicillin) extend coverage to some gram-negative bacteria such as salmonellae, *Haemophilus influenzae* (non–beta-lactamase producers), and *Escherichia coli*. Despite increasing resistance (beta-lactamase production), they remain useful against most enterococcal infections (usually with an aminoglycoside) and listerial infections (*Listeria monocytogenes*).

18. Name the antistaphylococcal penicillins.

Methicillin, nafcillin, oxacillin, cloxacillin, and others were developed to treat infections caused by penicillinase-producing staphylococci (hence penicillinase-resistant or antistaphylococcal penicillins). These agents are used almost exclusively to cover staphylococcal pathogens. Unfortunately, methicillin-resistant *S. aureus* (MRSA) isolates that are also resistant to all other members of this class have increasingly emerged (especially in hospitals).

19. How do the extended-spectrum penicillins differ from other penicillins?

The so-called extended-spectrum penicillins (carbenicillin, ticarcillin, mezlocillin, and piperacillin) increase the gram-negative coverage to include *Pseudomonas aeruginosa* (hence the name antipseudomonal penicillins) and *Bacteroides* species. Piperacillin and mezlocillin have better gram-positive (including enterococci) and anaerobic activity.

20. What are beta-lactamase inhibitors?

Clavulanic acid, sulbactam, and tazobactam inhibit many of the beta-lactamases that are produced by bacteria and destroy many beta-lactams (e.g., the penicillinase produced by staphylococci). When paired with certain beta-lactams (amoxicillin or ticarcillin + clavulanate, ampicillin + sulbactam, and piperacillin + tazobactam), they can restore antibacterial activity if they are effective against one or more beta-lactamases produced by the target bacteria.

21. How does the antibacterial spectrum of cephalosporins change from one generation to the next?

In general, as the generation increases, the gram-negative coverage increases and the gram-positive coverage decreases.

First-generation drugs (cephalexin, cefazolin, cephalothin, cephapirin, cephradine, cefadroxil) are active against many gram-positive organisms, including penicillinase-producing staphylococci; they also are effective against a limited number of gram-negative enterics (e.g., *E. coli*, indole-negative *Proteus mirabilis*).

Second-generation drugs (cefuroxime, cefaclor, cefamandole, cefprozil, loracarbef) expand coverage to some enteric and upper respiratory gram-negative organisms (*H. influenzae*, and *Moraxella catarrhalis*) and even some relatively penicillin-resistant pneumococci.

Third-generation drugs (cefotaxime, cefoperazone, ceftizoxime, ceftriaxone, ceftazidime, cefixime, cefpodoxime, ceftibuten) have broad gram-negative coverage due to increased resistance to beta-lactamases. Cefoperazone and ceftazidime even cover *P. aeruginosa*, but cefixime and ceftibuten relinquish almost all staphylococcal activity.

Fourth- and fifth-generation drugs are being studied and introduced (e.g., cefepime, which maintains antipseudomonal and gram-positive coverage and is less likely to induce beta-lactamase production). **Cephamycins** (cefoxitin, cefmetazole, cefotetan) are similar to second-generation cephalosporins but are more active against anaerobes, including *Bacteroides* species.

22. What are the carbapenems?

Imipenem and meropenem are carbapenems with extremely broad activity against gram-positive bacteria (but not MRSA), gram-negative bacteria (including *P. aeruginosa*), and anaerobes (including *Bacteroides* species). Imipenem is hydrolyzed in the kidney by renal dehydropeptidase to a toxic metabolite. To prevent tubular injury, imipenem is paired with cilastatin (a dehydropeptidase-1 inhibitor) as a fixed combination. Meropenem does not undergo hydrolysis and therefore does not need a drug such as cilastatin.

23. What is the primary spectrum of activity of the following antibiotics?
  1. **Aminoglycosides**
     - Aerobic gram-negative organisms
     - No antianaerobic activity
     - Enterococci: only gram-positive organisms for which aminoglycosides are considered the drug of choice (with either penicillin/ampicillin or vancomycin)
  2. **Aztreonam**
     - Aerobic gram-negative organisms, including *P. aeruginosa*
     - No gram-positive or antianaerobic activity
  3. **Clindamycin**
     - Gram-positive cocci and anaerobes
     - Active against many staphylococci (including penicillinase producers but not MRSA)
     - Drug of choice for anaerobic lung abscess and possibly invasive group A streptococcal infections
  4. **Metronidazole**
     - Anaerobic and protozoal infections
     - Excellent antianaerobic drug, including *Clostridium difficile*
     - Agent of choice for trichomoniasis, giardiasis, and amebiasis
     - Used in combination therapy against *Helicobacter pylori*
  5. **Quinolones**
     - Most gram-positive and gram-negative aerobes
     - Increasing resistance among MRSA and *P. aeruginosa*
     - Also cover many atypical organisms such as mycoplasmas and *Legionella* species (ofloxacin, grepafloxacin, and trovafloxacin have best antichlamydial activity)
     - Earlier agents (ciprofloxacin, ofloxacin, enoxacin, norfloxacin, lomefloxacin) have no antianaerobic activity
     - More recent additions (levofloxacin, sparfloxacin, grepafloxacin, trovafloxacin) better against anaerobes and increasingly penicillin-resistant pneumococci
  6. **Macrolides**
     - Clarithromycin and azithromycin extend erythromycin coverage to include more respiratory pathogens (especially *H. influenzae*)
     - Both have excellent activity against *Mycobacterium avium* complex (MAC)
     - Clarithromycin is used against *H. pylori* and azithromycin as single-dose therapy for uncomplicated chlamydial infections
  7. **Vancomycin**
     - Essentially *all* gram-positive and *only* gram-positive organisms, with rare exceptions

24. Which antibiotics are most likely to be associated with photosensitivity?
   1. **Sulfonamides** (trimethoprim to lesser degree): especially common in HIV infection, in which desensitization has a role.
   2. **Tetracyclines:** reported infrequently with doxycycline, which is used more commonly as a travel drug (chemoprophylaxis against malaria, leptospirosis, typhus fever, and traveler's diarrhea in tropical areas); sunscreen advised.
   3. **Quinolones:** although reported with all the members of this family, sparfloxacin carries a special warning about avoiding exposure to direct or indirect sunlight or sunlamps during and up to 5 days after the last dose (sunscreens do not help). Lomefloxacin is also a frequent cause (2.5%); evening dose (given once daily) decreases this potential reaction. Trovafloxacin (0.03%) and others have a low potential.
   4. **Azithromycin:** rare but may be prolonged with long half-life.

25. Which antibiotics have been associated with ototoxicity?
   1. **Aminoglycosides:** increased with coadministration of loop diuretics (e.g., furosemide) and in setting of increased "noise." Risk factors include renal insufficiency and increased plasma

levels. High-frequency loss occurs first (4000-8000 cycles). Avoid if possible in blind or elderly patients and in certain occupations (e.g., pilot).

2. **Erythromycin:** transient deafness, usually reversible, especially in patients with decreased renal or hepatic function given high dose (> 4 gm/day) intravenously. Document monitoring and discontinue with symptoms.

3. **Clarithromycin:** isolated postmarketing reports of hearing loss, which is usually reversible; chiefly in elderly women.

4. **Azithromycin:** transient deafness reported with high daily doses (> 600 mg/day).

5. **Vancomycin:** controversial with only a few dozen cases of hearing loss being reported; most patients have renal dysfunction or preexisting hearing loss or receive concomitant treatment with an ototoxic drug.

6. **Minocycline:** vestibular dysfunction (dizziness, ataxia, nausea and vomiting) has been seen in up to 20% of patients taking minocycline, especially women; decreased hearing has been reported only rarely.

26. Which antibiotics are associated with a disulfiram-like reaction with concomitant use of alcohol?

A disulfiram-like reaction (tachycardia, flushing, headaches, abdominal cramps, nausea, vomiting, and diarrhea) may be seen with concomitant use of alcohol and the following antibiotics:

1. **Metronidazole:** alcoholic beverages should not be consumed during therapy or for at least 3 days afterward; should not be given to patients who have taken disulfiram within the past 2 weeks to avoid acute toxic psychosis.

2. **Beta-lactams with the methylthiotetrazole (MTT) side chain**, including cefamandole, cefotetan, cefmetazole, cefoperazone, and moxalactam. These drugs also cause hypoprothrombinemia (prevented or treated with vitamin K)—another MTT association.

3. **Chloramphenicol:** minor disulfiram reactions have been reported.

27. List the antibiotics with the greatest potential for causing chemical phlebitis.

1. Nafcillin and to a lesser degree methicillin and oxacillin; extravasation may result in tissue necrosis.

2. Cephalothin/cephapirin (up to 20%)

3. Cefepime (about 10%). Other beta-lactams (including ampicillin/sulbactam, antipseudomonal penicillins such as ticarcillin with or without clavulanate, piperacillin, aztreonam, cefotaxime, ceftizoxime) are associated with phlebitis (2–5%).

4. Vancomycin

5. Erythromycin

6. Tetracyclines—may be used for chemical pleurodesis (intense pain and fever)

7. Clindamycin

28. Name the antibiotic known for each of the following color associations.

1. **Yellow babies**

   Sulfonamides pass the placenta and are excreted in milk; they can displace bilirubin from albumin, leading to kernicterus; therefore, they should not be used in newborns or in women near term.

2. **Yellow adults**

   A number of antibiotics may cause hepatitis, such as oxacillin and especially intravenous tetracycline given at dosages over 2 gm/day (may be fatal). The combination of amoxicillin and clavulanate given to elderly men for over 2 weeks causes a cholestatic hepatitis with reversible jaundice often 1–4 weeks after therapy has been stopped. Erythromycin estolate may cause intrahepatic cholestasis in adults (1 in 1,000) but not in children. Ceftriaxone may cause pseudocholelithiasis secondary to biliary sludging (demonstrated by ultrasound in 50% of cases but symptomatic in only 9%). Biliary sludging is more likely with high doses (> 2 gm/day), total parenteral nutrition (TPN), and poor oral intake.

Symptoms have led to cholecystectomy. Novobiocin (use fairly limited, e.g., MRSA carriage) may cause yellowing of the skin, sclerae, and plasma secondary to a yellow pigmented metabolite and is not hyperbilirubinemia.

3. **Gray babies**
   Progressive ashen-gray cyanosis appearing 3–4 days after high-dose chloramphenicol produces the gray baby syndrome. The syndrome is associated with a high mortality rate (40%) and is due to high serum concentrations of unconjugated drug secondary to immature hepatic and renal function.

4. **Red neck syndrome**
   Rapid infusion of vancomycin may cause flushing of the upper body (histamine-mediated rash), which is not an allergic reaction and usually resolves when the infusion rate is slowed, with or without an antihistamine drug. Teicoplanin (another anti–gram-positive agent) causes this syndrome less commonly.

5. **Brown-black thyroid**
   When given for prolonged periods, tetracyclines may produce brown-black microscopic discoloration of the thyroid glands. Minocycline may cause pigmentation and discoloration (often purplish) of the skin (especially in scars), mucous membranes, and new bone.

6. **Coffee-colored urine**
   Darkening of the urine has been reported in approximately 1 patient in 100,000 taking metronidazole and is probably secondary to a harmless metabolite.

7. **Red lobster syndrome**
   Rifampin causes a red-orange discoloration of urine, tears, and sweat (stains soft contact lens or implants). An overdose may produce the generalized reddening that denotes the red-lobster syndrome.

8. **Discolored teeth**
   Tetracyclines cause darkening (brown to greenish) of developing teeth. Ciprofloxacin has caused green teeth when given to premature babies.

9. **Loss of red/green perception**
   High doses of ethambutol (a primary antimycobacterial agent) may cause optic neuritis manifested clinically as decreased visual acuity, central scotomata, and loss of red/green color perception.

29. **Which antibiotics should be avoided in pregnancy?**
   - **Aminoglycosides**—possible eighth nerve toxicity in fetus.
   - **Erythromycin**—potentially hepatotoxic in women receiving high doses intravenously.
   - **Tetracyclines**—tooth and bone problems for infant and hepatotoxicity for mother.
   - **Sulfonamides**—kernicterus in newborn if given close to term.
   - **Quinolones**—potential for arthropathy.
   - **Clarithromycin**—teratogenic potential.

30. **List the major nephrotoxic antibiotics and the associated renal problem.**
   - **Aminoglycosides**—proximal tubular necrosis.
   - **Methicillin** (and other penicillins)—acute interstitial nephritis may occur in up to 1 in 6 patients receiving prolonged high dose (> 200 mg/kg/day); it also may cause acute hemorrhagic cystitis.
   - **Demeclocycline**—nephrogenic diabetes insipidus.
   - **Sulfonamides**—obstructive nephropathy.
   - **Tetracycline** (outdated preparation and its degradation products)—Fanconi syndrome (reversible proximal renal tubular dysfunction with renal glucosuria, hyperphosphaturia).
   - **Antipseudomonal penicillins** (carbenicillin, ticarcillin, piperacillin, mezlocillin) and other penicillins—hypokalemic alkalosis (penicillin moiety acts as a nonreabsorbed anion within the nephron).
   - **Penicillins and sulfonamides**—hypersensitivity glomerular damage.

31. Which antibiotics have been associated with hyperkalemia? Hypokalemia?

Hyperkalemia: intravenous aqueous, crystalline penicillin K+ if given in high doses with renal insufficiency; trimethoprim blocks distal renal tubular reabsorption of sodium and secretion of potassium and may cause a reversible hyperkalemia; prominently reported in HIV patients receiving high doses of trimethoprim/sulfamethoxazole for treatment of *Pneumocystis carinii* pneumonia (as many as 21% of patients).

Hypokalemia: various penicillins (especially the antipseudomonal agents) may act as nonreabsorbed anions in the kidney, leading to hypokalemia; high-dose nafcillin (200–300 mg/kg/day).

32. Which antibiotics are more likely to cause seizures?

- **Imipenem.** Probably overemphasized with typical dose (0.5 gm every 6 hr) but present in up to 10% of patients receiving high doses (1.0 gm every 6 hr). Dose needs to be decreased in elderly patients with decreased renal function, cerebrovascular disease, or seizure disorders. Meropenem (another carbapenem) is less likely to cause seizures.
- **Intravenous aqueous penicillin.** All penicillins (as well as other beta-lactams) may cause CNS irritability if plasma levels are high (large doses or renal insufficiency). Examples: high-dose cephalothin (300 mg/kg/day) in patients with renal failure or cefazolin, if given intraventricularly. In the days of limited antibiotic choice, clinicians would titrate penicillin to seizure activity and then decrease the dose, especially in the treatment of endocarditis.
- **Quinolones.** All are inhibitors of gamma aminobutyric acid (GABA) but infrequently cause seizures.
- **Metronidazole.** In addition to infrequent seizures, metronidazole also may induce an aseptic meningitis-like picture.

33. Which antibiotics have been most commonly implicated in *Clostridium difficile* diarrhea?

Although most antibiotics have been implicated, ampicillin, cephalosporins, and clindamycin are most often cited (this entity was first described in 1977 in association with clindamycin). For disease to occur, the following conditions are required: (1) colonization with *C. difficile*, (2) antibiotic use, and (3) *C. difficile* toxin production. Of interest, agents such as aminoglycosides and aztreonam appear to pose a lesser risk.

34. What are the clinical and laboratory predictors of *C. difficile* diarrhea?

Fecal leukocytes, semiformed stool, antibiotic use, and onset of diarrhea more than 6 days after initiation of antibiotics help to predict *C. difficile* diarrhea.

35. What are the diagnostic tests for *C. difficile*?

1. **Tissue culture**—excellent specificity, but results require 18–48 hours and lab expertise in tissue culture.

2. **Electroimmunoassay (EIA)**—relatively good sensitivity, rapid (4 hours), and does not require tissue culture.

3. **Latex agglutination**—rapid but with poor sensitivity because it assays a nonspecific protein.

4. **Fecal leukocytes**—rapid, inexpensive, good screening tool; moderately sensitive but not specific.

5. **Colonoscopy**—rapid, definitive diagnosis but invasive, insensitive, and expensive.

6. **Polymerase chain reaction (PCR)**—rapid and useful in epidemic outbreaks (potentially identifies toxic strains) but not automated or standardized.

36. What is the therapy for *C. difficile* diarrhea?

Nonspecific measures include stopping the implicated antibiotic, initiating fluid repletion and electrolyte correction, instituting enteric isolation in hospitalized patients, and avoiding antiperistaltic agents. Specific therapy (if symptoms are severe or persist for > 48 hours) include:

- Oral metronidazole (preferred agent), 250–500 mg 4 times/day for 7–14 days, or vancomycin, 125 mg 4 times/day for 7–14 days.
- Parenteral metronidazole (500 mg IV every 6–8 hr only until oral drug can be tolerated) or high-dose oral vancomycin (500 mg 4 times/day for refractory cases) also may be used.

37. How often does *C. difficile* diarrhea relapse after initial therapy?

About 10–20% of patients relapse. Multiple relapses may be treated with oral vancomycin or metronidazole for 10–14 days followed by a 3-week course of cholestyramine (4-gm packet 3 times/day with or without lactobacillus at a dose 1 gm orally 4 times/day) or vancomycin, 125 mg orally every other day for 1 month.

38. What class of antibacterials has the most frequent drug–drug interactions?

The erythromycin group (erythromycin and newer macrolides) has the most frequent drug–drug interactions. Examples include the following:

1. **Nonsedating antihistamines.** Erythromycin and clarithromycin, when taken concomitantly with terfenadine or astemizole, may result in increased Q-T intervals, torsades de pointes, or ventricular arrhythmias (rare cases of death with erythromycin and terfenadine).

2. **Theophylline.** High doses of erythromycin may result in high serum levels of theophylline and theophylline toxicity.

3. **Digoxin.** Coadministration of erythromycin and digoxin may result in elevated digoxin serum levels.

4. **Oral anticoagulants.** Anticoagulation may be increased, especially in the elderly.

5. **Ergotamine.** Acute ergot toxicity (with severe peripheral vasospasm and dysesthesia) may result from concomitant use of erythromycin and ergotamine/dihydroergotamine.

6. **Benzodiazepines.** Erythromycin has been reported to decrease the clearance of triazolam and midazolam and thus increase their pharmacologic effect.

7. **Drugs metabolized by the cytochrome P450 system.** Elevated serum concentrations of the following drugs have been reported when administered concurrently with erythromycin: carbamazepine, cyclosporine, hexobarbital, phenytoin, alfentanil, disopyramide, lovastatin, and bromocriptine.

39. Which class of antibiotics should be used with caution when neuromuscular blockage may be a clinically important adverse effect?

Rarely the use of aminoglycosides may worsen neurologic problems in patients being weaned from mechanical ventilators; patients with myasthenia gravis, botulism, or parkinsonism; and adults with hypomagnesemia. In addition, clindamycin infrequently has been reported to potentiate neuromuscular blockage.

40. Which penicillin preparations increase the potential for bleeding?

The extended-spectrum penicillins (e.g., carbenicillin, ticarcillin) interfere with platelet aggregation and are associated with a bleeding diathesis in some patients. This effect is most frequently seen in elderly patients with renal insufficiency or recent surgery, and it seems to be potentiated by aspirin or NSAIDS. Carbenicillin and ticarcillin are associated with this problem more frequently than piperacillin or mezlocillin.

41. Which beta-lactam antibiotic may be used in patients with an allergy to other beta-lactams (penicillins and cephalosporins)?

Aztreonam, a monobactam that has only gram-negative aerobic activity; it does not cover gram-positive aerobes or anaerobes. Of interest, aztreonam shares the same side chain as ceftazidime, and there may be cross-reactivity between thee two agents. Be careful with aztreonam in patients with severe ceftazidime allergy.

42. Which antibiotic induces an almost universal rash when given to a patient with infectious mononucleosis?

The classic association is ampicillin and a maculopapular, nonurticarial (nonpenicillin-allergic) rash in 65–100% of patients with acute infectious mononucleosis (usually related to Epstein-Barr virus but occasionally to cytomegalovirus).Of interest, the rash may occur with other aminopenicillins (amoxicillin and bacampicillin) and when they are given in other settings (e.g., 90% of patients with chronic lymphocytic leukemia, 15–20% of patients receiving concurrent allopurinol).

43. What unique rheumatologic and orthopedic complication has been associated with quinolone use?

Tendinitis and tendon rupture have been reported with most of the quinolones, and all now carry a warning as mandated by the FDA (report any cases at 1-800-FDA-1088). The important points about this adverse effect include the following:
- More common with chronic use
- Most common in Achilles tendon, followed by shoulder and hand
- More common in men, elderly people, and patients taking steroids
- Treatment: discontinuation of quinolone and rest

44. Which oral cephalosporin has been associated with a serum sickness-like reaction?

Cefaclor may cause a serum sickness-like reaction in 0.1–0.5% of patients, especially those receiving multiple courses. The reaction is characterized by arthralgias and rash (including erythema multiforme) but not lymphadenopathy, proteinuria, or immune complex formation. Because loracarbef is chemically similar to cefaclor, similar reactions have been reported with its use.

45. Which antibiotic has been most often associated with erosive esophagitis?

Doxycycline—although most tetracyclines can result in esophageal ulcerations. Esophagitis is a direct chemical effect (pH = 2.5) that occurs more commonly if the patient takes doxycycline at bedtime without adequate liquid. The problem is exacerbated with any kind of esophageal motility disorder. Substernal chest pain may result, awaken the patient, and occasion an emergency department visit to rule out more severe causes of chest pain. A history is critical.

46. Which urinary antibiotic has been associated with chronic pulmonary fibrosis?

Nitrofurantoin. Use for long-term suppression of urinary tract infection may result in chronic desquamative interstitial pneumonia with fibrosis.

47. What is the Jarisch-Herxheimer reaction? Which antibiotics most often cause it?

The Jarisch-Herxheimer reaction is an acute, systemic febrile reaction accompanied by headache, myalgia, tachycardia, hyperventilation, vasodilatation with flushing, and mild hypotension. It may occur within the first 24 hours (usually within 1–2 hours) after the initial treatment of syphilis with effective antibiotics, especially penicillin. The reaction is common among patients with early syphilis (occurring in 70–90% of patients with secondary syphilis) but may happen in any stage. Patients should be advised of this possible adverse reaction, which may last 12–24 hours. It is self-limited and may be treated with antipyretics. The degree of severity varies. The reaction may be clinically important in cardiovascular syphilis and neurosyphilis; steroids may favorably modify the symptoms (probably from inhibition of the release of heat-stable pyrogen). The reaction may induce early labor or cause fetal distress among pregnant women, but this concern should not prevent or delay therapy.

48. What is Hoigne's syndrome? Which antibiotics can induce it?

Hoigne's syndrome is an acute, nonallergic psychiatric reaction to penicillins, particularly the depot penicillins (procaine or benzathine penicillin). Hoigne's syndrome may include fear of death, confusion, acoustic and visual hallucinations, and possibly palpitations, tachycardia, and cyanosis. Rarely seizures or generalized twitching may occur. Symptoms usually subside within several minutes to an hour, and no specific treatment is indicated. Although the exact cause of Hoigne's syndrome has not been established, it historically has been associated most often with procaine penicillin (hence the procaine-reaction theory); however, it also has been reported, albeit rarely, with benzathine penicillin and amoxicillin.

ANTIFUNGAL AGENTS

49. Which drug is the traditional mainstay of therapy for invasive fungal disease?

Amphotericin B has been the gold standard for antifungal therapy with the broadest spectrum of activity of all antifungal agents. It covers most yeasts (e.g., *Candida* species, *Cryptococcus neoformans*), dimorphic fungi (e.g., *Blastomyces dermatitidis, Histoplasma capsulatum, Coccidioides immitis, Sporothrix* species), and filamentous fungi (*Aspergillus* species and zygomycetes). Amphotericin B resistance, although still rare in *Candida* species other than *C. lusitaniae*, is more common in emerging pathogens such as *Fusarium* species, *Trichosporon beigelii, Malassezia furfur,* and *Pseudallescharia boydii*. The introduction of other agents (including azoles, which are easier to administer, and newer formulations of amphotericin B that are less toxic) may change the traditional approach to antifungal therapy.

50. How is nonlipid amphotericin B administered?

Intravenous and oral preparations are available. Intramuscular administration is not recommended because of severe local irritation and poor absorption. The oral preparation has less than 5% bioavailability and is useful only as a topical therapy (e.g., oral candidiasis).

51. Why must IV amphotericin B be administered only in neutral dextrose solutions?

Amphotericin B is poorly water-soluble and formulated as a colloidal suspension with sodium deoxycholate. The presence of salts or an acidic pH causes aggregation of the colloid; to avoid precipitation, it should be prepared in electrolyte-free 5% dextrose in water at 0.1 µg/ml. Despite earlier custom, it is *not* necessary to protect amphotericin B from light.

52. What helps to prevent or treat the following amphotericin B-related problems?

1. **Chills and fever.** Severe rigors respond to meperidine (25–50 mg IV). Dantrolene also may be useful in some patients.

2. **Nephrotoxicity.** Avoid concurrent administration of potentially nephrotoxic agents and infuse the patient with 500 ml of normal saline over 30 minutes immediately before amphotericin B administration. The total daily dose should not exceed 1.5 mg/kg.

3. **Hypokalemia.** Amiloride, 10 mg orally twice daily, throughout the course of amphotericin B is recommended to prevent hypokalemia. It should be withheld for potassium levels > 5 mEq/L or with creatinine levels > 2.5 times baseline.

53. How rapidly can amphotericin B be infused?

The standard infusion period has been 4–6 hours. Except in selected patients (e.g., those with renal insufficiency or cardiac disease who are at risk for hyperkalemia and tachyarrhythmias), infusion of amphotericin B over 2 hours may be acceptable. More rapid administration (< 2 hours) should not be used routinely.

54. What are the lipid formulations of amphotericin B?

1. **ABLC** (amphotericin B lipid complex—Abelcet): ribbonlike structures containing bilayered membranes formed by combining a 7:3 molar ratio of dimyristoylphosphatidylcholine and dimyristoylphosphatidylglycerol with amphotericin B.

2. **ABCD** (amphotericin B colloidal dispersion—Amphotec): disklike structures of cholesteryl sulfate complexed with amphotericin B.

3. **L-AMB** (liposomal amphotericin B—AmBisome): small unilamellar vesicles made up of a bilayered membrane of hydrogenated soy phosphatidylcholine and distearoylphosphatidylglycerol stabilized with cholesterol in a 2:0.8:1 ratio combined with amphotericin B.

55. What are the potential advantages of the "lipid" formulations of amphotericin?

1. **Less toxicity.** All of the preparations appear to be preferentially accumulated in organs of the reticuloendothelial system as opposed to the kidney. This allows the use of higher doses (up to 5 + mg/kg/day) with the potential for less nephrotoxicity.

2. **Improvement in therapeutic index.** The higher tissue concentrations and larger volume of distribution translate into usefulness in invasive fungal infections in patients who have failed or who are intolerant of standard amphotericin. The high cost of the lipid formulations detracts from their usefulness as first-line therapy.

56. What are the oral azole antifungal agents?

Ketoconazole (an imidazole because of having 2 nitrogens in the 5-member azole ring; introduced at the beginning of 1980) and fluconazole and itraconazole (both triazoles because of having 3 nitrogens in the azole ring; introduced in the early 1990s) are the oral azole antifungal drugs. They have fungistatic, broad-spectrum activity that includes the organisms causing the major endemic mycoses (histoplasmosis, blastomycosis, and coccidioidomycosis) plus most yeasts and filamentous fungi. Miconazole is another azole available in topical (primarily for *Candida albicans* vaginitis) and intravenous (for patients critically ill with *Pseudallescharia boydii* infections) preparations.

57. How do azole antifungal agents work?

The azole antifungal drugs affect plasma membranes. They inhibit C-14 demethylation of lanosterol, thereby causing ergosterol depletion and accumulation of aberrant sterols in the membrane. The membrane is then more vulnerable to further damage, and the activity of several membrane-bound enzymes (e.g., those associated with nutrient transport and chitin synthesis) is altered.

58. Which oral azole agent is the only one with substantial activity against *Aspergillus* species?

Itraconazole is the only presently available azole with clinical activity against *Aspergillus* infections. Voriconazole is a new azole with potent (fungistatic) in vitro activity against fungi, including resistant strains. At therapeutic doses it is fungicidal against *Aspergillus* spp.

59. Which oral azoles may be associated with therapeutic failure when taken with an agent that increases gastric pH?

Ketoconazole and itraconazole. Absorption of ketoconazole and itraconazole is reduced by 40–95% in the presence of achlorhydria or hypochlorhydria (e.g., ketoconazole must be converted to the hydrochloride salt). Therefore, they are best administered without drugs that may decrease gastric acidity. This rule applies less to itraconazole than ketoconazole (e.g., absorption of itraconazole is reduced by antacids but not much by H2 blockers). Some acid-reducing agents may be given 2 hours after azole administration, but azole absorption may not be reliable. In addition, a number of medical conditions have been associated with decreased absorption. These agents and conditions include:

1. Antacids
2. H2 blockers (e.g., cimetidine, ranitidine, famotidine, nizatidine)
3. Proton-pump inhibitors (omeprazole, lansoprazole)
4. Sucralfate (ketoconazole only)
5. Didanosine (requires alkaline environment for absorption)
6. Conditions: AIDS, aging, gastric surgery, continuous ambulatory peritoneal dialysis, acute leukemia, transplant recipients

60. What can the physician and patient do to increase the absorption of the ketoconazole or itraconazole?

1. Because the presence of food enhances gastric acidity, ketoconazole and itraconazole should always be taken with a meal. Because absorption of fluconazole is less pH-dependent, it may be taken with or without meals or by patients receiving acid-reducing medications.

2. Acidic beverages (cola drinks) increase the absorption of ketoconazole and itraconazole and should be encouraged.

3. Itraconazole is available as a capsule or solution. The solution formulation is better absorbed (providing 60% greater bioavailability than the capsule, with or without food) and may be preferred in certain situations (e.g., candidal esophagitis in a patient with AIDS for topical effect and increased absorption).

4. Achlorhydric patients may dissolve ketoconazole in 4 ml of 0.2 N hydrochloric acid and carefully drink it through a straw.

61. Among the oral azoles, which agent achieves excellent penetration into cerebrospinal fluid (CSF) and concentration in the urine?

Fluconazole. Ketoconazole and itraconazole are minimally distributed in CSF and excreted in the urine. Both are metabolized almost entirely by the liver and do not need dosage modification with renal failure. Fluconazole is water-soluble and bound minimally to plasma proteins; it achieves excellent penetration of CSF (hence its effectiveness in cryptococcal meningitis) and other sites often inaccessible to drugs (e.g., eye). Almost 80% of a dose of fluconazole is excreted unchanged in the urine (hence its use in urinary tract infections and the necessity for dose reduction with renal insufficiency). Unlike ketoconazole and itraconazole, fluconazole also may be given intravenously.

62. Among the oral azoles, which agent inhibits steroidogenesis? What effects have been documented?

Ketoconazole. Ketoconazole (but not fluconazole or itraconazole at recommended doses) may reversibly inhibit the synthesis of testosterone (and therefore estradiol) and cortisol, resulting in a variety of endocrine disturbances: gynecomastia, oligospermia, loss of libido, impotence, menstrual irregularities, and adrenal insufficiency (rare Addison crisis). Of interest, blockage of steroidogenesis may be useful in precocious puberty and with "tumors that produce humors" (e.g., carcinomas with ectopic hormone syndromes).

63. Which three drugs are contraindicated with either ketoconazole or itraconazole because they have been associated with serious cardiovascular events, including death, ventricular tachycardia, and torsades de pointes?

Cisapride and the nonsedating antihistamines terfenadine and astemizole should not be co-administered with either ketoconazole or itraconazole, which are potent inhibitors of the cytochrome P450 3A enzyme system and may raise plasma concentrations of drugs metabolized by this pathway (such as terfenadine, astemizole, and cisapride). Ketoconazole also is associated with increased plasma concentrations of coadministered cyclosporine, warfarin, phenytoin, sulfonylurea drugs, midazolam, triazolam, and other drugs.

64. Flucytosine toxicity (especially dose-related bone marrow toxicity and enterocolitis) can be minimized by monitoring levels and keeping the serum concentration below what level?

Toxicity is much less when serum concentrations are kept below 100 µg/ml; some experts even recommend staying below 60 µg/ml. Flucytosine (not to be confused with fluconazole) has limited antifungal activity (*Candida* species and *Cryptococcus neoformans*) and should never be used alone because of the rapid development of resistance.

65. What treatments are available for fungal nail infections (onychomycosis)?

1. **Griseofulvin:** successful in only 25% of toenail and 75% of fingernail disease. It is poorly tolerated (headaches, nausea, abdominal pain, sun sensitivity) and must be continued until the nail has grown out normally (about 6 months for fingernails and 12–18 months for toenails).

2. **Ketoconazole:** no more effective than griseofulvin; hepatotoxicity (occurring in 1 in 10,000 patients) restricts its use.

3. **Fluconazole:** when combined with urea nail avulsion, fluconazole may be given weekly (150 to 300 mg) for nine months.

4. **Itraconazole:** may be given by two dosage schedules: (1) fixed dosage of 200 mg/day for 12 weeks for toenail disease and 6 weeks for fingernail disease and (2) pulse dosage of 200 mg twice daily for 1 week, given 1 week per month for 2–3 months for fingernails and 3–4 months for toenail disease.

5. **Terbinafine:** as effective as itraconazole when given 250 mg daily for 6 weeks for fingernail infection and 12 weeks for toenail disease.

ANTIVIRAL AGENTS

66. What are the antiherpetic drugs?

The antiherpetic agents are best grouped according to their clinical antiviral activity:

1. Active primarily against herpes simplex viruses 1 and 2 (HSV-1, HSV-2) and varicella zoster virus (VZV):
   • Acyclovir—topical, oral, and intravenous preparations
   • Valacyclovir or valaciclovir (international spelling)—oral
   • Famciclovir—oral (and topical as penciclovir)
2. Active primarily against cytomegalovirus:
   • Ganciclovir—oral, intravenous, intraocular
   • Cidofovir—intravenous (topical)
   • Foscarnet—intravenous (intraocular)

67. Which of the antiherpetic drugs are prodrugs?

Valacyclovir and famciclovir. Valacyclovir (an L-valyl ester of acyclovir) is converted into acyclovir through single passage in the intestines and liver. Acyclovir from valacyclovir is 3–5 times more bioavailable than oral acyclovir; therefore, oral valacyclovir provides acyclovir levels in the blood obtained only by intravenous acyclovir. Famciclovir undergoes rapid biotransformation into the active antiviral compound penciclovir. An oral prodrug of ganciclovir is under study (valganciclovir).

68. What virus-encoded enzyme is necessary for initial uptake and monophosphorylation of acyclovir and penciclovir?

Thymidine kinase. As an example, thymidine kinase converts acyclovir into its monophosphate derivative. Subsequent diphosphorylation and triphosphorylation are catalyzed by cellular enzymes, resulting in acyclovir triphosphate concentrations that are 40–100 times higher in virus-infected cells than in uninfected cells. The triphosphate compound then inhibits viral DNA synthesis. Herpesviruses can develop resistance through mutations in the viral gene encoding thymidine kinase. Acyclovir-resistant HSV and VZV (through generation of thymidine kinase-deficient mutants or selection of mutants possessing a thymidine kinase that is unable to phosphorylate acyclovir) are also resistant to valacyclovir, famciclovir (and thus penciclovir), and ganciclovir. Cytomegalovirus (CMV) lacks a virus-specific thymidine kinase and is resistant to acyclovir and penciclovir. CMV has an enzyme with putative protein kinase activity that is able to phosphorylate ganciclovir but not acyclovir or penciclovir; thus, ganciclovir is active against CMV.

69. Which agents are useful against resistant HSV and VZV infections?

On rare occasions isolates of HSV and VZV become resistant to the standard antiherpetic drugs (acyclovir and penciclovir), usually by altering their thymidine kinase. Resistance is most common in the setting of chronic treatment (often intermittent) of herpetic infections in immunosuppressed populations. Foscarnet and cidofovir are the agents of choice in such infections. Ganciclovir is not active unless the mechanism of resistance is different from alteration of thymidine kinase. For example, cidofovir is phosphorylated to its active form by cellular enzymes and does not need thymidine kinase. Therefore, resistant HSV and VZV isolates may still be susceptible to cidofovir. Foscarnet inhibits DNA polymerase directly and does not depend on conversion to an active form by thymidine kinase, as in the case of acyclovir and ganciclovir.

70. How safe is acyclovir?

Oral acyclovir, which has a bioavailability of 15–30%, is remarkably safe, even when taken chronically (e.g., for suppression of recurrent genital herpes). Rarely, oral acyclovir (more commonly high intravenous doses) has been associated with neurotoxicity, including agitation, disorientation, tremors, hallucinations, seizures, and coma (encephalopathy syndrome). The concurrent use of cimetidine or probenecid may decrease renal clearance and increase the plasma concentration of acyclovir, thus increasing the risk of toxicity. Nephrotoxicity also has been reported, especially in patients given large doses of acyclovir by rapid intravenous infusion; slow infusion and adequate hydration reduce the risk of renal dysfunction. Although acyclovir crosses the placenta, no increase in risk to the mother or fetus has been documented when it is administered during pregnancy. An *Acyclovir in Pregnancy Registry* is maintained by Glaxo Wellcome.

71. What unique side effect has been reported with high doses of valacyclovir in some severely immunocompromised patients?

Thrombotic thrombocytopenic purpura/hemolytic uremic syndrome has been reported. The active compound, acyclovir, has a remarkably safe track record orally, even when taken chronically. In addition, one controlled comparison of valacyclovir with acyclovir for the prevention of CMV infection in patients with advanced AIDS was stopped early because of a higher mortality rate in patients treated with high-dose valacyclovir.

72. What is the major adverse effect of intravenous ganciclovir?

Intravenous ganciclovir has been associated with myelosuppression, as reflected primarily by granulocytopenia and thrombocytopenia. It is therefore dangerous to administer ganciclovir with other drugs (e.g., zidovudine) that also cause hematologic toxicity. Granulocytopenia due to ganciclovir can be prevented with concomitant administration of recombinant granulocyte colony-stimulating factor (G-CSF) or granulocyte-macrophage colony-stimulating factor (GM-CSF).

73. What are the two major toxicities of foscarnet?

1. **Nephrotoxicity.** A 2- to 3-fold increase in serum creatinine levels occurs on average in 45% of patients receiving foscarnet, often in the second week. Coadministration of other nephrotoxic drugs should be avoided. Nephrotoxicity is usually reversible and can be reduced by dosage adjustment and adequate hydration. Almost 90% of a foscarnet dose is excreted in the urine.

2. **Electrolyte disturbances.** Changes in calcium (hypercalcemia and hypocalcemia), magnesium (hypomagnesemia), and potassium (hypokalemia) occur in 15–43% of patients. Either hyperphosphatemia or hypophosphatemia occurs in 6–8%. Ten percent to 28% of foscarnet is deposited in bone, where it may remain for months. Regular monitoring of electrolytes is necessary to avoid clinical toxicity.

74. Name a unique adverse genital effect of foscarnet.

Genital ulceration is an increasingly recognized adverse effect of foscarnet use:

1. It usually is heralded by dysuria and penile burning.
2. It occurs more commonly in men than women.
3. It most frequently occurs during induction use of foscarnet.
4. It usually presents clinically as periurethral or glans ulceration(s).
5. It probably represents a contact or chemical dermatitis due to the high concentration of foscarnet in the urine.
6. It resolves rapidly after discontinuation of foscarnet.

75. What are the advantages and disadvantages of cidofovir as a parenteral antiviral agent?

Advantages:

1. Inhibition of DNA polymerase, preventing DNA synthesis that does not depend on viral kinases

2. Broad-spectrum activity against HSV, VZV, CMV, and other viruses (e.g., Epstein-Barr virus, herpesvirus 6, adenovirus, hepatitis B virus), including thymidine kinase-resistant strains and some foscarnet-resistant strains

3. Ease of administration with doses given once weekly for 2 weeks, then every 2 weeks; no central catheter is required (peripheral stick every other week with 2 week drug-free period).

Disadvantage:

1. Nephrotoxicity.

76. What makes cidofovir nephrotoxicity so special?

1. It occurs in the majority of patients (53%).

2. Acute renal failure may occur after only a few doses.

3. It results in proximal tubular cell damage and metabolic acidosis, the early signs of which are proteinuria and glycosuria.

4. The drug is contraindicated with any nephrotoxicity (creatinine > 1.5 mg/dl).

77. In order to reduce cidofovir-associated nephrotoxicity, which 2 agents are administered concurrently?

1. **Probenecid:** 2 gm 3 hr before and 1 gm 2 and 8 hr after infusion; blocks renal tubular secretion by decreasing uptake in proximal tubules; may be dose-limiting in 5% of patients due to adverse effects, including nausea, fever, alopecia, myalgia, and rash (caution with history of hypersensitivity to sulfa-containing drugs)

2. **Normal saline:** 1 L over 1–2 hr immediately before and a second liter during or after infusion.

78. What antiviral agents have activity against influenza viruses?

Both amantadine and rimantadine are effective against influenza A, but not against other influenza strains (such as the common influenza B and rare influenza C). They can be used in two ways:

1. Prophylaxis against influenza A infection is used seasonally, after exposure or in outbreak setting with or without egg allergy vaccine, and as chemoprophylaxis in nonimmunized persons in the following groups:

   • > 65 years of age
   • Residents of chronic care facilities (e.g., nursing homes) that house patients with chronic medical conditions
   • Patients (adults and children) with chronic pulmonary or cardiovascular disorders (e.g., asthma)
   • Patients with chronic metabolic disorders, renal failure, hemoglobinopathies, or immunosuppression
   • Children on chronic aspirin therapy (risk of Reye's syndrome)

2. Treatment of influenza A infection: start within 48 hours of illness onset; used for a total of 3–5 days (stopped 48–72 hours after disappearance of symptoms).

A sialic acid analog, zanamivir, is a selective inhibitor of both influenza A and B and has been effective when used both intranasally and by inhalation. Vaccination remains the first line of defense against influenza.

79. What drugs are active against hepatitis B virus (HBV) infections?

Interferon alpha (5–10 million U 3 times/wk subcutaneously or intramuscularly for 4–6 months) has been used in the treatment of chronic HBV infections with only moderate success.

Both famciclovir, an antiherpetic agent, and lamivudine, an antiretroviral agent, have anti-HBV activity and may be useful in the future.

80. Name at least two viral infections for which ribavirin is acceptable treatment in the United States.

In respiratory syncytial virus (RSV) infections (RSV bronchiolitis and pneumonia, usually in hospitalized children) and chronic hepatitis C virus (HCV) infections, ribavirin has been used orally, intravenously, and by aerosol (as in the case of RSV infections). In HCV infections, it is used in combination with interferon alpha. Worldwide it has been used in many other viral infections, including hemorrhagic fever with renal syndrome (HFRS) measles, acute hepatitis, and others.

81. Name the most common adverse effects of interferons.

1. A flu-like syndrome that develops in almost all patients (98%), dominated by fatigue (89%) and myalgia (73%) and minimized by bedtime administration.

2. Myelosuppression (one-half of the patients with leukopenia and one-third each with anemia and thrombocytopenia) especially with concurrent myelosuppressive drugs (e.g., zidovudine).

3. Neurotoxicity (headache, dizziness, depression) mandates use with caution in severe psychiatric disorders.

4. Gastrointestinal problems (anorexia in almost one-half and diarrhea in one-third).

5. Others, including alopecia, increased thyroid-stimulating hormone, autoimmune thyroid disorders.

BIBLIOGRAPHY

Antbacterial Agents
1. Arky R: Physicians' Desk Reference, 52 ed. Medical Economics Company, Montvale, NJ, 1998.
2. Gold HS, Moellering RC: Antimicrobial drug resistance. N Engl J Med 335:1445–1453, 1996.
3. Graeme KA, Pollack CV: Antibiotic use in the emergency department. II: The aminoglycosides, macrolides, tetracyclines, sulfa drugs, and urinary antiseptics. J Emerg Med 14:361–371, 1996.
4. Hessen MT, Kaye D: Principles of selection and use of antibacterial agents. Infect Dis Clin North Am 9:531–545, 1995.
5. Hoigne R, Zoppi M, Sonntag R: Penicillins. In Dukes MNG (ed): Myler's Side Effects of Drugs, 12th ed. Amsterdam, Elsevier, 1992, pp 608–609.
6. Levison ME: Pharmacodynamics of antimicrobial agents. Infect Dis Clin North Am 9:483–495, 1995.
7. Livornese LL, Benz RL, Ingerman MJ, Santoro J: Antibacterial agents in renal failure. Infect Dis Clin North Am 9:591–614, 1995.
8. Manabe YC, Vinetz JM, Moore RD, et al: *Clostridium difficile* colitis: An efficient clinical approach to diagnosis. Ann Intern Med 123:835–840, 1995.
9. Papastamelos AG, Tunkel AR: Antibacterial agents in infections of the central nervous system and eye. Infect Dis Clin North Am 9:615–637, 1995.
10. Pollack ES, Pollack CV: Antibiotic use in the emergency department. I: The penicillins and cephalosporins. J Emerg Med 14:213–222, 1996.
11. Rybak MJ, McGrath BJ: Combination antimicrobial therapy for bacterial infections. Drugs 52:390–405, 1996.
12. Schmidt J, Pollack C: Antibiotic use in the emergency department. III: The quinolones, new beta lactams, beta lactams combination agents and miscellaneous antibiotics. J Emerg Med 14:483–496, 1996.
13. Schwab JC, Mandell GL: The importance of penetration of antimicrobial agents into cells. Infect Dis Clin North Am 3:461–467, 1989.
14. Shibl AM, Pechere JC, Ramadan MA: Postantibiotic effect and host–bacteria interactions. J Antimicrob Chemother 36:885–887, 1995.
15. Stell IM, Ojo OA: Amoxycillin-induced hallucinations—a variant of Hoigne's syndrome? Br J Clin Pract 50:279, 1996.
16. Urban AW, Craig WA: Daily dosage of aminoglycosides. Curr Clin Top Infect Dis 17:236–255, 1997.
17. Young EJ, Weingarten NM, Baughn RE, et al: Studies on the pathogenesis of the Jarisch-Herxheimer reaction. J Infect Dis 146:606–615, 1982.

Antifungal Agents
18. Bodey GP: Azole antifungal agents. Clin Infect Dis 14(Suppl 1):S161–S191, 1992.
19. Bonn D: New antifungals make mayhem for mycoses. Lancet 350:870, 1997.

20. Como JA, Dismukes WE: Oral azole drugs as systemic antifungal therapy. N Engl J Med 330:263–272, 1994.
21. Drutz DJ: Rapid infusion of amphotericin B: Is it safe, effective, and wise? Am J Med 93:119–120, 1992.
22. Gallis HA: Amphotericin B: A commentary on its role as an antifungal agent and as a comparative agent in clinical trials. Clin Infect Dis 22(Suppl 2):S145–S147, 1996.
23. Georgopapdadkou NH, Walsh TJ: Antifungal agents: Chemotherapeutic targets and immunologic strategies. Antimicrobiol Agents Chemother 40:279–291, 1996.
24. Graybill JR: Lipid formulations for amphotericin B: Does the emperor need new clothes? Ann Intern Med 124:921–923, 1996.
25. Hiemenz JW, Walsh TJ: Lipid formulations of amphotericin B: Recent progress and future directions. Clin Infect Dis 22(Suppl 2):S133–S144, 1996.
26. Kauffman CA: Role of azoles in antifungal therapy. Clin Infect Dis 22(Suppl 2):S148–S153, 1996.
27. Peacock JE, Herrington DA, Cruz JM: Amphotericin B therapy: Past, present, and future. Infect Dis Clin Pract 2:81–93, 1993.

Antiviral Agents
28. Borden EC: Interferons—expanding therapeutic roles. N Engl J Med 326:1491–1493,1992.
29. Crumpacker CS: Ganciclovir. N Engl J Med 335:721–729, 1996.
30. Hayden FG, Osterhaus AD, Treanor JJ, et al: Efficacy and safety of the neuraminidase inhibitor zanamivir in the treatment of influenza virus infections. N Engl J Med 337:874–880, 1997.
31. Lavoie SR, Starr SE, Tyring S. Rating the new antivirals. Int Med 20:49–55, 1996.
32. Valacyclovir. Med Lett Drugs Ther 38:3–4, 1996.
33. Wagstaff AJ, Bryson HM. Foscarnet: A reappraisal. Drugs 48:199–226, 1994.
34. Whitley RJ, Gnann JW: Acyclovir: A decade later. N Engl J Med 327:782–787, 1992.

V. Bacterial Infections

21. CLINICAL CONSIDERATIONS IN GRAM-POSITIVE INFECTIONS

Mireya A. Wessolossky, M.D., and Jennifer S. Daly, M.D.

1. What are the common clinical infections caused by *Streptococcus pneumoniae*?
• Otitis media
• Sinusitis
• Lower respiratory infections (bronchitis, pneumonia, empyema)
• Meningitis
• Bacteremia/sepsis (including pyarthrosis, endocarditis)

2. What is the incidence of penicillin-resistant *S. pneumoniae* in the United States?
Once rare in the United States, the incidence of penicillin-resistant pneumococci has increased in the past decade. Incidence varies by region but is increasing in many areas, and the number of regions reporting resistant isolates has increased. The Centers for Disease Control and Prevention (CDC) has reported areas in the United States where the incidence of penicillin-resistant *S. pneumoniae* is as high as 30%. In other countries, notably Spain, Hungary, Australia, South Africa, and Israel, the incidence is even higher. The chief factors responsible for the development of resistance are thought to be selective pressure exerted by antibiotic use, including excessive length of therapy, use of broad-spectrum agents, and unjustified administration of antibiotics. To detect penicillin resistance, laboratories need to use a 1-μg oxacillin disk test or perform a quantitative minimal inhibitory concentration (MIC). If *S. pneumoniae* is resistant by these tests, further testing against extended-spectrum cephalosporins, vancomycin, or other antibiotics is warranted.

3. How should we treat *S. pneumoniae*? Can infection be prevented?
Penicillin (PCN) is the drug of choice for penicillin-susceptible *S. pneumoniae*. For penicillin-resistant *S. pneumoniae*, a third-generation cephalosporin (e.g., ceftriaxone, cefotaxime, or ceftizoxime) or high-dose PCN is indicated, depending on the site of infection and level of PCN resistance. In patients with pneumonia or bacteremic pneumonia, PCN can be used against PCN-susceptible strains and possibly those of intermediate susceptibility (MIC 0.1–1.0 μg/ml). In patients with meningitis, high doses of third-generation cephalosporins (i.e., ceftriaxone, cefotaxime) plus vancomycin should be administered until results of susceptibility tests are available. Even when this regimen is used, some authorities recommend a second lumbar puncture 24–48 hours after beginning therapy to document response. In cases of high-level resistance (MIC > 1.0 μg/ml), vancomycin is the drug of choice (synergy has been reported when used with ceftriaxone). If the organism is found susceptible, a quinolone, clindamycin, or imipenem also may be used.

A vaccine for the 23 serotypes of *S. pneumoniae* is available but has been underutilized. The vaccine is recommended by the Advisory Committee on Immunization Practices (ACIP) for all persons > 65 years of age and for persons > 2 years of age who have certain predisposition for pneumococcal diseases (e.g., anatomic or functional asplenia, HIV infection, immunosuppressive chemotherapy). Unfortunately, the only available pneumococcal vaccine is a polysaccharide vaccine, not adequately immunogenic in young children, and is not recommended for use in children < 2 years of age, even if they are at risk for pneumococcal infections. Global curtailment of antibiotic use for marginal indications could reduce the selective pressure for drug-resistant organisms and prevent emergence of resistant strains.

4. How severe are pneumococcal infections? Are the resistant strains of *S. pneumoniae* more virulent than penicillin-susceptible strains?

Despite the use of antibiotics, patients continue to die of overwhelming pneumococcal infection. Many such patients are apparently normal hosts. Case-fatality rates vary by age, exposure to antibiotics, and underlying illnesses. For high-risk patients (see question 3), mortality rates have been reported to be > 40% for bacteremia and 55% for meningitis, despite appropriate antimicrobial therapy.

Clinical studies support the idea that both penicillin-resistant and penicillin-susceptible strains are equally virulent. In immunocompromised hosts the clinical presentation and outcome may be worse than in normal hosts, but outcome is not related to antibiotic susceptibility of the infecting strain.

5. What are the *Staphylococcus* spp.? How are they identified?

The two major clinically important groups of *Staphylococcus* spp. are differentiated in the laboratory by the coagulase test, the ability to clot plasma. Coagulase-positive staphylococci (e.g., *S. aureus*) are almost always pathogens, and coagulase-negative staphylococci (*S. epidermidis, S. saprophyticus, S. haemolyticus, S. warneri, S. lugdunensis*, among others) are often culture contaminants. The coagulase-negative strains are gaining greater importance as true pathogens, especially in patients with indwelling prosthetic devices or plastic vascular access catheters.

6. What infections are caused by *Staphylococcus* spp.?

Organism	Carrier	Infections
Coagulase-positive staphylococci (*S. aureus*)	Skin Nasopharynx Vagina	Skin: folliculitis, impetigo, furuncles, cellulitis, carbuncles, postoperative wound infections. Deep infections: endocarditis, meningitis, arthritis, pneumonia, osteomyelitis, pyomyositis, sepsis, and multiple organ failure. Toxin-mediated disease: food poisoning, scalded skin syndrome, toxic shock syndrome.
Coagulase-negative staphylococci (*S. epidermidis* and others)	Skin Ear canal Genitourinary tract Mucosal membranes	Indwelling foreign bodies' infections: prosthetic cardiac valves, permanent pacemaker wires and electrodes, vascular grafts, cerebrospinal fluid shunts, peritoneal dialysis catheters, prosthetic joints, intravenous catheters. Urinary tract infection: nosocomial (*S. epidermidis*); outpatient women (*S. saprophyticus*). Other: postoperative endophthalmitis, native valve endocarditis, osteomyelitis.

7. How do you treat a patient with a serious infection due to coagulase-negative staphylococci (e.g., osteomyelitis, prosthetic valve endocarditis)?

Vancomycin is considered the drug of choice in combination with an aminoglycoside and rifampin to treat prosthetic valve endocarditis, cerebral spinal fluid (CSF) shunt infections, and vascular graft infections. Surgical replacement of the graft or prosthetic material, along with drainage of any local abscess, is required in patients with prosthetic joints or vascular graft infections. CSF shunt and chronic ambulatory peritoneal dialysis catheter infections may be treated without catheter removal, but in case of a treatment failure, retreatment and catheter removal are required. Bacteremia in immunocompromised patients often is related to colonization of the long-term indwelling catheters. Therapy includes removal of the catheter, if feasible. When catheter removal is problematic, intravenous vancomycin alone may be successful.

8. What does MRSA mean? How do you treat serious staphylococcal infections?

MRSA means methicillin-resistant *Staphylococcus aureus*. When tested in the laboratory, *S. aureus* has two patterns of susceptibility that dictate the therapy: susceptible or resistant to methicillin. Resistance to methicillin implies resistance to all beta-lactam antibiotics, including penicillins, cephalosporins, carbapenems, and beta-lactamase inhibitor/beta-lactam combinations. For the treatment of infections due to MRSA, intravenous vancomycin is the drug of choice. In deep infection, such as endocarditis or osteomyelitis, depending on the susceptibility of the patient's organisms, a combination of vancomycin plus an aminoglycoside, rifampin, or trimethoprim-sulfamethoxazole has been used. Patients with an infection due to methicillin-susceptible strain (MSSA) are treated with penicillinase-resistant penicillins, such as nafcillin, oxacillin or, in case of a penicillin-allergic patient, first-generation cephalosporins (i.e., cefazolin). If the patient is allergic to all beta-lactam agents, vancomycin, clindamycin, or macrolides (i.e., erythromycin) are the drugs of choice.

9. How do you isolate patients with MRSA? How do you decolonize a patient with MRSA?

MRSA has become a major nosocomial pathogen in tertiary hospitals, long-term care facilities, and even community hospitals. Rapid detection of MRSA, prompt implementation of barrier precautions, and prospective surveillance are essential components of a successful control program. Barrier isolation precautions (e.g., use of a single room off a ward, masks for those in close proximity to the patient, gloves if patient or infective material is to be touched, and gowns if soiling is likely), particularly strict hand-washing, are the most effective methods of restricting the nosocomial spread of MRSA. Eradication of nasal carriage of MRSA among patients and health workers has been tried during epidemics. Mupirocin is a novel topical antibiotic with excellent antibacterial activity against staphylococci, including MRSA. Intranasal administration of calcium mupirocin has achieved excellent results in the eradication of nasal carriage of MRSA, producing an associated reduction in MRSA outbreaks in a variety of clinical settings, including neonatal nurseries, hemodialysis, cardiothoracic surgery, and familial staphylococcal infections. All patients who are known carriers of MRSA should be placed on barrier isolation precautions upon admission to a health care facility, unless appropriate screening tests have shown them to be free of MRSA. At home, carriers apparently are not a source of infection to healthy family members and friends.

10. How do you recognize, classify, and group streptococci?

Streptococci are gram-positive, catalase-negative organisms that grow in pairs or chains of varying lengths. Most grow both aerobically and anaerobically (facultatively) with variable nutritional requirements. This heterogeneous group of organisms has no single accepted classification system. Routinely, classification depends on a combination of (1) patterns of hemolysis in the blood agar plates (α, β, γ hemolysis); (2) antigenic differences in cell wall carbohydrates (A to H and K to V in the Lancefield scheme for the β-hemolytic strains); (3) biochemical reactions; and (4) growth characteristics.

The α-hemolytic strains, which produce partial hemolysis and cause a greenish discoloration in the culture medium, are called viridans (green, from Latin) streptococci. This group (including *S. intermedius*, *S. anginosus*, *S. bovis*, *S. sanguis*, *S. salivarius*, and *S. mutans*) contains many strains that normally inhabit the human respiratory and gastrointestinal tracts. *S. pneumoniae* is α-hemolytic and technically belongs to this group but usually is considered separately because of its virulence.

The β-hemolytic strains produce hemolysins, causing a colorless zone of hemolysis around the colonies on blood agar plates. These species are the most pathogenic for humans and include *S. pyogenes* (group A streptococci), and *S. agalactiae* (group B streptococci).

The γ-hemolytic strains do not produce detectable hemolysis on sheep blood agar plates. In the past enterococci were placed in the genus *Streptococcus* and are usually nonhemolytic.

Although the grouping system developed by Rebecca Lancefield in 1933 was initially used only for β-hemolytic streptococci, it has been extended to some strains with other types of

hemolysis. Certain α- and γ-hemolytic strains also contain group-specific antigens. The α-hemolytic *S. bovis* has a group D antigen, some α-hemolytic and γ-hemolytic streptococci have group
F antigen, and members of the recently designated new genus, *Enterococcus* (known before as
group D streptococci), possess the group D antigen.

11. What infections are caused by streptococci in humans?

Subgroup	Species	Clinical Features
A	*S. pyogenes*	Pharyngitis, tonsillitis, otitis media, scarlet fever, erysipelas, cellulitis, impetigo, pneumonia, puerperal endometritis, septicemia, necrotizing fasciitis Delayed nonsuppurative sequelae: acute rheumatic fever, acute glomerulonephritis
B	*S. agalactiae*	Puerperal sepsis, chorioamnionitis, neonatal sepsis and meningitis, cellulitis, endocarditis, bacteremia
C, F, G	*S. dysgalactiae* *S. equisimilis* *S. zooepidemicus*	Upper respiratory infections, cellulitis, wound (especially intraabdominal) infections, septicemia, endocarditis, deep-tissue infections
D (nonenterococcal)	*S. bovis* *S. equinus*	Genitourinary tract infections, wound infections, endocarditis
S. milleri group	*S. intermedius* *S. constellatus* *S. anginosus*	Purulent infections, odontogenic infections, brain abscesses, liver abscesses, cholangitis, endocarditis, subcutaneous abscesses, cellulitis

12. What organisms are called "flesh-eating bacteria"? Why? How do we treat patients with this infection?

S. pyogenes, or group A streptococcus, can cause necrotizing fasciitis and has been dubbed
the "flesh-eating bacteria" by the tabloid press. These infections are characterized by a sudden
onset of severe pain in deep tissues, with development of rapidly progressive necrotizing skin and
subcutaneous infection that advances to frank gangrene and death if untreated. A key component
of treatment is surgery, which may need to be extensive and repetitive, to debride necrotic tissue.
Most cases have been reported in previously healthy adults, who experience concomitant severe
systemic illness, such as septic shock, respiratory, hepatic and/or renal insufficiency, and disseminated intravascular coagulopathy.

S. pyogenes produces pyrogenic exotoxins types A, B, and C, which help in the destruction
of tissue. Streptococcus exotoxin type A is believed to be responsible for the streptococcal toxic
shock syndrome. Another pathogenic factor of the streptococci is the M protein, a cell membrane
macromolecule that is one of the major virulence antigens. Strains rich in this protein are resistant to phagocytosis by polymorphonuclear leukocytes.

In addition to prompt surgical debridement in cases of necrotizing fasciitis, the therapeutic
management of severe group A streptococcal infections requires high doses of intravenous antibiotics. Penicillin G traditionally has been the agent of choice, because there is no high-level resistance among the group A streptococci. Patients allergic to penicillin may be treated with a
first-generation cephalosporin, vancomycin, or clindamycin.

Recently, clindamycin has been recommended in addition to penicillin for all patients.
Experimental evidence indicates that clindamycin may be more effective than penicillin at inhibiting these organisms when they are present in a high inoculum and not dividing rapidly.
Evidence comes from in vitro observation of the "Eagle effect" as well as animal models. Harry
Eagle first showed that streptococci present at high inoculum ($> 10^7$) are very slowly killed by
penicillin. Animal models suggest that clindamycin with its inhibition of protein synthesis has
greater activity than penicillin against organisms in a stationary phase of growth and may reduce
production of toxins, and tumor necrosis factor (TNF). Ceftriaxone may have better affinity

than penicillin G for streptococcal penicillin-binding proteins, and may be preferable to penicillin in treatment of necrotizing fasciitis. Based on these experimental results, clindamycin should be used either with penicillin or ceftriaxone. Clindamycin alone is not recommended because some strains are resistant, especially in regions where macrolides are used extensively in outpatients.

13. How many cases of group A, C, or G streptococcal infection cause the sounding of the infection control "alarm"?

One. Any nosocomial (especially in a postoperative, or burn patients, postpartum women, or newborns) group A, C, or G streptococcal infection warrants infection control investigation. Outbreaks of nosocomial group A, C, or G streptococci infections have resulted in the designation of these infections as a locally reportable disease. Outbreak investigation includes obtaining throat, rectal, and vaginal cultures to detect group A, C, or G streptococci in the health care workers involved with the index case. All streptococcal isolates should be saved for typing. The management of a health care worker suspected as a source of group A, C, or G streptococcal nosocomial infections includes treatment with antibiotics and removal from duty until posttherapy cultures reveal elimination of carriage. If only the throat culture is positive, treatment with 1.2 million units of benzathine penicillin intramuscularly has been recommended. For vaginal carriers, oral penicillin is given; for rectal carriers, oral penicillin or vancomycin is used. Group A streptococcus ordinarily is spread by direct person-to-person contact, most likely via droplets of saliva or nasal secretions. Because of the potential for spread of serious group A streptococci disease, barrier protection is necessary when health care workers are exposed to wound exudates from infected patients.

14. Why do group A streptococci cause nonsuppurative sequelae, such as rheumatic fever and glomerulonephritis?

Acute rheumatic fever (ARF) and acute glomerulonephritis (AGN) are late sequelae of previous streptococcal infection of the pharynx (ARF and AGN) or skin (AGN). Not all streptococcal strains cause these nonsuppurative sequelae, and not all human carriers of these strains develop the disease. Unknown host and bacterial factors (e.g., human HLA antigen, strain virulence) may trigger the sequelae.

Evidence links specific peptides of the streptococcal M protein molecule with human tissues. Epitopes of streptococcal M proteins share antigenic determinants with cardiac myosin, sarcolemmal membrane proteins, synovial membranes, articular cartilage, and human glomerular basement membrane. The apparent reason for the immune phenomenon after group A streptococcal infection is the cross-reactivity between streptococcal constituents and specific human tissues. This cross-reactivity elicits an immunologically mediated injury to target organs, such as heart, kidney, and joints.

15. What are the risk factors for perinatal group B streptococcal infection? How can it be prevented?

Group B streptococcus (GBS) is a leading cause of serious neonatal infection (meningitis and sepsis). Most neonatal GBS infections can be prevented through the use of intrapartum antimicrobial prophylaxis in women who are at increased risk for transmitting the infection to their newborns. However, despite demonstrated effectiveness of intrapartum antibiotic prophylaxis, prevention strategies have not been implemented widely or consistently, and the incidence of neonatal GBS disease has not declined. The CDC recommends the use of one of two prevention strategies:

1. Identify women by screening or
2. Give prophylaxis to women with risk factors.

In the first strategy, intrapartum antibiotic prophylaxis is offered to women who are identified as GBS carriers through prenatal screening cultures collected at 35–37 weeks' gestation and who develop one of the following conditions: rupture of membranes > 12 hours before delivery, premature onset of labor or rupture of membranes at < 37 weeks' gestation, maternal fever (> 37.5°C) during labor, history of previous delivery of an infant with GBS disease, and multiple-gestation pregnancy.

In the second strategy, intrapartum antibiotic prophylaxis is provided to women whose colonization for GBS is unknown, but who develop one or more risk conditions as above.

16. What are the infectious caused by *Enterococcus* spp.? How are they treated?

Most Common	*Treatment**
Urinary tract infection	Penicillin, ampicillin, amoxicillin
	Vancomycin
	Nitrofurantoin
	Fluoroquinolones
Bacteremia/endocarditis	High-dose ampicillin or penicillin + aminoglycoside[†]
	Vancomycin + aminoglycoside[†]
Intraabdominal and	Ampicillin or penicillin with or without aminoglycoside[†]
pelvic infections	(plus another drug active against anaerobes)

* Treatment of enterococcal infections should be guided by susceptibility testing.

[†] Use of this agent should be guided by the results of high-level susceptibility testing. This testing predicts whether synergistic killing will occur with the combination of an aminoglycoside and a cell-wall active agent. In some centers up to 30% of hospital-acquired strains are resistant to high levels of aminoglycosides, making bactericidal therapy impossible to achieve.

Less common infections due to enterococci include wound and soft tissue infections, meningitis, neonatal sepsis, and pneumonia (extremely rare; only in patients with a debilitating illness). Most clinical isolates of enterococci are *E. faecalis*, which accounts for 80–90% of the organisms recovered in clinical specimens. *E. faecium*, which is more resistant to antibiotics, accounts for 5–10% of isolates at most institutions. Other species occasionally isolated are *E. durans*, *E. avium*, *E. casseliflavus*, *E. gallinarum*, *E. raffinosus*, and *E. hirae*. The most striking attribute of enterococci is their relative and absolute resistance to a variety of antibiotics. Because both intrinsic and acquired resistance occurs, susceptibility testing is critical to direct the therapy.

17. What does VRE mean? What are the mechanisms of resistance?

VRE means **v**ancomycin-**r**esistant **e**nterococci. Vancomycin inhibits bacterial cell wall synthesis but at an earlier step than β-lactams. Vancomycin is a large and rigid molecule that forms complexes with the peptidyl-D-alanyl-D-alanine termini of peptidoglycan precursors at the cell wall surface, preventing cell wall synthesis by hindering the process of new wall formation. Resistance to vancomycin occurs when organisms synthesize precursors that have decreased affinity for vancomycin. This resistance is plasmid-mediated. Plasmids encode enzymatic mechanisms to alter the peptidoglycan biosynthetic pathway and transfer resistance by infusing genetic material into a susceptible enterococcus.

Most strains of VRE are *E. faecium*, which is intrinsically resistant to tobramycin—a fact that has made gentamicin the aminoglycoside of choice for combination bactericidal therapy. However, many VRE isolates demonstrate high levels of resistance to all aminoglycosides, including gentamicin. This resistance arises from production of enzymes that modify, by phosphorylation and acetylation, the aminoglycoside molecule, making it inactive. This resistance is mediated either by a plasmid-encoded gene or genetic material on the bacterial chromosome. A few of gentamicin-resistant isolates remain susceptible to high levels of streptomycin, making streptomycin useful for a few patients.

VRE infections typically are seen in hospitalized patients. The spectrum of illness includes asymptomatic colonization, device-related infections, and clinically serious infections similar to those in patients with ordinary enterococci (see question 16). The lack of an effective agent may make the infections incurable with medical therapy. Risk factors for VRE infection have been defined in various case–control studies: gastrointestinal colonization with VRE, advanced age, severe underlying illness, immunosuppression, ICU residence, surgery (especially gastrointestinal, cardiothoracic, transplantation), invasive devices, and exposure to third-generation cephalosporins, vancomycin, or antibiotics effective against anaerobic organisms.

18. What infection control measures are needed in cases of VRE colonization or infection?

In response to the alarming increase in VRE infections and limited antimicrobial therapy options, the Hospital Infection Control Practices Advisory Committee (HICPAC) has suggested the following measures to prevent further transmission:

1. **Education.** Hospital staff and personnel need to be educated on the seriousness of this infection, modes of transmission, and strategies for prevention.

2. **Early detection and reporting by the clinical microbiology laboratory**. Periodic surveillance cultures (stool or a rectal swab) of patients in hospital units in which VRE has been a problem may be used to detect carriers of VRE. Periodic susceptibility testing of enterococcal isolates from all specimens and all hospital units should be performed to detect resistance before it becomes widespread in an institution (see question 17).

3. **Prevention and control of nosocomial transmission.** Hospitals should implement strict contact isolation precaution (similar to those used for patients colonized or infected with MRSA), including placing VRE-infected or VRE-colonized patients in single rooms or in the same room as other patients with VRE; wearing gloves and gowns when entering the room of infected patients; and dedicated use of noncritical items (e.g., stethoscopes and thermometers) in a single patient or a cohort of patients. Signs in front of the room should announce and explain precaution measures.

4. **Preventing excessive vancomycin use.** Because prior vancomycin use may be a risk factor for colonization and infection with VRE, inappropriate or indiscriminate use of vancomycin should be discouraged, especially via the oral route.

CONTROVERSIES

19. Is MRSA more virulent than MSSA?

For: In a meticulous 30-month prospective study of MRSA colonization in a long-term care facility, Muder and colleagues showed that asymptomatic colonization with MRSA was 4 times more likely to lead to staphylococcal infection than either colonization with MSSA or no staphylococcal colonization. Another study demonstrated that patients with MRSA colonization have a higher rate of infection than those not colonized.

Against: Studies in the 1980s suggest that clinical presentations and outcomes do not differ significantly between two groups of patients with infections due to MRSA and MSSA. Recently, a retrospective study by Hershow and colleagues found no greater intrinsic virulence of MRSA in a teaching hospital.

20. How do we treat VRE infections?

Despite the lack of effective antimicrobial agents, few patients have died of infections due to this organism, probably because of its relatively low virulence. Patients with VRE line-related bacteremia may be cured simply by removal of the intravenous devices. Surgical site infections, soft tissue infections, and abscesses may be managed by surgical debridement and drainage without specific antimicrobial agents. Urinary tract infection due to VRE may resolve spontaneously or respond to oral agents, such as nitrofurantoin, amoxicillin, or fluoroquinolones; removal of indwelling bladder catheters is necessary. Available agents to which the organism is susceptible can be tried, although monotherapy with a fluoroquinolone, novobiocin, or tetracycline is often associated with rapid development of resistance. Quinupristin/dalfopristin (Synercid) has been used in compassionate-use protocols and is under formal investigation. Several other antimicrobial agents are at an early stage of development, but their usefulness has not yet been established.

21. Should we worry about the development of vancomycin resistance in *S. aureus*?

For: Conjugative transfer of vancomycin resistance from *E. faecalis* to *S. aureus* has been reported under laboratory conditions. This transfer has been observed both in vitro and in vivo on the skin of mice. The emergence of vancomycin-resistant strains of coagulase-negative staphylococci raises concern that such resistance will appear in *S. aureus*. Laboratories need to remain vigilant. Indeed, reports of *S. aureus* with an intermediate susceptibility (8–16 µg/ml) to vancomycin have already been received from Japan and the United States. Edmond and colleagues have offered proposals that may be used as starting points for the development of formal guidelines for the isolation of colonized and infected patients and for microbiology laboratory precautions to control *S. aureus* if it becomes resistant to vancomycin.

Against: Leclercq and colleagues were not able to transfer vancomycin resistance from enterococci to *S. aureus*. To date, no isolates of high-level vancomycin-resistant (> 32 µg/ml) *S. aureus* have been recovered from clinical specimens worldwide.

BIBLIOGRAPHY

1. Bisno AL, Stevens DL: Streptococcal infections of skin and soft tissues. N Engl J Med 334:240–245, 1996.
2. Carratala J, Marron A, Fernandez-Sevilla A, et al: Treatment of penicillin-resistant pneumococcal bacteremia in neutropenic patients with cancer. Clin Infect Dis 24(2):148–152, 1997.
3. Centers for Disease Control and Prevention: Defining the public health impact of drug-resistant *Streptococcus pneumoniae:* Report of a working group. MMWR 45(Supplement), 1996.
4. Centers for Disease Control and Prevention: Prevention of perinatal group B streptococcal disease: A public health perspective. MMWR 45(7):1–24, 1996.
5. Edmond MB, Ober JF, Weinbaum DL, et al: Vancomycin-resistant *Enterococcus faecium* bacteremia: Risk factors for infection. Clin Infect Dis 20:1126–1133, 1995.
6. Edmond MB, Wenzel RP, Pasculle AW: Vancomycin-resistant *Staphylococcus aureus:* Perspectives on measures needed for control. Ann Intern Med 124:329–334, 1996.
7. Hershow R, Khayr W, Smith N: A comparison of clinical virulence of nosocomially acquired methicillin-resistant and methicillin-sensitive *Staphylococcus aureus* infections in a university hospital. Infect Control Hosp Epidemiol 13:587–593, 1992.
8. Hospital Infection Control Practices Advisory Committee (HICPAC): Recommendations for preventing the spread of vancomycin resistance. Infect Control Hosp Epidemiol 16(2):105–113, 1995.
9. Hudson I: The efficacy of intranasal mupirocin in the prevention of staphylococcal infections: A review of recent experience [see comments]. J Hosp Infect 27(2):81–98, 1994.
10. Leclercq R, Courvalin P: Resistance to glycopeptides in enterococci. Clin Infect Dis 24:545–554, 1997.
11. Leclercq R, Derlot E, Weber M, et al: Transferable vancomycin and teicoplanin resistance in *Enterococcus faecium.* Antimicrob Agents Chemother 33:10–15, 1989.
12. Muder R, Brennen C, Wagener M, et al: Methicillin-resistant staphylococcal colonization and infection in a long-term care facility. Ann Intern Med 114:107–112, 1991.
13. Mulhausen P, Harrell L, Weinberger M, et al: Contrasting methicillin-resistant *Staphylococcus aureus* colonization in Veterans Affairs and community nursing homes. Am J Med 100:24–31, 1996.
14. Noble WC, Virani Z, Cree RGA: Co-transfer of vancomycin and other resistance genes from *Enterococcus faecalis* NCTC 12201 to *Staphylococcus aureus.* FEMS Microbiol Lett 93:195–198, 1992.
15. Pallares R, Linares J, Vadillo M, et al: Resistance to penicillin and cephalosporin and mortality from severe pneumococcal pneumonia in Barcelona, Spain. N Engl J Med 333:474–480, 1995.
16. Quagliarello VJ, Scheld WM: Treatment of bacterial meningitis. N Engl J Med 336:706–716, 1997.
17. Ramage L, Green K, Pyskir D, Simor AE: An outbreak of fatal nosocomial infections due to group A streptococcus on a medical ward. Infect Control Hosp Epidemiol 17:429–431, 1996.
18. Stevens DL, Bryant AE, Hackett SP: Antibiotic effects on bacterial viability, toxin production, and host response. Clin Infect Dis 20(Suppl 2):S154–S157, 1995.
19. Stevens DL, Gibbons AE, Bergstrom R, Winn V: The Eagle effect revisited: Efficacy of clindamycin, erythromycin, and penicillin in the treatment of streptococcal myositis. J Infect Dis 158:23–28, 1988.
20. Wetzel R: Prevention and Control of Nosocomial Infections, 2nd ed. Baltimore, Williams & Wilkins, 1992.

22. CLINICAL CONSIDERATIONS IN GRAM-NEGATIVE INFECTIONS

Cheryl K. McDonald, M.D., and Nancy E. Madinger, M.D.

1. What are some common lactose-fermenting gram-negative bacilli?

Gram-negative bacilli represent an enormous and diverse group of organisms and require a variety of phenotypic tests for accurate identification. One useful characteristic is fermentation of lactose, which helps to subdivide the family Enterobacteriaceae. *Enterobacter, Klebsiella, Escherichia,* and some *Citrobacter* spp. typically are lactose-fermenters (exceptions exist). *Salmonella, Shigella, Proteus,* and *Serratia* spp. do not ferment lactose. Organisms that do not utilize carbohydrates, such as *Pseudomonas* and *Acinetobacter* spp., appear to be non-lactose-fermenters on screening agar such as MacConkey, while in fact these organisms belong to the nonfermenting group.

2. What is the rationale for combination therapy in serious gram-negative infections?

1. **Synergistic killing** has been clearly demonstrated in vitro with the combination of a cell wall active agent (penicillin or cephalosporin) and an aminoglycoside for many gram-negative rods, including *Pseudomonas aeruginosa, Klebsiella pneumoniae, Serratia marcescens,* and *Escherichia coli.* Synergy is not completely predictable for any given organism or with any particular antimicrobial combination.

2. **Preventing the emergence of resistance** is theoretically attractive; however, no clear data indicate that combination therapy accomplishes this goal for gram-negative rod infections. Many experts advocate dual combination therapy for organisms such as *P. aeruginosa,* particularly in compromised hosts or for sites where antimicrobials have poor penetration.

3. What is the best therapy for a serious infection due to an *Enterobacter* species which is sensitive to third-generation cephalosporins?

Enterobacter spp. have a chromosomal gene encoding for a broad-spectrum cephalosporinase that hydrolyzes cephalosporins and penicillins and is resistant to β-lactamase inhibitors. This gene (*AmpC*) is usually regulated; that is, production is low at baseline, then markedly increases on exposure to cephalosporins (i.e., induction). Mutations in the regulatory gene occur frequently; thus, within a given bacterial population a few organisms may express large amounts of the cephalosporinase at all times. Third-generation cephalosporins are poor inducers of the gene but excellent selectors for mutants. Treatment failures may occur in up to 20% of bacteremias. It is appropriate to avoid third-generation cephalosporins in treating serious *Enterobacter* spp. infections. Alternative therapies include single or combination therapy with carbapenems, quinolones, trimethoprim-sulfamethoxazole, and aminoglycosides.

4. Name two unusual localized skin/soft-tissue infections due to *P. aeruginosa* that occur in normal hosts and the clinical scenario associated with each.

Tennis shoe cellulitis. Patients who have a puncture wound through the sole of the tennis shoe may become infected with *P. aeruginosa.* Empiric therapy should include antimicrobials effective against this organism.

Hot tub folliculitis. Several outbreaks of diffuse maculopapular pruritic folliculitis have been associated with *P. aeruginosa.* For the most part, the rashes are self-limited and do not require therapy. In immunocompromised patients, lesions may progress to ecthyma gangrenosum and therefore should be treated. There have been two reports of progressive disease in children, and although treatment is not usually recommended, infections in children should be followed carefully in the absence of therapy.

5. Which gram-negative infection is intrinsically resistant to imipenem? What is the best treatment?

Stenotrophomonas (Xanthomonas) maltophilia produces a β-lactamase that hydrolyzes carbapenems. Stenotrophomonal infections commonly arise in patients who have received imipenem for prolonged periods. The best antibiotic treatment is either trimethoprim-sulfamethoxazole or ticarcillin-clavulanate.

6. What are the three most common types of *E. coli* that produce diarrhea and the clinical syndrome associated with each?

1. **Enterotoxigenic *E. coli* (ETEC)** makes secretory toxins that produce watery diarrhea via a mechanism similar to that of cholera. ETEC is the cause of most traveler's diarrhea.

2. **Enteropathogenic *E. coli* (EPEC)** may attach to the gut epithelial surface, producing fever, vomiting, and diarrhea with prominent mucus. EPEC is most common in infants.

3. A subset of **enterohemorrhagic *E. coli* (EHEC)** may possess cytotoxins (shiga-like toxins), resulting in bloody diarrhea without stool leukocytes and often without fever. These strains are often serotype 0157:H7. Patients may develop hemolytic-uremic syndrome or thrombotic thrombocytopenic purpura (adults).

Numerous other types of *E. coli* are associated with diarrhea, including enteroinvasive (EIEC) strains that cause dysentery similar to *Shigella* sp.

7. Why are neonates prone to infection with *E. coli*, capsular type K1?

The K1 capsule of *E. coli* is a polymer of N-acetyl neuraminic acid, which is poorly immunogenic probably because it closely resembles compounds found in embryonic tissue. Studies have shown increased colonization of pregnant women with K1 strains. In a neonatal rat model, gastrointestinal colonization of the neonate with this strain often leads to bacteremia and meningitis, providing evidence for a possible mechanism for the same entity in human neonates.

8. Which two gram-negative rods have been most commonly associated with transfusion-related sepsis outbreaks? How does this occur?

1. *Yersinia enterocolitica* has been associated with fatal sepsis after transfusion of contaminated packed red blood cells. It is thought that the donor patient is asymptomatically bacteremic or recovering from a mild gastrointestinal illness. These bacteria are able to proliferate quite well at 4°C, producing a high bacterial and endotoxin burden that is then infused into the patient.

2. *Pseudomonas fluorescens* also has been associated with posttransfusion sepsis. This bacterium, rarely a pathogen in other settings, is thought to be introduced to the bag by skin contamination. Like *Y. enterocolitica*, *P. fluorescens* proliferates well at 4°C, producing an overwhelming burden of endotoxin that is then infused into the patient.

9. Which gram-negative bacilli are associated with Reiter's syndrome?

Postdysenteric Reiter's syndrome develops from a few days to a few months after infections with *Salmonella*, *Shigella*, *Yersinia*, and *Campylobacter* spp. As with posturethritis Reiter's syndrome, there is a high association with HLA B27 positivity. Up to 10–30% of adults with *Yersinia* infections in Scandinavia suffer from postdysenteric Reiter's syndrome.

10. What are the four most common clinical syndromes associated with *Salmonella* spp. infection?

1. **Gastroenteritis.** Symptoms typically develop 48 hours after ingestion of contaminated food or water. This clinical syndrome typically consists of watery, nonbloody diarrhea with fecal leukocytes, fever, and abdominal pain. Any species other than *S. typhi* may cause this syndrome, although outbreaks from egg-contaminated products are associated with *S. enteritidis*.

2. **Bacteremia without gastrointestinal symptoms.** These infections are often due to infection of an intravascular source, such as atherosclerotic plaques or aneurysms. Although classically associated with *S. choleraesuis* or *S. dublin*, any species may cause this syndrome. Because

of the propensity to infect plaques, transient bacteremias in middle-aged and elderly patients should receive antimicrobial therapy.

3. **Enteric fever.** Patients with enteric fever have severe constitutional symptoms and fever and may have any of the following: a faint rash with characteristic rose spots, diarrhea, neuropsychiatric symptoms, relative bradycardia, and hepatosplenomegaly. The syndrome is caused either by *S. typhi* (typhoid fever) or *S. paratyphi* (paratyphoid fever).

4. **Carrier state.** A small percentage of patients chronically shed *Salmonella* spp. from their gastrointestinal tract after infection. This entity is more common after infection with *S. typhi* than after infection with nontyphi species.

11. For which disease syndromes involving nontyphi *Salmonella* spp. are antibiotic therapies appropriate?

Antimicrobial therapy is not indicated for immunocompetent patients with gastroenteritis due to nontyphi *Salmonella* spp. Such therapy neither alters the course of the clinical symptoms nor reduces subsequent chronic carriage. Some studies have suggested a higher rate of relapse in patients who receive antibiotics. However, treatment is recommended for selected patients at higher risk of developing bacteremia or metastatic complications. Neonates, for example, are at a higher risk of developing bacteremia and meningitis and should receive antibiotics for *Salmonella* spp. gastroenteritis. Similarly, patients with atherosclerosis, structural cardiovascular abnormalities, or prosthesis should be treated. Immunosuppressed patients, such as patients with AIDS or organ transplants, may have recurrent bacteremia and should receive therapy.

12. Which gram-negative infection is associated with Guillain-Barré syndrome?

Antecedent gastrointestinal infection with *Campylobacter jejuni* has been reported in up to 26% of patients with Guillain-Barré syndrome (GBS). Compared with other patients with GBS, patients with GBS after *Campylobacter* sp. infection are more likely to have a pure motor syndrome, slow recovery, and severe residual disability.

13. Which gram-negative bacillus may cause a disease that mimics pulmonary tuberculosis? In what part of the world is this disease endemic?

Melioidosis, caused by *Burkholderia (Pseudomonas) pseudomallei*, may produce a latent infection that can present as cavitary pneumonia years after primary exposure. Other clinical presentations include acute suppurative lymphangitis, acute septicemia, and chronic suppurative infections of various organs. This organism is endemic in Southeast Asia.

14. What is the clinically significant difference in treatment of *Proteus mirabilis* versus *Proteus vulgaris* infections?

Proteus mirabilis tends to be susceptible to a broad range of antibiotics, including first generation cephalosporins. The other *Proteus* species, including *P. vulgaris*, tend to be much more resistant to antibiotics such as aminoglycosides and first- and second-generation cephalosporins. *P. mirabilis* is the only indole-negative species of *Proteus*. A rapid spot indole may help direct therapy before speciation and susceptibility test results.

15. What is the role of *Proteus* sp. infections in nephrolithiasis?

Proteus species have a urease enzyme that splits urea into ammonium hydroxide, thereby alkalinizing the urine and promoting formations of struvite stones. Obstruction of urinary outflow by the stones may further contribute to chronic infection.

16. What is Lemiere's syndrome?

Lemiere's syndrome is the name given to septic thrombophlebitis of the internal jugular vein, usually due to the anaerobic gram-negative rod, *Fusobacterium necrophorum*. The syndrome usually follows a nonspecific upper respiratory infection, and the patient presents with fever and lateral neck tenderness. Evidence of septic emboli to the lungs may be present on chest radiography.

17. The patient is found to have a *Klebsiella* sp. infection resistant to ceftazidime but susceptible to cefotetan. What is the explanation? What is the appropriate therapy?

The *Klebsiella* sp. is producing an extended spectrum β-lactamase (ESBL), which hydrolyzes third-generation cephalosporins more easily than second-generation cephalosporins. Use of the second-generation cephalosporin is controversial despite in vitro susceptibility. An appropriate alternative is the new fourth-generation cephalosporin, cefepime, which is less susceptible to hydrolysis by β-lactamase.

18. What is the significance of isolating *Burkholderia (Pseudomonas) cepacia* from the sputum of patients with cystic fibrosis?

Patients with cystic fibrosis, unlike healthy patients, are susceptible to colonization and disease with this often highly resistant organism. Transmission has been clearly documented between patients with cystic fibrosis in hospitals and social settings such as cystic fibrosis camps. Mortality rates are significantly higher in colonized vs. noncolonized patients. Because of the difficulty in treating this organism, colonization may constitute a relative contraindication to lung transplantation at some centers.

19. Which two gram-negative rods are associated with cellulitis after water exposure?

1. *Vibrio vulnificus* may cause cellulitis after salt water exposure. Ingestion of raw oysters also may predispose to infection. Patients with cirrhosis are especially prone to dissemination and poor outcomes after infection.

2. *Aeromonas hydrophila* cellulitis may follow exposure to fresh water. Local infections have been reported after leech application.

20. Which gram-negative rods are characteristically associated with dog, cat, and human bites, respectively? Which antibiotics are appropriate to cover these pathogens?

Cat bites are typically associated with local infection due to *Pasteurella multocida*, which colonizes the mouths of up to 70% of cats.

Dog bites have been associated with infection due to *Capnocytophaga canimorsus* (previously called dysgonic fermenter 2 [DF-2]). Infection may result in a fatal sepsis syndrome in patients who are immunocompromised or asplenic. A second species, *C. cynodegmi* (previously called DF-2–like organisms), is less commonly associated with dog bites and thus far appears to cause only localized disease.

Human bites may be complicated by infection with the gram-negative bacillus, *Eikenella corrodens*, a common mouth flora bacteria in humans.

Although each of the above gram-negative rods is usually susceptible to penicillin or amoxicillin, bite wound infections are often accompanied by anaerobic bacteria. Thus, amoxicillin-clavulanic acid is generally the antibiotic of choice for outpatient therapy of such infections.

BIBLIOGRAPHY

1. Agger WA, Marden A: *Pseudomonas aeruginosa* infections of intact skin. Clin Infect Dis 20:302–308, 1995.
2. Chow JW, Fine MJ, Shales DM, et al: *Enterobacter* bacteremia: Clinical features and emergence of antibiotic resistance during therapy. Ann Intern Med 115:585–590, 1991.
3. Fang FC, Madinger NE: Resistant nosocomial gram-negative bacillary pathogens: *Acinetobacter baumannii, Xanthomonas maltophilia*, and *Pseudomonas cepacia*. Curr Clin Top Infect Dis 16:52–83, 1996.
4. Goldberg MB, Rubin RH: The spectrum of *Salmonella* infection. Infect Dis Clin North Am 2:571–598, 1988.
5. Goldstein EJ: Bite wounds and infection. Clin Infect Dis 14:633–638, 1992.
6. Leelarasamee A, Bovornkitti S: Melioidosis: Review and update. Rev Infect Dis 12:413–425, 1989.
7. Levine MM: *Escherichia coli* that cause diarrhea: Enterotoxigenic, enteropathogenic, enteroinvasive, enterohemorrhagic, and enteroadherent. J Infect Dis 155: 377–389, 1987.
8. Rees JH, Soudain SE, Gregson NA, Hughes RA: *Campylobacter jejuni* infection and Guillain-Barré syndrome. N Engl J Med 333:1374–1379, 1995.
9. Sanders CC, Sanders WE: Beta-lactam resistance in gram-negative bacteria: Global trends and clinical impact. Clin Infect Dis 824–839, 1992.

VI. Mycobacterial Infections

23. TUBERCULOSIS: THE WHITE PLAGUE REVISITED

John H. Hammer, M.D., and David L. Cohn, M.D.

1. What is the cause of tuberculosis?

Mycobacterium tuberculosis is a strictly aerobic, non–spore-forming, slow-growing (doubling time: 12–18 hours), nonmotile bacteria; its only natural reservoir is humans. Unlike other mycobacteria, infection is transmissible from person to person via aerosolized pulmonary secretions; transmission generally occurs through prolonged exposure in a relatively closed space. If infection results in disease, the course tends to be chronic and indolent. Rapid progression to fulminant disease may result if the host is immunocompromised. The host's cell-mediated immune response is primarily responsible for containment of infection and disease.

2 What does the term *acid-fast* mean in reference to tuberculosis?

Microbiologically, once the organisms are stained, they resist destaining with acid-alcohol treatment and are therefore referred to as acid-fast bacilli (AFB). This retention is theoretically due to the complexing of the carbolfuschin stain with mycolic acids present in the waxy cell wall. When the organism is cultured on complex solid media (Löwenstein-Jensen or Middlebrook 7H10 agar) at 37°C, opaque colonies are usually visible in 3–6 weeks. The time to positive culture may be halved by use of the radiometric (BACTEC) method with Middlebrook 7H12 (liquid) medium.

3. What is the incidence of tuberculosis in the United States?

In 1995 there were 22,860 cases of tuberculosis (TB) with an incidence of 8.7 cases per 100,000 population. The incidence has declined steadily since 1953, when there were 84,304 cases (53 cases/100,000), with the exception of a much publicized hump in late 1980s to early 1990s, which peaked in 1993 with 26,673 cases (10.5 cases/100,000). This increase was due largely to cases of TB in HIV-infected persons and changes within the federal and local public health infrastructure. Incidence rates by state in 1995 varied from 0.7/100,000 (Vermont) to 16.9/100,000 (New York). States with above average rates (> 8.7/100,000) included New York, California, Hawaii, Alaska, Texas, and all southern states except North Carolina, Virginia, West Virginia, and Kentucky. Mortality rates have remained fairly constant over the past decade at 0.6–0.8 deaths/100,000 population.

4. What is the incidence of TB worldwide?

In 1990 an estimated 8 million cases of tuberculosis (TB) resulted in approximately 3 million deaths. Ninety-five percent of these cases and 98% of the deaths occurred in developing countries, where 80% of cases involved persons between 15 and 59 years of age. According to a 1989 report from the World Health Organization, approximately 1.3 million cases and 450,000 deaths occurred in children younger than 15 years in developing countries. It is predicted that the 1990s will see approximately 90 million new cases of TB with an estimated 30 million deaths (if global control maintains its current level). TB is the most common preventable infectious disease in adults in the world.

5. What is the impact of HIV infection on global tuberculosis?

If the above picture is not bleak enough, consider the interaction of HIV and TB worldwide. Conservative calculations in 1994 estimated that 5.6 million people were coinfected with HIV and *M. tuberculosis*. Although an estimated 80,000 coinfected persons lived in North America, the majority (3.8 million) lived in sub-Saharan Africa, where the incidence of TB in some resource-poor countries has doubled or tripled. It is estimated that 20% of TB cases in sub-Saharan Africa are directly attributable to HIV. In many African countries HIV seroprevalence is greater than 50% among patients with TB. Asia contains almost two-thirds of the world's population infected with *M. tuberculosis*. The spread of HIV in Southeast Asia in the 1990s has been relentless, and its association with TB is both predictable and sobering. In northern Thailand, for example, HIV seroprevalence in patients with TB increased from 5% in 1989 to 26% in 1992. It is likely that this trend will continue into the foreseeable future.

In many developing countries TB has emerged as the most common opportunistic disease associated with HIV infection. Up to 72% of patients with AIDS in Africa, 24–28% of patients in Brazil and Mexico, and more than 50% of patients in India and Thailand have had clinical TB during the course of HIV infection.

6. What is multidrug-resistant tuberculosis (MDR-TB)?

MDR-TB is defined as TB that is resistant to more than one drug—right? Almost. Because the two most potent drugs used to treat TB are isoniazid (INH) and rifampin, MDR-TB conventionally refers to strains that are resistant to *both* drugs (with or without resistance to other first-line drugs).

7. How common is antimycobacterial drug resistance in the United States?

The incidence of drug resistance in the United States varies by both geographic distribution and demographic characteristics. In 1991 the Centers for Disease Control and Prevention conducted a nationwide survey to determine patterns of antituberculosis drug resistance and found MDR-TB in 3.5% of cases, with resistance to INH and/or rifampin in 9.5% of cases. New York City accounted for 61.4% of the nation's MDR-TB cases, which occurred during several outbreaks, largely in HIV-infected patients. When compared with the population-based rate in white Americans, the relative risk of MDR-TB in white New Yorkers was 39; in Hispanics, 299; in Asian/Pacific Islanders, 421; and in blacks, 701.

A 1995 survey of cases of tuberculosis treated in 8 relatively urban counties bordering Mexico found an MDR prevalence of 0.3% in U.S.-born whites, 1.1% in U.S.-born Hispanics, and 2.3% in foreign-born Hispanics. The prevalence of INH resistance was 3.9%, 7.2%, and 6.6%, respectively.

8. Which areas of the world are known to have a high prevalence of antimycobacterial drug resistance?

Representative studies of drug resistance patterns in the developing world are difficult to find. Many studies fail to differentiate between primary resistance (resistance in a patient who has received no therapy) and acquired resistance (history of previous drug therapy). From an epidemiologic standpoint this difference is significant. The general model is emergence of drug resistance in areas that are affluent enough to afford antituberculous drugs but have no effective TB control program. The resultant misuse of drugs (improper prescribing practices, nonadhrerence to prescribed regimens, availability of agents in the private market leading to inappropriate monotherapy) inevitably leads to drug resistance within a given area. Over the past 15 years the prevalence of primary resistance to at least two drugs (not INH and rifampin) of greater than 5% has been described in Benin, Ghana, Mali, Zaire, China (Beijing), India (Gujarat), Korea, Pakistan (Karachi), Saudi Arabia (Taif), Turkey (Istanbul), Haiti, Puerto Rico, and New York City. Of note, if acquired resistance is included, prevalence rates of greater than 40% have been recorded in Mauritania, Korea, Saudi Arabia, and the Philippines (Manila).

9. What is BCG? What is the rationale for its use?

The bacille Calmette-Guérin (BCG) vaccine was derived by in vitro attenuation of an isolate of *M. bovis* (the pathogenic species in cattle) and was first given to humans in 1921. Since that time, despite much controversy about the vaccine's efficacy and mechanism of action, BCG has become the most commonly used vaccine worldwide. Multiple field studies of vaccine efficacy have generally revealed decreasing benefit in populations nearer the equator (unfortunately, in the very areas that could use an effective vaccine). Theoretically, these populations have more consistent exposure to endogenous nontuberculous mycobacteria, thereby generating a natural cross-immunity to TB that overshadows any apparent benefit of BCG. The vaccine's mechanism of action is thought to be related to the development of delayed-type hypersensitivity, but its true effect is unknown. It appears to reduce uniformly the incidence of TB meningitis and other forms of disseminated TB in children but is less impressive in the prevention of pulmonary disease in adults. This finding has led to the speculation that it is more effective in inducing protection against the hematogenous spread of tubercle bacilli than in inducing local protection in the lungs.

10. What is a positive PPD? What is its significance?

Purified protein derivative (PPD) is manufactured by killing *M. tuberculosis* in culture, then concentrating and precipitating the culture filtrate. All lots are standardized for biologic activity with respect to a particular lot of tuberculin (PPD-S) kept in Copenhagen. Five tuberculin units (TU) or 0.1 ml is injected intradermally, and the diameter of induration is read at 48–72 hours. Although still widely used, "control" injections to test for anergy are of marginal benefit. A positive PPD (also known as tuberculin-positive), as defined below, indicates past or present infection with TB and varies by risk for infection.

Definition of Positive PPD

≥ 5 mm	≥ 10 mm	≥ 15 mm
Contacts of infectious cases	Infants and children under 4 years of age	People not in high-risk groups or high-risk environments
Fibrotic lesions on chest radiograph	Foreign-born people from high-prevalence areas	People 35 years of age or older with history of exposure in the past 2 years
HIV infection or other immunosuppression	Medically underserved, low-income populations	
	Other at-risk populations (e.g., health care workers, residents of long-term care facilities)	
	People younger than 35 yr with history of exposure in the past 2 years	

11. To what do we attribute PPD reactions that are smaller than the prescribed cut-off?

Generally, insignificant reactions are attributed to exposure to endogenous nontuberculous mycobacteria (or atypical mycobacteria), including prior BCG vaccination.

12. What is the difference between tuberculosis infection and disease?

Tuberculosis infection refers to the process beginning with exposure, in which the patient is inoculated with the bacteria (usually via the lungs), followed by lymphatic uptake of infected macrophages and then hematogenous dissemination of the bacteria. In a normal host, the infection is contained by a predominantly cell-mediated response that results in a positive skin test with PPD challenge—usually detectable within 8–12 weeks of infection. This entire process is usually asymptomatic. Tuberculosis disease occurs in 10–20% of infected persons (3–5% in the first year after infection) and refers to progressive infection poorly contained by host defense mechanisms associated with symptoms determined by the site of disease. This process most commonly occurs in lung parenchyma as a progressive infiltrative and cavitating process but also may occur virtually anywhere. Lymph nodes, bones and joints, kidneys, and the central nervous system are the most common extrapulmonary sites of infection. The distinction between infection and disease has important disease control and therapeutic implications.

13. How is tuberculosis transmitted from person to person?

Although transmission has been described via aerosols (laboratory accident, wound irrigation), direct inoculation (needle stick), and placental transfer, these routes are exceedingly rare. The major (essentially only) route of transmission is via airborne **droplet nuclei** produced by a coughing, sneezing, speaking, or singing person with pulmonary or upper airway disease. Droplet nuclei are microscopic droplets (1–3 microns) that can contain hundreds of bacilli. They are capable of remaining suspended in the air for prolonged periods and are quickly dispersed with air flow. Their small size permits passage past the mucociliary blanket into the alveoli, where the process of infection begins. Patients with tuberculosis who are smear-positive and/or have cavities on chest radiograph are more infectious to others because they exhale a greater number of organisms than those who are smear-negative or do not have cavities.

14. Under what circumstances should one consider placing a patient with "possible TB" in respiratory isolation when admitted to the hospital?

The first step in treating and containing the spread of TB is to consider the diagnosis. Screening criteria for a given health care system should be based on the prevalence and characteristics of TB in the area served. For the individual patient, risk factors should be considered for both infection and progression to disease:

- Risk factors for **infection:** prior TB or PPD positivity, family, or exposure history, country or region of birth and residence, age, socioeconomic status (homeless?)
- Risk factors for **progression** to disease: HIV infection, silicosis, and other medical conditions or therapies associated with immunosuppression (e.g., diabetes mellitus, lymphoma, cancer chemotherapy)

Symptoms suggestive of active TB include:
- Cough of at least three weeks' duration (with or without hemoptysis)
- Constitutional symptoms such as night sweats, weight loss, anorexia, and fever

Radiographic findings suggestive of TB include:
- Upper lobe infiltrate(s) with or without cavitation in the "normal" host
- Hilar adenopathy, pleural effusion, and parenchymal infiltrates in either upper or lower lobes in the HIV-infected/immunosuppressed host

If a given patient is hospitalized with risk factors, symptoms, and radiographic findings suggestive of active pulmonary TB, respiratory isolation should be strongly considered pending examination of serial sputa for acid-fast bacilli.

15. What isolation precautions should be taken for a patient with non-pulmonary tuberculosis?

As described above, the prime mode of transmission of TB is via droplet nuclei released from a patient with respiratory tract disease. If a patient with nonpulmonary TB has no signs or symptoms of pulmonary disease (no cough, normal chest radiograph), respiratory isolation is not generally indicated. However, contact isolation and masking in manipulating an open tuberculous wound or sinus tract are prudent.

16. When should one consider hospital admission for a patient with suspected active tuberculosis?

If the patient presents to or can be reliably referred to an effective TB control program, active tuberculosis can generally be managed on an outpatient basis. The program should be able to obtain background information efficiently, screen all household, work, and other contacts who may be at risk for infection, and initiate and follow through with a course of directly observed therapy. Reliable access to a laboratory that can process and read an AFB smear, grow and identify the organism, and determine drug susceptibilities is also critical. Potential indications for hospital admission include:

- Acutely ill or unstable patients with or without an established diagnosis (including most HIV-infected patients).
- Patients in whom noncompliance with follow-up or drug therapy is likely to become an issue (including acutely intoxicated patients or those with a history of noncompliance).
- Patients with an unstable home or social situation (which may lead to noncompliance as well as to the exposure of additional persons; the classic example is a homeless shelter).

Note: Patients with active pulmonary TB have most likely been infectious for some time and have already exposed people with whom they have shared relatively closed spaces. The public health objective at the time of initial evaluation is to prevent the exposure of additional persons (potentially including hospital patients and employees) and to screen people already exposed for disease and infection (such as household contacts).

17. What is Pott's disease?

Pott's disease of the spine, or tuberculous spondylitis, refers to infection of the vertebral bodies as a result of hematogenous dissemination (usually with initial infection), contiguous disease, or lymphatic spread from pleural disease. It most commonly affects the lower thoracic spine and presents as chronic back pain without systemic symptoms. If the disease is allowed to progress, destruction of contiguous vertebral bodies with intervening disc obliteration ensues, resulting in a tender spine prominence or gibbus. Paralysis and/or sinus tract formation may follow without treatment. In developing countries children and elderly people are most commonly affected, whereas in developed countries Pott's disease primarily affects the elderly.

18. What is miliary TB?

Miliary TB refers to pulmonary TB with a classic radiographic pattern of soft nodules, 2–3 mm in diameter, involving all lung fields. The term *miliary* is derived from this appearance, which early observers likened to millet seeds scattered throughout the lungs. In actuality this process represents hematogenous dissemination of a poorly contained infection with small tuberculous abscesses usually found throughout the body. It is generally seen in immunocompromised (e.g., HIV-infected) hosts.

19. What are the clinical manifestations of tuberculosis in HIV-infected patients?

The deleterious effects of HIV infection on cell-mediated immunity result in a high rate of reactivation in persons previously infected with *M. tuberculosis* and also predisposes to reinfection with new strains of tuberculosis. In addition, the clinical manifestations of TB may be atypical, especially in patients in the late stages of HIV infection. Extrapulmonary TB with or without pulmonary disease occurs in 25–75% of patients, especially lymphatic, central nervous system, and miliary forms. Widely disseminated TB in association with sepsis syndrome also has been seen. Chest radiographic abnormalities may be unusual, with mediastinal or hilar lymphadenopathy, lower lobe interstitial infiltrates, and pleural effusions.

20. When should drug therapy be initiated for infection? With what drug(s)?

Because tuberculosis infection is asymptomatic, it is revealed by skin-test conversion.

For tuberculin-positive immunocompetent patients:

- With an unknown exposure history or known exposure to isoniazid (INH)-sensitive organisms: isoniazid preventive therapy (IPT), including INH 300 mg plus vitamin B6, 50 mg/day for 6 months (normal chest radiograph) or 12 months (abnormal chest radiograph consistent with past tuberculosis and negative sputum smear).
- With known exposure to INH-resistant organisms: rifampin, 300 mg/day, or rifampin plus ethambutol, 15 mg/kg/day for 12 months.
- With known exposure to MDR-TB: no treatment with careful observation or empiric use of pyrazinamide, 20 mg/kg, plus ethambutol, 15 mg/kg/day, or pyrazinamide plus a fluoroquinolone.

For HIV-infected patients:
- Who is tuberculin-positive or has a documented history of a positive skin test with no known exposure to drug-resistant organisms: IPT for 12 months.
- Who is anergic and a known contact of drug-sensitive TB: IPT (12-month course).
- Who is tuberculin-positive after exposure to INH-resistant organisms: 12-month course of rifampin or rifampin/ethambutol (as above).
- Who has been exposed to MDR-TB with a high likelihood of infection (skin test conversion or anergic): pyrazinamide/ethambutol or pyrazinamide/fluoroquinolone combination (as above) for 12 months.

21. When should drug therapy be initiated for suspected active tuberculosis?

The timing of initiation of therapy for TB generally depends on one's index of suspicion for disease. If a sputum/tissue specimen is smear-positive for acid-fast bacilli, therapy with a 3–4 drug regimen (see below) should begin as soon as one is assured that an adequate specimen has been saved for culture with subsequent identification and susceptibility testing. If initial specimens are smear-negative, one must consider additional factors such as the patient's risk for infection, exposure history, clinical presentation, radiographic findings, and adequacy of the sputum/tissue specimen and examination. Regardless of whether therapy is initiated, specimen culture should be in progress. In the case of pulmonary TB, an adequately obtained and examined sputum that is smear-negative may be somewhat reassuring, because the patient is unlikely to be highly infectious. But if the index of suspicion is high because of risk factors and clinical presentation or if the prospects for compliance with follow-up are low, empiric therapy pending culture results may be considered.

22. Which antituberculous drugs are safe in pregnancy and lactation?

This question is asked fairly often by obstetricians and family physicians. Untreated TB presents a far greater risk to both the mother and her fetus than does treatment of the disease. Conversely, maternal TB is not an indication for therapeutic abortion. INH (with pyridoxine), rifampin, and ethambutol are thought to be safe in pregnancy. These drugs cross the placenta but have not been shown to have teratogenic effects. Because its teratogenic effects are unknown, pyrazinamide is not generally used in the United States (but it is used in other countries). Streptomycin is the only antituberculous drug documented to have harmful effects on the fetus (interference with ear development that may result in congenital deafness) and should not be used. Because of the scant information about other, second-line drugs, they should be avoided if possible.

As for lactation, due to the fact that only small concentrations of antituberculosis drugs reach the breast milk, nursing should not be discouraged. Conversely, drugs in the breast milk should not be considered effective treatment for disease, or as adequate preventive therapy, in the nursing infant.

23. What drug regimen should be initiated for active pulmonary disease? What course of therapy is recommended once the tuberculosis is determined to be drug-sensitive?

Because of outbreaks of MDR-TB and the growing problem of or potential for drug-resistant TB in many geographic areas, in 1993 the Centers for Disease Control and Prevention updated its treatment recommendations. Initial treatment for all patients should consist of four drugs, including isoniazid (INH), rifampin (RIF), and pyrazinamide (PZA) with ethambutol (EMB) or streptomycin (SM). All drugs are given orally except streptomycin, a parenteral agent. When community rates of INH resistance are known to be less than 4%, three drugs (INH, RIF and PZA) may be used initially. If organisms are found to be susceptible by antimicrobial susceptibility testing (now recommended for all patients), isoniazid and rifampin alone can be used after 8 weeks of initial four-drug therapy and continued for an additional 16 weeks to complete a 6-month regimen in immunocompetent patients.

In HIV-infected patients, the CDC recommends that the usual 6 months of total therapy be extended if the patient's clinical or microbiologic response is slow or suboptimal. The widespread use of protease inhibitors in HIV-infected patients presents potential difficulties because the hepatic metabolism of protease inhibitors tends to interfere with the metabolism of rifampin (and vice versa). When these agents are coadministered, rifampin levels (and potential toxicities) are increased, whereas protease inhibitor levels fall, potentially leading to decreased efficacy and emergence of HIV resistance. Although several possible treatment options for this scenario have been generally outlined, discussion of their relative merits and drawbacks is beyond the scope of this chapter.

It is now widely acknowledged that a major cause of drug-resistant TB and treatment failure is patient noncompliance with therapy; therefore, directly observed therapy (DOT) should be considered for all patients. To facilitate the delivery of DOT, several options using twice-weekly and thrice-weekly dosing after 0–8 weeks of daily therapy have been deemed acceptable. These options are summarized below:

Initial Treatment of Tuberculosis

Option 1
    8 weeks: INH, RIF, PZA, and EMB or SM daily*
    16 weeks: INH, RIF daily or 2-3 times/wk[†]

Option 2
    2 weeks: INH, RIF, PZA, and EMB or SM daily*
    6 weeks: INH, RIF, PZA, and EMB or SM 2 times/wk[†]
    16 weeks: INH, RIF 2 times/wk

Option 3
    24 weeks: INH, RIF, PZA, and EMB or SM 3 times/wk

For HIV-infected patients, use options 1, 2, or 3, but regimens may be longer than 6 months if culture conversion is delayed. Consider directly observed therapy in all patients, using regimens administered 2 or 3 times/wk.
* When INH resistance is known to be <4%, INH, RIF, and PZA may be used for initial therapy.
[†] Change to INH and RIF alone after 8 weeks when susceptibility to INH and RIF has been demonstrated.

Note: Patients found to have INH resistance should be treated with at least three other first-line agents for 6–9 months (for HIV-infected patients, 9–12 months). Patients with MDR-TB should be treated for 18–24 months with at least 3 or 4 agents to which the organism is susceptible. Above all, always remember the credo: Do *not* add a single drug to a failing regimen, because the added agent will soon be lost.

24. Why can we treat tuberculosis infection with one agent, whereas multiple drugs are necessary to treat tuberculosis disease?

When one thinks of tuberculosis infection, one should think of initial inoculation followed by a transitory hematogenous shower of organisms that is quickly subdued by the host immune system. This process has already come and gone by the time the skin test converts and therapy is initiated. Because there are no signs or symptoms of disease (the chest radiograph is "negative"), we are empirically treating a small focus of infection waiting for the right time to reactivate. Because both isoniazid and rifampin are extremely active against tuberculosis, either one as a single agent should be able to treat a small, occult infection. The prolonged course of therapy is prescribed because of the slowed doubling time of organisms in a resting state.

In active tuberculosis disease (e.g., cavitary pulmonary disease), poorly controlled infection involves billions of organisms multiplying at variable rates. Multiple agents are needed to kill rapidly a large number of organisms. In addition, because the spontaneous point mutation rate conferring resistance to a given drug is approximately one organism in one million, what is likely to happen if we give a single agent to the unfortunate patient? Within several weeks we will have managed to select for organisms that are resistant to the drug, and we will never be able to use it for this patient again. The same principle applies to the aforementioned credo (see question 23) about adding drugs to a failing regimen. Herein lies the principle for treating active disease with multiple agents. After 8 weeks of therapy, the disease burden has been decreased to the point that the two highly active agents, isoniazid and rifampin, can be used for the remaining course of therapy, provided that the initial organisms are susceptible, to kill slowly growing "persisters".

Imagine what would happen if the patient is given a two-month supply of pills with specific instructions and subsequently decides to stop one drug because "it wasn't working" and takes another once weekly "because it upsets my stomach," giving the extra pills to a friend "because she had a cough." Voila—we have acquired drug resistance.

25. When should directly observed therapy be used?

In the early 1990s, it was apparent that the battle against TB in the United States was being lost. The two major markers of this failure were the increasing incidence of TB and the rising prevalence of drug resistance. These findings were particularly striking in the inner cities. Although 6–9-month drug regimens had proven efficacy in curing TB, high rates of treatment failure jeopardized patient welfare and allowed patients to transmit infection to others, thus creating a growing public health risk. It was known that treatment nonadherence rates with self-administered therapy were at least 30% (and higher in some populations). It was also known that professionals are consistently unable to distinguish compliant from noncompliant patients in advance. Only with the widespread institution of directly observed therapy (DOT) were rising inner city rates of TB and MDR-TB curbed. DOT simply refers to the practice of giving patients their pills and seeing that they are swallowed. DOT can be accomplished by a nurse or aide in a given clinic (or at the patient's home or place of work).

A cost-analysis compared a directly observed 62-dose (twice-weekly therapy for the last 16 weeks) regimen to a daily self-administered regimen, factoring in drug and nursing costs along with laboratory and radiology costs. The analysis found that a course of therapy using DOT was $51 less expensive than a course of self-administered therapy ($561 vs. $612). The potential costs of a failed regimen, including retreatment, potential drug resistance, and possible infection of contacts, were not factored into the analysis.

Who should receive DOT? Given the potential risks of noncompliance with self-administered therapy and the fact that noncompliance cannot be reliably predicted by professionals, it has been recommended that all patients with drug-sensitive tuberculosis receive largely intermittent DOT. As of 1993, only 10–12% of patients with tuberculosis in the United States were treated with DOT. We have a long way to go.

BIBLIOGRAPHY

1. American Thoracic Society/Centers for Disease Control and Prevention: Treatment of tuberculosis and tuberculosis infection in adults and children. Am J Respir Crit Care Med 149:1359–1374, 1994.
2. Barnes PF, Bloch AB, Davidson PT, Snider DE: Tuberculosis in patients with human immunodeficiency virus infection. N Engl J Med 324:1644–1650, 1991.
3. Bloch AB, Cauthen GM, Onorato IM, et al: Nationwide survey of drug-resistant tuberculosis in the United States. JAMA 271:665–671, 1994.
4. Centers for Disease Control and Prevention: Screening for tuberculosis and tuberculous infection in high-risk populations and the use of preventative therapy for tuberculous infection in the United States. MMWR 39(RR-8):1–12, 1990.
5. Cohn DL, Bustreo F, Raviglione MC: Drug-resistant tuberculosis: Review of the worldwide situation and the WHO/IUATLD global surveillance project. Clin Infect Dis 24(Suppl l):S121–130, 1997.
6. Raviglione MC, Snider DE, Kochi A: Global epidemiology of tuberculosis. JAMA 273:220–226, 1995.

24. MYCOBACTERIA OTHER THAN TUBERCULOSIS

Nina J. Karlin, M.D.

1. What organisms are represented by MOTT?

MOTT stands for "mycobacteria other than tuberculosis," including:

M. avium complex	*M. kansasii*	*M. chelonei*	*M. simiae*
M. marinum	*M. fortuitum*	*M. ulcerans*	*M. haemophilum*
M. scrofulaceum	*M. szulgai*	*M. xenopi*	

2. What type of person is at risk for MOTT infections?

MOTT occurs most commonly in immunocompromised patients, e.g., those with HIV infection. Others at particular risk include patients with underlying disease such as chronic obstructive pulmonary disease (COPD), malignancy, prior *M. tuberculosis* infection, bronchiectasis, emphysema, chronic aspergillosis, achalasia, and silicosis. It also may be found in persons with impaired cell-mediated immunity and occasionally in patients with an intact immune function.

3. What are the clinical and radiographic features of pulmonary MOTT infection?

Clinical features include chronic and productive cough, dyspnea, hemoptysis, fever, malaise, weight loss, and fatigue. Clinical pulmonary infection occurs when organisms gain access to the lower respiratory tract in a susceptible host. **Radiographic features** include upper lobe cavitation, lower lobe nodules, solitary pulmonary nodules, lower lobe infiltrates, and/or abscess formation.

4. If you are clever enough to think someone has MOTT, how would you prove it?

Diagnosis is based on the isolation of the particular organism in a patient with an appropriate clinical syndrome. Identification of the organism is key because signs, symptoms, and radiographic findings are neither sensitive nor specific for MOTT. Specimens submitted for culture should be inoculated onto solid and broth media. Solid media detect growth in 2–4 weeks and broth media in 1 week. Because most local hospital laboratories are usually not properly equipped, the majority of isolates are sent to state health departments for speciation. Newer methods for identification not yet widely used (but on the horizon) include thin-layer chromatography, gas–liquid chromatography, high-pressure liquid chromatography, and amplification of mycobacterial DNA via polymerase chain reaction (PCR).

5. What are the rapidly growing mycobacteria?

Rapidly growing mycobacteria include *M. abscessus*, *M. smegmatis*, *M. fortuitum*, and *M. chelonae* and grow well in only 1–3 days on standard mycobacteria media. With the exception of *M. fortuitum* and *M. chelonae*, most of these organisms are saprophytes and do not have an association with human disease. They have been isolated from municipal water, contaminated aquariums, marine life, and domestic animals. Human infections are usually acquired by accidental trauma, surgery, or injection.

6. What clinical syndromes do the rapidly growing mycobacteria cause?

The rapidly growing mycobacteria most commonly cause skin and soft tissue infections (pyogenic abscesses and ulceration) via a penetrating wound or foreign body. Lung disease occurs infrequently. Less common infections include lymphadenitis, osteomyelitis, mediastinitis, endocarditis, meningitis, and peritonitis. Infections are more commonly seen in patients with severe underlying diseases (lymphoma/leukemia, collagen-vascular disease, hemodialysis-associated renal failure) or patients receiving immunosuppressive therapy.

7. How are rapidly growing mycobacteria infections treated?

Treatment includes surgical removal of all involved tissue (if possible) as well as appropriate antibiotic coverage for 2–4 weeks. Because these organisms are highly resistant to typical anti-tuberculosis drugs, sensitivity testing should be performed. Recommended treatment consists of amikacin (10–15 mg/kg/day) and cefoxitin (200 mg/kg/day) for 6 months. Clarithromycin, 500 mg 2 times/day for 6 months, is an alternate regimen. Less serious infections can be treated with sulfa-methoxazole (3 gm/day) or doxycycline (200 mg/day) for 2–4 months. In patients with extensive tissue or organ involvement and patients who are more immunocompromised, three or more drugs may be used for a more prolonged course. Antibiotic susceptibilities are not uniform within this group; therapy should be guided by the individual organism and the results of susceptibility testing.

8. What does "MAC" mean? Where are these organisms found?

MAC stands for *Mycobacterium avium* complex, which includes both *M. avium* and *M. intracellulare* (*M. scrofulaceum* is occasionally grouped with MAC.). Of all the MOTT organisms, these two cause pulmonary or disseminated disease with the greatest frequency. Ubiquitous in the environment, MAC is found in soil, water, dairy products, house dust, and both domestic and wild animals. In one New York County, MAC was isolated from 32% of random water samples. Aerosolized organisms cause infection after gaining access to the lower respiratory tract. Of interest, the disease has a high prevalence in the southeastern United States, Texas, Louisiana, Pacific Northwest, and north central plains. In coastal areas, MAC may be aerosolized from brackish water by wave action. Furthermore, MAC has been found with greater frequency in females with scoliosis, decreased anteroposterior diameter, and mitral valve prolapse.

9. What underlying pulmonary diseases are commonly associated with MAC infection?

The usual suspects are COPD, previous primary TB infection, bronchogenic carcinoma, bronchiectasis, pulmonary fibrosis, and pneumoconioses, all of which predispose to MAC infection.

10. How is the diagnosis of MAC established? Why is it important to distinguish between colonization and infection?

Diagnosis requires isolation of the organism along with appropriate clinical and pathologic features. Identification of MAC in the sputum does *not* constitute definitive disease. However, the presence of cavities not attributed to another disease process (TB or fungal infection) and more than two sputum or bronchial washing specimens with moderate-to-heavy growth of MAC indicate infection. For patients with noncavitary lung disease, the diagnosis can be established if more than two sputum samples produce moderate-to-heavy growth on culture and if the sputum cultures fail to convert to negative with 2 weeks of antimycobacterial treatment. Finally, the diagnosis also can be established if the organism is isolated from tissue and appropriate histopathologic changes are noted.

Distinction between infection and colonization needs to be made because of the therapeutic implications. Simple colonization is more likely if MOTT is sporadically isolated from the patient's sputum, if radiographic findings are stable, and if systemic symptoms are minimal.

11. What are the clinical and radiologic manifestations of MAC in non-AIDS patients?

Clinical manifestations may include any of the following: productive cough, hemoptysis, low-grade fevers, weight loss, superficial lymphadenitis, extrapulmonary dissemination (uncommon), and cutaneous disease (ulcers, abscesses, ecthyma, panniculitis). There are three categories of **radiographic findings**: (1) cavities (smaller and thinner walled than tuberculosis); (2) patchy or nodular upper-lobe infiltrates without cavities, and (3) isolated pulmonary nodules. Of interest, a subset of patients with noncavitary infiltrates includes middle-aged women with a high incidence of middle lobe and lingular infiltrates.

12. What are the clinical and radiologic manifestations of MAC in patients with AIDS?

Because the gastrointestinal tract is the most likely portal of entry in patients with AIDS, common symptoms include diarrhea, abdominal pain, malabsorption, anorexia, weight loss, and hepatomegaly or splenomegaly. Fever and night sweats also may occur, and dissemination to blood, bone marrow, lymph nodes, liver, and spleen is common. MAC from the sputum is usually a colonizer (because lungs are usually not involved). When MAC is truly pathogenic in the lungs, diffuse interstitial infiltrates and/or nodular lesions may be seen on the chest radiograph.

13. What are several striking features of MAC infection in patients with AIDS?

Prominent features include: (1) large bacillary population, (2) little tissue reaction with no granulomatous response, (3) blood as the most frequent source of positive cultures, and (4) increased frequency of gastrointestinal tract involvement.

14. What is the treatment of MAC pulmonary disease in non-AIDS patients?

Treatment is difficult because of resistance to antimycobacterial medications. Treatment may consist of 3–4 antituberculous drugs, including rifampin, ethambutol, streptomycin, ciprofloxacin, clofazimine, and clarithromycin. Rifampin decreases the serum levels of clarithromycin when the two drugs are given together. MAC is often resistant to isoniazid and pyrazinamide. For progressive disease, ethionamide or cycloserine may be added. If disease is limited or localized, resection of the involved lobe combined with pharmacologic treatment is advocated. Surgery should be pursued after the patient's sputum culture has converted to negative. New drug regimens are undergoing testing, and an infectious disease specialist may be able to help with the latest recommended therapies.

15. What is the treatment of disseminated MAC in patients with AIDS?

Treatment is still under investigation, but a reasonable initial regimen with three agents is (1) clarithromycin (500 mg 2 times/day), (2) ethambutol (15 mg/kg/day), and (3) a third drug:
- Clofazimine (100 mg/day), *or*
- Rifampin (600 mg/day), *or*
- Ciprofloxacin (500 mg 2 times/day)

Toxicity, possible drug interactions, and patient compliance must be closely watched. Optimal length of therapy is unknown (lifelong therapy is advocated by many wise people).

16. What is the recommended prophylaxis against MAC in patients with AIDS? When should it be initiated?

MAC is the third most common opportunistic disease affecting persons with AIDS in the United States. Recommended prophylaxis regimens include:
- Azithromycin (1200 mg once weekly)
- Rifabutin (300 mg/day)
- Clarithromycin (250 mg 2 times/day)

Rifabutin (300 mg/day) *plus* weekly azithromycin is most effective but not as well tolerated. Prophylaxis should be initiated when the CD4 count drops below 75/ml in patients who have had opportunistic infections or below 50/ml in patients without prior opportunistic infections.

17. Where is *M. kansasii* found, and what are the natural reservoirs?

It is found in midwestern states, Texas, Louisiana, and Florida; it has been recovered from water, cattle, and swine.

18. What are the signs, symptoms, and radiologic findings of *M. kansasii* pulmonary disease?

Signs and symptoms are vague and nonspecific: cough, fever, and malaise. In patients who are severely immunocompromised, infection of extrapulmonary tissues may occur rarely: osteomyelitis, tenosynovitis, and lymphadenitis. Radiologic findings include upper-lobe cavitary disease. The cavities have thinner walls and less surrounding infiltration than is seen with tuberculosis. Pleural thickening adjacent to parenchymal disease may sometimes be seen.

19. What distinguishes *M. kansasii* from other types of MOTT?

M. kansasii is distinguished by production of a yellow-orange pigment in the growing colonies upon exposure to light. Another such photochromogenic mycobacteria is *M. marinum*.

At 25° C, *M. szulgai* is also photochromogenic. However, at 37° C *M. szulgai* is scotochromogenic, producing pale yellow colonies whether exposed to light or not. *M. scrofulaceum* produces a pigment in the dark and is also classified as a scotochromogen. MAC produces little or no pigment, in the presence or absence of light (nonphotochromogenic).

Characteristics of Pigment Production by Mycobacteria Colonies

MYCOBACTERIA	PIGMENT PRODUCED IN THE DARK	PIGMENT PRODUCED ON LIGHT EXPOSURE	PHOTOREACTIVITY
M. kansasii	No	Yellow to orange	Photochromogenic
M. marinum	No	Yellow to orange	Photochromogenic
M. simiae	No	Yes	Photochromogenic
M. szulgai, at 25° C	No	Yellow to orange	Photochromogenic
M. szulgai, at 37° C	Pale yellow	Pale yellow	Scotochromogenic
M. scrofulaceum	Yes	Yes	Scotochromogenic
M. gordonae	Yes	Yes	Scotochromogenic

Nonpigmented or only lightly pigmented mycobacteria include: *M. tuberculosis, M. bovis, M. ulcerans, M. fortuitum, M. chelonei.*

20. How do you diagnose *M. kansasii*? What is the treatment?

Diagnosis is established by multiple isolates (at least 3) along with radiographic abnormalities. The same criteria for diagnosis described for MAC apply to *M. kansasii*. Sometimes a lung biopsy or bronchoscopy may be necessary. Unlike MAC, *M. kansasii* responds well to the usual antituberculosis drugs. Treatment should include isoniazid (300 mg/day), rifampin (600 mg/day), and ethambutol (25 mg/kg/day) for 18–24 months. Streptomycin (15 mg/kg/day) may be added for the initial 2–3 months of treatment.

21. Give at least one noteworthy fact about the other MOTT that occasionally cause disease in humans.

M. xenopi: causes lung disease; has been isolated from hot water taps within hospitals.

M. szulgai: associated with infection of lung, skin, olecranon bursa, bone, and cervical lymph nodes.

M. scrofulaceum: causes scrofula (granulomatous lymph node) disease (most common in children ages 1–3 yr); may cause lung disease.

M. marinum: infection follows trauma in swimming pools or aquariums or from fish spines or nips by crustaceans; causes "swimming pool granuloma" (cutaneous ulcers and abscesses).

M. simiae: isolated from monkeys and tap water; infects patients with a history of bronchopulmonary disease.

M. haemophilum: causes subcutaneous nodules in HIV-infected patients.

M. genavese: produces disease that mimics disseminated MAC in HIV-infected patients.

The following species are occasionally isolated from clinical specimens but are usually regarded as environmental contaminants. Still, they sometimes cause disease in humans: *M. gordonae, M. terrae, M. asiaticum, M. gastri, M. flavescens, M. thermoresistibile, M. paratuberculosis.*

BIBLIOGRAPHY

1. Boggs DS: The changing spectrum of pulmonary infections due to nontuberculous mycobacteria. J Okla State Med Assoc 88:373–382, 1995.
2. Havlin DV, Dubé MP, Sattler FR, et al: Prophylaxis against disseminated *Mycobacterium avium* complex with weekly azithromycin, daily rifabutin, or both. N Engl J Med 335:392–398, 1996.
3. Hoffner SE: Pulmonary infections caused by less frequently encountered slow-growing environmental mycobacteria. Eur J Clin Microbiol Inf Dis 13:937–941, 1994.
4. Murray JF, Nadel JA (eds): Textbook of Respiratory Medicine, 2nd ed. Philadelphia, W.B. Saunders, 1994.
5. Williams D: *Mycobacterium avium* complex pulmonary disease (MAC-PD) in middle-aged women. Pulmon Crit Care Update 11(20):2–8,1996.

VII. Fungal Infections

25. CANDIDIASIS

Sammi Dali, M.D., and Stephanie Stafford, D.O.

1. How important is candidiasis in the hospital setting?

Candida spp. is currently the sixth most common nosocomial pathogen overall; it was promoted from seventh place in a study done by the Centers for Disease Control and Prevention in the 1980s. In the intensive care setting in the 1980s *Candida* spp. was found to be the fourth most common pathogen, accounting for 10% of all bloodstream infections and 25% of urinary tract infections. In the 1990s the frequency of nosocomial candidemia has increased 500% in large teaching hospitals, 219% in small teaching hospitals, and 370% in large nonteaching hospitals. In the past 15 years, the rate of increase in nosocomial candidal infections has exceeded all pathogens except coagulase-negative staphylococci.

2. What factors predispose patients to candidal infections?

Candida spp. becomes pathogenic when normal defense mechanisms are disrupted by conditions such as diabetes mellitus, malignancy, chronic granulomatous disease, malnutrition, and premature birth. Iatrogenic causes include the use of broad-spectrum antibiotics, intravenous and Foley catheters, corticosteroids or cytotoxic medications, and hyperalimentation containing high concentrations of glucose. Burns, surgical wounds, and IV drug abuse also promote candidal infections. Basically, patients are at risk if natural barriers (skin or mucous membranes, disruption of normal flora, neutropenia, and/or cell-mediated immunity) are impaired.

3. How many species of *Candida* have been identified? Which are the usual suspects when the fungus causes disease?

Over 100 species of *Candida* have been identified; however, only a few have been isolated in humans. *C. albicans* is the most common isolated cause of fungemia and hematogenously disseminated candidiasis. Other clear pathogens include *C. tropicalis*, *C. glabrata*, *C. parapsilosis*, *C. krusei*, and *C. lusitaniae*. Overall, 46% of invasive candidial infections are due to species other than *C. albicans*. It has been suggested that the emergence of species other than *C. albicans* is due to the selection of less susceptible species by antifungal agents such as fluconazole. A strong argument against this proposal was the increasing incidence of non-albicans candidal infections before the widespread use of azoles.

4. What is important about *C. tropicalis*?

Infection by *C. tropicalis* accounts for 12% of all hematogenous infections and is associated with a high mortality rate. In addition, it causes 32% of all fungal infections in patients undergoing bone marrow transplantation or with hematologic malignancies. It is second only to *C. albicans*, which is more lethal and more common in the same populations. Infection from the patient's endogenous organism predominate, but nosocomial infections also have been reported. Treatment outcome for *C. tropicalis* infections is equally effective with amphotericin B, flucytosine, or the triazoles. The synergistic fungicidal activity achieved by combination therapy with amphotericin B and flucytosine may be important in the treatment of *C. tropicalis* fungemia.

5. Why should you know about *C. glabrata*?

C. glabrata, the third most commonly isolated species, occurs more often among patients with solid tumors and nononcologic disorders than among patients with hematologic malignancies. Colonization of multiple sites precedes infection. Portals of entry include the respiratory tract, surgical wounds, and genitourinary tract. Optimal treatment is amphotericin B, because resistance to azoles has been documented. Increased colonization and infection are found in patients using azole antifungal prophylaxis. Mortality after infections with *C. glabrata* is high despite its low virulence, because most patients have a rapidly or ultimately fatal disease.

6. What is the fourth most commonly isolated *Candida* species?

The fourth most commonly isolated species is *Candida parapsilosis* (gotta love that name!), which is associated with invasive procedures, hyperalimentation, prosthetic devices, intravascular catheters, arterial pressure monitors, and ophthalmic irrigation solutions. It is a frequent colonizer of skin. Significant clinical manifestations include fungemia, endocarditis, septic arthritis, and peritonitis. Like *C. glabrata*, *C. parapsilosis* is found in patients with solid tumors and nononcologic diseases. In contrast to *C. tropicalis*, *C. parapsilosis* infection is usually due to an exogenous source. Infections are generally responsive to both fluconazole and amphotericin B. Because *C. parapsilosis* can form extensive biofilms on catheter surfaces, removal of infected catheters is imperative for effective treatment.

7. What is possibly the worst species of *Candida*?

C. krusei should be viewed as a significant pathogen. Fungemia most often develops in profoundly immunosuppressed patients with hematologic malignancy or bone marrow transplants and granulocytopenic patients with cancer who undergo antifungal prophylaxis with fluconazole. Clinically *C. krusei* fungemia appears similar to *C. tropicalis* with a high incidence of cutaneous lesions and endogenous infection from the gastrointestinal tract secondary to loss of mucosal integrity. *C. krusei* has shown resistance to fluconazole in vitro and is less sensitive to amphotericin B than *C. albicans*. Current treatment consists of high daily doses of amphotericin B or high doses of amphotericin B with flucytosine.

8. Which *Candida* species is the most fascinating?

Sixth in order of importance is *C. lusitaniae*. Infrequently isolated, it is still considered an important cause of nosocomial infections among immunocompromised patients. It is fascinating because it is an endogenous pathogen caused by a single strain unique to each individual. *C. lusitaniae* has been isolated from the respiratory tract, urine, and blood stream. Although it is resistant to fluconazole, its resistance or rapid development of resistance to amphotericin B appears to be its most ominous feature.

9. When should you suspect hematogenous candidiasis? What should you do about it?

The portals of entry for *Candida* spp. into the blood stream are mentioned in question two. Physicians should have a high index of suspicion in patients with colonization by candidal organism at multiple body sites and/or a fever unresponsive to broad-spectrum antibacterial agents. Work-up should include cultures of urine, wound drainage sites, throat, sputum, and stool, along with two sets of blood cultures daily for two days (perhaps longer if the patient continues to be febrile). A fundoscopic exam to identify retinitis (uncommonly found in neutropenic patients) is needed, and the skin should be inspected for lesions that can be biopsied. Treatment is variable, depending on the precise species isolated. Experimental use of granulocyte-macrophage colony-stimulating factor has been encouraging. White blood cell transfusions (although limited by the number of neutrophils that can be collected from healthy donors) shows promise, but clinical experience is limited.

10. In a patient with hematogenous candidiasis, can anything be done to improve the outcome?

Removal of central catheters eliminates potential sites of persistent infection. Some retrospective studies show that the replacement of all vascular lines before therapy is initiated or at the start of therapy shortens the duration of candidemia from 5.5 to 4.2 days. Other studies show no outcome improvement after removal of central venous catheters. As always, decisions to remove the catheters should be made on an individual basis.

11. What is the advantage of using lipid formulations of amphotericin B and nystatin in the treatment of hematogenous candidiasis?

Four polyene lipid formulations are currently available: amphotericin B lipid complex, amphotericin B colloidal suspension, liposomal amphotericin B, and a lipid formulation of nystatin. (Check the *Wall Street Journal* to see if another was released this week.) Studies suggest a superior therapeutic index and reduced nephrotoxicity compared with nonlipid formulations. Larger doses are required to obtain superior treatment results. These products are an attractive but expensive option for patients at increased risk of nephrotoxicity (e.g., patients taking concomitant cyclosporine A, FK506).

12. Is it possible to contract primary pneumonia caused by *Candida* species?

Yes. Primary candidal pneumonia is not uncommon in patients with myelosuppression, antimicrobial treatment, cytotoxic or steroid therapy, or altered mental status with or without aspiration. It is a life-threatening problem with an 84% mortality rate in patients with cancer. In some cases candidal pneumonia appears to represent a metastatic infection with no identifiable primary source, such as intermittent fungemia.

Tachypnea, fever, chest pain, cough, and sputum production have been reported. Radiographs show nonspecific patchy infiltrates. The only reliable diagnosis is histologic demonstration of *Candida* spp. in the lung tissue. Amphotericin B is the main therapy; it should be used for a minimum of 2 weeks after signs of infection have disappeared. Oral 5-fluorocytosine (100 mg/kg/day) has been added, but serum levels must be monitored. Surgical resection has been attempted with questionable benefits. Few data are available about the outcome of aggressively treated patients.

13. How does one contract, diagnose, and treat candidal arthritis?

Septic arthritis caused by *Candida* species is uncommon and has an unknown incidence. There are two separate clinical syndromes: (1) monoarticular arthritis, which is caused by direct intraarticular inoculation of fungi that inhabit the skin, and (2) mono- or polyarthritis as a complication of hematogenously disseminated candidiasis.

Monoarticular arthritis usually results from repeated injections of a joint, usually with corticosteroids. The steroids may damage the local defense and clearance mechanisms of a previously diseased joint. Arthroplasty is another cause of candidal arthritis. The clinical presentation is typical: pain with limited range of motion and joint swelling. Fever is present in only 11% of reported cases. The onset of symptoms has been reported as late as 2 years after the initial surgery. Synovial fluid analysis shows serosanguinous or purulent fluid with leukocyte counts ranging from 4,000–15,000/mm^3; polymorphonuclear cells predominate.

Hematogenous dissemination may be found in infants (mainly neonates) and is hospital-acquired in hosts with underlying illnesses, such as respiratory distress syndrome, aspiration pneumonia, and gastrointestinal defects, including gastroschisis, chronic diarrhea, malnutrition, necrotizing enterocolitis, and jaundice.

Metaphyseal osteomyelitis occurs concurrently with candidal arthritis in infants (unlike adults) and may spread through the bone via the metaphyseal vessels. The knees are the most commonly affected joints. Radiographs show joint effusion, punched-out lesions at the metaphysis, and a periosteal reaction. Hematogenous infection also may be seen in IV drug abusers and HIV-infected people. IV drug abusers have a predilection for fibrocartilaginous joints, such as the costochondrals, intervertebral discs, and sacroiliac joints. Anticandidal therapy with amphotericin B alone or in combination with 5-fluorocytosine is highly effective; surgical intervention is often required. Reduced joint function occurs in a low percentage of cases.

14. The risk of infection with *Candida* spp. increases with the number of sites of candidal colonization in immunosuppressed patients. What frequent site of candidal colonization has not been associated with an increased risk of candidal infection?

For reasons that are not clear, vaginal candidal colonizations and infections, although frequent in immunosuppressed patients, do not confer an increased risk of systemic infection.

15. In neutropenic patients with an indwelling central line and persistent fever despite antibiotics, a single positive blood culture for *Candida* spp. may be treated by removal of the offending indwelling catheter alone. True or false?

False. In neutropenic patients, even a single positive blood culture must be considered to represent significant infection with a high likelihood of dissemination. Systemic antifungal therapy should always be undertaken.

16. The laboratory reports that the yeast noted in a positive blood culture in the morning is "germ tube positive" in the afternoon. Does this finding narrow the diagnostic possibilities?

Yes. *C. albicans* produces a germ tube when incubated in an appropriate medium for 2–4 hr. *C. tropicalis* also may make a germ tube that is morphologically distinct from *C. albicans* and easily differentiated by experienced laboratory personnel. Other yeast recoverable from the blood, such as cryptococci and other non-albicans *Candida* spp., do not make germ tubes.

17. Summarize the antifungal susceptibilities of *Candida* species.

Usual Susceptibilities to Amphotericin B and Fluconazole

ORGANISM	AMPHOTERICIN B	FLUCONAZOLE
C. albicans	Yes	Yes
C. tropicalis	Yes (consider addition of 5-flucytosine)	No (especially when fluconazole has been used as prophylaxis)
C. parapsilosis	Yes	Yes
C. krusei	Yes	No
C. glabrata	Yes	Variable
C. lusitaniae	No (may develop resistance during therapy)	Yes (consider addition of 5-flucytosine)

CONTROVERSIES

18. Are immunodiagnostic methods useful for the diagnosis of candidal infections?

Clinical diagnosis relies on the direct detection, isolation, and identification of the fungus. Despite great research efforts, the detection of candidal antibodies in sera remains controversial. There are at least three limitations to this method of detection:

1. Methods of antigen preparation differ from lab to lab.
2. Results of tests differ from lab to lab, making comparison difficult.
3. Antibodies to *Candida* spp. often can be detected in the sera of patients without clinical candidiasis because *Candida* spp. is a ubiquitous component of the human microflora.

19. Despite the controversy, which immunodiagnostic method seems to be best?

The enzyme-linked immunosorbent assay (ELISA) to measure antibody to a purified cytoplasmic protein from *C. albicans* has proved to be a sensitive, inexpensive, and rapid method for the quantification of antibody titers that bypasses the limitations listed above. However, this serologic test is invasive; for this reason, salivary IgA levels have been investigated as a noninvasive method for candidal detection. The major problem is that levels of antibody titers are much lower in saliva than in blood and thus are less useful for quantification.

BIBLIOGRAPHY

1. Bodey GP: Disseminated candidiasis in neutropenic patients. Int J Infect Dis 1(Suppl 1):2–5, 1997.
2. Goldman M, Pottage JC, Weaver DC: *Candida krusei* fungemia. Medicine 72:143–151, 1993.
3. Harone E, Vartivarian S, Anaissie E, et al: Primary *Candida* pneumonia. Medicine 72:137–142, 1993.
4. Jeganathan S, Chan YC: Immunodiagnosis in oral candidiasis. Oral Surg Oral Med Oral Pathol 74:451–454, 1992.
5. Pfaller MA: Nosocomial candidiasis: Emerging species, reservoirs, and modes of transmission. Clin Infect Dis 22(Suppl 2):89–92, 1996.
6. Silveria LH, Cuellar ML, Citera G, et al: *Candida* arthritis. Rheum Dis Clin North Am 19:427–438, 1993.
7. Uzun O, Anaissie EJ: Problems and controversies in the management of hematogenous candidiasis. Clin Infect Dis 22(Suppl 2):95–101, 1996.

26. COCCIDIOIDOMYCOSIS

David P. Dooley, M.D.

1. What is coccidioidomycosis?

Coccidioidomycosis is a local (usually pulmonary) or disseminated infection with the fungus *Coccidioides immitis*, a normal inhabitant of the soil in the desert of the southwestern United States. Clinical syndromes are remarkably reminiscent of tuberculosis and similar to those caused by other dimorphic fungi.

2. How did the organism get its name?

The tissue form of *C. immitis*—the spherule with endospores—was thought to be a coccidial parasite when first discovered early in the century; when its true nature was discovered, the genus was named *Coccidioides*. *Immitis* is the Latin word meaning *severe*. Initially clinicians did not appreciate the asymptomatic or primary stage, and all known patients were morbidly or terminally ill.

3. What is a dimorphic fungus?

Dimorphic means of two bodies. *C. immitis* exists in nature in its mycelial form. Arthroconidia (spores) of the fungus break off and become airborne, either in dust or from fomites. When victims, human or animal, inhale this highly infectious form, the initial inoculation of the lung occurs. But at 37° C the organism's tissue grows as a yeastlike form (in this case, the spherule) that is not contagious. The dimorphism is exploited in the laboratory: the mycologist can definitively identify the mycelial isolate, initially grown at 30° C, by converting the fungus (that is, transferring it to broth at 37° C and observing its growth in the spherule form).

4. How does *C. immitis* compare with other dimorphic fungi and *Mycobacterium tuberculosis*?

The other classic dimorphic fungi include *Histoplasma capsulatum, Blastomyces dermatitidis, Sporothrix schenckii, Paracoccidioides brasiliensis,* and *Penicillium marneffei.*

Comparison of Coccidioides immitis, *Other Dimorphic Fungi, and* Mycobacterium tuberculosis

CHARACTERISTIC	C. IMMITIS	OTHER DIMORPHIC FUNGI	M. TUBER-CULOSIS
Primary pulmonary infection from inhalation of inoculum; local disease or occasional dissemination	+	+	+
Characteristic geography of exposures	+	+	–
Useful and available skin test	+	–	+
Serology important in diagosis and management	+	Histoplasmosis, paracoccidioidomycosis (latter not easily available)	–
Tissue and blood eosinophilia	Common	–	–
Disseminated disease commonly refractory to therapy	+	– (except in immuno-compromised patients)	–

5. What should I know about the microbiology of *C. immitis*?

- *C. immitis* grows fast (less than 1 week) on the appropriate fungal media. Whereas it used to take many days to identify the organism by either morphology or conversion (see above), it is now rapidly identified by DNA hybridization testing or (less safely) by exoantigen testing.
- Only the mycelial form with its arthroconidia (spores), as found in nature and on laboratory isolation plates, is infective. The tissue spherule phase is not infective; therefore, coccidioidomycosis is not typically contagious from person to person.
- Accidental laboratory inoculation is legendary and has been fatal. Alert the laboratory if you suspect that *C. immitis* may grow.

6. What illnesses does pulmonary coccidioidomycosis most closely mimic?

Acute coccidioidomycosis	Chronic coccidioidomycosis
Atypical pneumonias	Tuberculosis
Typical bacterial pneumonias	Atypical mycobacterial infection
	Nocardiosis
Nodular or cavitary coccidioidomycosis	Histoplasmosis
Aspiration pneumonia or abscess	Blastomycosis
Round pneumonia differential	Cryptococcosis
Solitary pulmonary nodule differential	Sporotrichosis
Vasculitis (especially Wegener's granulomatosis,	Postobstructive pneumonia
Churg-Strauss syndrome)	Carcinoma

7. What is valley fever?

Episodes of fever, arthralgias or arthritis (desert rheumatism), erythema nodosum (painful nodules, commonly on the shins), and erythema multiforme, in any combination, were commonly seen in the San Joaquin Valley. The syndrome was later shown to be caused by hypersensitivity phenomena to primary infection with *C. immitis*.

8. Who is at risk to acquire infection with *C. immitis*?

Essentially all patients with coccidioidomycosis have a history of at least a transient visit to endemic areas. Most patients have naive immunities, spend a great deal of time outdoors, and commonly remember exposure to much airborne dust. Frequently infected populations include:

- Military personnel, assigned from elsewhere to endemic areas
- Agricultural, construction, and oil-field workers
- Archaeology students on digs
- Participants in outdoor sports
- Sightseers (Reports of traveler's coccidioidomycosis, with presentation within weeks to months after return to the native state or country, are numerous.)
- Remote infection from fomites (e.g., factory workers handling cotton harvested in the Southwest) has occurred but is rare.

9. Where is the endemic area?

Most intensely endemic areas

Southern and central California

Southern Arizona and New Mexico

West Texas

Border states of Mexico

Less intense foci of infection (as determined by skin test prevalence among inhabitants) stretch from southern Utah and Nevada through Mexico to areas in Central and South America (especially Honduras, Guatemala, Colombia, and Venezuela).

10. Define the general clinical presentations of coccidioidomycosis and the associated laboratory results.

Presentations of Coccidioidomycosis

SYNDROME	TIMING OF COURSE	ADENOPATHY	SKIN TEST	IgM ANTIBODIES (TUBE PRECIPITIN)	IgG ANTIBODIES (COMPLEMENT FIXING)*
Acute pulmonary (± erythema nodosum)	Days to weeks after inhalation	Often hilar	Eventually	+	Low +; high + suggests possible dissemination
Persistent pneumonia, nodule or cavity	Weeks to months after inhalation	Occasionally hilar	+	+	Low +; high + suggests possible dissemination
Chronic progressive pneumonia (see figure below)	Progressive, since inhalation, over months to years	Occasionally hilar	+	Usually +	Usually +
Disseminated disease	Within months after inhalation, or with later immuno-compromise	Occasionally disseminated; liver/spleen involvement common	Often + (depends on extent of disease)	+ or −	Usually high (depends on extent of disease)
Local inoculation	Weeks after cutaneous inoculation	Regional	+	+	Usually −

* Low positive, 1:2 –1:4; high positive, ≥ 1:16

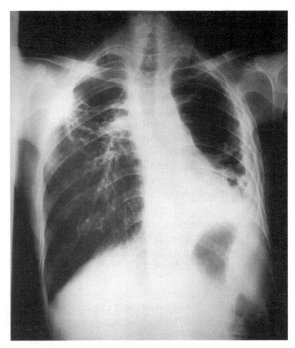

Chest radiograph of a 42-year-old man in whom chronic progressive coccidioidomycosis has destroyed the entire left lung and the upper lobe of the right lung. (Courtesy of Robert Longfield, M.D.)

11. Is any laboratory feature peculiar to coccidioidomycosis?

A minority of patients with acute coccidioidomycosis may have eosinophilia (> 8% of total white blood cells; often 10–20%), which may persist in disseminated disease. It is less common in chronic pulmonary coccidioidomycosis. Eosinophilia has been found in other body fluids, most significantly cerebrospinal fluid and pleural effusions. It will not be found, however, unless the disease is suspected and a Wright or Giemsa stain of the cellular components is requested specifically.

12. Does the pulmonary cavity of coccidioidomycosis have a defining characteristic?

A thin-walled cavity, appearing usually within months of the presumed primary infection (often developing from an antecedent infiltrate or nodule), is typical. Little surrounding infiltrate is evident, and the walls may be only a few millimeters thick. Histopathologic findings and computed tomography have indicated that coccidioidal infiltrates and cavities are often surrounded by satellite or daughter microabscesses, not evident on chest radiography. There is some basis, therefore, for the recommended practice of treating patients with antifungal therapy before and after an indicated resection (if the diagnosis is known) to minimize local surgical spillage of disease.

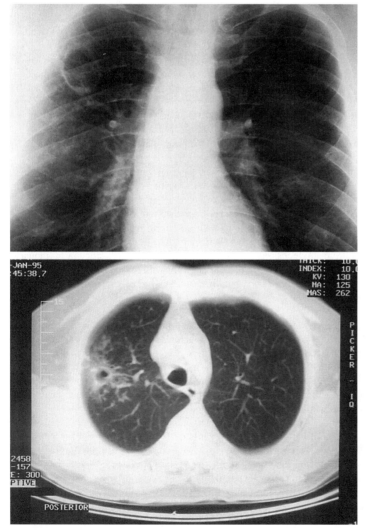

Right upper-lobe thin-walled cavity and associated infiltrate in a 60-year-old man with acute progressive coccidioidomycosis. (Courtesy of Robert Longfield, M.D.)

CT of same patient demonstrates cavity and extent of associated parenchymal disease. (Courtesy of Robert Longfield, M.D.)

13. List the most common and less common sites of involvement in disseminated disease.

Most common	Skin, subcutaneous tissues
	Meninges
	Bone and joint
Less common	Reticuloendothelial system (liver, spleen, lymph nodes)
(and often	Genitourinary tract (bladder, prostate, epididymis, salpinx)
clinically	Brain (coccidioma, often with meningitis)
silent)	Eye
	Larynx
	Pericardium
	Peritoneum, omentum (not lower gastrointestinal tract!)
	Kidney and adrenals

14. What is an adequate evaluation to exclude the presence of disseminated disease?

Any patient with a tissue or culture diagnosis of coccidioidomycosis or a suggestive clinical syndrome with supporting serologic data should at least receive a thorough history, review of systems, physical examination, and initial (baseline) serologic studies (if not already done). Further diagnostic efforts should be directed toward positive findings. A survey of bone (bone scan is ideal) and a cerebrospinal fluid examination (with complement fixation titer) are also recommended. Because of its ease, many recommend a culture of spun urinary sediment for *C. immitis* if the diagnosis is uncertain, although positive results may be seen in disease limited to the chest.

15. List the major risk factors for dissemination of disease in coccidioidomycosis.

- Male sex
- Race (roughly in descending order of risk): Filipino, African American, Mexican, American Indian, non-Filipino Asian, Caucasian
- Pregnancy (third more often than second trimester)
- Immunocompromise (e.g., AIDS, bone marrow transplant, solid organ transplant, steroid use)

16. Do skin lesions in coccidioidomycosis always represent disseminated disease?

Almost always. In rare cases of coccidioidomycosis due to primary inoculation, disease is limited to the skin lesion and regional adenopathy. Characteristics of this syndrome include a history of believable inoculation, single lesion, regional adenopathy, lack of evidence of pulmonary or disseminated disease, positive skin test, and presence of IgM with low or absent IgG (CF) antibodies. The lesion usually resolves on its own, but dissemination has been described. Treatment (probably with azoles) seems prudent.

17. What is the relationship between coccidioidomycosis and pregnancy?

Alone among the deep fungal infections and unlike tuberculosis, any stage of pregnancy predisposes to dissemination of coccidioidomycosis. The risk is increased in the second and especially third trimesters. Available therapy has markedly improved the prognosis for the mother (congenital disease does not seem to occur), and the previously formidable maternal mortality rate has diminished. Women with new infection are at high risk, but it is believed that the disease can also reactivate in women with antecedent disseminated disease.

18. The serologic tests are confusing. What do they mean? How are they used?

Only two types of antibodies are measured: (1) an IgM antibody to coccidioidin, measured by tube precipitin, immunodiffusion-tube precipitin, latex agglutination, or IgM–enzyme-linked immunosorbent (ELISA) assays, and (2) an IgG antibody to coccidioidin, measured by a formal complement fixation (CF), immunodiffusion-CF, or IgG ELISA assay.

The **IgM antibody tests** are positive in early disease and disappear within 3–4 months (they rarely rise to low positive levels in disseminated disease). Quantitation is meaningless and is not performed; the antibody is not found in cerebrospinal fluid. The **CF antibody** is quantitated and appears in low titer (~1:2 to 1:4) or not at all in early, controlled disease (acute primary coccidioidomycosis). It is present in high titer ($\geq$ 1:16) in many but not all patients with disseminated disease. The lesser the degree of dissemination (especially if only meningitis is present), the lower the titer. The CF antibody is measured in cerebrospinal fluid; with rare exceptions, any degree of positivity implies active meningeal disease.

High CF titers early in disease portend a poorer outcome (e.g., subsequent dissemination). Falling titers with therapy suggest the adequacy of the regimen. The height and direction of movement over time of CF titers in cerebrospinal fluid have the same implications for the therapy of meningitis as does the CF titer in the periphery.

19. What does a positive Spherulin skin test mean?

A positive skin test, defined as a 5-mm induration assessed at 24 hr and 48 hr after careful intradermal injection of commercially available Spherulin (Berkeley Biologicals, Berkeley, CA), is strong evidence for antecedent exposure and infection with *C. immitis* (*H. capsulatum* occasionally gives small positive reactions). The test is almost always positive in acute coccidioidomycosis (unless dissemination has already begun), variably positive in disseminated disease (depending on the extent of dissemination), and usually positive in the chronic pulmonary and local inoculation forms of disease. A positive skin test in a person with chronic endemic exposure to *C. immitis* (the population skin test positivity in many areas runs between 5–70%) is not surprising and is not helpful in determining the diagnosis.

20. When should a skin test be applied?

- When the previous skin test is known to be, or almost certainly was, negative and the current presentation may represent a skin test-converting acute infection with *C. immitis*.
- When the diagnosis is already known, serial skin testing can be helpful for prognostic purposes (conversion of a previously negative skin test to positive suggests improved control of disseminated disease, and vice versa).

21. What treatments are available for coccidioidomycosis?

Controlled trials have not compared any of the following agents. In general, **amphotericin B** is still considered the gold standard and should be used for severe or life-threatening disseminated or pulmonary disease. Although a total course of 1–2.5 gm is suggested, in reality therapy with this or any other agent is usually continued until both clinical symptoms and laboratory abnormalities resolve or stabilize (if ever). There is no experience yet with liposomal formulations of amphotericin B and human coccidioidomycosis.

Miconazole and ketoconazole are no longer alternatives because of toxicity or suboptimal efficacy. **Itraconazole and fluconazole** have shown moderate efficacy (50–80% initial response rates, but with appreciable relapse rates) in the treatment of chronic lung or nonmeningeal disseminated disease. Both are well tolerated at $\leq$ 400 mg/day each and are considered by many to be the first-choice drugs for less severe disease. Preliminary data suggest that early azole therapy for acute (primary) coccidioidomycosis may significantly reduce the incidence of subsequent complications (dissemination or chronic disease requiring therapy). No reported experience suggests that a combination of amphotericin B with an azole is more effective than therapy with either alone.

Almost no decision in the therapy of nonmeningeal coccidioidomycosis is easy (to treat or not to treat, choice of agent, how to follow responses, when to stop therapy), and it is recommended that the approach include consultation with an infectious disease specialist.

22. Compare meningeal coccidioidomycosis with meningeal tuberculosis.

The two have striking similarities but important differences, as indicated by the following table.

Comparison of Coccidioidal and Tuberculous Meningitis

FEATURE	COCCIDIOIDAL MENINGITIS	TUBERCULOUS MENINGITIS
Chronic meningitis presentation (gradual headache, nausea, lymphocytic pleocytosis in cerebrospinal fluid (CSF), hypoglycorrhachia, routine cultures negative)	+	+
Primarily basilar meningitis, complicated by hydrocephalus and vasculitis with strokes	+	+
Frank intracerebral involvement (rare)	+	+
Organisms found in CSF on culture	Rare	Common
Eosinophilia in CSF	Common	Rare if ever
Diagnosis by positive CSF specific antibody	+ (CF)	None available
Fatal if untreated	+	+
Treatment curative	Rare	Usual

23. How is meningeal coccidioidomycosis treated today?

No randomized trials have been performed. Before 1990, intrathecal amphotericin B was necessary to control the disease (along with varying doses of systemic drug, depending on the extent of extrameningeal disease). Most patients still needed life-long therapy to avoid relapses. This course was fraught with difficulty because the drug had to be given intrathecally, intracisternally, or (optimally) into the ventricle via an Ommaya reservoir. Toxicities were common. In the early 1990s trials demonstrated the usefulness of either itraconazole or fluconazole (both at 400 mg/day) for control of disease. Long-term control appears to be achieved at least as often as with amphotericin B, with fewer procedure- or device-related complications, fewer toxicities, and better patient and physician acceptance. Probably no patient should be considered cured, because discontinuation of therapy (even after years of normal clinical and laboratory parameters) is frequently followed by relapse. Whether higher doses of the azoles or various combinations of amphotericin B with an azole (sequential or simultaneous) may improve the rate of response is unknown. Meningeal coccidioidomycosis is potentially lethal even under optimal care. Decisions about initial or ongoing therapy are so hazardous that consultation with an infectious disease specialist should be obtained.

BIBLIOGRAPHY

1. Ampel NM, Dols CL, Galgiani JN: Coccidioidomycosis during human immunodeficiency virus infection: Results of a prospective study in a coccidioidal endemic area. Am J Med 94:235–240, 1993.
2. Caldwell J, Welch G, Johnson R, Einstein H: Evaluation of response to early azole treatment in primary coccidioidomycosis [abstract no. 43]. In Conference Program and Abstracts, Centennial Conference on Coccidioidomycosis. Fifth International Conference, Stanford University, August 1994.
3. Carroll GF, Haley LD, Brown JM: Primary cutaneous coccidioidomycosis. A review of the literature and a report of a new case. Arch Dermatol 113:933–936, 1977.
4. Catanzaro A, Galgiani JN, Levine BE, et al, for the NIAID Mycoses Study Group: Fluconazole in the treatment of chronic pulmonary and nonmeningeal disseminated coccidioidomycosis. Am J Med 98:249–256, 1995.
5. Dewsnup DH, Galgiani JN, Graybill JR, et al: Is it ever safe to stop azole therapy for *Coccidioides immitis* meningitis? Ann Intern Med 124:304–310, 1996.
6. Drutz DJ, Catanzaro A: Coccidioidomycosis (Parts I & II). Am Rev Respir Dis 117:559–585, 727–771, 1978.
7. Galgiani JN, Catanzaro A, Cloud GA, et al, for the NIAID-Mycoses Study Group: Fluconazole therapy for coccidioidal meningitis. Ann Intern Med 119:28–35, 1993.
8. Graybill JR, Stevens DA, Galgiani JN, et al, for the NAIAD [sic] Mycoses Study Group: Itraconazole treatment of coccidioidomycosis. Am J Med 89:282–290, 1990.
9. Peterson CM, Schuppert K, Kelly PC, Pappagianis D: Coccidioidomycosis and pregnancy. Obstet Gynecol Surv 48:149–156, 1993.
10. Tucker RM, Denning DW, Dupont B, Stevens DA: Itraconazole therapy for chronic coccidioidal meningitis. Ann Intern Med 112:108–112, 1990.

27. HISTOPLASMOSIS

Chandra Dommaraju, M.D., and E. Dale Everett, M.D.

1. How does one catch histoplasmosis?

Histoplasmosis is caused by a dimorphic fungus, *Histoplasma capsulatum*. It is present in soil and flourishes in soil that is "fertilized" with avian excrement. In addition, bats excrete *H. capsulatum* from their gut, resulting in contaminated guano in caves used as bat roosts. The infectious form is the mycelial phase, which produces conidia at ambient temperatures. Humans become infected when conidia become aerosolized such as during excavation or cleaning of chicken coops, and are inhaled. Rare reports of conjugal transmission suggest that under unusual circumstances the yeast form may be infectious to others.

2. What happens when a human acquires the infection?

From a clinical standpoint, usually nothing. Skin test surveys show that approximately 90% of infected persons are asymptomatic or have an illness so mild that they do not seek medical attention. Even if medical attention is sought, symptoms may be so nonspecific that the practitioner diagnoses a viral respiratory infection.

3. Something *must* happen in the lung—what is it?

Pathophysiologically, once the conidia enter an alveolus, temperature change and complex biochemical mechanisms result in conversion to a yeast. Despite the initial polymorphonuclear response, lymphatic and hematogenous dissemination may occur. Crucial to containment is development of cell-mediated host defense. The end result is granuloma formation and healing, usually with calcification.

4. What about the 10% who get sick?

Depending on the inoculum size and whether infection results from primary exposure or reexposure in a previously immune host, the incubation period ranges from 3–21 days. The clinical syndrome is nonspecific and usually consists of fever, headache, malaise, and a nonproductive cough. Severe cases may lead to hypoxemia and respiratory failure.

5. Can a chest radiograph help with the diagnosis?

If radiographic manifestations occur with acute pulmonary histoplasmosis, one of three patterns emerge:

1. Patchy infiltrates with or without hilar or mediastinal lymph node enlargement (sometimes regional lymph node enlargement occurs without an identifiable parenchymal lesion);
2. Nodular infiltrates; or
3. Miliary infiltrates.

Nodular infiltrates are thought to result from reexposure to a heavy inoculum in persons with some level of immunity, whereas miliary infiltrates are associated with reexposure in persons with a high level of immunity. Pleural effusions with acute pulmonary histoplasmosis are rare, and their presence should suggest another diagnosis. Cavitary lesions during acute histoplasmosis are also distinctly uncommon.

6. Are there other syndromes caused by histoplasmosis?

Of course there are or the question would not have been posed. Among the most serious illness caused by histoplasma is disseminated disease. Dissemination tends to occur in infants or immunocompromised people but can occur in people without apparent immunocompromise. The AIDS epidemic has led to increased numbers of cases of disseminated disease. Dissemination may occur with primary exposure or reactivation of a latent focus from previous exposure.

Disseminated disease has been divided into three clinical syndromes: chronic, subacute, and acute. The chronic form generally presents as a vague illness characterized by prolonged fatigue and weight loss. Fever and hepatosplenomegaly occur in only about one-third of patients. One helpful clue is the occurrence of mouth ulcers in 50–60% of patients with chronic disease. In the subacute variety, fever, weight loss, malaise, and hepatosplenomegaly are common. Evidence of concomitant pulmonary disease is rare. Acute disseminated disease is usually associated with fever, weight loss, cough, and shortness of breath. Patients often present within a few days to a few weeks after onset. Seen in young children, patients with Hodgkin's disease or lymphocytic leukemia, and patients receiving immunosuppressive drugs, the acute variety is now most commonly associated with AIDS. A septic shock presentation with multiorgan failure occurs in about 10% of cases. Adrenal insufficiency may be seen in all forms of disseminated disease, and adrenal function should be assessed in all patients.

Another relatively common syndrome is chronic pulmonary histoplasmosis. The clinical setting is a patient with underlying chronic obstructive pulmonary disease, most often an elderly man. Symptoms of increased cough, weight loss, malaise, and low-grade fever are present for several weeks to months. Radiographic findings are usually upper lobe (90%) fibronodular infiltrates, often accompanied by cavitary changes. The syndrome is clinically indistinguishable from reactivation tuberculosis or other granulomatous diseases.

Other clinical syndromes caused by histoplasmosis include mediastinal granulomatosis; solitary or multiple pulmonary nodules, which may be confused with malignancy; meningitis (usually chronic); pericarditis; arthritis; hemoptysis secondary to erosion of a calcified lymph node into a bronchus (broncholith); and progressive mediastinal fibrosis with obstruction of bronchi and/or large blood vessels (e.g., superior vena cava syndrome).

7. How can one confirm the diagnosis of histoplasmosis?

Sometimes with great difficulty. Diagnosis of histoplasmosis requires a high index of suspicion and recognition of the various syndromes it produces. Definitive diagnosis requires isolation and identification of the organism. Cultures, histologic examination, and antibody and antigen detection may contribute to establishing a diagnosis.

In acute pulmonary histoplasmosis, cultures are rarely positive. Strong support for the diagnosis may be obtained by antigen detection in the urine (approximately 75% of cases) or, more commonly, by detection of complement-fixing antibodies and/or antibodies by immunodiffusion (approximately 95% of cases). Detectable antibodies usually peak 4–6 weeks after onset of the illness and persist for several years.

In disseminated disease, examination of peripheral blood smears for intracellular organisms (which look like protozoa rather than typical yeast), fungal blood cultures, and biopsies and culture of tissues, especially mouth ulcers and bone marrow, frequently yield the diagnosis. Urinary antigen detection is an excellent means for diagnosing disseminated histoplasmosis.

For chronic pulmonary histoplasmosis repeated culture of expectorated sputum (up to a dozen sputum specimens) yields the diagnosis in about 75% of patients. Elevated complement-fixing antibodies ($\geq 1{:}32$) also strongly support the diagnosis, but some patients have lower titers. Detection of antigen in the urine may occur in up to 20% of patients with chronic pulmonary histoplasmosis.

8. When do patients need to be treated?

Patients with severe primary pulmonary disease benefit from a short course of amphotericin B (total dose = 500–1000 mg). Some prescribe concomitant corticosteroid treatment. Patients with pericarditis or arthritis usually do not require antifungal therapy but benefit from treatment with anti-inflammatory agents.

Left untreated, disseminated histoplasmosis is a fatal illness. Therefore, all patients require therapy. Amphotericin B is the cornerstone of therapy, particularly in patients with acute dissemination. In non-life-threatening disease, itraconazole can be used in a dose of 400 mg/day for 6–12 months, although there is less experience with itraconazole than with amphotericin. In the

AIDS population, the disease is usually controlled with 0.7 mg/kg/day (to a total dose of 1000 mg) of amphotericin intravenously, followed by itraconazole, 200 mg twice daily indefinitely. A less desirable means of therapy (because of logistics and complications) is therapy with amphotericin B to a total dose of 2 gm over several weeks, followed by 50–80 mg biweekly indefinitely.

The standard treatment for chronic pulmonary histoplasmosis is 35 mg/kg total dose of amphotericin over several weeks. Some success has been achieved with itraconazole, 200 mg twice daily for 6–12 months. Surgery for localized upper lobe disease may be considered, but many patients are not good candidates because of underlying chronic obstructive lung disease.

9. Why do birds, which are the frequent source of histoplasmosis, not get the disease?

The fungus is mycelial at 25–30° C and at 37° C becomes a yeast. The core temperature of birds (about 40° C) does not support the tissue disease-causing growth of yeast.

10. Why are skin tests for histoplasmosis generally a bad idea?

Skin tests usually are not helpful with diagnosis and, of greater importance, when done with histoplasmin may boost the serologic response in recipients, leading to false-positive results.

BIBLIOGRAPHY

1. Goodwin RA, Loyd JE, DesPrez RM: Histoplasmosis in normal hosts. Medicine 60:231–266, 1981.
2. Negroni R, Robles AM, Arochavala A, Taborda A: Itraconazole in human histoplasmosis. Mycoses 32:123–130, 1989.
3. McKinsey DS, Gupta MR, Riddler SA, et al: Long-term amphotericin B therapy for disseminated histoplasmosis in patients with the acute immunodeficiency syndrome (AIDS). Ann Intern Med 111:655–659, 1989.
4. Wheat J, Hafner R, Walfsohn M, et al: Prevention of relapse of histoplasmosis with itraconazole in patients with the acquired immunodeficiency syndrome. Ann Intern Med 118:610–616, 1993.
5. Wheat J, Hafner R, Korzan AH, et al: Itraconazole treatment of disseminated histoplasmosis in patients with the acquired immunodeficiency syndrome. Am J Med 98:336–342, 1995.
6. Dismukes W, Bradsher R, Cloud G, and others in the NIAID Mycoses Study Group: Itraconazole therapy for blastomycosis and histoplasmosis. Am J Med 93:489–497, 1992.
7. Wheat J: Histoplasmosis experience during outbreaks in Indianapolis and review of the literature. Medicine 76:339–354, 1997.

28. NORTH AMERICAN BLASTOMYCOSIS

Chandra Dommaraju, M.D., and E. Dale Everett, M.D.

1. Where and how does one acquire blastomycosis?

Blastomycosis is a fungal infection caused by *Blastomyces dermatitidis*, a dimorphic fungus. The agent is rarely isolated from the environment but is present in soil that contains large amounts of organic debris and animal excrement. The endemic areas in the United States are the upper midwestern, south central, and southeastern regions. The portal of entry is inhalation of aerosolized conidia into the lungs. The prevalence of infection is not known because of lack of an accurate screening test, such as a skin test antigen, that can be used to study populations. The incubation period has been reported to vary between 21–106 days with a median of 45 days.

2. What happens when a human is infected with *B. dermatitidis*?

Blastomycosis has not been as well studied as the other endemic fungal diseases (e.g., histoplasmosis, coccidioidomycosis). After inhalation of conidia, transformation from a mycelia to a yeast form occurs. Before the host can mount an immune response, the organism may disseminate to other organs through the lymphatic system and bloodstream. An immune response eventually develops, resulting in an influx of monocyte-derived macrophages and polymorphonuclear cells at the site of the infection. This influx produces the pyogranulomatous lesion distinctive for blastomycosis. Severity of infection varies from no symptoms to overwhelming fatal disease. Occasionally, persons may develop active disease from a latent focus that was acquired months to years earlier.

3. What kind of symptoms and disease do patients manifest?

Many—because the organism often disseminates during the primary infection. Almost any organ system may be involved. However, most patients seek medical attention for one of four problems:

1. Pulmonary manifestations
2. Nonhealing skin lesions
3. Bone lesions, often without pain, associated with subcutaneous swelling or a draining lesion
4. Symptoms related to the genitourinary tract

Chronic meningitis, brain abscesses, lymphadenopathy, splenic abscesses, orbital abscess, and laryngeal involvement are less common. Laryngeal involvement is noteworthy because the pseudoepitheliomatous hyperplasia induced by the infection may result in misdiagnosis as squamous cell carcinoma of the larynx.

4. If a patient has lung involvement, what can be expected?

Some patients lack pulmonary symptoms, but infiltrates, masses, or cavitary lesions may be discovered when chest radiographs are done for another reason. When patients are symptomatic, pulmonary blastomycosis generally is categorized into acute or chronic forms. With the acute syndrome, symptoms are similar to other acute pneumonias—fever, chills, and productive cough. Failure to respond to antibacterial agents may raise suspicion of fungal or mycobacterial infection, prompting studies that lead to the diagnosis of blastomycosis. Chronic disease may resemble lung carcinoma. Symptoms are often present for weeks to months and include cough, chest pain, hemoptysis, fever, night sweats, anorexia, and weight loss.

Severe acute pulmonary blastomycosis associated with adult respiratory distress syndrome and respiratory failure is uncommon but requires early diagnosis so that appropriate therapy can be instituted. Fortunately, examination of sputum or tracheal secretions reveals broad-based budding yeast and allows a prompt diagnosis.

5. Do chest radiographs help in the diagnosis of pulmonary blastomycosis?

Yes and no. The chest radiograph often shows abnormalities, but they are not sufficiently distinctive to be diagnostic of blastomycosis. Radiographic findings may include alveolar infiltrates; nodules; mass lesions that mimic malignancies; hilar, mediastinal, or paratracheal lymphadenopathy; fibronodular infiltrates; cavitary lesions; pleural effusion (uncommon); or miliary infiltrates. In contrast to histoplasmosis, calcification of blastomycosis lesions is uncommon.

6. What about extrapulmonary blastomycosis?

Cutaneous lesions are the most common extrapulmonary manifestation of blastomycosis. Skin lesions may be solitary or multiple and may occur with or without an active pulmonary focus. The lesions are generally slowly expanding ulcerative or verrucous lesions without systemic symptoms. Patients often receive several courses of antimicrobial agents or topical steroid therapy without benefit before the diagnosis is established. Lesions often are mistaken for basal cell or squamous cell carcinoma.

Bone lesions follow skin lesions in frequency. They often present with minimal-to-no pain; subcutaneous swelling or draining lesions may overlie the involved bone(s). Radiographically bone lesions are usually well-circumscribed lytic lesions. Juxtaarticular lesions may extend into joint spaces, resulting in infectious arthritis.

When the genitourinary tract is involved, the prostate is the most frequent site. Patients may present with obstructive symptoms, a tender prostate, or pyuria on urinalysis. Epididymal or testicular masses also may occur.

7. When blastomycosis occurs in immunocompromised patients, is the syndrome different?

Although blastomycosis occasionally infects patients with immunocompromise, for reasons that are unclear it is much less frequent than histoplasmosis, cryptococcosis, or coccidioidomycosis. Even in patients with AIDS cases are rare. When blastomycosis occurs in patients with AIDS, the CD4 count is usually below 200 cells/mm^3. In such patients, it appears to be a much more aggressive disease, with fulminating pulmonary disease or dissemination with a high incidence of central nervous system involvement. Early death is relatively common, but if patients live for longer than 1 month, control of the infection is possible.

8. How is the diagnosis established?

Because blastomycosis is relatively uncommon and has diverse presentations, it is often not recognized or considered in the differential diagnosis. Often the diagnosis is made serendipitously from scrapings of lesions, sputum examinations, or biopsies performed as part of the evaluation. Although definitive diagnosis requires isolation of the organism in cultures, the diagnosis can be made with confidence by histologic examination based on the unique size and characteristic appearance of the organism. At present, no serologic, skin test, or antigen detection method with sufficient sensitivity and specificity to support the diagnosis is commercially available.

9. What is the treatment of blastomycosis?

Before the development of azole antifungal drugs, amphotericin B was the cornerstone of therapy. It remains the drug of choice for severe illness. In such patients, amphotericin B at a daily dose of 0.7–1 mg/kg is suggested until the acute disease is controlled. Follow-up therapy with an oral azole may be used. In patients with nonmeningeal, non-life-threatening disease, ketoconazole has been used successfully. Because of efficacy and fewer side effects, itraconazole has largely replaced ketoconazole. The recommended dose of itraconazole is 200–400 mg/day for 6–12 months.

In patients with AIDS, it seems reasonable to administer a maintenance dose of itraconazole, perhaps 200 mg/day, indefinitely after acute disease is controlled with amphotericin. This recommendation is not as well substantiated as the maintenance therapy for histoplasmosis and cryptococcus.

BIBLIOGRAPHY

1. Bradsher RW: Blastomycosis. Clin Infect Dis 14(Suppl 1):S82–S90, 1992.
2. Cush R, Light RW, George RB: Clinical and roentgenographic manifestations of acute and chronic blastomycosis. Chest 69:345–349, 1976.
3. Davies SF, Sarosi GA: Blastomycosis. Eur J Clin Microbial Infect Dis 8:474–479, 1989.
4. Dismukes WE, Bradshear RW, Kauffman CA, et al: Itraconazole therapy for blastomycosis and histoplasmosis. Am J Med 93:489–497, 1992.
5. Eickenberg H, Amin M, Lich R Jr: Blastomycosis of the genitourinary tract. J Urol 113:650–652, 1975.
6. Meyer KC, McManus EJ, Maki D: Overwhelming pulmonary blastomycosis associated with the adult respiratory distress syndrome. New Engl J Med 329:1231–1236, 1993.
7. Pappas PG, Pottage JC, Powderly WG, et al: Blastomycosis in patients with the acquired immunodeficiency syndrome. Ann Intern Med 116:847–853, 1992.
8. Riegler HF, Goldstein LA, Belts RF: Blastomycosis osteomyelitis. Clin Orthop 100:225–231, 1974.
9. Bradsher RW: Histoplasmosis and blastomycosis. Clin Infect Dis 22(Suppl 2):5102–5111, 1996.

29. SPOROTRICHOSIS

George Winters, M.D.

1. What is sporotrichosis?

Sporotrichosis is an infection caused by *Sporothrix schenckii*, a dimorphic saprophytic fungus. It is less virulent than many other fungal pathogens, and infection is generally limited to the skin, although disseminated disease is seen. A primary pulmonary form has been reported in fewer than 100 cases.

2. Where is *Sporothrix* sp. found?

Sporothrix sp. is found worldwide in decaying wood and vegetable matter, soil, rose bushes, sphagnum moss, tree bark, and both wild and domestic animals. Most infections in the United States are found in Midwestern river valleys (especially the Mississippi and Missouri River valleys).

3. What is the pathogenesis of infection?

1. **Lymphocutaneous disease**, which accounts for 80% of all cases, is an occupational disease of farmers and gardeners. Infection follows direct inoculation of the organism via breaks in the skin, almost always in the upper extremities. The initial skin break is often a minor or unrecognized injury. Progressive lymphocutaneous disease evolves, although a small percentage of infections remain localized.

2. **Primary pulmonary disease** is thought to be secondary to inhalation or aspiration, although this mechanism has not been definitively proved. It generally occurs in patients with some underlying lung disturbance (e.g., chronic obstructive pulmonary disease or tobacco abuse).

4. What are the clinical manifestations of non-disseminated sporotrichosis?

1. **Lymphocutaneous disease.** Initially a subcutaneous nodule of dusky-red color develops and often ulcerates. Spread to regional lymphatics then follows, with red streaking in the skin and development of secondary nodules. The nodules may ulcerate and drain but do not cause pain. Spread beyond the skin and lymphatics is uncommon.

2. **Primary pulmonary disease** commonly presents as a low-grade indolent pulmonary infection with productive cough. Fever and weight loss are less common, and hemoptysis is rare. It often is asymptomatic, and discovered by routine chest radiograph.

5. How is the diagnosis made?

The clinical appearance of lymphocutaneous disease should suggest the diagnosis, especially in light of an appropriate exposure history. Culture of aspirated material confirms the diagnosis (any cultural isolation of *S. schenckii* is highly suggestive of infection, because the organism is an uncommon laboratory contaminant). Histopathologic examination reveals granulomatous lesions, often with a characteristic asteroid body, but does not confirm the diagnosis. The granulomatous lesions rarely reveal organisms, and the small, gram-positive, oval or cigar-shaped organisms are best seen when the usual acetone-ethanol decolorizer is replaced by 95% ethanol. Skin testing is not commercially available and does not confirm the diagnosis (because of cross-reactivity with other organisms and a 10% positive result in asymptomatic persons in endemic areas).

Serology tests have limited availability (agglutination appears to be the most satisfactory) but may be used to measure therapeutic efficacy. The absolute level of antibody does not correlate with duration of infection, and a negative titer does not exclude the diagnosis.

In pulmonary disease, bronchial washings and cultures are usually positive, whereas biopsies may not be helpful. The diagnosis often can be made solely on the basis of sputum culture.

Diagnosis of articular disease requires culture of synovial tissue or synovial fluid. Tissue culture is superior to synovial fluid culture alone; concomitant synovial tissue and fluid culture have the highest yield. Organisms are rarely found on histologic sections.

6. What is the differential diagnosis of lymphocutaneous nodules?
- Sporotrichosis
- Atypical mycobacterial infection
- Cutaneous nocardiosis
- Syphilis
- Pyoderma gangrenosum
- Leishmaniasis

7. What are the common chest radiographic findings of primary pulmonary disease?
Chest radiographic findings are highly variable. The most common finding is an apical fibro-cavitary lesion, which explains why pulmonary sporotrichosis is often mistaken for reinfection pulmonary tuberculosis or chronic pulmonary histoplasmosis. Cavitary lesions were found in 74% of patients with pulmonary disease; in 60% the finding was unilateral; and in 87% the upper lobe was involved. Alternate findings range from unilateral hilar adenopathy to single or multiple nodules and occasionally lobular infiltrates. Pleural effusions are exceedingly rare (three reported cases). Chest radiographs in disseminated disease with pulmonary involvement (as opposed to primary pulmonary disease) tend to show multiple pulmonary nodules or linear infiltrates and infrequently are cavitary.

8. What is the treatment of non-disseminated sporotrichosis?
1. **Lymphocutaneous disease.** Saturated solution of potassium iodide (SSKI) was the drug of choice for years and remains quite effective, but side effects limit its utility. Itraconazole is currently the drug of choice for lymphocutaneous disease at doses of 100–200 mg/day. It has achieved response rates greater than 90% and, although more expensive than SSKI, is tolerated much better. Ketoconazole is not effective. Fluconazole is significantly less effective than itraconazole and should be reserved for patients who cannot tolerate itraconazole. Amphotericin B may be necessary in deep infections, such as direct inoculation of the tendon sheath. Lymphocutaneous disease almost never relapses. Optimal length of therapy has not been well established, but therapy generally lasts 3–6 months. The major guidelines are to treat until all lesions have resolved and then continue for several months after clinical resolution.

2. **Primary pulmonary disease.** Responses of patients with pulmonary disease have been discouraging for all modalities. Amphotericin B has a cure rate of < 50% alone, although the rate is raised to 70–80% when amphotericin B is combined with surgical resection. In some series itraconazole has been as efficacious as amphotericin B at doses of 200 mg twice daily and may be used as first-line therapy in nonacutely ill patients. Treatment generally lasts 1–2 years. Acutely ill patients probably benefit from amphotericin B and may be changed to itraconazole for long-term therapy once they are clinically stable.

3. For **osteoarticular disease** without systemic involvement, the first-line therapy is itraconazole, 200 mg twice daily for 1–2 years.

9. Does heat therapy still play a role in the treatment of sporotrichosis?
Yes. Local heat brings symptomatic improvement to cutaneous disease. It also has effected cure in some pregnant women in whom it was desirable to avoid medications.

10. What are the features of disseminated sporotrichosis?
Disseminated sporotrichosis is rare and develops presumably through hematogenous spread. It is more common in alcoholics and other immunocompromised patients. Almost all cases of sporotrichosis in patients with AIDS are disseminated. The leukocyte count is usually normal, and a low-grade fever is found in only 30% of cases. Anorexia and weight loss are more common (60%). The sedimentation rate is usually elevated. Involved areas include:
1. Cutaneous and subcutaneous lesions (as described above) present in more than 90% of all cases of disseminated sporotrichosis.

2. Bone or articular lesions are seen in 80%. Bone involvement is generally confined to long bones near affected joints. Multiple joints are usually involved. The joint is painful and swollen, occasionally red, but rarely hot. The most common joint is the knee; ankle, wrist, and elbow are also commonly involved.

3. Pulmonary lesions are seen in only 20% of cases. Findings are distinct from primary pulmonary disease, as discussed above.

4. Central nervous system, genitourinary, and eye involvement have been described but are extremely rare.

11. What is the treatment of disseminated sporotrichosis?

Amphotericin B is clearly indicated for the treatment of central nervous system disease. In all other disseminated disease the best treatment is less clear. Recent studies have demonstrated the efficacy of itraconazole in disseminated disease, and because of its easier administration and fewer side effects, many people use it as the first-line agent. However, itraconazole is not approved by the Food and Drug Administration for treatment of sporotrichosis, and most physicians use amphotericin B in any acutely or seriously ill patient. Given the long length of therapy, itraconazole is a more attractive long-term agent. Patients may be switched from amphotericin B after initial improvement. Prognosis is guarded in disseminated disease, and surgical drainage is often necessary. Consultation with an infectious disease specialist is recommended.

In nonacutely ill patients with disseminated disease who are candidates for primary itraconazole therapy, the dose is 300 mg twice daily for 6 months and then 200 mg twice daily for long-term treatment. Therapy should continue for 1–2 years and should be lifelong in patients with AIDS because of an extremely high relapse rate. The total dose of amphotericin B in such cases should total at least 2 gm.

12. Are there any special instructions for taking itraconazole?

Itraconazole should be taken with food to increase its absorption (2–3-fold increase). Antacids, H_2 blockers, and omeprazole should be avoided because they interfere with absorption by decreasing gastric acidity. Doses of 200 mg or less can be given daily, but doses > 200 mg should be split into twice-daily dosing.

BIBLIOGRAPHY

1. Crout JE, Brewer NS, Tompkins RB: Sporotrichosis arthritis: Clinical features in seven patients. Ann Intern Med 86:294–297, 1977.
2. Kaufman CA: Old and new therapies for sporotrichosis. Clin Infect Dis 21:981–985, 1995.
3. Lynch PJ, Voorhees JJ, Harrell ER: Systemic sporotrichosis. Ann Intern Med 73:23–30, 1970.
4. Pluss JL, Opal SM: Pulmonary Sporotrichosis: Review of treatment and outcome. Medicine 65:143–153, 1986.
5. Wilson DE, Mann JJ, Bennett JE, Utz JP: Clinical features of extracutaneous sporotrichosis. Medicine 46:265–279, 1967.
6. Winn RE: Sporotrichosis. Infect Dis Clin North Am 2:899–911, 1988.

VIII. Parasitic Infections

30. IMPORTANT PARASITIC INFECTIONS IN THE UNITED STATES

Mary A. Marovich, M.D., and Ferric C. Fang, M.D.

1. What are the most important parasitic infections acquired in the United States?

Intestinal protozoa
Blastocystis hominis
Cryptosporidium parvum
Cyclospora cayetanensis
Dientamoeba fragilis
Entamoeba histolytica
Giardia lamblia
Isospora belli
Microsporidia

Extraintestinal protozoa
Acanthamoeba spp.
Babesia microti
Balamuthia mandrillaris
(*Entamoeba histolytica*) spp.
Leishmania spp.
Naegleria fowleri
Plasmodium vivax
Toxoplasma gondii
Trichomonas vaginalis
Trypanosoma cruzi

Intestinal nematodes
Anisakis spp.
Ascaris lumbricoides
Contracaecum spp.
Enterobius vermicularis
Necator americanus
Pseudoterranova spp.
Strongyloides stercoralis
Trichuris trichiura

Extraintestinal nematodes
Ancylostoma braziliense
Dirofilaria immitis
Toxocara spp.
Trichinella spiralis

Intestinal cestodes
Diphyllobothrium latum
Dipylidium caninum
Hymenolepis diminuta
Hymenolepis nana
Taenia saginata
Taenia solium

Extraintestinal cestodes
Echinococcus multilocularis

Extraintestinal trematodes
Fasciola hepatica

2. Has anyone survived primary amebic meningoencephalitis?

Yes, but survivors are rare. The free-living amoeba *Naegleria fowleri* inhabits fresh or brackish water throughout the world. Human infection most often results after swimming and is manifested by acute fulminant meningoencephalitis. Antimicrobial agents, including amphotericin B and rifampin, have been administered with occasional benefit, but most cases of primary amebic meningoencephalitis have been fatal. Recently, a leptomyxid amoeba designated *Balamuthia mandrillaris* has been reported to cause a somewhat similar clinical syndrome.

3. Which parasitic infection may present as gram-negative bacteremia or meningitis?

Strongyloides stercoralis hyperinfection syndrome may be associated with gram-negative bacteremia or meningitis. This ubiquitous, often asymptomatic, intestinal nematode infection can become life-threatening in patients with certain immunosuppressive conditions (corticosteroid usage, hematologic malignancy, or severe malnutrition). Proliferating larvae may migrate across the intestinal wall in enormous numbers, facilitating secondary dissemination of enteric bacterial flora. This parasite is endemic in parts of the southeastern U.S. and is also prevalent in chronically institutionalized people and immigrants from the developing world.

4. Should hydrogen peroxide be used to disinfect contact lenses?

No. Hydrogen peroxide does not kill the free-living amoeba *Acanthamoeba*. Heat-sterilization is preferred. *Acanthamoeba* sp. are important causative agents of keratitis and usually occur in people with improperly sterilized contact lenses. Effective treatment generally includes both surgical debridement and topical propamidine.

5. Which intraerythrocytic parasite can be cotransmitted with Lyme disease or ehrlichiosis?

Babesia microti, a protozoan parasite, can be transmitted by the same tick (*Ixodes scapularis*) that transmits the causative agents of Lyme disease and human granulocytic ehrlichiosis. Coinfection with *B. microti* and the Lyme disease spirochete *Borrelia burgdorferi* is associated with more severe symptoms than infection with *B. burgdorferi* alone. Most *B. microti* infections are subclinical, but elderly or asplenic people are more susceptible to disease. Symptomatic *B. microti* infections resemble malaria, with fever and hemolytic anemia. High levels of parasitemia may occur, but infection is rarely fatal. On inspection of the peripheral blood smear, the parasite may be seen as small ring forms within erythrocytes. A tetrad form resembling a Maltese cross is diagnostic. Babesiosis is classically described along the northeastern seaboard of the U.S. (e.g., Nantucket Island), but cases have been described in locales as geographically diverse as Georgia, Wisconsin, California, and Washington state.

6. How should *Trichomonas* vaginitis be treated during pregnancy?

Metronidazole probably remains the therapeutic agent of choice, despite some concern about mutagenicity and possible teratogenicity. Alternative agents for the treatment of *Trichomonas* vaginitis are less effective, and persistent vaginitis may precipitate preterm labor. Limited studies suggest that brief courses of metronidazole may be safely administered during pregnancy, particularly during the second and third trimesters.

7. Which parasitic diseases can be transmitted by blood transfusion or organ transplantation?

American trypanosomiasis (Chagas' disease), malaria, toxoplasmosis, leishmaniasis, and babesiosis.

8. Can *Cyclospora* infections be treated?

Yes. The coccidian protozoan parasite *Cyclospora cayetanensis* was previously referred to as *Cryptosporidium*-like, coccidian-like, or *Cyanobacterium*-like bodies (CLBs). In contrast to cryptosporidiosis, the prolonged diarrheal syndrome associated with *C. cayetanensis* can be rapidly ameliorated by treatment with trimethoprim-sulfamethoxazole.

9. Which parasite is frequently mistaken for lung cancer?

Dirofilaria immitis is a canine parasite (dog heartworm) that most often presents as a solitary pulmonary nodule when acquired by humans. This infection is often asymptomatic, but about one-half of afflicted patients complain of cough and chest pain. Like other filarial diseases, dirofilariasis is transmitted by mosquitoes. When humans are infected, the filarial larvae migrate to the right heart and pulmonary vasculature but cannot complete their life cycle. The dying larvae instigate local inflammatory responses in the lung. A definitive diagnosis requires excisional biopsy.

10. How often is cysticercosis acquired by ingesting undercooked pork?

Never. People ingesting measled pork (containing cysticerci) can become infected with the adult tapeworm, but cysticercosis is actually acquired by ingesting fecally contaminated food or water containing eggs of the pork tapeworm, *Taenia solium*. This was demonstrated during an outbreak of cysticercosis in an orthodox Jewish community in New York City, in which none of the afflicted people had ingested pork. Two household workers with evidence of *T. solium* infection were the most likely source of the outbreak. The most serious complication of cysticercosis is involvement of the central nervous system, which may cause seizures, meningitis, and hydrocephalus.

11. Are all strains of *Entamoeba histolytica* pathogenic?

No. There are two strains of *E. histolytica* with indistinguishable morphology, only one of which is pathogenic for humans. The nonpathogenic strain has recently been proposed as a separate species, *Entamoeba dispar*. Laboratory confirmation of amebiasis requires the presence of trophozoites or cysts in stool or tissue, or a positive serologic test. *E. dispar* infection does not induce serum antibodies. All *E. dispar* infections and most *E. histolytica* infections are asymptomatic, but *E. histolytica* may cause dysentery, intestinal mass lesions (amebomas), perianal ulceration, and visceral abscesses (especially in the liver).

12. Can parasites be acquired from sushi?

Yes. Anisakidosis (anisakiasis) is caused by ingesting larval nematodes of *Anisakis, Pseudoterranova,* or *Contracaecum* sp. in raw fish. The larvae attach to the gastric or intestinal wall, causing nausea and severe pain; visceral perforation occasionally occurs. Endoscopic or surgical resection is often required. Anisakidosis is entirely preventable by cooking or freezing fish before consumption. In some parts of the world (including the U.S.), consumption of raw fish can also result in infection with cestodes (*Diphyllobothrium latum* and *Sparganum proliferum*), intestinal trematodes (*Heterophyes, Metagonimus,* or *Nanophyetus* sp.), or other nematodes (*Gnathostoma* and *Eustrongylides* spp.).

13. Can leishmaniasis be acquired in the United States?

Yes. Although it is uncommon, infection with *Leishmania mexicana* has been acquired in Texas, where the sandfly vector (*Lutzomyia* sp.) exists. *Leishmania,* an intracellular parasite, can cause three distinct clinical syndromes: visceral, cutaneous, or mucocutaneous leishmaniasis. The disease manifestations are determined both by characteristics of the parasite and by the nature of the host immune response. Autochthonous leishmaniasis acquired in the U.S. has been limited to cutaneous involvement. Two recently identified risk groups for exogenous leishmaniasis encountered (but not acquired) in the U.S. are patients with AIDS and troops returning from the Persian Gulf.

14. Can intestinal microsporidiosis be diagnosed from routine stool ova and parasite studies?

No. Microsporidia (e.g., *Enterocytozoon, Encephalitozoon,* and *Septata* sp.) are intracellular parasites that can cause both intestinal and extraintestinal infection in immunocompromised patients, particularly in patients with AIDS. Although microsporidia may be visualized with Gram, Giemsa, acid-fast, or other routine staining protocols, detection in stool requires special chromotrope-based or fluorochrome-based methods.

15. Can *Giardia lamblia* be transmitted from person to person?

Yes. In fact, person-to-person transmission of *G. lamblia* is the second most common mode; waterborne transmission is the primary mode. Fecal-oral transmission of *G. lamblia* cysts typically occurs in settings of suboptimal hygiene, such as among young children in day care centers, chronically institutionalized people, and participants in oral-anal sexual activity.

16. How can the diagnosis of visceral larva migrans be confirmed?

The most useful confirmatory test is an enzyme-linked immunosorbent assay (ELISA) for serum antibodies to *Toxocara* sp. Diagnosis requires clinical correlation, because elevated titers are prevalent in some populations without clinical evidence of active infection. Visceral larva migrans is acquired by children when they ingest *Toxocara* eggs from environmental sources contaminated with dog or cat feces. Severe infections may be complicated by wheezing, hepatomegaly, fever, and eosinophilia. Most patients recover without specific treatment. Diethylcarbamazine, albendazole, and mebendazole have been administered but are of uncertain benefit.

17. Of the parasitic pathogens causing diarrhea in patients with AIDS, which are acid-fast on stool smears?

Isospora belli, Cyclospora cayetanensis (see question 8), and *Cryptosporidium parvum. Isospora, Cyclospora,* and *Cryptosporidium* spp. may be diagnosed by examination of acid-fast stained fecal material. The relative size of the oocysts facilitates species discrimination: *Isospora* sp. are typically 20–30 μm in diameter; *Cyclospora* sp., 8–10 μm; and *Cryptosporidium* sp., 4–6 μm. Each of these parasites can cause diarrhea, particularly in immunocompromised hosts. Extraintestinal involvement is sometimes seen with *Cryptosporidium* sp.

18. Is trichinosis acquired exclusively from pork?

No. Although human infection with *Trichinella spiralis* is usually acquired by ingesting inadequately cooked pork, trichinosis has occasionally resulted from ingestion of bear, wild boar, or walrus meat. Beef or horse meat inadvertently contaminated with infested pork has also been implicated.

19. What is the primary host of *Ascaris lumbricoides*?

Humans are the primary hosts of *A. lumbricoides*. This parasite is probably the most common human intestinal helminth; as much as one-fourth of the world's population is believed to be infected. Ascariasis is typically asymptomatic or causes mild symptoms of vague abdominal discomfort, but large worm burdens or aberrant migration may produce severe symptoms.

20. Which parasite can cause megaloblastic anemia?

Diphyllobothrium latum, the fish tapeworm, effectively competes with its human host for ingested vitamin B12. A small percentage of infected patients develop hematologic and neurologic manifestations of B12 deficiency.

21. Does a negative *Toxoplasma* serologic test exclude the diagnosis of toxoplasmic encephalitis in patients with AIDS?

No. Negative serology does not completely exclude the possibility of cerebral toxoplasmosis in patients with AIDS. However, a negative serologic test makes the diagnosis much less likely, because most cases of toxoplasmic encephalitis result from reactivation of latent infection. Although definitive diagnosis requires culture or direct demonstration of *Toxoplasma* in brain tissue by histopathologic or molecular methods, it is reasonable and appropriate to administer empiric antiparasitic therapy to seropositive patients with compatible clinical and radiologic features of toxoplasmic encephalitis, without obtaining a brain biopsy. Patients with HIV infection should have a screening *Toxoplasma* serologic test, and prophylaxis is recommended for seropositive patients with CD4 lymphocyte counts < 100/mm^3.

BIBLIOGRAPHY

1. Davis CE: Laboratory diagnosis of parasitic infections. In Isselbacher KJ, Braunwald E, Wilson JD, et al (eds): Harrison's Principles of Internal Medicine, 13th ed. New York, McGraw-Hill, 1994, pp 872–877.
2. Drugs for Parasitic Infections. Med Lett Drugs Ther 37:99–108, 1995.
3. Garcia LS, Bruckner DA: Diagnostic Medical Parasitology, 2nd ed. Washington, DC, American Society for Microbiology, 1993.
4. Goodgame RW: Understanding intestinal spore-forming protozoa: Cryptosporidia, Microsporidia, Isospora, and Cyclospora. Ann Intern Med 124:429–441, 1996.
5. Maguire JH, Keystone JS: Parasitic diseases. Infect Dis Clin North Am 7:467–738, 1993.
6. Mandell GL, Bennett JE, Dolin R (eds): Principles and Practice of Infectious Diseases, 4th ed. New York, Churchill Livingstone, 1995.

IX. Sexually Transmitted Diseases

31. URETHRITIS

Kristie J. Lowry, M.D.

1. What are the presenting signs and symptoms of urethritis in men?

Urethral discharge may be scant or heavy enough to stain undergarments. The drainage may be clear, mucopurulent, or frankly purulent; its color may be white, yellow-green, or brown. The patient may complain of dysuria at the meatus or anywhere along the shaft and/or pain, itching, frequency, urgency, or a feeling of heaviness in the genitals. The pain may persist between micturitions.

2. What is the laboratory diagnosis of urethritis?

The initial laboratory diagnosis includes a urethral smear showing ≥ 4 polymorphonuclear neutrophils (PMNs). However, up to 50% of all men with documented urethral infections have less than 4 PMN per oil immersion field. Even if only 1 PMN is present on the smear, infection should be considered present, and a work-up should proceed.

3. Name potential common infectious and noninfectious causes of urethritis.

Infectious causes of urethritis	Noninfectious causes of urethritis
Neisseria gonorrhoeae	Self-induced trauma from stripping (milking)
Chlamydia trachomatis	of urethra for fear of urethritis
Trichomonas vaginalis	Foreign object-induced trauma
Ureaplasma urealyticum	Systemic disease (Stevens-Johnson or Wegener's
	granulomatosis)
Herpes simplex virus (rare)	Reiter's syndrome
Mycoplasma genitalium (rare)	Spermicides

4. How is suspected urethritis initially evaluated?

The patient should undergo a directed history and physical exam. Underwear should be examined for staining, the entire genital area for lymphadenopathy or skin lesions, and the hair for nits. The testes and spermatic cord should be palpated for masses or tenderness. The meatus should be examined for dried crust, redness, or spontaneous discharge. A swab and Gram stain of expressed or spontaneous urethral discharge should then be performed. Nucleic acid hybridization for *N. gonorrhoeae* and *C. trachomatis* should be sent as well as culture for *U. urealyticum*. In addition to these studies, HIV and serum rapid plasma reagin (RPR) tests should be done to rule out HIV infection and syphilis.

5. What is the proper way to examine the urethra and process the collected specimen?

The foreskin should be retracted and the glans and meatus examined. If no discharge is present, the urethra should be gently stripped (milked) by placing the gloved thumb along the ventral surface of the base of the penis and the forefinger on the dorsum and then applying gentle pressure while moving toward the meatus. The specimen should be collected with a calcium alginate urethral swab. Cotton or wooden swabs should not be used because they may be toxic to fastidious organisms. The swab should be inserted into the urethra at least 2 cm. The swab should then be rolled on a slide (not smeared) to better preserve morphologic characteristics.

6. What is the the urine leukocyte esterase test? When is it applicable?

The urine leukocyte esterase test screens for an enzyme released from degraded white blood cells. Given the low sensitivity of this test for urethritis, routine screening is not warranted. However, it may have a role in asymptomatic contacts who refuse urethral swabbing or asymptomatic HIV-positive patients. Some clinicians believe that all adolescent males should be routinely screened with this inexpensive test to diagnose and eradicate the asymptomatic carrier state.

7. What four variables increase the probability of a positive urethral culture in both symptomatic and asymptomatic males?

1. Sexual contact with a known infected partner in the past month
2. Having ever used a condom
3. Five or more lifetime partners
4. More than one sexual partner in the past month

8. What diagnostic smears, cultures, or assays of urethral specimens are available for urethritis?

1. Gram stain smears for *N. gonorrhoeae* continue to be a quick, inexpensive and sensitive test for gonorrhea (GC) and are still recommended during initial screening. Because 5% of smears are negative in active infection, additional screening for GC should be performed when the Gram stain is negative.

2. Culture for GC remains the standard for diagnosis of gonococcal infections but is not performed as routinely as before. The drawbacks of culture include slow turn-around time (48–72 hr), requirement for a heavy inoculum, and failure of some fastidious strains to grow.

3. Culture for chlamydia is no longer routinely performed. Culture is time-consuming and requires special equipment and trained personnel not often available in small clinics.

4. Nucleic acid probes are a highly sensitive and specific test for both *N. gonorrhoeae* and *C. trachomatis*. They require trained lab personnel and special equipment (water bath and luminometer) but can be run in 2–3 hours. These tests are frequently used.

5. Enzyme immunoassay (EIA) tests are available for both chlamydia and GC. The tests are quick and easy to batch, however, the sensitivity is low (chlamydia: 72–95%) compared with culture. The EIA for GC is also less sensitive than culture and is associated with false-positive results. It should be used only in high-risk populations.

6. Polymerase chain reaction (PCR), a new test for chlamydia, is highly sensitive (100%) and specific (95+%). In some studies it is more sensitive than culture. PCR is expensive and requires trained personnel and special equipment. It may have a role in suspected chlamydia conjunctival infections, in which culture is only 50% sensitive.

7. Direct fluorescent antibody was the first nonculture chlamydia detection test. The test is quick to process (30–60 minutes) but has a low sensitivity (50–77%).

9. How does gonococcal urethritis differ from nongonococcal urethritis in terms of its clinical characteristics?

Clinical Distinction Between Gonococcal and Nongonococcal Urethritis

MANIFESTATIONS	GONOCOCCAL	NONGONOCOCCAL
Incubation period	2–7 days	10–21 days
Onset	Abrupt	Gradual
Discharge	Yellow, profuse	Thin, clear, watery
Dysuria	Moderate	Mild

10. What is the natural course of untreated gonococcal urethritis?

Seventy-five percent of men acquiring urethral gonorrhea develop symptoms abruptly within 4 days and 80–90% within 2 weeks. Patients frequently develop a thick yellow discharge with dysuria (71%). The symptoms gradually subside over a period of 1–3 months in 30–70% of patients, and 95% of untreated patients are free of symptoms after 6 months. It is unknown how many of these patients are asymptomatic carriers.

11. What are the potential complications of urethritis?

Both *C. trachomatis* and *N. gonorrhoeae* have been identified as causes of epididymitis, and 20–30% of men infected with either agent have documented asymptomatic prostatic involvement. Urethral stricture has been reported. *C. trachomatis* can infect the conjunctiva. Approximately 4% of patients with nongonococcal urethritis (NGU) have developed an oculogenital syndrome with conjunctivitis and NGU.

12. Define postgonococcal urethritis (PGU).

PGU is characterized by signs, symptoms, and laboratory evidence of urethritis developing 4–7 days after successful single-dose therapy for gonococcal urethritis. PGU is a manifestation of a dual urethral infection for which the nongonococcal portion was untreated. Chlamydia is recovered in up to 50% of cases of PGU.

13. What is the prevalence and clinical significance of trichomonal urethritis?

Trichomoniasis may be found in 5–60% of male patients presenting to sexually transmitted disease clinics. Most are symptomatic with dysuria and discharge (50–65%). The infection may persist for months if untreated. It occasionally is complicated by prostatitis. *Trichomonas* sp. rarely involves other genitourinary organs. A major concern is the risk of spread to a sexual partner.

14. When should patients be screened for trichomonal urethritis?

Patients with a recent history of exposure, symptomatic patients with a history of previous treatment for *Trichomonas* sp., or patients with a recurrent or persistent urethritis despite NGU therapy should be evaluated by wet mount and culture.

15. What is the current therapy for trichomonal urethritis?

Metronidazole, 2 gm single dose orally (better tolerated if dose is given over several hours)
   or
Metronidazole, 375–500 mg 2 times/day orally for 7 days

16. How does herpes simplex urethritis present?

Herpes simplex is isolated from the urethra in 30% of men during a primary genital infection. The dysuria is far worse than the urethral discharge, and few polymorphonuclear leukocytes are isolated on smear. Most patients with urethritis have genital lesions, but a small percentage do not.

17. Define Reiter's syndrome.

Reiter's syndrome is a clinical symptom complex that may include urethritis, arthritis, conjunctivitis, uveitis, and oral or penile ulcers secondary to a postinfectious host immune response. About 60–90% of patients carry the HLA-B27 histocompatibility antigen. Reiter's syndrome typically follows either sexually transmitted urethritis or bacterial gastroenteritis.

18. How is Reiter's syndrome treated?

Attempts to diagnose infective urethritis should be made and all active infections treated. However, if no infection is diagnosed, a 7-day course of doxycycline is prudent, given the frequency with which chlamydia is associated with Reiter's syndrome. Nonsteroidal antiinflammatory drugs are the most effective treatment for systemic inflammatory manifestations.

19. What are the four major goals in the clinical management of urethritis?

1. Accurate identification of the most likely causative agent
2. Prompt administration of effective antimicrobial therapy
3. Initiation of appropriate counseling
4. Notification and treatment of sexual partners

20. What are the current recommended treatments for gonococcal urethritis?

Gonococcal Therapy

First line:
Ceftriaxone, 125 mg IM single dose (in 1% lidocaine)
    plus
Doxycycline, 100 mg 2 times/day orally for 7 days
    (for possible coexistent chlamydial infection)

Alternatives include any of the following:
Cefixime, 400 mg single dose orally
Ciprofloxacin, 500 mg single dose orally
Ofloxacin, 400 mg single dose orally
Spectinomycin, 2 gm single dose IM
    with
Doxycycline, 100 mg 2 times/day orally for 7 days
    (for possible coexistent chlamydial infection)

21. What are the current recommended treatments for chlamydial urethritis?

Chlamydial Therapy

First line:
Doxycycline, 100 mg 2 times/day orally for 7 days
    or
Azithromycin, 1 gm single dose orally

Alternatives:
Ofloxacin, 300 mg 2 times/day orally for 7 days
    or
Erythromycin, 500 mg 4 times/day orally for 7 days

Pregnancy (any of the following):
Erythromycin, 500 mg 4 times/day orally for 7 days
Amoxicillin, 500 mg 3 times/day orally for 10 days
Azithromycin, 1 gm single dose orally

22. When should azithromycin be considered the drug of choice for chlamydial urethritis?

Azithromycin is highly effective (98%) for uncomplicated *C. trachomatis* urethritis but has a higher initial cost than doxycycline ($15–30 vs. $3). However, hypothetical cost analyses of the two drugs show that azithromycin may be cheaper in the long term because of treatment failure and complications of failure due to noncompliance in the doxycycline-treated group. Azithromycin should be given to all patients likely to be noncompliant. The most frequently noncompliant patients include referred contact patients or patients diagnosed with asymptomatic urethral infections.

23. Define the acute urethral syndrome in women.

Acute urethral syndrome in women includes dysuria, frequency, urgency, and/or nocturia without bacterial cystitis caused by a urethral STD.

24. How is the acute urethral syndrome diagnosed?

Patients often have failed empiric therapy for bacterial cystitis, and urine cultures have been negative. At this time urethral smears for Gram stain, wet prep, culture, and nucleic acid hybridization test to rule out gonococcal, chlamydial, and trichomonal infection should be performed.

BIBLIOGRAPHY

1. Borchardt KA, Al-Haraci S, Maida N: Prevalence of *Trichomonas vaginalis* in a male population by interview, wet mount microscopy, and the InPouch(TM) TV test. Genitourin Med 71:405–406, 1995.
2. Drugs for sexually transmitted diseases. Medical Lett 37:117–122, 1995.
3. Janier M, Lassua F, Casin I, et al: Male urethritis with and without discharge. Sex Transm Dis 22:244–252, 1995.
4. Johnson J, Neas B, Parker D: Screening for urethral infection in adolescent and young adult males. J Adolesc Health 14:356–361, 1993.
5. Kreiger JN: Trichomoniasis in men: Old issues and new data. Sex Transm Dis 22:83–96, 1994.
6. Martin DH, Mroczkowski TF, Dalu ZA: A controlled trial of azithromycin for the treatment of chlamydial urethritis and cervicitis. N Engl J Med 327:921–925, 1992.
7. McCormack WM, Rein MF: Urethritis. In Mandell GL, Bennett JE, Dolin R (eds): Principles and Practice of Infectious Diseases, 4th ed. New York, Churchill Livingstone, 1995, pp 1063–1074.
8. Patrick DM, Rekart ML, Knowles L: Unsatisfactory performance of the leukocyte esterase test of first voided urine for rapid diagnosis of urethritis. Genitourin Med 70:187–190, 1994.
9. Schmid GP, Fontanarosa PB: Evolving strategies for management of the nongonococcal urethritis syndrome. JAMA 274:577–579, 1995.
10. Shafer M, Schachter J, Moscicki A, et al: Urinary leukocyte esterase screening test for asymptomatic chlamydial and gonococcal infections in males. JAMA 262:2562–2566, 1989.

32. MANAGEMENT OF SYPHILIS

Edmund C. Tramont, M.D.

1. Why are the VDRL and RPR tests referred to as "nonspecific" serologic tests? What are they used for?

In any situation that involves chronic immune stimulation, antibodies to cardiolipin-choles-terol-lecithin may develop; hence, these antibodies are not specific for *Treponema pallidum*, the microorganism that causes syphilis. However, because the Venereal Disease Research Laboratory (VDRL) and rapid plasma reagin (RPR) tests are easy, quick, inexpensive, and virtually always positive in patients with untreated syphilis, they are used to screen for syphilis. Furthermore, because they are low-affinity antibodies, they disappear with successful therapy and consequently are used to gauge the success of therapy. Patients with early syphilis should become seronegative within 2 years and patients with late syphilis by 5 years. The old term for these nonspecific antibodies was *reagenic antibodies*.

2. What are the specific serologic tests for syphilis? What are they used for?

Specific serologic tests for syphilis refer to measurements of specific binding antibodies to *Treponema pallidum*; they are used to verify that a positive nonspecific test is caused by *T. pallidum*. The fluorescent treponemal antibody, absorbed (FTA-ABS) test is the oldest such test still in use today, but it is being slowly replaced by other simpler and more versatile tests, such as the *T. pallidum* hemagglutination (TPHA) test, microhemagglutination–*T. pallidum* (MHA–TP) test, and various newer enzyme-linked immunosorbent assays (ELISAs). These tests usually remain positive for the life of the patient but may revert to negative if appropriate treatment is instituted early in the disease.

3. When is a dark-field examination done?

A dark-field examination of scrapings from a syphilitic ulcer to directly visualize the spirochete is the most direct means of establishing the diagnosis in early disease. Specific fluorescent or immunoperoxidase antibodies also may be used to detect spirochetes.

4. When should a test for syphilis be done?

Syphilis should be ruled out whenever a patient has a sexually transmitted disease or is at risk for a sexually transmitted disease, including HIV infection, genital herpes, gonorrhea, nonspecific urethritis, and hepatitis B. Genital ulcer disease increases the relative risk of acquiring HIV by 1.5–7 fold. Syphilis also should be ruled out whenever patients present with a confusing diagnosis, especially with an unusual or difficult to characterize cancer or with unilateral hearing loss, uveitis or any unexplained neurologic problem. The incidence of syphilis is highest in the so-called core groups, especially prisoners and women drug abusers.

5. What are the "stages" of syphilis?

The so-called stages of clinical syphilis were used by past clinicians to estimate the length of time of infection, to describe particular clinical parameters, and to determine treatment modalities. They are less useful today. Primary syphilis refers to the presence of a chancre, which is usually a single, nonpainful ulcer at the site of inoculation (most often in the genital area). Secondary syphilis refers to the most florid stage, which coincides with the highest levels of spirochetemia and immune reactivity. Skin rashes are the most common manifestation. During this period the central nervous system (CNS) is invaded. Other manifestations may include condyloma lata, generalized lymphadenopathy, mucous patches, fever, malaise, pharyngitis, arthralgias, tinnitus, vertigo, and diplopia. During this stage, renal failure and tissue invasion that masquerade as cancer are also most common. These stages usually occur early (between 2 weeks and 3 months after inoculation) but never more than 4 years later. Latent syphilis refers to patients with a positive serology but no clinical manifestations. Any patient with neurologic signs or symptoms is considered to have neurosyphilis. Tertiary or late syphilis is a slowly progressive inflammatory disease that usually involves the CNS; involvement of the cardiovascular system and development of syphilitic granulomas (gummas) are rare today.

6. Why after 50 years is the antibiotic treatment of syphilis still controversial?

The controversy surrounds the level of risk that one is willing to take to ensure a cure. To understand that risk, the following points must be reconciled:

1. A spirochetemia that can seed any organ, including the CNS, develops soon after inoculation in 40% of cases.

2. The average doubling time of *T. pallidum* is over 30 hours, which requires a treponemicidal antibiotic level in the invaded tissues for at least 8 days.

3. Most people with a well-functioning immune system clear the infection; clearance is greatly enhanced with even low doses of appropriate antibiotics.

4. The manifestations of late syphilis are delayed by years, making it difficult to discern treatment failures from reinfection.

Clinicians on one side of the controversy believe that a regimen that probably ensures a treponemicidal level in the blood for more than 8 days is adequate treatment. Hence, depending on the stage or length of time of infection, treatment with 1–3 doses of 1.2 M units of benzathine penicillin intramuscularly is sufficient to cure most patients with early syphilis and 1.2 M units each week for 3 weeks is sufficient for neurosyphilis, late syphilis, or syphilis infection of unknown duration. They cite as proof the rarity of diagnosed neurosyphilis, the most difficult form to cure.

Clinicians on the other side of the controversy believe that because the CNS is invaded in 40% of cases and benzathine penicillin fails to reach treponemicidal levels in the CNS in over 90% of infected patients, the risk of treatment failure is too great and the possibility of late manifestations of neurosyphilis is too high. They cite (1) the relatively high incidence of cerebral vascular incidents (stroke) and psychological problems that result in the hospitalization of patients with positive specific serologic tests and (2) the many documented cases in the medical literature of treatment failures with benzathine penicillin. They recommend antibiotic regimens that are highly likely to achieve treponemicidal levels in the CNS for at least 10 days.

7. What antibiotic regimens achieve treponemicidal levels in the CNS?

The following antibiotic regimens have been reported to achieve treponemicidal levels in the CNS (in order of most studies reported):

1. Aqueous penicillin, 2–4 gm intravenously every 4 hours for 10 days

2. Amoxicillin, 3 gm, plus probenecid, 0.5 gm, orally twice daily for 10–14 days

3. Doxycycline, 2 gm orally twice daily for 21 days

4. Procaine penicillin, 2.4 M units/day intramuscularly, plus probenecid, 1 gm orally, for 10 days

5. Ceftriaxone, 1 gm diluted in 1% lidocaine intramuscularly for 10–14 days

8. What regimen(s) should be used when patient compliance is an issue?

Benzathine penicillin, 1.2 M units intramuscularly each week for 3 weeks, should be added to any of the above regimens.

9. Is syphilis more difficult to diagnose in HIV-infected persons?

Sometimes. HIV-infected persons have a dysfunctional immune system that can either delay a serologic response or give rise to a false-positive serologic response. In addition, a nonspecific serologic response (VDRL, RPR) can remain persistently elevated despite adequate treatment. Thus, the diagnosis of syphilis in this high-risk population can be problematic.

10. Is the clinical presentation altered in HIV-infected patients?

Sometimes. As with any patient with a dysfunctional immune system, HIV-infected persons often have a more florid clinical presentation and more extensive disease, including acute syphilitic meningitis and other manifestations of neurosyphilis, especially uveitis. The incidence or probability of neurosyphilis, however, does not appear to be increased in dually infected patients.

11. Do dually infected HIV patients require more aggressive treatment?

Yes. All dually infected persons should be treated with the same antibiotic regimen that is required for neurosyphilis (see above). Patients, however, have been cured with a single 1.2 M unit intramuscular injection of benzathine penicillin.

12. Should pregnant women be treated with the same regimens as nonpregnant women?

Yes. But as a precaution, the neonate also should be treated at birth with 50,000 units/kg/day intravenously in 2 divided doses for 10 days. The same dosage of procaine penicillin may be given, but it is quite painful. The probability of adverse reactions to penicillin is remote in neonates.

13. What abnormalities are present in the cerebrospinal fluid of patients with neurosyphilis?

Most patients have normal cerebrospinal fluid (CSF) parameters. A positive VDRL or RPR test of the CSF is diagnostic. Elevated protein and cell counts are the most common abnormal findings. However, if adequate doses of antibiotics are administered, examination of the CSF is not necessary unless there are clinical indications of CNS involvement.

14. When should congenital syphilis be considered?

Neonatal syphilis should be considered whenever the mother is infected, has been infected, or is at risk for infection, especially if she is a drug abuser or is or has been incarcerated. The clinical presentation is quite variable, but hepatosplenomegaly is the most prominent clinical feature.

15. What is the Jarisch-Herxheimer reaction?

The Jarisch-Herxheimer reaction is an acute systemic reaction that occurs 1–2 hours after initial treatment with effective antibiotics. It results from the rapid death and release of spirochetal antigens and is seen most often with penicillin treatment of secondary syphilis. One dose of 60 mg of prednisone intravenously dramatically aborts most instances.

BIBLIOGRAPHY

1. Reyes MP, Hunt N, Ostrea EM, et al: Maternal/congenital syphilis in a large tertiary-care urban hospital. Clin Infect Dis 17:1041–1046, 1992.
2. Royce RA, Sena A, Cates W, Cohen MS: Current concepts: Sexual transmission of HIV. N Engl J Med 336:1072–1078, 1997.
3. Swartz MN: Neurosyphilis. In Holmes K, Mardh P, Sparling PF, et al (eds): Sexually Transmitted Diseases, 2nd ed. New York, McGraw-Hill, 1990, pp 231–246.
4. Thin RN: Early syphilis in the adult. In Holmes K, Mardh P, Sparling PF, et al (eds): Sexually Transmitted Diseases, 2nd ed. New York, McGraw-Hill, 1990, pp 221–230.
5. Tomberlin MG, Holton PD, Owens JL, et al: Evaluation of neurosyphilis in human immunodeficiency virus-infected individuals. Clin Infect Dis 18:288–294, 1994.
6. Tramont EC: *Treponema pallidum* (syphilis). In Mandel G, Bennett J, Dolin R (eds): Principles and Practice of Infectious Diseases, 4th ed. New York, Churchill Livingstone, 1995, pp 2117–2133.

33. CLINICAL CONSIDERATIONS IN PELVIC INFLAMMATORY DISEASE

Susan L. Fraser, M.D.

1. What disorders comprise the spectrum of pelvic inflammatory disease (PID)?

PID is an inflammatory disorder of the female upper genital tract that may include any combination of endometritis, salpingitis, tuboovarian abscess (TOA), and pelvic peritonitis. PID is usually but not always sexually transmitted. Traditionally, infections arising from surgery or parturition are not included in the definition of PID.

2. What are the major risk factors for developing PID?

- Young age(< 25 yr)
- Early age at first intercourse
- Multiple sexual partners, especially more than one male partner in the past 30 days
- Lower socioeconomic status
- Unmarried status
- Sex during the previous menses
- Lack of birth control method
- Gravidity, parity, or spontaneous abortions > 1
- Presence of bacterial vaginosis
- History of sexually transmitted disease (STD)
- Known exposure to nongonococcal urethritis in the past 30 days
- Cigarette smoking
- Substance abuse
- Presence of an intrauterine device (especially if recently inserted)
- Douching

Oral contraceptive use and depot medroxyprogesterone are associated with a reduced incidence of PID, partly because of increased cervical mucus viscosity and reduced menstrual blood flow.

3. What organisms can be implicated in cases of PID?

Sexually transmitted organisms, especially *Neisseria gonorrhoeae* and *Chlamydia trachomatis*, are implicated in most cases. Other bacteria that may be part of the vaginal flora can also cause PID. These and some uncommon microorganisms that have been isolated from women with PID are listed below.

Organisms Implicated in PID

Sexually transmitted	*Neisseria gonorrhoeae, Chlamydia trachomatis*
Vaginal flora	
Gram-negative bacilli	*Gardnerella vaginalis, Haemophilus influenzae, Escherichia coli, Klebsiella* species, other enterobacteriaceae
Gram-positive cocci	*Streptococcus agalactiae* (group B streptococci), *Streptococcus pneumoniae, Streptococcus pyogenes* (group A streptococci), other *Streptococcus* spp., *Staphylococcus* and *Enterococcus* spp.
Anaerobes	*Bacteroides fragilis, Prevotella* sp., *Peptostreptococcus, Peptococcus,* and *Fusobacterium* spp.
Uncommon organisms	*Neisseria meningitidis; Actinomyces israelii; Mycobacterium tuberculosis* and other mycobacteria; dimorphic fungi, including *Blastomyces, Histoplasma* and *Coccidioides* spp.; *Salmonella* group Cl
Controversial or unsure	*Mycoplasma hominis, Ureaplasma urealyticum*

4. Of women with inadequately treated chlamydial or gonococcal cervicitis, how many will develop PID?

From 10–40% will develop PID.

5. Why do we no longer use penicillin or tetracycline to treat gonorrhea?

Over 30% of *N. gonorrhoeae* isolates in the United States are resistant to penicillin or tetracycline by plasmid or chromosomally mediated mechanisms. Resistance to spectinomycin and the fluoroquinolones has been reported, but resistance to ceftriaxone has not yet been seen.

6. How can the diagnosis of PID be made?

The diagnosis of PID is usually made on the basis of clinical grounds, including physical examination and laboratory findings. Signs and symptoms, some of which are mild or atypical. vary widely. This variation in presentation may create difficulties and delays in reaching the correct diagnosis; many cases of PID are not recognized. The positive predictive value of a clinical diagnosis of acute PID varies depending on epidemiologic characteristics and the clinical setting, with no single historical, physical, or laboratory finding that is both sensitive and specific. Even the gold standard, laparoscopy, which can be used to obtain a more accurate visual and a more complete bacteriologic diagnosis of TOA, salpingitis, or pelvic peritonitis, does not detect subtle inflammation of the fallopian tubes or endometritis.

7. What are the three minimal criteria for diagnosing PID?

Lower abdominal tenderness, adnexal tenderness, and cervical motion tenderness. If all three clinical criteria are present and no other cause is established for pelvic inflammation, empiric treatment of PID should be instituted.

8. What are the additional routine and elaborate criteria for diagnosing PID?

Additional criteria may be used to increase the specificity of the diagnosis, especially when a more elaborate diagnostic evaluation is warranted, for patients with severe clinical signs or for whom incorrect diagnosis and management may cause unnecessary morbidity. Routine criteria for diagnosing PID include an oral temperature > 38.3° C (100.9° F), abnormal cervical or vaginal discharge, elevated erythrocyte sedimentation rate, elevated C-reactive protein, and culture documentation of cervical infection with *N. gonorrhoeae* or *C. trachomatis*. The elaborate criteria for diagnosing PID include histopathologic evidence of endometritis on endometrial biopsy, TOA on sonography or other radiologic tests, and laparoscopic abnormalities consistent with PID.

9. List the major criteria used to determine whether a patient diagnosed with PID should be hospitalized.

- Fever greater than 38° C
- White blood cell count above 11,000/mm^3
- Uncertain diagnosis or failure to exclude surgical emergencies such as acute appendicitis and ectopic pregnancy
- Suspicion of TOA, pelvic abscess, or peritonitis
- Pregnancy (a sensitive pregnancy test should be performed on all patients suspected of having PID)
- Significantly lower expected compliance (e.g., adolescent patient, drug addiction)
- HIV infection
- Severity of illness or nausea and vomiting that preclude outpatient management
- Patient's inability to follow or tolerate an outpatient regimen
- Failure to respond clinically to outpatient therapy
- Inability to arrange clinical follow-up within 72 hours of starting antibiotic treatment
- IUD in place

10. How is PID different in HIV-infected patients?

PID in HIV-infected patients is more aggressive than in immunologically normal hosts, with a fatal course in some instances. Abdominal pain and leukocytosis may not be as remarkable, or leukopenia may be present. HIV-infected women are more likely to require surgical intervention. PID in the setting of HIV infection usually mandates hospitalization and aggressive therapy with intravenous antibiotics.

11. What is the differential diagnosis for PID?

Selected Differential Diagnosis for PID

Infectious disorders	Appendicitis, cystitis, pyelonephritis, diverticulitis, mesenteric lymphadenitis, inflammatory bowel disease, cholecystitis, gastroenteritis
Noninfectious disorders	Ectopic pregnancy, ovarian cyst, hemorrhagic or ruptured corpus luteum, ovarian torsion, endometriosis, irritable bowel syndrome, nephrolithiasis, adhesions, somatization, tumor

12. Name at least two antibiotic regimens that can be administered to hospitalized patients with PID.
- Cefoxitin, 2 gm IV every 6 hr (or cefotetan, 2 gm IV every 12 hr) plus doxycycline, 100 mg IV or orally every 12 hr. Continue this regimen for at least 48 hours after significant clinical improvement occurs; then give doxycycline, 100 mg 2 times/day orally, to complete a total of 14 days of therapy.
- Clindamycin, 600–900 mg IV every 8 hr, plus gentamicin, 2 mg/kg IV or IM loading dose followed by 1.5–1.7 mg/kg every 8 hr. Continue this regimen for at least 48 hours after significant clinical improvement occurs; then give doxycycline, 100 mg 2 times/day orally, or clindamycin, 450 mg 4 times/day orally, to complete a total of 14 days of therapy. If TOA is present and tests for *C. trachomatis* are negative, clindamycin is the preferred drug for continued therapy because of its anaerobic coverage. Therapeutic drug level monitoring of gentamicin is recommended, especially if it is administered longer than 48–72 hr. A single daily dose of gentamicin (5–7 mg/kg/day) is a consideration but has not been studied in women with PID.
- Other options include (1) ampicillin-sulbactam, 3 gm IV every 6 hr; ticarcillin-clavulanic acid, 3.1 gm IV every 6 hr; or piperacillin-tazobactam, 3.375 mg IV every 6 hr, plus doxycycline, 100 mg IV or orally every 12 hr; or (2) ofloxacin, 300–400 mg IV twice daily plus either IV clindamycin as above or metronidazole, 500 mg IV every 6 hr. Forty-eight hours after considerable clinical improvement is documented, these regimens can be changed to oral doxycycline, clindamycin, or metronidazole to complete a total of 14 days of therapy.

13. Is PID handled differently in a woman with an IUD in place?
Yes. Women with an IUD in place should be hospitalized and the IUD removed after antibiotic therapy is initiated. Although its removal may not be required for therapy to be effective, most experts consider the IUD to be contraindicated if previously associated with PID. If an IUD is in place and TOA is diagnosed, removal of the IUD should be delayed until definitive improvement on antimicrobial therapy has occurred, because septic shock has been associated with early removal of an IUD in this setting.

14. Which drugs have antimicrobial activity against *C. trachomatis*?
The tetracyclines, including tetracycline, doxycycline, and minocycline, and the macrolide antibiotics, including erythromycin, clarithromycin, and azithromycin, along with ofloxacin, chloramphenicol, and rifampin, have good activity against *C. trachomatis*. Intravenous but not oral clindamycin has been demonstrated to be active against *C. trachomatis*. Ciprofloxacin is *not* active against this organism.

15. List the potential outpatient regimens that can be used to treat PID.
- Cefoxitin, 2 gm IM, plus probenecid, 1 gm orally in a single dose concurrently, plus doxycycline, 100 mg 2 times/day orally for 14 days.
- Ceftriaxone, 250 mg IM or IV (or another third-generation cephalosporin such as cefotaxime or ceftizoxime IM) in a single dose, plus doxycycline, 100 mg 2 times/day orally for 14 days.

- Ofloxacin, 300–400 mg 2 times/day orally, plus either clindamycin, 300–450 mg 4 times/day orally, or metronidazole, 500 mg 2 times/day orally for 14 days.
- Amoxicillin-clavulanic acid, 500 mg 3 times/day orally, plus doxycycline, 100 mg 2 times/day orally, for 14 days.

16. What follow-up should you recommend for a patient treated for PID?

Hospitalized patients should improve within 3–5 days of initiating therapy, with a decrease in abdominal, uterine, adnexal, and cervical motion tenderness and normalization of temperature. If they do not improve, usually further diagnostic tests or surgical intervention are indicated. For outpatients, clinical improvement should be seen and documented at 72 hours after initiating therapy. Failure of initial therapy is indicated by persistent fever, rising white blood cell count, worsening of abdominal pain, or development of an adnexal mass. Within 7–10 days after completion of therapy, repeat screening should be performed for *C. trachomatis* and *N. gonorrhoeae*; some experts also recommend rescreening 4–6 weeks later.

17. How should the sex partners of women diagnosed with PID be managed?

Every attempt should be made to locate any or all of the sexual partners of women with PID. Even if asymptomatic, partners should be cultured and treated empirically with regimens effective against both *N. gonorrhoeae* and *C. trachomatis*, regardless of the apparent causes of PID or the pathogens isolated from the infected woman.

18. What is Fitz-Hugh–Curtis syndrome?

Fitz-Hugh–Curtis syndrome is a perihepatitis that may be associated with either *N. gonorrhoeae* or *C. trachomatis* salpingitis. Its manifestations include pleuritic right upper quadrant pain, referred right shoulder or back pain, and mild elevations of liver-associated enzymes. In the acute phase, a purulent exudate is present on the liver capsule. In the chronic phase, "violin-string" adhesions between the anterior surface of the liver and anterior abdominal wall can often be demonstrated at laparotomy or laparoscopy. The syndrome usually responds to appropriate antibiotic therapy.

19. What are the potential sequelae of PID?

- TOA
- Recurrent PID
- Chronic or recurrent abdominal and/or pelvic pain
- Dyspareunia
- Dysmenorrhea
- Adhesive disease
- Ectopic pregnancy
- Infertility

Women previously diagnosed with PID may have more hospital admissions for endometriosis and hysterectomy than normal controls.

20. What is the likelihood of developing infertility after an episode of PID?

With a first, severe episode of PID, up to 21% of women become infertile. Collective data suggest that 8–13% are infertile after one episode, 20–35% after two episodes, and 40–75% are infertile after a third episode of PID. If true TOA is present, only 7–14% of women will conceive after treatment.

21. How can PID be prevented?

Certain reproductive behaviors can be targeted for public health attention and education about risk reduction interventions, including postponement of one's sexual debut, limited numbers of sexual partners, use of barrier methods of contraception, avoidance of sexual intercourse during menses, early health care-seeking behavior; and, once PID is diagnosed, compliance with recommended therapy and treatment of sexual partners. Intrauterine devices should be selectively inserted into women at low risk for PID. Not douching may decrease the risk of PID.

CONTROVERSIES

22. Should all women diagnosed with PID be hospitalized?

For: At some point during the illness, almost all women meet at least one of the criteria listed in question 9 for hospitalization. Hospitalization ensures early compliance and follow-up, and complications or failure of therapy is detected more readily. In addition, aggressive initial therapy may reduce serious sequelae and preserve fertility.

Against: In the patient with early diagnosis, in whom compliance is likely and for whom follow-up can be arranged easily, hospitalization may not be mandated. The cost of inpatient therapy is significantly higher and may not change the ultimate outcome.

23. Do *Ureaplasma urealyticum* and *Mycoplasma hominis* cause PID?

Although both organisms have been isolated from the fallopian tubes in a modest number of women with PID, their causative role is less certain. However, it is now recognized that up to 50% of cases of acute PID may involve a number of organisms found in cervicovaginal and fecal flora, suggesting that *U. urealyticum* and *M. hominis* also may be implicated in certain cases.

BIBLIOGRAPHY

1. Centers for Disease Control and Prevention: 1993 sexually transmitted diseases treatment guidelines. MMWR 42(RR-14):75–81, 1993.
2. Mead PB: Infections of the female pelvis. In Mandell GL, Bennett JE, Dolin R (eds): Principles and Practice of Infectious Diseases, 4th ed. New York, Churchill Livingstone, 1995.
3. Newkirk GR: Pelvic inflammatory disease: A contemporary approach. Am Fam Physician 38:1127–1135, 1996.
4. Soper DE: Pelvic inflammatory disease. Infect Dis Clin North Am 8:821–840, 1994.
5. Washington E, Berg AO: Preventing and managing pelvic inflammatory disease: Key questions, practices, and evidence. J Fam Pract 43:283–293, 1996.

34. GENITAL WARTS AND BLISTERS: FRIENDS FOR LIFE

Christopher Parker, D.O., and Donald R. Skillman, M.D., FACP

1. Why group genital warts and blisters together?

Genital warts and blisters are sexually transmitted diseases generally caused by viruses. Viral infections are sometimes difficult or even impossible to cure. Thus the infection may be the patient's "friend" for the rest of his or her life.

2. What do classic genital blisters look like? What organisms cause them?

Small, grouped, vesicular, and painful lesions are caused by herpes simplex virus (HSV). Herpes originally meant "creep" and referred to any creeping vesicular skin disorder. Now herpes describes only diseases caused by herpesviruses. In men the lesions usually appear on the glans or shaft of the penis. The vulva, perineum, cervix, or vagina are generally infected in women. The vesicle may rupture so that the lesions appear ulcerative. A patient's first episode may be accompanied by systemic symptoms such as fever, malaise, myalgias, and tender inguinal adenopathy. Such infections usually improve in a few days to weeks, and if they recur, symptoms are usually not as severe as in the first episode.

3. Are the genital blisters exactly the same as a "cold sore" of the mouth?

Maybe. Herpes simplex viruses are subtyped as HSV-1 and HSV-2. The two types are clinically indistinguishable. HSV-2 causes the majority of primary genital infections (about 70–90%).

4. How do you establish the diagnosis of HSV?

In our experience, when people who have called you by your first name for years one day begin a question starting with "Doctor," you have almost made the diagnosis before identifying the characteristic lesions. The above-mentioned lesions in a sexually active patient are all that is usually needed to make the diagnosis. Laboratory confirmation of the clinical diagnosis is appropriate if the diagnosis is uncertain. Papanicolaou smear or Tzanck preparation showing multinucleated giant cells with intranuclear inclusions is relatively inexpensive but has a nearly 50% false-negative rate. Serologic assays documenting seroconversion are rarely clinically useful because a positive antibody test does not identify when infection was acquired. Thus, detection of viral antigen by immunologic methods or by isolation of virus in tissue culture is best.

5. Can HSV infection cause more than genital or oral lesions?

Yes. Herpesvirus infections can be associated with pharyngitis, aseptic meningitis, encephalitis, hepatitis, and proctitis. HSV infection can develop into vesicular lesions due to direct contact at any focal area (especially the finger, known as "herpetic whitlow"). Generalized or disseminated HSV disease (including visceral organ involvement) may occur in immunocompromised patients.

6. Can HSV infection be cured?

Unfortunately, no. Herpesviruses usually cause symptoms, then become dormant in a spinal nerve sensory ganglia, and later may become active and cause recurrent symptoms. While the patient is having symptoms, the infection may be treated with oral acyclovir, valacyclovir (prodrug of acyclovir), or famciclovir. Therapy has been shown to decrease the duration of viral shedding, to improve local and systemic symptoms, and to accelerate healing for patients with their first episode. For recurrent episodes, however, it shortens viral shedding and speeds healing by only 1–2 days.

7. When is suppressive antiviral therapy indicated in the treatment of HSV?

For patients with severe, frequent recurrences (> 6/year), the same drugs mentioned above have been shown to be safe and effective as suppressive therapy. Unfortunately, once suppressive therapy is stopped, most people continue to have recurrences.

8. What causes genital warts?

Warts are the other genital hazard caused by viral infection. They are generally caused by either human papillomavirus (HPV), also known as condyloma acuminata, or molluscum contagiosum virus (MCV). Condyloma lata are not true warts. They result from infection with the syphilis spirochete.

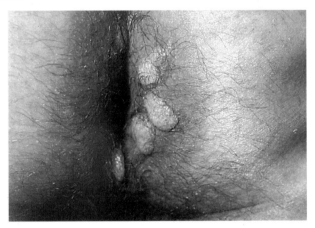

Condyloma lata. Note the nonverrucous nature of lesions seen in secondary syphilis.

9. How do you diagnose HPV infection?

Clinical diagnosis is possible if lesions are clearly visible. Classic condyloma acuminata are pigmented, sessile, or hyperplastic papules with pointed projections (see figure, at right). They are usually broad-based, pedunculated, and soft. They may occur by themselves or in clusters and vary in size from microscopic to several square centimeters when they merge to form plaques. The lesions may reach considerable size, especially with immunosuppression or during pregnancy and, on rare occasions, may mechanically impair normal child delivery. In men, the glans, corona, and shaft of the penis are common sites of infection (see figure, top of next page). Women are usually infected on the posterior introitus, cervix, and labia. The diagnosis of subclinical infection may be difficult.

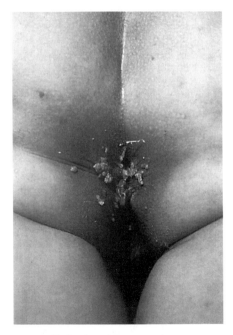

Perianal condyloma acuminata.

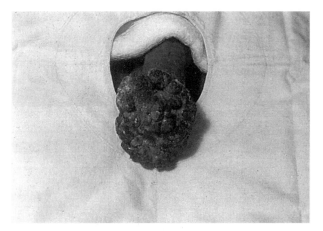

Severe condyloma acuminata involving the glans penis.

10. What is the best way to diagnose subclinical infection with HPV?

Lesions of the cervix are generally flat and difficult to identify clinically. The use of colposcopy and prior soaking of examined tissues with 3–5% acetic acid have expanded the clinical diagnostic spectrum of HPV. Even in men, acetic acid soaking and colposcopic examination have shown HPV-infected papules and macules to be up to two times more common than exophytic condylomas, particularly on the prepuce and scrotum.

11. Can HPV be treated?

Yes, but whether treatment leads to cure is debated. There is a 10–20% spontaneous remission rate for untreated lesions over 3–4 months. Optimal treatment has not been established. Current therapies do not always lead to eradication of HPV or prevent transmission of infection. No current evidence indicates that treatment changes the uncommon development of neoplasia.

12. Who should receive treatment for HPV?

Before treatment begins, the goals of therapy, alternatives, costs, and potential side effects should be discussed because efficacy of all methods is variable and relatively low. The principal reasons for treatment include cosmetic improvement, relief of local symptoms, alleviation of adverse psychological impact, and restoration of normal physiologic function.

13. If you decide to treat HPV, what are the options?

Currently available therapeutic regimens focus on elimination of lesions. Topical agents are locally cytotoxic and have substantial relapse rates. Examples include podophyllin compounds, trichloroacetic acid, and fluorouracil. Surgical and electrocautery relapse rates are no better, and patients may require anesthesia for these procedures. Expensive new methods include carbon dioxide laser or interferon therapy, but they have no definite advantage over other treatments. Cryotherapy with nitrous oxide or liquid nitrogen remains the recommended treatment if you consider cost, efficacy, recurrence rates, and adverse effects.

Treatment	Efficacy*	Treatment	Efficacy*
Cryotherapy	50–100%	Electrosurgery	80–90%
Podophyllin	20–40%	CO_2 laser	80–90%
Podophyllotoxin	45–58%	Interferons α and β	35–60%
Surgery	Up to 66%		

* Efficacy is defined in various articles as "cure," "no relapse in 12 months," or "absence of visible lesions."

14. Are there any long-term complications of HPV infection?

Yes. Localized symptomatic infections are socially stigmatizing and at least inconvenient for one's sex life. In addition, there is a strong association with genital and anorectal neoplasia. Heterosexual men and women with a history of anogenital warts have a 30-fold increased risk of neoplastic disease compared with control populations. HPV 16 and HPV 18 account for over 80% of the cervical cancers in the United States.

15. How do you diagnose and treat *Molluscum contagiosum*?

MCV is a benign and self-limited condition, and the diagnosis is usually straightforward. Lesions are smooth, round, pear- to skin-colored papules of varying size. Although they range from 1–15 mm in diameter, most are 3–5 mm. Lesions are often umbilicated and usually occur in symmetrical crops on opposed skin surfaces. The same therapy as HPV can be used to prevent further spread or for cosmetic reasons. Individual lesions may resolve within 2 months but are often replaced by new lesions.

16. Can genital warts and blisters be completely asymptomatic?

Yes. Although itching, burning, pain, and tenderness are noted with anogenital warts, about three-fourths are asymptomatic. As many as 15% of adults may be excreting HSV-1 or HSV-2 at any given time, depending on the population studied. Prostitutes may have especially high rates of HSV-2 excretion because shedding is related to sexual activity.

17. Are there effective protective measures?

Yes. Like other sexually transmitted diseases, abstinence is universally accepted as the best protective method. Condoms can protect both the user and sexual partner if used correctly. Health care workers should wear gloves when examining a patient's genitals.

18. Are genital warts and blisters sometimes a nosocomial infection?

Yes. HSV can be a neonatal infection acquired from the infected mother during delivery. It also may be given to others via direct contact to skin (herpetic whitlow). Nosocomial transmission is also possible with HPV because infectious virus can be recovered from the fumes released from lesions during treatment with CO_2 laser or electrocoagulation.

19. Are these infections reportable to the CDC?

No. Reporting is not mandatory, but you may report them if you wish.

CONTROVERSY

20. Should sexual partners of patients with genital warts or blisters be notified and evaluated?

Common sense says that you should quickly notify the sexual contacts of persons with STDs. However, patient confidentiality rights and the privacy act prevent such disclosure.

BIBLIOGRAPHY

1. Handsfield HH: Recent developments in STDs: II. Viral and other syndromes. Hosp Pract 27:175–182, 187, 191–192, 1992.
2. Mandell GL, Bennett JE, Dolin R (eds): Principles and Practice of Infectious Diseases, 4th ed. New York, Churchill Livingstone, 1995.
3. McCance, DJ: Human papillomaviruses. Infect Dis Clin North Am 8:751–767, 1994.
4. Ordoukhanian E, Lane AT: Warts and molluscum contagiosum. Beware of treatments worse than the disease. Postgrad Med 101:223–226, 229–232, 235, 1997.
5 Sargent SJ: The "other" sexually transmitted diseases. Chlamydial, herpes simplex virus, and human papillomavirus infections. Postgrad Med 91:359–377, 1992.

35. INFECTIOUS VAGINITIS

Lonnie Empey, M.D., and Arthur Herpolsheimer, M.D.

1. What microorganism is predominantly responsible for maintaining the vaginal ecosystem?
Lactobacillus species accounts for 95% of vaginal microorganisms. *Lactobacillus acidophilus* maintains the vaginal pH at 3.8–4.2 from the production of lactic acid. Lactobacilli also suppress the growth of the gram-negative and gram-positive facultative and obligate anaerobes via the production of hydrogen peroxide.

2. What organisms make up the normal vaginal flora?
Facultative organisms: lactobacilli, corynebacteria, streptococci, *Staphylococcus epidermidis*, *Gardnerella vaginalis*
Anaerobic organisms: peptostreptococci, peptococci, anaerobic lactobacilli, *Bacteroides* spp.

3. What are the three most common infectious causes of vaginitis and their predisposing risk factors?

Infection	Pathogens	Predisposing factors	
Bacterial vaginosis	*Gardnerella vaginalis* *Mycoplasma hominis* Anaerobes	Pregnancy Lactation Use of intrauterine device (IUD)	Sexual activity Multiple sexual partners (probably not STD)
Vaginal candidiasis	*Candida albicans* *Candida tropicalis* *Candida glabrata*	Antibiotic use Oral contraceptive use Pregnancy	Diabetes Sexual activity
Trichomoniasis	*Trichomonas vaginalis*	Sexual activity Multiple sexual partners Pregnancy Menopause	Vaginal discharge/ dysuria Black or Asian race STDs

STD = sexually transmitted disease.

4. What clinical and laboratory findings are associated with three most common causes of infectious vaginitis?

Clinical and Laboratory Findings

FEATURES	NORMAL	BACTERIAL VAGINOSIS	CANDIDIASIS	TRICHOMONIASIS
Symptoms				
Discharge	0	0–++	0–++	+–+++
Pruritus	0	0–+	+–+++	0–+++
Dysuria	0	0	0–++	0–+
Dyspareunia	0	0	0–++	0–+
Characteristics of discharge				
Amount	0–+	0–++	0–++	+–+++
Consistency	Curdy	Homogeneous	Curdy or thrush	Homogeneous
Color	White or slate	Gray	White or slate	Gray or greenish
Odor	0	+–++	0	+–+++
pH	3.8–4.2	5.0–5.5	4.0–5.0	5.5–5.8

(Table continued on following page.)

183

Clinical and Laboratory Findings (Continued)

FEATURES	NORMAL	BACTERIAL VAGINOSIS	CANDIDIASIS	TRICHOMONIASIS
Laboratory findings				
Wet mount				
Clue cells	0	+	0	0
Trichomonads	0	0	0	+
Spores and filaments	0	0	+	0
Leukocytes	0–+	0–+	+–+++	++++
Bacteria	Large rods	Small rods	Large rods	Mixed

5. What office laboratory techniques should be used in the diagnosis of vaginitis?

- Microscopic saline wet mount examination for the presence of "clue cells," trichomonads, leukocytes, and *Lactobacillus* sp.
- KOH test (performed by combining small vaginal specimen with 10% potassium hydroxide) and checking "whiff" test for fishy odor; then examine under light microscopy for pseudohyphae.
- pH determination by applying vaginal discharge on pH paper with pH range of 3.0–5.5.

6. What factors play a role in determining vaginal pH? Do changes in vaginal pH increase susceptibility to infection?

- Chronologic/gynecologic age
- Oral contraceptive use
- Phase of menstrual cycle/menstrual bleeding
- Pregnancy
- Vaginal douching
- Intercourse
- Race

Vaginal pH does influence vaginal infections. An alkaline environment enhances the growth of *Trichomonas vaginalis* and the adherence of bacteria to the vaginal epithelial cells.

7. What are clue cells?

Clue cells are vaginal epithelial cells seen on microscopy. Oval-shaped bacteria attach and surround the cell. The organisms responsible are *Gardnerella vaginalis* and *Mobiluncus* species.

8. What clinical and laboratory criteria are needed to establish the diagnosis of bacterial vaginosis?

The diagnosis of bacterial vaginosis requires the presence of 3 of the 4 following criteria (Amsel criteria):

- Homogenous noninflammatory discharge (minimal white blood cells)
- Vaginal pH >4.5
- Clue cells
- Positive whiff test for fishy odor when alkaline KOH solution is added to smear

9. List three unusual manifestations of bacterial vaginosis.

- Vaginitis emphysematosa characterized by multiple gas-filled cystoid spaces in vaginal and cervical mucosa
- Septicemia
- Posthysterectomy vaginal cuff cellulitis

10. Once the diagnosis of bacterial vaginosis is made, is it necessary to treat the sexual partner?

Cotreatment of the sexual partner is common in cases of refractory bacterial vaginosis. However, it has not been shown to improve the cure rate or to reduce the incidence of recurrence.

11. How prevalent is vulvovaginal candidiasis?

Of the estimated 10 million visits to physicians' offices each year for vaginitis, 20–25% are due to vulvovaginal candidiasis. An estimated 75% of women experience at least one episode of vulvovaginal candidiasis during their lifetime, and 40–50% of these women have at least one recurrence. Probably fewer than 5% of women develop recurrent vulvovaginal candidiasis.

12. What drugs are available for the treatment of vulvovaginal candidiasis? How do they work?

The polyene antifungal agent family. The antifungal medication nystatin, discovered in the late 1940s, comes from the *Actinomyces* species isolated from soil samples from a dairy farm in New York state; hence the name (**New York STAT**e). Nystatin is a tetraene macrolide produced by *Streptomyces noursei* that induces excessive fungal cell wall permeability. Not currently recommended because of the necessarily long duration of therapy.

Imidazole derivatives. Miconazole, clotrimazole, terconazole, econazole, and butoconazole are synthetically derived by various pharmaceutical companies. They biochemically inhibit the membrane cytochrome P-450 of fungal cells. This inhibition results in alteration of cell wall permeability with a lethal loss of cytoplasmic material and ions.

13. How should treatment of vulvovaginal candidiasis be stratified?

Acute vulvovaginal candidiasis in nonpregnant and pregnant women. Topical agents should be considered as first-line therapy. Clotrimazole, 500 mg intravaginally, may be most appropriate for mild or uncomplicated vulvovaginal candidiasis. Recent studies have shown single-dose oral fluconazole, 150–300 mg, to be effective.

Recurrent vulvovaginal candidiasis in nonpregnant women. Identify and treat predisposing factors (pregnancy, uncontrolled diabetes mellitus or estrogen or corticosteroid use, antibiotic use, tight-fitting/synthetic clothing, douching and vaginal perfumes, identification of HIV infection). Oral ketoconazole (100 mg/day for 6 months), fluconazole (150 mg orally once monthly), and topical clotrimazole used weekly may be effective. Because of the controversy surrounding the dosage; duration and route of administration for the treatment of recurrent vulvovaginal candidiasis, continued studies are needed. Alternative treatment is to use a 6-month maintenance regimen of fluconazole, 100 mg once weekly.

Acute/recurrent vulvovaginal candidiasis in women infected with HIV. Treatment regimens are controversial because of the development of resistant strains of *Candida* sp. in patients treated for prior oropharyngeal candidiasis.

14. What single-dose therapeutic regimen has been shown to treat uncomplicated vaginal candidiasis effectively?

Fluconazole, at a single dose of 150 mg orally, was shown to be as efficacious as intravaginal clotrimazole for 7 days, oral ketoconazole for 5 days, and a single intravaginal dose of miconazole and econazole.

15. What treatment is most effective in curing vaginitis due to *Torulopsis*?

Although *Candida* sp. is the most common cause of yeast vaginitis, *T. glabrata* accounts for 10–15% of all vaginal yeast infections. Conventional antimycotic treatments, including azoles, are less effective in vitro against *T. glabrata* than *C. albicans*. An effective treatment is vaginal boric acid (600 mg/day for 14 days), which results in clinical improvement or cure in 81% of cases and mycologic eradication in 77% of cases.

16. Are patients infected with HIV at increased risk for vaginal candidiasis?

Yes. HIV-infected women are at higher risk for both vaginal and oral candidiasis. Recent studies have shown that prophylaxis with fluconazole (200 mg once a week) is useful in the management of HIV-infected women at risk for recurrent mucosal candidiasis.

17. Once treated, can women reliably self-diagnose vulvovaginal candidiasis?

Only 35% of women previously given a clinical diagnosis of vulvovaginal candidiasis were able to identify correctly a classic case scenario. Prior diagnosis, however, appeared to have some positive effect on self-diagnosis; only 11% of women who had never received a diagnosis of vulvovaginal candidiasis were able to diagnose correctly the classic case scenario.

18. What treatment regimens are available for patients with bacterial vaginosis?
- Metronidazole, 500 mg orally 2 times/day for 7 days
- Metronidazole, 2 gm as a single dose
- Accepted alternative therapy when metronidazole is contraindicated: clindamycin, 300 mg orally 2 times/day for 7 days
- Intravaginal clindamycin and intravaginal metronidazole may be effective alternatives with fewer side effects than the current recommendations; studies are currently ongoing.

19. What are the treatment options for patients diagnosed with refractory trichomoniasis?

Resistance Level	Metronidazole Regimen
Marginal	Retreatment with standard dose: 250 mg 3 times/day for 7 days Alternative therapy: metronidazole, 2 gm as a single dose
Low	2 gm/day for 3–5 days
Moderate	2–2.5 gm in divided doses daily for 7–10 days
High	3–3.5 gm/day for 14–18 days Alternative therapy: 2 gm IV every 6–8 hr for 3 days

20. Once the diagnosis of trichomoniasis is made, is it necessary to treat the male partner?

Because in most cases the male partner is also infected and because fewer than 20% of men harboring the organism have symptoms, he should be treated along with the woman.

ZEBRAS

21. Patients with a foul vaginal discharge and a history of ulcerative lesions of the colon may have what amebic cause of vaginitis?

Entamoeba histolytica. The cyst can be seen on Papanicolaou smear and wet mount preparations. Also check the stool for the cyst or trophozoites.

22. What common childhood anal-rectal irritation can cause vaginal pruritus and irritation?

Enterobius vermicularis (pinworm). Evaluation is performed by placing cellophane tape over the rectum for 30 seconds in the morning and examining the removed tape for pinworms.

23. What organism commonly seen in Egypt and Africa can cause vaginal irritation, bleeding, and foul discharge with papilloma-like lesions of the cervix?

Schistosoma haematobium. The urine and feces as well as the Papanicolaou smear should be evaluated for the presence of schistosomal eggs.

CONTROVERSIES

24. Is ingestion of yogurt containing *Lactobacillus acidophilus* a prophylactic therapy for candidal vaginitis?

Based on recent studies evaluating the concentration of viable lactobacilli and the competitive disadvantage to their survival in the gut, it appears as though prophylactic treatment for vaginal candidiasis with yogurt is not effective.

BIBLIOGRAPHY

1. American College of Obstetricians and Gynecologists: Vaginitis. ACOG Tech Bull 226, 1996.
2. Amsel R, Totten PA, Spiegel CA, et al: Nonspecific vaginitis: Diagnostic criteria and epidemiologic associations. Am J Med 74:14–22, 1983.
3. Burnhill MS: Infectious vulvovaginitis. In Monif GRG (ed): Infectious Diseases in Obstetrics and Gynecology: Problem Areas: Gynecology. Omaha, IDI Publications, 1993, p 412.
4. Drutz DJ: Lactobacillus prophylaxis for candida vaginitis. Ann Intern Med 116:419–420, 1992.
5. Ernest JM : Topical antifungal agents. Obstet Gynecol Clin North Am 19:587–607, 1992.
6. Ferris DG, Delke C, Litaker MS: Women's use of over-the-counter antifungal medications for gynecologic symptoms. J Fam Prac 45:595, 1996.
7. Ferris DG, Hendrich J, Payne PM, et al: Office laboratory diagnosis of vaginitis. J Fam Prac 41(6):575–581, 1995.
8. Goode MA, Grauer K, Gums JG: Infectious vaginitis: Selecting therapy and preventing recurrence. Postgrad Med 96:85–99, 1994.
9. Hammill HA: Normal vaginal flora in relation to vaginitis. Obstet Gynecol Clin North Am 16:329–336, 1989.
10. Hammill HA: Unusual causes of vaginitis. Obest Gynecol Clin North Am 16:337–345, 1989.
11. Joesoef MR, Schmid GP: Bacterial vaginosis: Review of treatment options and potential clinical indications for therapy. Clin Infect Dis 20:S72, 1995.
12. Lossick JG, Kent HL: Trichomoniasis: Trends in diagnosis and management. Am J Obstet Gynecol 165:1217–1222, 1991.
13. Majeroni BA: New concepts in bacterial vaginosis. Am Fam Physician 44:1215–1219, 1991.
14. Reed BD, Eyler A: Vaginal Infections: Diagnosis and management. Am Fam Physician 47:1805–1816, 1993.
15. Reef SE, Levine WC, McNeil MM, et al: Treatment options for vulvovaginal candidiasis, 1993. Clin Infect Dis 20:S80–S90, 1995.
16. Rhoads JL, Wright DC, Redfield RR, Burke DS. Chronic vaginal candidiasis in women with human immunodeficiency virus infection. JAMA 257:3105–3107, 1987.
17. Schuman P, Capps L, Peng G, et al: Weekly fluconazole for the prevention of mucosal candidiasis in women with HIV infection. Ann Intern Med 126:689–696, 1997.
18. Sobel JD, Brooker D, Stein GE, et al: Single dose fluconazole compared with conventional clotrimazole topical therapy of candida vaginitis. Am J Obstet Gynecol 172:1263–1268, 1995.
19. Sobel JD, Chaim W: Treatment of *Torulopsis glabrata* vaginitis: Retrospective review of boric acid therapy. Clin Infect Dis 24:649, 1997.
20. Stevens-Simon C, Jamison J, McGregor J, Douglas JM: Racial variation in vaginal pH among healthy sexually active adolescents. Sex Trans Dis 21:168–172, 1994.

X. Bone and Joint Infections

36. BONE AND PERIARTICULAR INFECTIONS
Raymond J. Enzenauer, M.D., FACP

OSTEOMYELITIS

1. How are bone infections classified etiologically?

According to the Waldvogel system, bone infections are classified as hematogenous osteomyelitis or osteomyelitis secondary to a contiguous focus of infection. Contiguous focus osteomyelitis is subdivided into disease with or without vascular insufficiency.

2. What are presenting signs and symptoms of osteomyelitis?

Patients often present with localized warmth, swelling, and pain in the involved area. Constitutional symptoms and signs of bacteremia, such as fever, chills, and night sweats, may be present in the acute phase but are usually absent in the chronic phase. Signs and symptoms in the chronic phase include abscess and bacteremia.

3. What is the differential diagnosis of osteomyelitis?

Malignant and benign tumors, including Ewing's sarcomas, osteosarcomas, fibrous histiocytomas, fibrosarcomas, lymphomas, and benign giant cell bone cysts, may be confused with osteomyelitis. Other diseases that can be confused with osteomyelitis include leukemia with bony infiltrates, bone infarcts secondary to sickle cell anemia or other hemoglobinopathies, noninfected nonunions, and old trauma. The correct diagnosis is usually based on histology and culture results.

4. What is the treatment for osteomyelitis?

Intravenous antibiotics are the treatment of choice for osteomyelitis. Except for hematogenous osteomyelitis, in which positive blood or joint fluid cultures may suffice, antibiotic treatment should be based on meticulous bone cultures taken at debridement surgery or from deep bone biopsy. If possible, cultures should be obtained before antibiotics are initiated or after the patient has been taken off antibiotic therapy for at least 24 hours. Sinus cultures are not reliable for predicting gram-negative organisms that cause osteomyelitis.

After cultures are obtained, parenteral antibiotics to cover the suspected pathogens should be initiated. Once the organism is identified, the antibiotic can be selected by appropriate sensitivity methods. Because of the vascular nature of pediatric bone, pediatric osteomyelitis usually can be managed with antibiotics alone. Most patients require 4–6 weeks of antibiotic therapy, parenteral and oral. The usual recommendation is 2 weeks of parenteral antibiotic therapy followed by 4 weeks of oral antibiotics.

5. What microorganisms are the most common causes of osteomyelitis?

Staphylococci and streptococci predominate in both hematogenous and contiguous focus osteomyelitis. Infants and children also may be infected with *Escherichia coli* and *Haemophilus* spp., whereas adults have an increased incidence of other gram-negative infections.

Staphylococcus aureus	27%	Other gram-negative organisms	20%
Other gram-positive organisms	5%	Polymicrobial infection	33%
Pseudomonas aeruginosa	15%		

6. What imaging studies are useful in the diagnosis and treatment of osteomyelitis?

Roentgenograms may show osteopenia, scalloping, thinning of cortical bone, or loss of trabecular architecture in cancellous bone. A sequestrum is radiodense relative to normal bone. Periosteal elevation may be present as well as soft-tissue swelling in patients with an abscess or cellulitis. Plain radiographs are 60% sensitive and 81% specific but may not show changes in the acute stages of osteomyelitis.

Radionuclide scans, computerized tomography (CT), or magnetic resonance imaging (MRI) may be obtained when the diagnosis of osteomyelitis is equivocal or to help gauge the extent of bone and soft tissue infection. In general, they are not necessary for long-bone osteomyelitis. However, in suspected vertebral osteomyelitis, technetium polyphosphate and MRI scans may be useful. MRI is also useful in distinguishing diabetic osteopathy from infection. The MRI scan enhances with the T2-weighted or STIR images in the presence of infection.

Sensitivities and Specificities of Radiologic Examination for Osteomyelitis

TEST	SENSITIVITY (%)	SPECIFICITY (%)
Magnetic resonance imaging	77–79	53–100
Technetium-99	61–100	25–70
Indium-111	80	29
Radiographs	60	81

7. What are the goals of surgical management of osteomyelitis?
- Adequate drainage
- Extensive debridement of all necrotic tissue
- Obliteraton of dead spaces
- Adequate soft tissue coverage

The goal of debridement is to leave healthy, viable tissue. Adequate debridement may leave a large bony defect termed *dead space*. The goal of dead space management is to replace dead bone and scar tissue with durable vascularized tissue.

8. What is the most commonly involved site for hematogenously acquired osteomyelitis in adults? In children?

In adults, vertebrae; in children, metaphyses of long bones.

9. What are the symptoms of vertebral osteomyelitis?

Neck or back pain/stiffness	> 90% (50% over 3 months)
Limited back motion	15%
Positive straight leg sign	15%

10. What are the signs of vertebral osteomyelitis?

Fever (50%) and peripheral leukocytosis (40%).

11. What factors predispose to vertebral osteomyelitis?

Male predominance	2:1
Intravenous drug abuse	6:1
Blunt spine trauma	10–20%
Diabetes mellitus	19%

12. What are the usual sites of vertebral osteomyelitis?

Lumbar spine	> 50% (lower > upper)
Thoracic spine	35%
Cervical spine	< 15%
Sacral spine	Increased incidence with pressure sores

13. What is the prognosis of pyogenic vertebral osteomyelitis?

Prognosis is good with early diagnosis and treatment. Mortality in the antibiotic era is < 5%. Residual neurologic deficit is < 7%. Poor prognosis is associated with advanced age and diabetes. Mortality and neurologic complications are actually decreased in intravenous drug abusers.

14. What is the usual source of infection in patients with vertebral osteomyelitis?

Mnemonic: **SPINEDIS** (spine disease)

S = **S**urgery (of spine or disc)
P = **P**ulmonary infection
I = **I**ntravenous drug abuse
N = **N**ephrologic disease (genitourinary tract: 30%)
E = **E**ndocarditis
D = **D**ental work
I = **I**nfected vascular site
S = **S**oft tissue infection

SEPTIC BURSITIS

15. What are the demographics of septic bursitis?

Septic bursitis is most commonly seen in manual laborers (e.g., gardeners, carpenters, plumbers). The median age is 47 years; up to 100% of patients are men.

16. What are the most common symptoms of septic bursitis?

Bursal swelling (100%) and bursal pain (92%).

17. What other signs and symptoms are associated with septic bursitis?

Fever of 38.2–38.9° C (35%), cellulitis (74–89%), regional adenopathy (25%), and limb edema (11%).

18. What is the pathogenesis of septic bursitis?

Repetitive trauma to the affected limb or sustained pressure on the knees or elbows is seen in 85% of cases. Evidence of skin breakage with laceration, abrasion, or draining sinus is seen in 45% of cases. Predisposition to trauma, be it accidental direct blows, inadvertent repetitive minor blows, or unnoticed constant pressure, appears to be the common denominator when occupations and other related disorders are taken into account.

19. What is the bacterial cause of septic bursitis?

The overwhelming majority (78–96%) of septic bursitis is due to *Staphylococcus aureus*. Approximately 2% is due to group A beta-hemolytic streptococci and 2% to *Staphylococcus epidermidis*.

20. What are the results of the typical bursal fluid analysis in septic bursitis?

Mean bursal fluid cell count is 77,000 cells/mm^3 (range: 1500–418,000) with a polymorphonuclear neutrophil predominance (52–98%). Bursal fluid glucose is low (< 60 mg/dl), in sharp contrast to traumatic bursitis. Bacteria are seen on Gram stain in only 65% of culture-positive bursal fluids. Bursal leukocyte count in culture-positive fluids is > 1000 per mm^3.

21. What are the associated laboratory abnormalities in septic bursitis?

• Peripheral blood leukocyte count is elevated above 10,000 in 56% of patients.
• The mean erythrocyte sedimentation rate (ESR) is 43 mm/hr (range: 10–106 mm/hr).

22. True or false: Infection of the prepatellar or olecranon bursa does not imply involvement of its respective joint.

True. This point has therapeutic and prognostic import. In contrast, septic arthritis of the knee involves a popliteal (Baker's) cyst.

23. How can septic bursitis be distinguished from septic arthritis clinically?

The patient with a bursal infection usually presents with the affected limb held in partial flexion. Joint motion, including rotation, is usually painless in septic bursitis, except with full flexion and extension, which stretches and compresses the bursae. In contrast, septic arthritis produces pain with joint motion.

24. Which bursae are commonly involved with septic bursitis?

Olecranon bursae (63%) and prepatellar bursae (27%).

25. What is the treatment of septic bursitis?

Septic bursitis is treated with antibiotics. Some patients may be treated with oral antibiotics despite acute onset of symptoms; however, oral therapy may fail in two-thirds of cases. Patients with systemic symptoms, underlying bursal disease, or high bursal fluid leukocyte count may be candidates for intravenous antibiotic therapy. Initial treatment should include a semisynthetic penicillinase-resistant penicillin or a cephalosporin. For curative therapy, antibiotics should be continued for 5 days after achievement of bursal fluid sterility. Severe infections may require longer duration of treatment than moderate infections, and higher doses of antimicrobial agents given intravenously may shorten the duration of necessary therapy. The value of surgical drainage compared with repeated aspirations of the bursa is unknown. In most patients, bursal fluid becomes sterile in less than 1 week (mean: 4.3 days).

SEPTIC DISCITIS

26. Discitis after lumbar disc surgery is rare. In the event of increasing pain postoperatively, what two types of spondylodiscitis must be suspected?

Septic discitis and avascular necrosis of the adjacent edge of the vertebrae or aseptic (chemical) discitis.

27. What parameters are useful to distinguish the two?

ESR, C-reactive protein (increased with septic discitis), and percutaneous discal biopsy.

28. What is the treatment for postoperative discitis?

For septic discitis, antibiotic therapy must be used until the levels of C-reactive protein are reduced. For aseptic discitis, rest and physical therapy should be initiated.

29. What is the major symptom of septic discitis?

Localized back pain is the most common complaint. Most patients with lumbar discitis also have symptoms of sciatica.

30. Which laboratory tests are useful in septic discitis?

The leukocyte count and ESR often are elevated, although normal values may be seen.

31. What is the most serious potential complication of septic discitis?

Paraplegia may develop in up to 40% of patients.

32. What are the radiographic findings of septic discitis?

The earliest radiographic change is a decrease in the vertebral height of the affected intervertebral disc space. The degree of disc narrowing is variable and may not correlate with subsequent progression of disease. The second sign, seen in 2–3 months, is progressive sclerosis of the sub-chondral bone with an increase in density of the adjacent areas of the vertebral bodies on either side of the affected disc.

BIBLIOGRAPHY

1. Aliabadi P, Nikpoor N: Imaging osteomyelitis. Arthritis Rheum 37:617–622, 1994.
2. Fouquet B, Goupille P, Jalliot F, et al: Discitis after lumbar disc surgery. Features of "aseptic" and "septic" forms. Spine 17:356–358, 1992.
3. Gentry LO: Antibiotic therapy for osteomyelitis. Infect Dis Clin North Am 4:485–499, 1990.
4. Hawkins BJ, Langerman RJ, Calhoun JH: Osteomyelitis. Bull Rheum Dis 43:4–7, 1994.
5. Ho G, Tice AD, Kaplan SR: Septic bursitis in the prepatellar and olecranon bursae. Ann Intern Med 89:21–27, 1978.
6. Ho G, Su EY: Antibiotic therapy of septic bursitis. Arthritis Rheum 24:905–911, 1981.
7. Laughlin RT, Sinha A, Calhoun JH, Mader JT: Osteomyelitis. Curr Opin Rheumatol 6:401–407, 1994.
8. Raddatz DA, Hoffman GS, Franck WA: Septic bursitis: Presentation, treatment and prognosis. J Rheumatol 14:1160–1163, 1987.
9. Rosenthall L: Radionuclide investigation of osteomyelitis. Curr Opin Radiol 4:62–69, 1992.
10. Sapico FL, Montgomerie JZ: Vertebral osteomyelitis. Infect Dis Clin North Am 4:539–550, 1990.
11. Zimmermann B, Mikolich DJ, Ho G: Septic bursitis. Semin Arthritis Rheum 24:391–410, 1995.

37. INFECTIONS OF NONVASCULAR IMPLANTED DEVICES

Stephanie L. Marglin, M.D., and Richard T. Ellison III, M.D.

1. What nonvascular devices are at risk of infection?

A prosthetic nonvascular device is an artificial device that is placed in the body and not associated with the vascular system. Examples include the following:

1. Artificial joints
2. Cerebrospinal fluid (CSF) ventriculoperitoneal shunts
3. Ommaya reservoirs
4. Continuous ambulatory peritoneal dialysis catheters
5. Intraocular lens
6. Intravenous drug infusion implants
7. Breast implants
8. Penile prostheses
9. Mesh for hernia repair
10. Implantable cardiac defibrillators

Placement of these devices requires a surgical procedure with incision into the skin. Infections of essentially all devices have been reported.

2. When do protheses become infected?

The timing of prosthetic device infections can be divided into four categories:

1. Early infections usually originate during surgery or insertion of the device and are due to high-grade bacterial pathogens (*Staphylococcus aureus*, group A streptococci, and nosocomial gram-negative bacilli) that are introduced perioperatively or as a result of concurrent nosocomial bacteremia.

2. The second period of risk extends up to 8–9 months after device insertion. Infection in this period is also due to organisms that contaminate the device during surgical implantation. The infecting organisms most typically are relatively indolent and usually consist of normal skin flora. The primary pathogens are coagulase-negative staphylococci. There have been rare outbreaks of infections with unusual organisms, such as atypical mycobacteria, that contaminated devices before implantation.

3. A late infection is usually from hematogenous spread and may develop many months to years after surgery. The offending organisms also may originate from skin flora but more likely disseminate from a separate infection.

4. Finally, devices that undergo manipulation (e.g., ventriculoperitoneal shunt or dialysis catheters) may become infected at the time of manipulation.

Device infections have a peak incidence somewhere between 3 and 6 months, with rare infections developing years later (see figure, top of next page). The vast majority of infections take place in the middle period, and the primary pathogens are coagulase-negative staphylococci.

3. How do prostheses become infected?

Select bacteria have the capacity to adhere to and colonize prosthetic devices. Initial adhesion is accomplished by hydrophobic interaction, electrostatic attraction, and van der Waals forces. Subsequently, bacteria (such as coagulase-negative staphylococci) associated with infection produce an extracellular slime that competes with serum and tissue proteins in coating the surface of foreign materials. Extracellular slime interferes with host defense mechanisms by inhibiting bacterial uptake and opsonization by neutrophils. The slime also may protect the bacteria by acting as a penetration barrier against antibiotics.

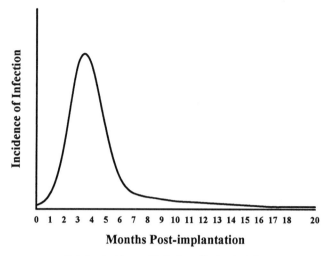

Relative incidence of infection after implantation.

4. Which organisms infect a prosthetic device?

The principal pathogens found depend in part on the time after placement. However, the most common organisms to infect a prosthesis are coagulase-negative staphylococci, which are part of the normal skin flora and usually contaminate the surface of the device during surgical implantation. Infections with these bacteria tend to develop within 3–6 months after implantation but occasionally are noted either earlier or later. *S. aureus* is also a common infecting organism. Along with streptococcal species, it may cause early infection as well as late infection via hematogenous spread. Gram-negative bacilli, a rare cause of late infections, may be associated with immediate postoperative infections or infections originating from gastrointestinal or urinary sources.

5. How are prosthetic device infections best treated?

The best treatment is usually removal of the prosthesis followed by a course of antibiotics. Unfortunately, it is not always feasible to remove the device. In such situations, the physician may try to treat with antibiotic coverage alone, with the knowledge that treatment often results in failure. The choice of antibiotic agent depends on the infecting organism. The antibiotic agents used to treat device infections are preferably bactericidal or fungicidal, particularly if treatment is attempted with the prosthesis left in place. In addition, adequate antibiotic concentration must be achievable at the site of infection. For instance, intraocular infections often do not respond to systemic antimicrobial therapy because of inadequate antibiotic penetration into the vitreous. Intravitreal injection may be quite effective in such cases.

6. What are the symptoms of prosthetic joint infection?

Patients with infected prosthetic joints often present with complaints of increasing pain in the area of the joint. Erythema and fevers often accompany the pain. Some patients have purulent drainage from the incision site. Many patients have only decreased range of motion of the joint.

7. When do prosthetic joints become infected?

The infectious process may be acute, subacute, or chronic. In the subacute phase, the infection usually occurs within 3 months of the surgery and is most likely related to the surgical procedure. A chronic infection may take months to years to develop and is usually due to seeding of the joint from a previous indolent nosocomial or new hematogenous infection. A late infection may also be due to trauma of the prosthetic joint long after the original surgery.

8. Who is at risk for getting infection?
Risk factors for infection of prosthetic joints include the following:
1. Prior surgery at the site of the prosthesis
2. Corticosteroid treatment
3. Diabetes mellitus
4. Poor nutritional status
5. Obesity
6. Extremely advanced age

9. How do you diagnose prosthetic joint infection?
Suspect infection in patients with erythema, pain, decreased range of motion, sinus tract with purulent drainage, or loosening of the joint itself. An elevated white blood cell count and sedimentation rate also suggest infection but are not diagnostic. Radiographic abnormalities may be found, including abnormal lucencies, changes in position of prosthetic components, cement fractures, and periosteal reactions. Such changes are evident in only about 50% of cases.

Prosthetic joint infection is diagnosed microbiologically. Aspiration of the joint fluid or culture of the tissue should be performed. Organisms are seen on approximately 30% of Gram stains, and cultures are positive in 85–98% of cases. Depending on the clinician's suspicion, cultures may be held for several weeks to determine the presence of slow-growing organisms such as mycobacteria or *Brucella* spp.

10. What organisms infect prosthetic joints?
The most common pathogens that infect joints are the staphylococcal species that are part of normal skin flora. Coagulase-negative staphylococci are implicated in about 35% of cases and *S. aureus* in about 20%.

In about 20–40% of cases bacteremia or hematogenous spread leads to prosthetic joint infection. Implicated pathogens depend on the distant infection. For example, a patient with pyogenic skin infection may seed the joint with organisms such as *S. aureus* or group A streptococcal species. Patients with urinary tract infection may develop an enterococcal or gram-negative bacillus infection, and patients with abdominal sepsis may develop infecetion with gram-negative bacilli, enterococci, or anaerobes (e.g., *Bacteroides fragilis*).

Mycobacteria have also been seen in prosthetic joint infections. These organisms are difficult to grow on routine media in the laboratory, and the physician with clinical suspicion of this infection should alert the microbiology lab.

11. What is the treatment of prosthetic joint infections?
Most studies agree that the best method of treatment of prosthetic joint infections is to remove the prosthetic joint. Antibiotic therapy should then be based on the organism's susceptibilities. Because of possible concurrent osteomyelitis, the selected agents should have bactericidal activity, and therapy should be prolonged. A typical course is at least 6 weeks.

Conservative treatment includes surgical removal of the prosthesis and a 6-week course of antibiotics. After the full course of antibiotics is completed, the patient should be observed for a variable period before a new device is implanted. This approach hopefully ensures total eradication of the pathogen.

An alternative approach is removal of the prosthesis, thorough debridement, and immediate insertion of a new device, using an antibiotic-impregnated cement. A prolonged course of antibiotics follows. At present the optimal approach remains undetermined, and treatment must be adapted to the individual patient. The major risk of early reimplantation is infection of the new prosthetic device. This risk is counterbalanced by more rapid restoration of joint function. Early mobility may be preferable in the treatment of an infected knee prosthesis; prolonged delay in reimplantation of the device is associated with increased scar function and ultimately decreased joint mobility.

Choice of antibiotics should be based on the organism involved. If results of the Gram stain and culture are unknown, empiric treatment for the most likely pathogen should be based on the clinical scenario. If a gram-positive organism is suspected, the physician may want to use an antibiotic, such as vancomycin, that adequately covers most staphylococcal species until susceptibilities are determined. If anaerobes are suspected, clindamycin is a good choice for coverage. If gram-negative rods are the causative pathogen and susceptibilities are unknown, therapeutic options may include a third-generation cephalosporin or an antipseudomonal penicillin; a carbapenem with or without an aminoglycoside; or a fluoroquinolone. When susceptibilities are known, the antibiotic should be changed accordingly. Attention to antibiotic susceptibilities provided by the friendly microbiology lab for gram-negative organisms in your institution may greatly assist in the choice of empiric therapy.

12. Should patients with prosthetic joints receive prophylactic antibiotics for dental procedures?

Whether patients with prosthetic joints should take antibiotics when they undergo a procedure, such as dental work, that causes transient bacteremia has been somewhat controversial. Many physicians fear that the resultant bacteremia will lead to a prosthetic joint infection. A few cases of infection have been documented after dental procedures; however, it has not been proved that the procedures caused the infections. The invading bacteria in this setting would be normal host mouth flora, including viridans streptococci, diphtheroids, and peptostreptococci. The most common bacteria to infect prosthetic joints are the staphylococci species, which account for a small percentage of oral flora (< 0.05%). Therefore, the likelihood of getting a prosthetic joint infection with coagulase-negative staphylococci from a dental procedure is very small. Infection with viridans streptococci occurs rarely.

13. What are symptoms and signs of infections in continuous ambulatory peritoneal dialysis (CAPD) catheters?

Patients with CAPD catheter infections often present with abdominal pain, fevers, chills, nausea, and vomiting. The abdominal pain ranges from vague and mild to diffuse and severe in association with abdominal distention. Patients have an elevated white blood cell count, and the dialysate is usually cloudy. Erythema may be seen at the site of catheter insertion in the skin.

14. What pathogens commonly infect CAPD catheters?

Most CAPD infections arise from direct contamination of the catheter. Rarely infections may have an intraabdominal origin, such as diverticulitis. Thus, most infections are unimicrobial. The common organisms are coagulase-negative staphylococci and *S. aureus*, which account for 70% of infections. Such infections tend to be mild, especially with coagulase-negative staphylococci. Other potential pathogens include *Escherichia coli*, *Klebsiella* sp., *Enterobacter* sp., *Pseudomonas* sp., and *Proteus* sp. These organisms cause more severe illness with higher morbidity and mortality rates. Although they usually develop from the skin, a possible intraabdominal origin should be considered, especially when the infection is polymicrobial. Although not as common, *Candida albicans* and mycobacteria also may cause CAPD catheter infection.

15. How is the diagnosis of dialysate infection made?

The most important way of diagnosing CAPD infection is Gram stain and culture of cloudy dialysate fluid. Gram stain is positive in up to 50% of cases of infection. The leukocyte count of the dialysate is usually greater than $100/mm^3$ and more often greater than $500/mm^3$ with a predominance of neutrophils.

16. What is the treatment of CAPD catheter infection?

The symptoms are usually mild, and the infection often is treated on an outpatient basis. Choice of antibiotics is based on susceptibilities of the offending organism. Antibiotics may be mixed with dialysate and given intraperitoneally. Some clinicians choose to give antibiotics intravenously as well. If the organism has not been identified, empiric therapy with vancomycin and an aminoglycoside or extended-spectrum cephalosporin should be started to cover both staphylococci and gram-negative rods until the treatment can be narrowed. The prognosis is usually quite good, and the patient should show clinical improvement within 3 days of the initiation of therapy. The catheter usually does not need to be removed.

17. What circumstances require removal of the peritoneal dialysis catheter?
1. Persistent skin infection at the catheter site
2. Fungal, fecal, or mycobacterial infection
3. Persistent peritonitis
4. Recurrence of infection with the same organism
5. Catheter malfunction

18. How does a central nervous system shunt become infected?
1. Direct colonization usually during surgery
2. Hematogenous spread
3. Contamination of the distal end of the shunt

Most infections occur within 3 months of surgery and involve coagulase-negative staphylococci, which suggest contamination during surgery. The rest of the infections depend on the type of shunt placed. Ventriculoatrial (VA) shunts may be infected at the atrial end with bloodborne organisms. Ventriculoperitoneal (VP) shunt infection often involves enteric bacteria and enterococci, presumably from an intestinal origin.

19. How do patients with shunt infections present clinically?
Some patients present with symptoms typical of meningitis—headache, fever, neck stiffness, and photophobia. A VP shunt infection may present with abdominal pain and be associated with peritonitis, bowel obstruction, appendicitis, or perforation. A VA shunt infection may present as bacteremia and include pulmonary embolus, hypocomplementemia, and immune complex production. Rarely VA shunt infection presents as an immune complex-mediated glomerulonephritis.

20. What is the treatment for CNS shunt infections?
Treatment depends on the infecting organism. The most likely involved bacteria are coagulase-negative staphylococci. In this case, treatment with vancomycin plus rifampin or trimethoprim-sulfamethoxazole with removal of the shunt system is considered the gold standard. However, when the involved bacteria are not slime-producing, it is thought that high-dose antibiotic therapy against the bacteria is sufficient. Externalization of the distal end of the shunt followed by 2–3 weeks of intraventricular and systemic antibiotics has also been successful. After treatment, the distal end of the shunt is replaced.

BIBLIOGRAPHY

1. Bennett J, Brachman P: In Hospital Infections, 3rd ed. Boston, Little, Brown, 1992.
2. Brause B: Infections with prostheses in bones and joints. In Mandell GL, Douglas RG, Bennett JE (eds): Principles and Practice of Infectious Diseases. New York, Churchill Livingstone, 1995, pp 1051–1055.
3. Cardner P, Sadigh M, Leipzig T: CNS shunt infections. In Gorbach SL, Bartlett JG, Blacklow NR (eds): Infectious Diseases. Philadelphia, W.B. Saunders, 1992, pp 1188–1193.
4. Graevenitz A, Amsterdam D: Microbiological aspects of peritonitis associated with continuous ambulatory peritoneal dialysis. Clin Microbiol Rev 5:36–48, 1992.
5. Jansen B, Peters G: Foreign body associated infection. J Antimicrob Chemother 32(Suppl A):69–75, 1993.
6. Karchmer AW: Approach to the patient with infection in a prosthetic device. In Gorbach S, Bartlett J, Blacklow N (eds): Infectious Diseases. Philadelphia, W.B. Saunders, 1992, pp 1374–1384.
7. Morissette I, Gourdeau M, Francoeur J: CSF shunt infections: A fifteen-year experience with emphasis on management and outcome. Canad J Neurol Sci 20:118–122, 1993.
8. Rupp M, Archer G: Coagulase-Negative Staphylococci: Pathogens Associated with Medical Progress. Clin Infect Dis 19:231-245, 1994.
9. Wahl M: Myths of dental-induced prosthetic joint infections. Clin Infect Dis 20:1420–1425, 1995.

38. INFECTIOUS ARTHRITIS

Raymond J. Enzenauer, M.D., FACP

BACTERIAL ARTHRITIS

Nongonococcal Arthritis

1. What is the most common route of infection in bacterial arthritis?

Most cases of bacterial arthritis develop when bacteria reach the joint via the hematogenous route; infections preceding joint involvement may or may not be clinically apparent. Other routes of infection include direct inoculation during diagnostic or therapeutic arthrocentesis or arthroscopies and contiguous infection during the course of osteomyelitis, cellulitis, abscesses, tenosynovitis, or septic bursitis.

2. What are the clinical manifestations of bacterial arthritis?

About 80% of patients present with monoarthritis, most commonly involving the knee. Most patients also have constitutional symptoms of fever, chills, and malaise. Local signs of inflammation are generally present in the affected joint(s); pain, usually severe and incapacitating, is a cardinal clinical manifestation.

3. Discuss the microbiology of bacterial arthritis.

The microbiology of septic arthritis is governed by the age of the patient.

In **infants and neonates**, *Staphylococcus aureus* accounts for 80% of cases of bacterial arthritis. A smaller proportion of bacterial arthritis results from other gram-positive organisms, particularly group B streptococci, and gram-negative organisms, mainly *Pseudomonas aeruginosa* and other coliforms.

In **children younger than 2 years**, *Haemophilus influenzae* was the most common isolate in bacterial arthritis. The incidence has decreased since the introduction of an effective vaccine. Pneumococci have become increasingly common.

In **children 2 years of age and older**, *S. aureus* is the most common pathogen. A few cases of bacterial arthritis in children have been attributed to a variety of gram-positive and gram-negative organisms.

In **adults**, after the exclusion of gonococcal arthritis, *S. aureus* is the most common organism encountered in bacterial arthritis (55%). Streptococcal species are seen in one-fourth of patients (27%), gram-negative bacilli in 14%, and miscellaneous pathogens in 4%. Coagulase-negative staphylococci remain common pathogens, mainly in prosthetic joints. Infections due to gram-negative organisms usually occur in adults with some predisposing factor.

4. What patient populations are at increased risk for bacterial arthritis?

Intravenous drug users are at increased risk for typical and atypical bacterial arthritis, including gram-negative bacterial arthritis. They are also at increased risk for involvement of joints that are rarely the target of infection, such as the sternoclavicular joint, sacroiliac joint, manubriosternal joint, and symphysis pubis.

Patients with severe erosive, destructive, long-standing rheumatoid arthritis (RA) are more likely to develop bacterial arthritis than rheumatoid patients with less severe disease. Various factors predispose patients with RA to bacterial arthritis, including their overall health status, comorbid diseases (such as diabetes), chronic administration of corticosteroids and cytotoxic drugs, and intraarticular use of corticosteroids.

Patients with prosthetic joints are predisposed to both early and late bacterial arthritis involving the joint prosthesis. Early (< 12 months) postoperative infections may be caused by

Staphylococcus epidermidis or anaerobes. Late (> 12 months) infections may be due to either gram-positive or gram-negative organisms.

Immunocompromised patients, including old and very old patients with multiple organ system involvement, patients with organ transplants, and patients with nonmalignant disorders treated with immunosuppressants (i.e., lupus nephritis) are at increased risk of bacterial arthritis. Immunocompromised patients are also at increased risk for polymicrobial, polyarticular bacterial arthritis. Although patients infected with the human immunodeficiency virus (HIV) are at increased risk for infection, bacterial arthritis is relatively uncommon, unless the patient is also an intravenous drug user.

5. What joints are most commonly involved in adults with nongonococcal bacterial arthritis?

The knee is the most commonly involved joint (54% of cases). Other commonly involved joints include:

Hip	16%	Hand	4%
Shoulder	8%	Foot	4%
Wrist	8%	Elbow	3%
Ankle	7%		

6. How is the diagnosis of bacterial arthritis made?

The single most important diagnostic procedure in patients suspected of having infectious arthritis is arthrocentesis. In patients with cellulitis or clinical evidence of skin infection, arthrocentesis should be performed away from the area of skin involvement. In patients with polyarticular involvement, all joints should be tapped.

Synovial fluid (SF) should be gram-stained and cultured, and leukocyte count with differential should be obtained. A high leukocyte count (usually > 50,000/μl) with a predominance of polymorphonuclear neutrophils (> 90%) is characteristic of bacterial arthritis. (*Note:* Similar findings are reported in the "pseudoseptic" arthritis associated with rheumatoid arthritis and other arthritides.) SF glucose level is significantly lower than serum glucose, and SF protein levels are high in bacterial arthritis. Note that SF glucose and protein findings are similar in patients with active rheumatoid arthritis alone.

7. How are synovial effusions categorized?

Synovial effusions are categorized as class I (noninflammatory), class II (inflammatory), and class III (septic). Distinguishing features are summarized in the table below.

Gross Examination	Normal	Class I	Class II	Class III
Volume (ml) (knee)	< 3.5	> 3.5	> 3.5	> 3.5
Viscosity	High	High	Low	Variable
Color	Colorless	Straw	Yellow	Variable
White blood cells (mm^3)	< 200	200–2000	2000–75,000	> 75,000
Polymorphonuclear neutrophils (%)	< 25	< 25	> 50	> 75
Culture	Negative	Negative	Negative	Positive
Mucin clot	Firm	Firm	Friable	Friable
Glucose	= blood	= blood	< 50 mg/dl lower than blood	> 50 mg/dl lower than blood

8. What are the optimal imaging studies in bacterial arthritis?

- Conventional radiographs are rarely of diagnostic value because they are normal during the first few days of infection. They are usually obtained at baseline for future reference.

- Technetium scintography and/or computed tomography may be useful in the study of patients suspected of sacroiliac or sternoclavicular joint involvement.
- Magnetic resonance imaging is the method of choice for patients with hip pain of sudden onset and patients with suspected deep-seated bone or joint infections.

9. What is the differential diagnosis of bacterial arthritis?

The differential diagnosis varies according to the age of the patient and other clinical variables. In children and young adults with polyarticular involvement, the diagnoses of acute rheumatic fever, Lyme disease, Kawasaki disease, and viral infections (i.e., parvovirus, hepatitis B, rubella) should be entertained.

In all older adults, the diagnosis of crystal-induced arthritis should be entertained and ruled out by polarized microscopy of the synovial fluid. Other diagnoses to be considered include "pseudoseptic" arthritis, infectious arthritis caused by other pathogens (e.g., mycobacteria, *Brucella* sp.), and reactive arthritis.

10. What is the treatment of bacterial arthritis?

1. **Antibiotics.** Patients suspected of having bacterial arthritis should be treated accordingly until bacteriologic studies are completed. Before identification of a presumptive organism by Gram stain, antibiotics should be used judiciously to cover the most likely pathogens. In very ill patients, treatment of both gram-positive and gram-negative organisms is indicated pending identification. Nafcillin or other penicillinase-resistant synthetic penicillins are the drugs of choice; when methicillin-resistant *Staphylococcus aureus* is a concern, vancomycin is a reasonable alternative. Gram-negative organisms are usually well covered with a third-generation cephalosporin, quinolone, or aminoglycoside. If the offending organism is not identified but the patient responds to a combined antibiotic regimen, this regimen should be continued. If the microorganism is identified, the treatment should be guided by the antibiotic sensitivity of the bacterial isolate.

Parenteral antibiotics are recommended for no less than 4 weeks. Shorter courses of parenteral antibiotics followed by oral antibiotics have been used in children with good results. Long-term administration of oral antibiotics is recommended in patients with protracted bone and joint infections (i.e., prosthetic joints).

2. **Drainage.** Close-needle drainage of the affected joint is recommended on a daily basis until the SF becomes sterile or the effusion is minimal. Prompt reaccumulation of large amounts of SF may be due to lack of antibiotic sensitivity, presence of more than one organism, or loculation of SF in the joint cavity. Surgical drainage is indicated in all cases of hip involvement, in joints that do not respond to antibiotic therapy, in joints with loculated effusions, and in joints anatomically altered by underlying pathology. Surgical drainage can be performed either arthroscopically or by open arthrotomy.

3. **Joint immobiliatoin/mobilization.** Joint immobilization is recommended only for patients with incapacitating pain. Mobilization of the affected joint through its range of motion, both passively and actively, should be encouraged.

Gonococcal Arthritis

11. What is the prevalence of disseminated gonococcal infection (DGI)?

DGI is a common illness with an estimated prevalence of 0.5–3%.

12. What percentage of all septic arthritis is gonococcal?

Gonococcal arthritis is the most frequent type of septic arthritis among young adults, accounting for up to two-thirds of the cases of septic arthritis and tenosynovitis in North America.

13. True or false: DGI is always preceded by symptomatic mucosal infection.

False. Although DGI is always preceded by mucosal infection with *Neisseria gonorrhoeae*, usually involving the endocervix or urethra, pharynx, or rectum, the infection may or may not be symptomatic. Most patients who develop DGI have asymptomatic primary gonococcal infection of the genitourinary (GU) tract.

14. Describe the "typical" arthritis of DGI.

The most common symptom of DGI is the acute onset of oligo- or polyarthralgia in a diffuse, migratory, or additive pattern; it peaks within a few days of onset. Fewer than 50% of patients develop true arthritis. Most cases are monoarthritis, but in some patients oligo- or polyarthritis develops. Any joint may be involved, but the knees, wrists, hands, and ankles are usually affected.

15. Describe the tenosynovitis of DGI.

Two-thirds of patients with DGI develop tenosynovitis with or without arthritis. Tenosynovitis commonly affects the wrists, fingers, ankles, or toes.

16. Describe the skin involvement of DGI.

Skin involvement, although easily overlooked, may be seen in two-thirds of patients with DGI. Most lesions are painless, and patients may be unaware of them. The lesions are generally few in number; they are found most commonly on the extremities and trunk and rarely on the face, palms, or soles. They usually present as macules, papules, or pustules on an erythematous base; however, vesicular, bullous, and erythema nodosum-like or erythema multiforme-like lesions have been described. Skin lesions typically resolve with or without treatment.

17. What distinguishes the bacteremic form from the suppurative form of DGI?

The **bacteremic** form is characterized by tenosynovitis, dermatitis, fever, and chills. When true arthritis is present, the effusion is sparse and usually culture-negative. Blood cultures are more often positive in this form, but the percentage is still less than 50%.

In the less common **suppurative** form, arthritis is the major manifestation and the joint effusions are larger and purulent. Joint fluid cultures may be positive (< 50%), but blood cultures usually are not. Dermatitis may be present but is less common than in the bacteremic form.

18. Who gets DGI?

Although in the preantibiotic era DGI was more common in males, females are now affected 4 times more commonly than males.

19. What are risk factors for DGI?

- Recent menstruation (within 1 week) and pregnancy or the initial postpartum period increase the risk of dissemination from the genitourinary tract. Fifty percent of females with DGI have one of these two risk factors.
- Promiscuous homosexual men with asymptomatic pharyngeal or rectal involvement are also at increased risk.
- Other less common risk factors include inherited deficiencies of the terminal components of complement C5–C8 (especially C8) as well as other complement component deficiencies (including C3 and C4).

Although most patients with DGI are young and otherwise healthy, DGI also may be seen in the elderly and in children as well as in patients with other connective tissue disorders such as systemic lupus erythematosus, rheumatoid arthritis, and Reiter's syndrome. DGI also has been reported in the setting of other infections, including *Mycobacterium avium* complex (MAC) and HIV.

20. What is the differential diagnosis of DGI?

The differential diagnosis of arthritis-dermatitis is extensive. Major differential diagnoses include Reiter's syndrome, nongonococcal septic arthritis, bacterial endocarditis, hepatitis B infection, rheumatic fever, and juvenile rheumatoid arthritis (in children).

21. What is the treatment of DGI?

1. Because in a significant number of patients DGI may be due to penicillin-resistant strains, the initial recommended therapy is a third-generation cephalosporin, such as ceftriaxone, 1 gm intramuscularly or intravenously every 24 hr; ceftizoxime, 1 gm intramuscularly or intravenously every 8 hr; or cefotaxime, 1 gm intravenously every 8 hr. Ampicillin, 1 gm intravenously every 6 hr, may be substituted for the cephalosporins when penicillin sensitivity has been demonstrated on culture.

2. Parenteral therapy should be continued until symptoms of DGI resolve or clinical improvement is evident (usually 2–4 days). Oral antibiotics may then be substituted: amoxicillin, 500 mg, with clavulanate, 125 mg, 3 times/day; cefuroxime axetil, 500 mg 2 times/day; or ciprofloxacin, 500 mg 2 times/day (contraindicated in pregnancy). Therapy is continued for 7 days. In patients in whom cultures show penicillin resistance, cefixime, 400 mg orally 2 times/day, or cefuroxime axetil, 500 mg orally 2 times/day, may be used for 7 days after initial symptoms have subsided.

3. Unless there is evidence that chlamydial infection is not concomitantly present, doxycycline, 100 mg orally 2 times/day, should also be used for 7 days. In pregnant patients erythromycin base, 500 mg/day, should be used.

4. In penicillin-allergic patients, initial therapy for DGI is spectinomycin, 2 gm intramuscularly every 12 hr. When symptoms resolve, spectinomycin may be replaced by ciprofloxacin, 500 mg orally 2 times/day for 7 days.

Lyme Arthritis

22. What is the best clinical marker for Lyme disease?

The initial skin lesion, erythema chronica migrans (ECM), is the best clinical marker; it occurs in 60–80% of patients.

23. What are the three clinical stages of Lyme disease?

Lyme disease is often divided into clinical stages for the purpose of description. Stages 1 and 2 generally encompass the first weeks to months of disease, with stage 3 occurring several months to years into the disease. A patient infected with *Borrelia burgdorferi* may proceed through all stages of disease, be completely asymptomatic, or present with stage 2 or 3 disease without having symptomatic earlier stage disease.

Stage 1: Early localized infection. Low-grade fever, minor constitutional symptoms, and local adenopathy may be seen. Alternatively, patients may feel completely well. ECM, the pathognomonic skin lesion, occurs at the site of the tick bite 3–32 days (mean: 7 days) after the bite. The lesion starts as a small erythematous macule or papule and gradually expands to a diameter of 3–68 cm (mean: 15 cm). The lesion is warm to touch and mildly symptomatic with burning or pruritus in about one-half of patients. Thus, 20–40% of patients in whom ECM was not reported may have had asymptomatic lesions in inconspicuous locations.

Stage 2: Early disseminated infection. Days to weeks into the illness the organism may disseminate widely to multiple organ systems. *B. burgdorferi* has been cultured from skin, blood, and cerebrospinal fluid. Musculoskeletal symptoms are typically migratory, lasting hours to days in any single location and involving both articular and periarticular structures. Most commonly pain without swelling occurs at only one or a few sites at a time. Both large and small joints may be involved.

Stage 3: Late (persistent) infection. Sixty-two percent of patients develop frank arthritis at a mean of 6 months after disease onset. The typical pattern is an intermittent, inflammatory mono- or oligoarthritis involving predominantly large joints; the knee is involved at some point in nearly all cases. A symmetric small joint pattern resembling rheumatoid arthritis is rare and, when it does occur, transient.

Initial episodes of Lyme arthritis during the first year, although often dramatic with large effusions, are usually brief, lasting days to a few weeks. When arthritis persists into the second and third year it usually occurs in one or perhaps two large joints, with the knee involved in the vast majority of cases. Episodes at this point may last months. With each passing year, arthritis resolves in 10–20% of patients. Ten percent of untreated patients with joint involvement develop chronic Lyme arthritis, which is defined as at least one episode of continual joint inflammation lasting 1 year or longer. Chronic Lyme arthritis has been associated with an increased frequency of the class II major histocompatibility complex alleles HLA-DR4 and HLA-DR2.

24. How is Lyme arthritis diagnosed?

The diagnosis of Lyme arthritis depends mainly on serologic techniques that detect antibodies to the spirochete. An IgM antibody response usually develops by 2–4 weeks after the onset of ECM. An IgG response is seen by 4–8 weeks. The IgM response generally fades after several months. In cases with ongoing active disease, especially arthritis, IgG titers tend to remain high and reactivity to multiple spirochetal polypeptides is seen. In successfully treated or spontaneously resolving disease, specific IgG levels typically decline slowly over months to years, eventually reaching a steady state of low-level positivity.

An enzyme-linked immunosorbent assay (ELISA) is more sensitive and specific than the original indirect immunofluorescence assay. Unfortunately, serologic testing has not been standardized, and interlaboratory and even intralaboratory variation continues to be a problem. False-negative and false-positive results must always be considered. False-negative results may be seen (1) in the early weeks of infection before development of a detectable IgM antibody response; (2) occasionally in patients with late disease who received treatment early in the course of disease, presumably blunting the development of a normal humoral response; and (3) rarely in patients in whom antibody titers have diminished over time. False-positive results are seen in patients with other spirochetal infections, Rocky Mountain spotted fever, echovirus infection, varicella infection, or various autoimmune diseases as well as in healthy individuals.

Direct detection of cellular components of *B. burgdorferi* by polymerase chain reaction (PCR) has been reported from cerebrospinal fluid, urine, joint fluid, skin, and serum of patients with Lyme disease.

25. What is the treatment for Lyme disease and Lyme arthritis?

Early disease (without carditis or frank neurologic involvement) may be treated orally with doxycycline or amoxicillin for 10–30 days, depending on the severity of illness and clinical response. Major sequelae, such as arthritis, are seen only rarely after early treatment and indicate treatment failure.

Late disease (arthritis) may be treated with a course of oral therapy, doxycycline, 100 mg 2 times/day for 30 days, or amoxicillin and probenecid, 500 mg each 4 times/day for 30 days. Intravenous therapy with ceftriaxone, 2 gm/day for 14 days, should be considered for nonresponders. Clinical response to therapy may be slow, especially where arthritis has become persistent, with a decrease in inflammation over weeks to months. In cases of persistent arthritis, other therapeutic options include corticosteroid injection and synovectomy.

NONBACTERIAL ARTHRITIS

Mycobacterial Arthritis

26. What is the typical presentation of tuberculous arthritis?

Mycobacterial infections generally produce a chronic monoarticular arthritis in 90% of patients. Elderly patients may have more systemic symptoms, more foci of extraarticular tuberculosis, and more involvement of non–weight-bearing joints. Knees may be affected in 30% but non–weight-bearing joints may be involved in 39% of patients.

27. Which nontuberculous mycobacteria can cause granulomatous synovitis?

Mycobacterium kansasii, marinum, gordonae, avium-intracellulare, chelonei, or *fortuitum*. These species produce an infection in the hand or wrists in patients with nonpenetrating trauma.

28. How is mycobacterial arthritis definitively diagnosed?

A history of tuberculous infection or exposure may suggest the diagnosis. Purified protein derivative (PPD) and anergy testing are usually positive for exposure. Synovial fluid (SF) culture may be positive in 79% of cases; yield is increased by multiple aspirations with SF culture. Definitive diagnosis is made by synovial biopsy, which shows chronic inflammation with granuloma formation and giant cells with positive tissue culture in 90% of cases.

29. What is the incidence of skeletal tuberculosis among all patients with tuberculosis ?

Skeletal tuberculosis is an infrequent form of the disease, accounting for 1–5% of all cases.

30. Of all cases of musculoskeletal tuberculosis, what percent is articular and what percent is osseous?

66% articular and 33% osseous.

31. What is Poncet's disease?

Poncet's disease is characterized by polyarthritis during acute tuberculous infection in which no mycobacterial involvement can be found and no other known cause of polyarthritis detected. It is an entity distinct from tuberculous arthritis, which is usually monoarticular and caused by direct tuberculin infection. Poncet's disease remains a diagnosis of exclusion. The arthritis responds to antituberculous and antiinflammatory drugs.

32. What is Pott's disease?

Tuberculous spondylitis. First described by Percival Pott in 1779, this disease presents in its classic form as a paraplegia with accompanying kyphotic deformity of the spine. In the United States, paraplegia may develop in 7–10% of patients with Pott's disease. Approximately 90% of patients with Pott's disease have a positive tuberculin skin test. Radiographically, 50% of patients with tuberculous spondylitis have chest radiographs that are negative for active or inactive pulmonary tuberculosis. The lower thoracic and upper lumbar vertebrae are the most frequent sites.

Fungal Arthritis

33. What is the most common cause of fungal arthritis?

Sporothrix schenckii is the most frequently reported infection of the joint because it is found worldwide in warm, moist environments. Most patients have contact with moist soil or do labor-intensive work.

34. What are other reported causes of fungal arthritis?

Joint infections are uncommonly seen as a manifestation of coccidioidomycosis, blastomycosis, histoplasmosis, candidiasis, and infection with dermatiaceous fungi.

35. What are the demographic and diagnostic highlights of fungal arthritis?

Worldwide distribution
Compromised host
Occupational hazard
Monoarthritis (usually) or oligoarthritis
Osteomyelitis (common)
Delayed diagnosis (common)
Often requires direct visualization of the organism in synovial fluid, membrane, or both for accurate diagnosis.

36. Which cause of fungal arthritis is usually diagnosed in synovial fluid culture and rarely requires tissue diagnosis?

Candidal arthritis.

37. True or false: Most patients with fungal arthritis have systemic symptoms.

False. In most patients with fungal arthritis, systemic symptoms are not present. In fact, local heat is rarely present; thus, diagnosis of an infectious cause is delayed. Asymmetric chronic involvement of any joint should lead to examination of fluid and synovial tissue for both mycobacteria and fungi.

38. What factors predispose to fungal arthritis?

- Diabetes
- Malignancies associated with immunologic disequilibrium
- Sarcoidosis
- Malnutrition
- Prematurity
- Prolonged use of broad-spectrum antibiotics
- Use of intravenous or Foley catheters
- Corticosteroid or cytotoxic therapy
- Hyperalimentation with high glucose concentrations
- Traumatized skin (burns, surgical wounds)
- Intravenous drug abuse

39. What is the treatment for fungal arthritis?

A combination of medical and surgical therapy seems to be the most common modality of treatment. Amphotericin B continues to be the drug of choice at intravenous dosages of 0.3–0.7 mg/kg/day. A total dose of 1–3 gm is given over 6–10 weeks. On rare occasions, in patients with candidal arthritis, 5-fluorocytosine (5-FC) is administered orally in 4 divided doses per day for a total of 150 mg/kg/day, along with amphotericin B. 5-FC should not be used alone because of the rapid emergence of resistance. Intraarticular amphotericin B may be a useful adjunctive therapy in infections that are limited to the joint capsule and not disseminated. Other therapeutic options include the azoles: ketoconazole, 400–800 mg/day; fluconazole, 200–400 mg/day; or itraconazole, 200–400 mg/day. Surgical treatment, mainly joint drainage, is important, particularly in prosthetic fungal infection.

Viral Arthritis

40. What viral agents are commonly associated with arthritis? Which patients are characteristically involved with each?

Rubella	Adult females
Hepatitis B	Patients in preicteric phase
Mumps	Adult males
Lymphocytic choriomeningitis virus	Adults with aseptic meningitis
Parvovirus	Adults with erythema infectiosum

Virus	*Frequency of Arthritis*
Parvovirus B19	50% adults (women 60%, men 30%), 5% children
Hepatitis B virus	Arthritis, 10%; arthralgia, 25%
Rubella virus	15–30% adult women; children and men, less often
Rubella vaccine	15% adult women, 1–5% children
Alphavirus	Most adults with clinical infection
Mumps virus	0.4% (males more often than females)
Adenovirus	Case reports
Cytomegalovirus	Case reports
Epstein-Barr virus	Case reports
Herpes simplex virus type I	Case reports
Varicella zoster virus	Case reports
Lymphocytic choriomeningitis virus	Case reports
Coxsackieviruses	Case reports
Echoviruses	Case reports
Hepatitis A virus	Case reports, arthralgias 11%
Smallpox virus	0.25–0.5%, 2–5% children

41. What are the arthropod-borne viral arthritides?

Ross River virus (Australia)   Chikungunya (East Africa, India)
Ockelbo virus (Sweden)   O'nyong-nyong (East Africa)

42. Describe the acute arthritis of rubella infection.

Rubella infection is associated with polyarthritis in female adults, usually within 7 days of the eruption. Small joints of the hands are frequently involved with less frequent involvement of the wrists and knees. SF has a mononuclear predominance, and the virus is rarely recovered in SF. The course is usually self-limited, although symptoms may persist longer than 1 month in some patients. Men develop arthralgias but have arthritis less commonly than women. The arthritis also may be seen in women receiving rubella vaccine, but it is a milder syndrome with arthralgias rather than arthritis.

43. Describe the arthritis associated with acute parvovirus B19 infection.

Arthralgias are seen in 5% of children under 10 years of age, with joint swelling in 3%. Joint pain and swelling occur in 12% and 5% of adolescent patients, respectively. However, joint pain occurs in 77% and joint swelling in 60% of adults 20 years of age or older. The arthritis of adults with parvo infection is an acute, moderately severe, symmetrical polyarthritis that usually starts in the hands or knees and quickly spreads (1–2 days) to involve the wrists, ankles, feet, elbows, and shoulders. Distribution of joint involvement and its symmetry may suggest a diagnosis of rheumatoid arthritis. Many patients have morning stiffness for longer than 1 hour.

44. What are the commonly affected joints in adults with parvo arthritis infection?

Metacarpophalangeal joints (MCPs)	75%	Wrists	55%
Proximal interphalangeal joints (PIPs)	75%	Ankles	40%
Knees	65%		

45. How can chronic parvo B19 arthropathy be distinguished from classic rheumatoid arthritis?

The absence of rheumatoid nodules or joint destruction helps to distinguish B19 arthropathy from classic, erosive rheumatoid arthritis (RA). Fifty percent of patients meet the criteria for RA established by the American College of Rheumatology. A positive rheumatoid factor and the subtlety of skin eruptions in adults may make it difficult to differentiate between B19 arthropathy and early RA. Fewer than 50% of patients report a history of rash.

46. What is the presumed pathogenesis of parvo arthropathy?

The arthropathy is presumably immunologically mediated, because its onset is coincident with the first appearance of circulating antibodies.

47. What is the most useful serologic test to diagnose parvovirus arthropathy?

IgM serology is the most useful diagnostic modality in most cases of rheumatologic importance. IgG becomes detectable within several days after IgM and persists for years and probably for life. Patients with chronic hematologic disorders or immunocompromised patients may have an unpredictable antibody response. Tests for B19 DNA or viral antigens are most useful in such patients. The most sensitive assays for detecting B19 DNA are hybridization assays and polymerase chain reaction. Parvovirus B19 DNA also has been isolated from synovial fluid.

Failure to obtain human parvovirus B19 serologic testing at presentation may leave the diagnostic IgM antibody response undetected and result in failure to diagnose B19 arthropathy in patients in whom joint symptoms persist.

48. What is the outcome of parvo B19 arthropathy?

Improvement is generally noted within 2 weeks, but some symptoms may remain for months, or, in rare cases, years.

49. What other rheumatic diseases are associated with parvo B19 infection?

There have been numerous reports of serologically confirmed parvo B19 associated with nonthrombocytopenic purpura, including Henoch-Schönlein purpura. Rare reports of necrotizing vasculitis, resembling polyarteritis nodosa and Wegener's granulomatosis, have been described; all cases responded to intravenous gammaglobulin. A lupus-like syndrome also has been reported in a patient with thrombocytopenia, neutropenia, hypocomplementemia, rash, and arthritis. Transient rheumatoid factor and antinuclear antibody positivity may be seen.

50. What rheumatic syndromes are associated with chronic hepatitis B or C infection?

About 50% of patients with polyarteritis nodosa (PAN) have serologic evidence of hepatitis B infection, and about 50–70% of patients with type II mixed cryoglobulinemia have serologic evidence of infection with hepatitis B or C. Hepatitis B surface antigen has been documented in cryoprecipitate in patients with cryoglobulinemia.

PROSTHETIC JOINT INFECTION

51. What is the infection rate of total joint replacement?

The combination of ultra clean air, antibiotics, and exhaust ventilated suites have made it possible to limit the infection rate in total joint arthroplasty to 0.5% or less.

52. What is the incidence of infection in total joint arthroplasty?

An infection rate of 0.5%, when universally attained, translates into 1250–2500 new cases of infection each year.

53. Describe the classification of infection after joint replacement proposed by the Mayo Clinic.

Stage 1	Infections occur in the first 3 months after surgery.
Stage 2	Infections occur between 3 months and 2 years after surgery.
Stage 3	Late; infections occur after 2 years.

54. Discuss the microbiology of infected joint replacements.

In 70% of cases only single pathogens can be identified; mixed and sterile cultures are identified in 15% each of remaining cases. The dominance of staphylococcal species has major implications for prophylaxis.

Organism	% Cases
Staphylococcus aureus	30
Staphylococcus epidermidis	14–35
Other gram-positive organisms	10
Gram-negative organisms	15
Anaerobes	7–9

55. List the host factors increasing the risk of infection in joint replacement.

- Previous local surgery
- Previous sepsis
- Remote infection at the time of surgery
- Diabetes mellitus
- Rheumatoid arthritis

56. What is the major source of infection in total joint arthroplasty?

Wound contamination derived from operating room air through dispersal of bacteria on desquamated skin (only 5–15% from the patient's own skin).

57. Specify the incidence and predominant organisms of hematogenous infection of joint implants.

Incidence: 0.1–0.7%.

Predominant organisms: *Staphylococcus aureus* (50%), *Staphylococcus epidermidis* (10%), other gram-positive organisms (11–23%), gram-negative organisms (21–24%), and anaerobes (2–8%).

58. What are the putative sources of hematogenous infection in total joint replacement?

The mnemonic **BBLOODS** may be helpful:

B	**B**owel (gastrointestinal tract)
BL	**BL**adder (urinary tract)
O	**O**ropharynx
O	**O**ther
D	**D**ental work
S	**S**kin/**S**oft tissue

59. Total joint infection can be difficult to distinguish from aseptic loosening because both may present with pain alone. What procedures help to distinguish between the two?

Joint aspiration helps to confirm infection in 60% of patients and tissue biopsy in 80%. Elevated acute phase reactants (erythrocyte sedimentation rate, C-reactive protein) and positive indium 111-labeled leukocyte studies are more suggestive of an infected joint prosthesis.

60. What principles underlie the management of infected total joint replacement?

1. Microbiologic diagnosis
2. Assessment and modification of the host
3. Anatomic definition of local disease
4. Antibiotic therapy
5. Surgical debridement of the implant, cement, scar, and granulation tissue
6. Obliteration of debridement cavity
7. Restoration of functional stability

CONTROVERSIES

61. Should patients with prosthetic joints receive antibiotic prophylaxis for dental work?

Prophylactic antibiotics have been recommended in all patients undergoing dental work. Others have argued that when one considers the risk of death from an infected total joint replacement, cost of revision arthroplasty, and apparent risk of infecting a total joint in the absence of dental sepsis, a small margin emerges in favor of avoiding routine antibiotic prophylaxis. A small increase in infection risk—for example, when a systemic condition predisposes to infection—would alter the balance.

62. List the suggested indications for antibiotic prophylaxis in patients with prosthetic joints.

1. Oropharyngeal procedures
   • All dental procedures likely to cause gingival bleeding
   • Bronchoscopy, tonsillectomy, adenoidectomy
2. Genitourinary and gastrointestinal tract procedures
   • Surgery or instrumentation of genitourinary tract, cystoscopy, prostatic manipulation
   • Surgery or instrumentation of genitourinary/biliary tract, endoscopic biopsy
3. Surgical procedures on any infected or contaminated tissues

63. What antibiotic regimen is recommended when antibiotic prophylaxis is considered in patients with indwelling joint prostheses?

Prophylactic use of antibiotics in patients with indwelling joint prostheses is similar to that in patients with prosthetic cardiac valves. Although no study is available to determine the adequacy of prophylactic antibiotic regimens, the following guidelines have been proposed:

Oropharyngeal procedures
- Procaine penicillin G, 1.2 million units intramuscularly 30–60 min before procedure; then penicillin V, 500 mg orally every 6 hr for 8 doses.
- In patients allergic to penicillin: clindamycin, 600 mg intramuscularly or intravenously 60 min before procedure, then 300 mg orally every 6 hr for 8 doses *or* cefazolin, 1.0 gm intramuscularly or intravenously 30–60 min before procedure, then cephradine, 500 mg orally every 6 hr for 8 doses

Genitourinary and gastrointestinal tract procedures (begininng 30–60 min before procedure)
- Procaine penicillin G, 2.4 million units intramuscularly every 8 hr for 3 doses
    or
- Ampicillin, 1.0 gm intramuscularly or intravenously every 8 hr for 3 doses, + gentamicin, 1.0 mg/kg (not to exceed 80 mg) intramuscularly or intravenously every 8 hr for 3 doses
    or
- Streptomycin, 1.0 gm intramuscularly every 12 hr for 2 doses
- In patients allergic to penicillin (beginning 30–60 min before procedure): vancomycin, 1.0 gm intravenously (over 30–60 min) every 12 hr for 2 doses + streptomycin, 1.0 gm intramuscularly every 12 hr for 2 doses

Surgical procedures on infected or contaminated tissues
Regimen depends on anticipated pathogens; for example, for *Staphylococcus aureus*:
- Nafcillin, 2.0 gm intravenously 30–50 min before procedure, then dicloxacillin, 500 mg orally every 6 hr for 8 doses
    or
- Cefazolin, 1.0 gm intramuscularly or intravenously 30–60 min before procedure, then cephradine, 500 mg orally every 6 hr for 8 doses
    or
- Clindamycin, 600 mg intramuscularly or intravenously 30–60 min before procedure, then 300 mg orally every 6 hr for 8 doses

BIBLIOGRAPHY

1. Brause BD: Infected total knee replacement. Diagnostic, therapeutic, and prophylactic considerations. Orthop Clin North Am 13:245–249, 1982.
2. Cuellar ML, Silveira LH, Citera G, et al: Other fungal arthritides. Rheum Dis Clin North Am 19:439–455, 1993.
3. Espinoza LR (ed): Infectious arthritis. Rheum Dis Clin North Am 19:279-513, 1993 [special issue].
4. Finkel TH, Torok TJ, Ferguson JF, et al: Chronic parvovirus B19 infection and systemic necrotising vasculitis: Opportunistic infection or aetiological agent? Lancet 343:1255–1258, 1994.
5. Gillespie WJ: Infection in total joint replacement. Infect Dis Clin North Am 4:465–484, 1990.
6. Kalish RA, Knopf AN, Gary GW, Canoso JJ: Lupus-like presentation of human parvovirus B19 infection. J Rheumatol 19:169–171, 1992.
7. Moreland LW, Koopman WJ: Infection as a cause of arthritis. Curr Opin Rheumatol 3:639–649, 1991.
8. Smith CA: Virus-related arthritis, excluding human immunodeficiency virus. Curr Opin Rheumatol 2:635–641, 1990.
9. Smith JW. Infectious arthritis. Infect Dis Clin North Am 4:523–538, 1990.
10. Torok TJ: Parvo B19 and human disease. Adv Intern Med 37:431–455, 1992.

39. RHEUMATIC SYNDROMES ASSOCIATED WITH INFECTIOUS DISEASES

Raymond J. Enzenauer, M.D., FACP

REACTIVE ARTHRITIS

1. Define reactive arthritis.

The acute, inflammatory sterile arthritis that develops days to weeks after infection at a remote site is known as reactive arthritis.

2. How long has reactive arthritis been clinically recognized?

The association of inflammatory sterile arthritis with infection has been recognized for at least 500 years. The earliest report appears to be the case of a man with knee arthritis and "gonorrhoea" described by Van Forest in 1507. Musgrave described a similar case in England in 1703. Descriptions by Salle (1781), Hunter (1786), and Cooper (1824) suggest that by the end of the 18th century the concept that genital infection may give rise to arthritis involving the knees and feet was gaining widespread acceptance.

3. What are the primary triggering infections associated with reactive arthritis?

Reactive arthritis is generally triggered by either an enteric or urethral infection. Triggering infections may be asymptomatic in 26–36% of patients.

Many enteric organisms have been implicated, but *Shigella* (especially *S. flexneri*), *Salmonella* (especially *S. typhimurium*), certain subtypes of *Yersinia*, and *Campylobacter* spp. are most often cultured. Case reports of reactive arthritis have been described in association with *Clostridium difficile, Blastocystis hominis, Brucella abortus, Vibrio parahaemolyticus,* enteropathogenic *Escherichia coli,* giardiasis, *Hafnia alvei,* cryptosporidia, and certain intestinal parasites such as *Entamoeba histolytica, Taenia saginata,* and *Strongyloides stercoralis.*

Urethral infection, often contracted sexually, also may cause reactive arthritis. *Chlamydia trachomatis* (about 50% of cases) and *Ureaplasma urealyticum* are the primary venereal pathogens. Reactive arthritis following gonorrhea is most likely due to concomitant nongonococcal urethritis.

4. Describe the signs and symptoms associated with reactive arthritis.

Inflammatory arthritis begins 7–30 days after intestinal or genital infection. Typically it is an asymmetric oligoarthritis (an average of three affected joints) and primarily involves the articulations of the lower extremities. The knee is the most commonly affected joint, often with massive effusions containing > 100 cc of fluid. Axial skeleton involvement, which occurs in many patients, is independent of the activity of peripheral arthritis. The usual complaint is low back pain, which often is worse on wakening and gradually improves throughout the day. Joint involvement in B27-associated reactive arthritis may include the following clinical features:

- Asymmetric distribution
- Predilection for large joints
- Joints involved in rapid succession
- Lower extremities affected (80–90% of cases)
- Upper extremities affected (about 50%)
- Oligoarthritis
- Enthesopathy (insertional tendonitis) (30–50%)
- Low back pain (20–30%)

5. Define enthesopathy.

Enthesopathy is the inflammation at ligament-bone junctions that is a distinctive feature of reactive arthritis. Typical sites include the insertion of the fibrous joint capsule, tendons, and/or ligaments into subchondral bone and periarticular periosteum. Because of the extraordinary quantity of these sites, pain may be widespread. Common sites of enthesopathy include the insertion of the plantar fascia, insertion of the Achilles tendon, tibial tuberosity, and medial and lateral epicondyles of the elbow. Most often physical examination reveals only local tenderness at insertion sites. Occasionally, impressive swelling and erythema are seen.

6. What is dactylitis?

Patients with reactive arthritis often develop peculiar swelling of the entire digit (either fingers or toes), which is graphically denoted as a "sausage digit" because of its appearance. The appropriate term is dactylitis. It is distinguished from simple arthritis by the recognition that swelling and tenderness extend beyond the confines of the synovium along the bone between the interphalangeal joints, particularly on the dorsal aspect of the digit.

7. What is "lover's heel"?

Another characteristic location for enthesopathy is the foot. Inflammation at the insertion of the plantar fascia into the calcaneus causes "lover's heel."

8. How do articular manifestations differ among triggering organisms?

The prevalence of joint disease seems to be higher for enteric infections than for venereally acquired disease (about 3% vs. 1%, respectively). Relapse of arthritis, however, is greater in venereally acquired than in enteric reactive arthritis (50% vs. 20%, respectively). The prevalence of back involvement, the mean number of joints affected, and the degree of enthesopathy appear to be the same for all triggering organisms.

9. What features are similar in postenteric and postvenereal reactive arthritis?

- Strong association with HLA-B27.
- Reactive arthritis develops in only a minority (about 2%; 20% of B27-positives) of people with potentially arthritogenic infection.
- Interval of 1–2 weeks between triggering infection and development of arthritis.
- Disease usually has a self-limiting course.
- Antibiotic therapy may have no distinct effect on the course of disease.
- The clinical picture of arthritis is considerably uniform regardless of triggering infection.
- Extraarticular manifestations are common.
- Laboratory tests are nonspecific and indicate only acute inflammation.
- Most patients are seronegative for rheumatoid factors.

10. What is the natural history of reactive arthritis?

At 1 year, over 80% of patients are symptom-free. By 5 years after the initial attack, however, 50% have a relapse significant enough to interfere with employment. One-half of these patients, or 25% of the total, have severely disabling disease.

11. What are the common extraarticular manifestations of reactive arthritis?

Mucocutaneous, ocular, and cardiac abnormalities are seen in association with reactive arthritis. The most common **mucocutaneous lesion** is keratoderma blennorrhagica (KDB), in which heaped-up scaling lesions appear on the palms and soles of the feet. Histologically they are indistinguishable from psoriasis. KDB is mainly seen in postvenereal Reiter's syndrome. Circinate balanitis is a hyperkeratotic lesion at the junction of the glans and shaft of the circumcised penis, often with a serpiginous, circumferential distribution. It is seen in 25% of men with Reiter's syndrome. Erythema nodosum is occasionally observed in association with *Yersinia* infection. Except for erythema nodosum, mucocutaneous lesions are primarily a feature of venereally acquired disease!

Ocular disease includes conjunctivitis, which, although described as part of the classic triad of Reiter's syndrome, occurs in less than one-third of patients. Acute anterior uveitis, which occurs in less than 5% of patients, may be either unilateral or bilateral and represents an ophthalmologic emergency.

Rare forms of **cardiac involvement** include myocarditis, conduction abnormalities (including complete heart block), and a distinctive aortic root lesion leading to aortic dilation and aortic valve insufficiency.

12. What are the genetic associations of reactive arthritis?

Possession of a Y chromosome is a major risk factor for venereally acquired reactive arthritis, which exhibits a male-to-female ratio of 10:1. Although there is a male predominance with enteric-associated disease, the discordance is much less. This may reflect the fact that genital inflammation (cervicitis) in women is frequently overlooked; as a result, women may be underrepresented in the category of venereally acquired reactive arthritis.

The other major genetic contribution to reactive arthritis is the presence of the HLA-B27 haplotype. Although present in only 6–8% of most Caucasian populations, 80% of patients with reactive arthritis have this class I major histocompatibility antigen. In addition, HLA-B27–positive patients with reactive arthritis are more likely to have more severe disease with multiple relapses.

13. What is the proposed mechanism of disease in reactive arthritis?

Reactive arthritis is believed to represent an aberrant immune response in a genetically susceptible person. Only arthritogenic strains can stimulate an immune response in susceptible people. In addition, the HLA-B27 haplotype cannot be the sole requirement for abnormal response, which may be a closely linked gene or subtype of HLA-B27 not yet serologically defined. Trapped bacterial antigens (documented in some cases of reactive arthritis) or cross-reacting synovial epitopes may result in persistent synovial inflammation.

14. Although cultures are negative, what intraarticular bacterial antigens have been identified in inflamed joints of patients with reactive arthritis?

Chlamydia trachomatis, Yersinia pseudotuberculosis, Yersinia enterocolitica, Salmonella enteritidis/typhi, and *Shigella flexneri.* The pathogenic significance of intraarticular bacterial antigens remains unclear. Immunohistochemistry does not allow determination of whether bacterial antigen is present within the joint as viable organisms or degraded antigens.

15. What is the potential significance of bacterial antigen within the joint?

Several bacterial components, including lipase, outer membrane proteins, and cell wall preparations, have been shown to induce inflammation in experimental systems. If bacterial antigens in the joint are critical in the initiation of arthritis, it is possible that persistence of antigen also contributes to persistence of arthritis.

16. What is the treatment for reactive arthritis?

The major treatment of reactive arthritis is nonsteroidal antiinflammatory drugs (NSAIDs). Aspirin is usually ineffective in reactive arthritis. Intraarticular corticosteroid injection may be useful when symptoms are severe and do not respond to NSAID treatment. Oral corticosteroids are seldom helpful and should be avoided. Arthritis symptoms that persist or recur may be treated with various slow-acting antirheumatic drugs, including sulfasalazine, azathioprine, and methotrexate. HIV disease must be ruled out before initiation of immunosuppressive therapy. Skin and ocular disease usually can be managed with topical steroids.

17. Discuss the use of antibiotics in reactive arthritis.

Because of the high likelihood of coincident chlamydial or ureaplasmal infection in venereally acquired reactive arthritis, a 7-day course of tetracycline is indicated for a new patient and his or her sexual partner. Longer treatment (3 months) has been reported to decrease the duration of illness in patients with *Chlamydia*-triggered reactive arthritis. Enteric pathogens should be eliminated with antibiotics when appropriate.

18. What is the prognosis of reactive arthritis?

Reactive arthritis has a self-limiting course, although the acute attack may last up to 1 year. Two-thirds of patients complain of mild joint symptoms and/or low back pain many years after the initial attack. A substantial minority of patients report recurrences, which are more frequent in the postvenereal form of disease, probably because of the tendency for nongonococcal urethritis to recur and because of repeated genital infections in sexually active people.

19. How is reactive arthritis diagnosed?

The diagnosis of reactive arthritis is based on (1) a typical clinical picture and (2) laboratory evidence of a triggering infection. Enteric bacteria usually can be cultured from stools within the first 2 weeks after onset of symptoms. In patients with uroarthritis, it is important to search for *Chlamydia* sp. and gonococci.

20. What is the differential diagnosis of reactive arthritis?

The differential diagnosis is usually easy to make. The most important diseases to be considered are rheumatoid arthritis, rheumatic fever, acute bacterial septic arthritis, psoriatic arthritis, and crystal synovitis.

21. Who was Dr. Hans Reiter?

Dr. Hans Reiter was a Prussian army physician. His relatively obscure case report (in 1916) of a young soldier who developed postdysenteric arthritis focused the attention of the medical community on the syndrome that now bears his name.

22. What is the classic triad of Reiter's syndrome?

The classic triad of Reiter's syndrome is arthritis, urethritis, and conjunctivitis. Reiter's syndrome is the best known subtype of reactive arthritis.

23. What is meant by the term incomplete Reiter's syndrome?

If the entire triad is not present, the term incomplete Reiter's syndrome is used.

24. Describe the use of antibiotics in the treatment of Reiter's syndrome.

Antibiotic treatment with tetracycline or erythromycin has been shown to reduce the incidence of postvenereal arthritis. In addition, a 3-month course of tetracycline decreases significantly the duration of illness in patients with *Chlamydia*-triggered reactive arthritis.

25. What famous explorer is believed to have suffered from Reiter's syndrome?

Christopher Columbus.

26. What is a Reiter's cell?

A Reiter's cell is a macrophage containing polymorphonuclear leukocytes; it was described 30 years ago as a specific finding in the synovial fluid of patients with Reiter's syndrome.

27. What laboratory testing *must* be completed for all patients with newly diagnosed Reiter's syndrome?

HIV testing must be completed. Both HIV infection and Reiter's syndrome are venereal diseases. In addition, cases of HIV-associated Reiter's syndrome have developed into full-blown AIDS soon after the initiation of immunosuppressive therapy with methotrexate for Reiter's syndrome.

ACUTE RHEUMATIC FEVER

28. Define acute rheumatic fever (ARF).

Rheumatic fever is an inflammatory disease induced by an antecedent group A beta-hemolytic streptococcal pharyngitis.

29. What are the common manifestations of ARF?

Carditis and acute polyarthritis are the most common manifestations. Chorea, erythema marginatum, and subcutaneous nodules are less frequent.

30. What is the incidence of ARF in streptococcal infection?

Early studies indicated that ARF occurred in 3% of patients with severe streptococcal pharyngitis and less than 0.1% with mild cases. This rate has remained relatively unchanged both in frequency and severity.

31. Only certain serotypes of streptococci have been associated with outbreaks of ARF. What are the rheumatogenic strains of streptococci?

A relatively small number of M serotypes (types 5, 14, 18, and 24) have been implicated in outbreaks of rheumatic fever. Streptococcal strains that cause nephritis (type M55) rarely cause ARF.

32. What sites of streptococcal infection cause ARF?

ARF is the result of an antecedent group A beta-hemolytic streptococcal *pharyngeal* infection. Other sites of infection do not cause ARF.

33. What is the incidence of symptomatic pharyngitis in ARF?

In outbreaks of ARF, at least 50% (33–74%) of patients had no history of pharyngitis.

34. What is the latent period between infection and onset of ARF?

3-4 weeks. This latent period persists even for repeated attacks!

35. What is the genetic susceptibility to ARF?

Numerous studies have documented no association of class I HLA antigens with ARF. In contrast to the lack of definitive association with HLA-DR antigens, a strong relationship with Ia-like B cell alloantigens has been documented. The B cell allotype 883 was detected in 50–75% of patients compared with 15% of controls.

36. What is the presumed pathogenesis of ARF?

Molecular mimicry. Humoral and cellular immune responses directed at various group A streptococcal antigens cross-react with a number of human antigens. Immune complexes may be important in the development of some manifestations.

37. What are the clinical features of ARF?

The clinical features depend on the age of the patient. In children and adolescents, polyarthritis and carditis predominate; chorea, rash, and nodules are less common. In adults, polyarthritis is usually the only major manifestation.

38. What are the revised Jones criteria for the diagnosis of ARF?

ARF is diagnosed in the presence of two major criteria or one major plus two minor criteria, together with evidence of prior group A streptococcal infection.

Major criteria	Minor criteria
Carditis	Fever
Polyarthritis	Arthralgia
Chorea	Previous rheumatic fever or rheumatic heart disease
Erythema marginatum	
Subcutaneous nodules	

Supporting evidence of preceding streptococcal infection
- Increased levels of antistreptolysin O or other streptococcal antibodies
- Positive throat culture for group A beta-hemolytic streptococci
- Recent scarlet fever

39. What are the five major clinical manifestations of ARF? Which is the only one that will not eventually disappear without treatment?

Carditis, polyarthritis, chorea, erythema marginatum, and subcutaneous nodules. Carditis is the only manifestation that will not resolve without treatment.

40. Describe the carditis of ARF.

The carditis of ARF is a pancarditis because the three layers of the heart are affected. Pancarditis distinguishes ARF from other systemic rheumatic diseases.

41. True of false: pericarditis can be an isolated finding in ARF.

False. Pericarditis in ARF is almost never an isolated finding. When it does occur, other causes must be excluded.

42. What are the clinical findings of myocarditis in ARF?

Myocarditis frequently leads to heart failure. Auscultation demonstrates persistent tachycardia with a gallop rhythm, even when the patient is afebrile.

43. What is the major physical finding of carditis in ARF?

In practically all patients with rheumatic carditis, auscultation discloses a murmur!

44. What is the most common valvular lesion in ARF?

Mitral regurgitation is the most common valvular lesion. A distinctive feature of ARF is the involvement of two or even three valves. Fusion of valvular leaves during the healing process leads to stenosis. A significant number of patients without evidence of valvular involvement during the acute phase present with mitral stenosis after 10–20 years.

45. What are useful tools to aid in the diagnosis of rheumatic carditis?

Chest radiographs and electrocardiograms aid in defining the enlargement of cardiac chambers and the conduction block associated with myocarditis. Echocardiograms help to assess the presence of pericardial effusion and extent of valvular disease.

46. Describe the arthritis of ARF.

The arthritis is acute in onset and migratory. Large joints, particularly the knees, elbows, ankles, and wrists, are the most frequently involved. In rare cases, the small joints of the hands and feet are affected.

47. What is Jaccoud's arthropathy?

Jaccoud's arthropathy is a chronic deforming arthritis of the hands caused by capsular and periarticular fibrosis; it is described particularly in patients who have had several acute episodes of rheumatic fever.

48. What is the treatment of the arthritis of ARF?

A distinctive feature of ARF is its dramatic response to aspirin and other nonsteroidal antiinflammatory medication. Improvement is noted within 24 hours of attaining therapeutic blood levels.

49. Describe the subcutaneous nodules of ARF.

Nearly 20% of patients have small subcutaneous nodules located primarily over bony prominences of the spinal column or surrounding the joints. They are smaller than 0.5 cm and painless.

Subcutaneous nodules appear only in patients with carditis, and their presence heralds severe carditis.

50. Histologically, what do the subcutaneous nodules resemble?

Rheumatoid nodules.

51. Describe the chorea of ARF.

Chorea primarily affects female adolescents. It is characterized by purposeless uncoordinated movements of the extremities that preclude normal writing. Inappropriate facial grimaces are a frequent feature. Inappropriate movements are more apparent with anxiety and disappear during sleep. Chorea may be the only clinical evidence of disease. Chorea is a benign manifestation of ARF; symptoms resolve completely without neurologic sequelae.

52. Describe the rash of ARF.

Erythema marginatum is the rarest of the major signs of ARF (< 5% of cases). It is characterized by a nonpruritic, evanescent pink eruption with irregular but well-demarcated borders, located primarily on the trunk. Individual lesions appear and disappear rapidly over a period of a few hours. Like nodules, EM is seen only in patients with carditis.

53. What laboratory parameters are helpful in the diagnosis of ARF?

When ARF is suspected, a search for streptococcal antibodies is indicated. The most commonly used test is antistreptolysin O (ASO); a titer > 250 is considered abnormal. The high prevalence of such titers among the general population limits its value. Antideoxyribonucleotidase B (anti-DNAse B) is the test of choice; combined with ASO, sensitivity increases to 95%. Significant antibody titers to other streptococcal enzymes, including streptokinase, hyaluronidase, and diphosphopyridine dinucleotidase, are present in most of the remaining patients. A commercially available Latex agglutination test (Streptozyme), designed to study all of these antibodies in one reaction, is not recommended.

Acute phase reactants are uniformly abnormal in ARF except in cases of pure chorea. Both erythrocyte sedimentation rate (ESR) and C-reactive protein (CRP) are useful parameters of disease activity and minor criteria for diagnosis. ESR is often > 100 mm/hr (range: 46–155) and returns to normal over 12 weeks of treatment with antiinflammatory agents. ESR may be normal at the onset of chorea!

54. What is the differential diagnosis of ARF?

Reactive arthritis, gonococcal arthritis, adult or juvenile rheumatoid arthritis, adult-onset Still's disease, systemic lupus erythematosus, Takayasu's arteritis, Kawasaki's disease, primary antiphospholipid syndrome, subacute bacterial endocarditis, viral infections (coxsackie, parvovirus), and Lyme disease.

55. What is the standard treatment of ARF?

Bed rest and high doses of aspirin (50–100 mg/kg/day) or other nonsteroidal antiinflammatory drugs approved by the Food and Drug Administration for use in children. Duration of therapy is guided by the expected course of disease. Because 90% of cases resolve within 12 weeks, gradual reduction of antiinflammatory agents after 8 weeks is prudent. Symptoms and an increase in ESR will recur if the disease has not yet run its course.

In severe carditis, prednisone (1 mg/kg/day) is frequently used. No controlled studies demonstrate the superiority of prednisone over aspirin.

In chorea, haloperidol or other tranquilizers (particularly phenobarbital) are used. Both patient and family should be reassured that chorea does not lead to intellectual sequelae. Treatment should be maintained for the duration of the attack, usually < 2 months, and tapered slowly to avoid flare.

56. What is the difference between primary and secondary prevention in the treatment of ARF?

Primary prevention is the avoidance of disease by adequate treatment of streptococcal pharyngeal infection. Clinical features include febrile sore throat and dysphagia. Cough and rhinorrhea are not suggestive of streptococcal pharyngitis. A throat culture should be taken to confirm the diagnosis. The best treatment is "one-shot" intervention with a single intramuscular injection of benzathine penicillin—600,000 units in children, 1.2 million units in adults. Other schemes (10-day course of oral antibiotics) are effective but run the risk of noncompliance.

In patients who have already suffered ARF, **secondary prevention** should be instituted with a program of monthly (or every 3 weeks) injection of benzathine penicillin. The importance of a strongly founded diagnosis of ARF cannot be overstated, because the patient must submit to therapy for several years. The duration of secondary prevention is controversial. Some authors recommend life-long prevention if carditis has been severe. If not, the program can be stopped after the school years. Some authors suggest secondary prevention for 5 years after the last attack in patients younger than 18 years with rheumatic fever. Continuous prophylaxis is recommended to patients frequently exposed to streptococcal disease (e.g. school teachers).

57. When is recurrence of ARF most likely?

Recurrences of ARF are more likely in patients with carditis at onset, particularly those who develop rheumatic heart disease. Recurrences are more common during the first 2 years after the acute event. The tendency to suffer recurrences declines with time.

BIBLIOGRAPHY

1. Aho K, Leirisalo-Repo M, Repo H: Reactive arthritis. Clin Rheum Dis 11:25–39, 1985.
2. Amigo M-C, Martinez-Lavin M, Reyes PA: Acute rheumatic fever. Rheum Dis Clin North Am 19:333–350, 1993.
3. Bardin T, Enel C, Cornelis F, et al: Antibiotic treatment of venereal disease and Reiter's syndrome in a Greenland population. Arthritis Rheum 35:190–194, 1992.
4. Hoenig LJ: The arthritis of Christopher Columbus. Arch Intern Med 152:274–277, 1992.
5. Hughes RA, Keat AC: Reiter's syndrome and reactive arthritis: A current view. Semin Arthritis Rheum 24:190–210, 1994.
6. Kaye BR: Rheumatologic manifestations of infection with human immunodeficiency virus (HIV). Ann Intern Med 111:158–167, 1989.
7. Keat A: Reiter's syndrome and reactive arthritis in perspective. N Engl J Med 309:1606–1614, 1983.
8. Kvein TK, Glennas A, Melby K, et al: Reactive arthritis: Incidence, triggering agents, and clinical presentation. J Rheumatol 21:115–122, 1994.
9. Lauhio A, Leirisalo-Repo M, Lahdevirta J, et al: Double-blind, placebo-controlled study of three-month treatment with lymecycline in reactive arthritis, with special reference to *Chlamydia* arthritis. Arthritis Rheum 34:6–14, 1991.
10. Pope RM: Rheumatic fever in the 1990s. Bull Rheum Dis 38:1–8, 1989.
11. Silveira LH, Gutierrez F, Scopelitis E, et al: Chlamydia-induced reactive arthritis. Rheum Dis Clin North Am 19:351–362, 1993.
12. Stollerman GH, Markowitz M, Taranta A, et al: Jones criteria (revised) for guidance in the diagnosis of rheumatic fever. Circulation 32:664–668, 1965.
13. Wald ER: Acute rheumatic fever. Curr Probl Pediatr 23:264–270, 1993.

XI. Gastrointestinal Infections

40. INFECTIOUS HEPATITIS

Jason D. Maguire, M.D.

1. What are the infectious causes of hepatitis?

Viral	Bacterial	Parasitic	Fungal
Hepatitis A, B, C, D, E	Gram-negative sepsis	Schistosomiasis	Histoplasmosis
Epstein-Barr infection	Streptococcal pneumonia	Fascioliasis	Coccidioidomycosis
Cytomegalovirus	Brucellosis	Capillariasis	Candidiasis
infection	Legionellosis	Visceral larva migrans	
Herpes zoster	Plague		
Herpes simplex	Tularemia		
Yellow fever	Melioidosis		
Measles	Granuloma inguinale		
Rubeola	Listeriosis		
Rubella	Bartonellosis		
Coxsackie B infection	Leptospirosis		
Adenovirus infection	Syphilis		
	Query (or Q) fever		
	Tuberculosis		
	Leprosy		

Most cases of infectious hepatitis are due to hepatitis A, B, C, D, and E. Although other agents can be linked to elevations of liver-associated enzymes, they are not major causes of acute or chronic infectious hepatitis. With the exception of yellow fever and leptospirosis, they are rarely associated with jaundice. In addition, infection with hepatitis A, B, C, D, and E viruses usually is limited to the liver, whereas the other agents generally involve multiple organ systems. This chapter focuses on infections causes by hepatitis A, B, C, D, and E viruses.

2. How prevalent is viral hepatitis? Who is at risk?

Infection with **hepatitis A virus** (HAV) is underreported because of the high number of asymptomatic cases. Prevalence is high in underdeveloped and developing nations because of overcrowding and poor sanitary conditions. Cases occur primarily in children, whereas most cases in developed countries occur in adults who have traveled to endemic areas or have other risk factors such as male homosexuality and bisexuality, frequent shellfish ingestion, institutionalization, and child day care contact. Prevalence in the United States was as high as 70% in middle-class white Americans by serology at age 50 through the 1970s but has declined over the past 20 years. In temperate zones the incidence is highest in the fall and early winter, whereas in tropical climates cases are more frequent during the rainy season.

Worldwide estimates of infection with **hepatitis B virus** (HBV) range between 300–400 million people. Only 7% of the United States population is positive by serology at age 50. Prevalence based on blood donor screening is regional with rates < 0.1% in northern Europe, North America, and Australia; 5% in southern Europe, Mediterranean countries, and Central and South America; and > 20% in Africa, Asia, and the Pacific. HBV is endemic in closed institutions, such as prisons and mental institutions, and more prevalent in adults living in urban communities with poor socio-economic conditions. Intravenous drug users, male homosexuals and bisexuals, and adults with numerous sexual partners are also at high risk for infection. Once prevalent in frequent blood product recipients, such as dialysis patients and hemophiliacs, cases are declining in countries that test blood products for HBV. In the United States, chronic carrier rates are at 1% overall with higher rates in certain subpopulations (6% in male homosexuals and 7% in intravenous drug users).

The worldwide incidence of infection with **hepatitis C virus** (HCV) is unknown because of the high percentage of asymptomatic cases and limited availability of recently developed diagnostic tests. The incidence in the United States is estimated at 0.2–0.6% based on serologic screening. HCV infection is primarily a complication of blood product administration, accounting for more than 90% of all cases of transfusion-associated viral hepatitis in countries that now screen blood for HBV. With more recent testing of blood for HCV, rates continue to decline, leaving intravenous drug use as the primary parenteral route of transmission (one-third of all cases). Perinatal transmission and accidental needlestick infections are rare. Still, one-third to one-half of all cases are considered community-acquired with no known risk factors.

Because the **hepatitis D virus** (HDV) depends on HBV surface antigen to produce its structural protein shell, HDV infection occurs in similar settings. Worldwide prevalence is estimated at 15 million; endemic nonparenteral transmission has been documented in central Africa, the Middle East, Mediterranean countries, and southern Italy. Pockets of frequent epidemics are found in central Africa and the Amazon Basin. In North America and western Europe cases are more sporadic and associated with parenteral and sexual transmission; risk factors are similar to those for HBV infection. However, cases in male homosexuals and health care workers are extremely rare, and the number of cases in blood product recipients continues to decline because of screening for HBV.

Infection with **hepatitis E virus** (HEV) primarily occurs in young adults with highest rates in pregnant women. Although first described in India, outbreaks have occurred in Russia, Nepal, Myanmar (formerly Burma), the Middle East, Southeast Asia, Pakistan, China, central Africa, Peru, and Mexico. Only six imported cases have been reported in the United States from 1989–1992.

3. How is viral hepatitis transmitted?

HAV and **HEV** are transmitted by the fecal-oral route. HEV infection is more commonly due to fecal contamination of common source drinking water than ingestion of contaminated food. Although waterborne HAV outbreaks have been reported, they are uncommon in areas with piped and treated water. HEV infection is not prevalent in developed nations for the same reason. HAV is primarily transmitted by person-to-person contact, as in day care centers, closed institutions, and male homosexual and bisexual practices that may increase chances of fecal-oral contact. Foodborne HAV is generally due to contamination of food by infected food handlers who do not adequately wash their hands after defecation or by ingestion of inadequately cooked shellfish from polluted water sources. HAV is rarely transmitted by the parenteral route; parenteral transmission has not been described for HEV.

HBV has been isolated from blood, saliva, vaginal fluids, semen, colostrum, and breast milk with occasional reports from urine, bile, feces, sweat, and tears. Parenteral transmission by injection or contact with contaminated blood products remains the primary mode in the United States. Sexual and other intimate contact are also routes of infection. Worldwide, the primary mode of transmission is vertical (mother to child during childbirth) with transmission rates as high as 60% in China and Southeast Asia. The risk increases in mothers with a history of vertical transmission, development of acute infection from the second trimester through 2 months after delivery, and high surface antigen or e antigen levels in maternal blood during pregnancy. Surface antigen and e antigen are indirect markers of viral load and ongoing viral replication, respectively. In utero transmission is rare, and infection occurs by blood mixing between mother and child at the time of birth. In the United States, HBV is predominantly transmitted through contact with contaminated blood during surgical and dental procedures and use of contaminated instruments for immunization, unlawful intravenous drug use, tattooing, body piercing, acupuncture, and shaving. In the tropics, transmission also has been associated with scarification, blood letting, ritual circumcision, and repeated bloodsucking arthropod bites in endemic areas. Intrafamilial transmission also has been well documented in the absence of sexual or vertical transmission; saliva is the speculated culprit.

HCV and **HDV** infections follow similar parenteral transmission modes to HBV. Although the incidence of HCV infection appears to be higher in male homosexuals, adults with multiple sexual partners, and sexual partners of HCV-infected patients, sexual transmission does not appear to be as efficient as with HBV. Studies have demonstrated antibodies to HCV in 0–35% of the sexual partners of HCV-infected patients. In addition, vertical transmission of HCV is relatively uncommon unless the mother has coinfection with HIV. Intrafamilial spread of HCV occurs by unknown mechanisms at rates of 5–7%.

4. What are the incubation periods for viral hepatitis?

HAV: 3–5 wk	HCV: 6–7 wk	HEV: 2–8 wk
HBV: 8–24 wk	HDV: unknown	

5. How do patients with acute infectious viral hepatitis present?

Acute hepatitis is clinically similar for all five viral agents. Patients with clinically apparent HAV infection generally note a 3–10-day preicteric phase marked by nonspecific symptoms such as fever, chills, anorexia, headache, malaise, arthralgias and myalgias, nausea and vomiting, and achy right upper quadrant abdominal discomfort. A small percentage of patients also may have a virus–antibody immune complex-mediated rash and a migratory polyarticular arthritis that resolves with the onset of jaundice. This presentation is more common with acute HBV infection (10–20%) than with HAV infection. Fever generally resolves with onset of the icteric phase, which is marked by darkened urine, clay-colored stool, and jaundice with pruritus. Patients often note rapid improvement in symptoms with the onset of jaundice, which persists for 2 weeks. When symptomatic, children usually exhibit mild or absent preicteric symptoms and a shorter icteric phase. Clinically apparent icteric HAV infection accounts for only 20–50% of all HAV cases. HBV and HCV infection present similarly to HAV infection but generally have a more insidious onset. The percentage of clinically inapparent HBV and HCV cases is even higher than reported for HAV infection, and most cases of HCV remain undiagnosed until unexplained liver-associated enzyme abnormalities on routine blood work are investigated. Less than 30% of all HCV cases present with symptoms, and less than 50% have jaundice. Because HDV replication relies on HBV helper function, HDV infection generally occurs in the setting of either acute coinfection with HBV or, more commonly, superinfection in previously asymptomatic HBV carriers. HEV typically causes an acute, self-limited illness with complete recovery. Only 25% of patients are icteric.

6. Do all patients recover after an episode of acute viral hepatitis?

The overall mortality rate for acute icteric viral hepatitis is 1%, but it is higher in the elderly and may vary with the agent.

Viral agent	Overall mortality
HAV	< 0.1%
HBV	0.1%
HCV	Rare
HDV	2–20%
HEV	< 1%

Mortality is generally associated with the development of fulminant hepatitis marked by acute liver failure and encephalopathy. Fulminant hepatitis usually occurs within 8 weeks of onset of jaundice but may occur as late as 12 weeks. Because of high worldwide prevalence, HBV accounts for a large portion of cases of fulminant hepatitis (30–60%); 30–40% of patients with fulminant HBV have concomitant HDV infection. HDV mortality rates are higher in the setting of superinfection of a chronic HBV carrier with underlying liver damage. In most cases of HBV and HDV coinfection, mortality rates are less than 5% because the majority of patients clear the HBV infection, making HDV replication impossible. Although overall mortality rates for HEV infection are low, they may be as high as 10–20% in pregnant women, particularly in the third trimester. Patients who survive acute HAV and HEV infection make complete recoveries, whereas patients with acute HBV, HDV, and HCV infection may develop persistent infection that results in chronic liver damage.

7. How are patients with acute viral hepatitis managed?

No specific therapies are available, and care is primarily supportive with goals of symptom relief, minimization of liver damage, and early transplant referral in fulminant cases. Hospitalization is usually required only when oral hydration is not feasible or when early liver failure is suspected based on prolonged prothrombin time. Alcohol avoidance, rest, low fat diet, and avoidance of potentially hepatotoxic mediations are advocated. Alpha interferon has not been efficacious in trials involving acute HBV infection. Beta interferon reduces the incidence of chronic infection when administered to patients with acute HCV infection, but data are limited to a small number of patients.

8. Corticosteroids have been helpful in the treatment of acute alcoholic hepatitis. What is their role in acute viral hepatitis?

In general, they should not be used and have not been shown to shorten the course of illness or to reduce the risk of development of fulminant hepatitis. Conversely, they have been documented to prolong illness, increase relapse, and increase the incidence of the chronic carrier state for HBV. Corticosteroids, however, may be used in cases of HAV infection complicated by prolonged intrahepatic cholestasis to quicken resolution of jaundice and its associated symptoms.

9. Since clinical manifestations are similar for all five agents, how are they distinguished for diagnosis?

HAV. Although virus can be demonstrated in the feces by enzyme immunoassay, radioimmunoassay, and electronmicroscopy, these methods of diagnosis are not commonly used because viral shredding rapidly declines with the onset of jaundice—the stage at which most patients present. Anti-HAV IgM is usually present in the serum at the time of clinical presentation, peaking at 4 weeks and waning by 4–5 months. Presence of IgM in a patient's serum is diagnostic of acute infection. IgG is often detectable at the time of presentation and persists in the serum indefinitely. Consequently, IgG is not helpful in diagnosing acute infection and in the absence of IgM may reflect only past infection.

HBV. HBV surface antigen persists during the acute phase and chronic carrier states but clears with convalescence. HBV e antigen usually wanes soon after clinically apparent infection in uncomplicated cases but may persist indefinitely in the chronic carrier state as a marker of active viral replication. HBV e antigen antibody usually appears with onset of symptoms and disappears by 6 months in uncomplicated cases but may remain detectable in the chronic carrier state. HBV core antibody IgM wanes after a few months; IgG persists indefinitely. HBV core antibody IgG is therefore the most reliable marker of present or past infection and serves as an excellent screening test for HBV exposure. In uncomplicated cases, HBV surface antibody appears late in convalescence and usually persists indefinitely but sometimes wanes to undetectable

Time to Appearance in Patient's Serum of Markers of HBV Infection

	TIME IN WEEKS									
	12*	10	8	6	4	2	0†	2	4	6 → 20
HBV surface antigen			xxxxxxxxxxxxxxxxxxxx							
HBV e antigen			xxxxx							
HBV core antibody				xxxxxxxxxxxxxxxxxxx						
HBV e antigen antibody							xxxxxxxxxxxxxxx			
HBV surface antibody										xxx

* Exposure to virus.
† Onset of chemical hepatitis or jaundice

levels. Surface antibody is not detectable in patients who progress to the chronic carrier state. Presence of surface antigen and core antibody IgG and absence of surface antibody are the most common serologic pattern observed in the serum of chronic carriers.

HCV. Screening with enzyme-linked immunosorbent assay (ELISA) to detect anti-HCV antibodies unfortunately has a low specificity (high false-positive rate). Polymerase chain reaction (PCR) techniques for detection of viral RNA are highly sensitive and specific but may not be available in all clinical settings. Second-generation enzyme immunoassays (EIAs) are more sensitive and specific than the first-generation ELISAs. Because recombinant immunoblot assays (RIBA) are more specific than current ELISAs, they are are recommended to confirm diagnosis of HCV infection in patients with positive ELISA. False-positive HCV ELISA results may be seen in autoimmune hepatitis, primary biliary cirrhosis, and hypergammaglobulinemia. False-negative HCV ELISA results may be due to a 3-month delay in antibody production by infected hosts. Suspected cases should be retested at 3 and 6 months.

HDV. Delta antigen appears early in infection, then disappears. Anti-delta antigen antibodies in acute infection may be delayed, short-lived, or present in extremely low titers. Significantly elevated titers are usually a marker of chronic HDV infection.

HEV. Antibodies to HEV develop early in the course of infection and are easily measured with an enzyme immunoassay using antigen derived from a recombinant DNA system. With a specificity of 100%, a positive test confirms diagnosis.

10. Should all markers be ordered for all patients with suspected viral hepatitis?

No. A good starting point includes anti-HAV IgM, HBV surface antigen, HBV core antibody IgM, and HCV ELISA. Diagnosis may be established with these four tests. A positive HAV IgM establishes the diagnosis of acute HAV infection. Because HBV surface antigen can be present in both acute infection and the chronic carrier state, a positive HBV core antibody IgM confirms acute infection, whereas a negative IgM suggests either an exacerbation of chronic HBV or superinfection with HDV. Evaluation for HDV should be limited to patients with HBV surface antigen and demographics placing them at risk for HDV infection. HEV serology should be obtained only for patients with reasonable exposure histories.

11. What is chronic viral hepatitis?

This term generally refers to viral hepatitis lasting more than 6 months and is limited to a small number of patients with HBV infection, patients with HDV infection in the face of chronic HBV infection, and a high proportion of patients with HCV infection. Most patients are either asymptomatic or mildly symptomatic, but reactivation may result in fulminant hepatitis. **Chronic carrier state** is a term used primarily for patients with chronically detectable HBV surface antigen in the blood, which may or may not be associated with histologic hepatitis. Chronic hepatitis due to any of these three agents is frequently categorized based on pathologic changes in the liver. In **chronic persistent hepatitis**, inflammatory changes and fibrosis are confined primarily to the portal areas. When these changes extend into the surrounding lobules, the term **chronic active hepatitis** is used and indicates more aggressive hepatitis with a poorer prognosis. The spectrum of damage varies from patient to patient.

12. How often does chronic viral hepatitis occur, how is it diagnosed, and what are the long-term effects?

The chronic carrier state of HBV infection is more common in males and more likely when acute infection is asymptomatic, particularly when acquired in childhood. Although only 5–10% of infected adults develop the chronic carrier state, 20–50% of infected infants and children become chronic carriers. Diagnosis is usually confirmed when surface antigen is present in the serum for more than 6 months. Although the combined presence of abnormal liver-associated enzymes and HBV surface antigenemia is suggestive, definitive diagnosis usually requires biopsy to eliminate other possible causes; not all chronic HBV carriers develop chronic hepatitis. HBV infection remains the most prevalent cause of cirrhosis worldwide, affecting an estimated 5%. Chronic HDV infection occurs in < 5% of cases when coinfecting with HBV because most cases of HBV infection do not proceed to the chronic carrier state. However, when HDV superinfection occurs, the incidence of chronicity is 50%. Chronic HDV infection is more aggressive than either HBV or HCV alone; > 70% of patients develop cirrhosis within 10 years. HCV more than any other cause of viral hepatitis has a propensity for chronicity; 40–50% of all infected patients suffer chronic liver damage.

13. What are the complications of chronic viral hepatitis other than cirrhosis?

Both chronic HBV and HCV infections are strongly correlated with development of hepatocellular carcinoma. The prevalence is higher in male patients and patients with macronodular cirrhosis.

14. What treatments are available for chronic viral hepatitis?

Of all agents studied, alpha interferon is the most promising. Most studies with HBV have shown response rates of 25–50% with long-term remission rates of 20–30%. The primary measures of effectiveness are reduction or normalization of liver-associated enzyme levels in the blood, histologic improvement on liver biopsy, and reduction or loss of markers of viral replications (surface antigen and e antigen). Response rates for patients with HCV are measured similarly, except viral replication is monitored by PCR detection of HCV RNA. Response rates have been around 45% with 18-month regimens and 30% with 6-month regimens. Remission rates 6 months after treatment range between 10 and 25%, indicating that treatment is less effective for HCV than HBV. Current recommended regimens are 5 million units subcutaneously each day for 4 months in HBV-infected patients and 3 million units subcutaneously 3 times/week for 12–18 months in HCV-infected patients.

15. Response rates seem rather low. Are all patients treated with interferon?

No. Because the correlation between symptoms and severity of disease is weak, the decision to treat is usually based on the severity of liver-associated enzyme abnormalities and liver histology. Patient willingness to undergo liver biopsy as well as a risk-benefit assessment must be taken into account. Factors include the patient's ability to self-administer medication, comply with the regimen, comprehend the implications of both disease and treatment, and tolerate prolonged therapy that may have severe debilitating side effects, including headache, fever, myalgias, arthralgias, malaise, neutropenia, and thrombocytopenia.

16. Should patients with chronic viral hepatitis be screened for hepatocellular carcinoma?

Studies of patients with chronic HBV and HCV infection suggest that 5–8% have hepatocellular carcinoma at the time of initial presentation with an additional 5% developing carcinoma over a 10-year period. Patients with severe chronic active hepatitis and/or cirrhosis have a higher incidence of carcinoma. Liver biopsy of all patients with chronic viral hepatitis may be indicated to establish risk for development of carcinoma. Most experts currently recommend screening in select high-risk patients with ultrasound and serum alpha-fetoprotein every 3 months.

17. When is a liver biopsy indicated?

Although not typically helpful in acute hepatitis, liver biopsy may be helpful in the evaluation of chronic hepatitis under certain circumstances:
- To eliminate other diagnoses, such as Wilson's disease or hemochromatosis
- To clarify diagnosis when more than one cause is in contest
- To direct and monitor alpha interferon treatment
- To establish risk for development of carcinoma and need for screening

18. How should occupational exposure to possible HBV and HCV be managed in health care workers?

Occupational exposures include contact of the eyes, mouth, or other mucous membranes, broken skin, or blood (by needlestick or laceration) with blood or other potentially infected material. The risk of HBV transmission after a needlestick injury appears to correlate with the presence or absence of e antigen in the contact source; infection rates range from 2% with e antigen-negative sources to 40% with e antigen-containing sources. The risk through other exposures, such as mucous membrane or broken skin, has not been quantified but is minimal. Optimally, both the patient source and exposed worker should be tested for the presence of HBV surface antigen and antibody as well as HIV antibody. If the source is surface antigen-negative, the risk of HBV transmission is zero.

Even previously vaccinated exposed people should be tested for the presence of surface antibody because titers may be at unprotective levels or may have waned. When exposure has occurred, as measured by the presence of surface antigen in the source's blood, the exposed person need not be treated if he or she has surface antibody titers ≥ 10 International Units (IU)/ml. Previously vaccinated exposed persons with unknown titers or titers < 10 IU/ml should be administered a booster dose. In addition, HBV hyperimmune globulin should be administered if the person has not had a documented response to prior vaccination by titer > 10 IU/ml. Hyperimmune globulin should also be administered along with the primary vaccination series in exposed persons not previously vaccinated. Prior nonresponders are not revaccinated but should be given a second dose of hyperimmune globulin 1 month later. The exposed person should be followed with repeat serologic studies over time but not before 6 months if he or she has received HBV hyperimmune globulin, which interferes with the ability to detect true response to active immunization.

The risks for occupational exposure to HCV are not well established, but with needlestick injuries transmission ranges between 3–10%. Immune globin prophylaxis has not proved efficacious, nor has prophylactic alpha interferon therapy. Once HCV has been documented in the source, the exposed person should be followed with HCV ELISA testing at the time of exposure and again in 6–9 months to guide management if infection has occurred.

19. How can we prevent and control the spread of infection?

The primary mode is by avoidance of the risk factors previously described for all agents, especially improvement of community sanitation conditions to minimize the spread of HAV and HEV.

20. Can medical therapies help to reduce the transmission of HAV?

Yes. Because viral shedding occurs late in incubation and during early prodrome with rapid decline at the onset of jaundice when most patients present for care, strict isolation at this point is generally ineffectual. Most close contacts have already been exposed. Within 14 days of exposure, close contacts and family members of active cases can be passively immunized with intramuscular human immune globin. This may not prevent infection but frequently attenuates symptoms and often prevents development of clinical disease. The dosage is 2 IU/kg body weight and is doubled for pregnant contacts and patients with underlying liver disease. Passive immunization is also offered to travelers of all ages to HAV endemic regions and affords protection from 3 months at 2 IU/kg to 6 months at 6 IU/kg.

Since 1995, immune globin has been in short supply and remains difficult to obtain for prophylaxis in travelers. Fortunately, with the recent approval by the Food and Drug Administration of two inactivated HAV vaccines that provide long-term protection, the need for immune globin is declining except in cases of contact exposures. In addition to travelers, vaccination is now recommended for children over the age of 2 years in high-prevalence communities, homosexual and bisexual men, intravenous drug users, day care and institution workers, food handlers, and sewage workers. Highly effective when administered 2 weeks before expected exposure, a booster is recommended at 6 months to confer long-term immunity. Five-year efficacy is documented, and evaluation for more prolonged immunity continues. When given concomitantly with other vaccines, HAV vaccine remains safe as well as immunogenic. Safety in pregnancy has not been fully evaluated, but the use of immune globin should still be considered in pregnant women traveling to HAV endemic areas.

21. Should providers be concerned about the transmission of HCV with administration of intramuscular immune globin?

No. Previously reported cases of HCV infection associated with immune globin resulted from intravenous preparations. HCV has not been linked to intramuscular preparations, which are tested for syphilis, HBV surface antigen, HCV antibody, and HIV antibody.

22. Can immunizations be given for any of the other agents of viral hepatitis?

Unfortunately, no vaccines or effective immune serum preparations are available for the prevention of HCV, HDV, or HEV. As previously mentioned, HBV preparations are available. Passive immunization with HBV hyperimmune globulin (HBIG) prepared from pooled plasma with high titers of HBV surface antibody is also recommended at doses of 200–500 IU in conjunction with active immunization for regular sexual contacts of patients with acute HBV infection and infants born to infected mothers. For single exposures, administration optimally should occur within 48 hours of exposure. For perinatal prevention, HBIG should be given within 12 hours of birth at the same time as the first dose of HBV vaccine; it has 90% efficacy in preventing mother-to-child transmission. Active immunization with either of the two available recombinant viral antigen preparations is recommended for hemodialysis patients, spouses and sexual contacts of active HBV cases, health care providers of high-risk patients, lab workers, dentists and ancillary staff involved in direct patient care, and high-risk community members. The most recent vaccine recommendations from the Centers for Disease Control and Prevention include all newborns and all unvaccinated children under the age of 11 who are considered at high risk (Alaskans, Pacific Islanders, and children of first-generation immigrants from countries where HBV has intermediate-to-high endemicity). Both vaccines are given at 0, 1, and 6 months. Postvaccination antibody testing is not generally recommended but should be considered in persons whose management depends on knowing their titer. Examples include health care providers at risk for occupational exposure, dialysis patients, and infants of HBV surface antigen-positive mothers. Immunization is safe during pregnancy and compatible with other concomitantly administered vaccines.

23. Are hepatitis A, B, C, D, and E the only viral causes of significant viral hepatitis?

No. A recent review of patients in Saudi Arabia with acute infectious hepatitis failed to demonstrate hepatitis A, B, C, D, or E as the causative agent in 13% of patients presenting with the classic viral hepatitis syndrome. The proposed sixth agent was implicated in patients from the Middle East, Sub-Saharan Africa, and the Indian subcontinent but was most prevalent in people traveling in the Far East. Studies to identify this agent are ongoing.

BIBLIOGRAPHY

1. Curely SA, Izzo F, et al: Identification and screening of 416 patients with chronic hepatitis at high risk to develop hepatocellular carcinoma. Ann Surg 222:375–383, 1995.
2. Gerberding JL: Management of occupational exposures to blood-borne viruses. N Engl J Med 332:444–451, 1995.
3. Ghabrah TM, Strickland GT, et al: Acute viral hepatitis in Saudi Arabia: Seroepidemiological analysis, risk factors, clinical manifestations, and evidence for a sixth hepatitis agent. Clin Infect Dis 21:621–627, 1995.
4. Goodman RA: Licensure of inactivated hepatitis A vaccine and recommendations for use among international travelers. MMWR 44:559–560, 1995.
5. Goodman RA: Update: Recommendations to prevent hepatitis B virus transmission—United States. MMWR 44:574–575, 1995.
6. Goodman RA: Prevention of perinatal hepatitis B through enhanced case management—Connecticut, 1994–1995, and United States, 1994. MMWR 45:584–587, 1996.
7. Iwarson S, Norkrans G, Wejestal R: Hepatitis C: Natural history of a unique infection. Clin Infect Dis 20:1361–1370, 1995.
8. Omata M, Yokosuku O, et al: Resolution of acute hepatitis C after therapy with natural beta interferon. Lancet 338:914–915, 1991.
9. Poynard T, Bedossa P, et al: A comparison of three interferon alfa-2b regimens for the long-term treatment of chronic non-A, non-B hepatitis. N Engl J Med 332:1457–1462, 1995.
10. Purdy MA, Krawczynski K: Hepatitis E. Gastroenterol Clin North Am 23:537–546, 1994.
11. Tong MJ, Neveen SE, et al: Clinical outcomes after transfusion-associated hepatitis C. N Engl J Med 332:1463–1466, 1995.
12. Thompson RF: Travel and Routine Immunizations: A Practical Guide for the Medical Office. Milwaukee, Shoreland Medical Marketing, 1996.
13. Unoura M, Kaneko S, et al: High-risk groups and screening strategies for early detection of hepatocellular carcinoma in patients with chronic liver disease. Hepatogastroenterology 40:305–310, 1993.

41. FOOD POISONING

Sammi Dali, M.D., and Donald R. Skillman, M.D., FACP

1. How common is food poisoning?

Food poisoning is a major and frequently underestimated cause of morbidity in the United States. On average, 18,335 cases are reported to the Centers for Disease Control and Prevention annually. When unreported cases and unidentified agents are included, it is estimated that there are about 12.6 million cases/year, with a possible cost of $8.4 billion annually.

2. How is food poisoning classified?

Food poisoning can be classified according to the predominant symptoms produced:
- Nausea and vomiting
- Noninflammatory diarrhea
- Inflammatory diarrhea
- Neurologic symptoms
- Systemic or miscellaneous symptoms

3. How important is *Staphylococcus aureus* as a cause of food poisoning in the United States? What are the signs and symptoms?

S. aureus is the third most common food poisoning agent, with an average of 600 cases per year. Symptoms are self-limited; therefore, the true incidence is likely much higher. Nausea, vomiting, and abdominal pain are followed by diarrhea beginning 1–6 hours after ingestion. Fever is rare. The toxins responsible for this syndrome are staphylococcal enterotoxins A through E, with A implicated in 55% of cases. These enterotoxins are heat-stable and cause a net increase in the secretion of water and electrolytes from the intestinal wall. Vomiting is caused by stimulation of enteric autonomic sensory neurons.

4. What food poisoning syndrome is related to *Bacillus cereus*?

B. cereus causes an acute emetic syndrome 1–6 hours after ingestion of contaminated food. The syndrome begins as nausea, vomiting, and abdominal pain and resolves in approximately 10 hours. Poisoning is related to heat stable toxins present in fried rice, usually prepared in Chinese restaurants and take-out establishments. The food often has been inadequately refrigerated and is heavily contaminated with the bacteria.

5. How important is *Clostridium perfringens* food poisoning in the United States? How is it diagnosed?

C. perfringens ranks fourth as a cause of documented food-borne disease in the United States. It produces two types of food poisoning syndromes:

Type A poisoning usually causes a 24-hour illness and is seen mainly in Western countries. Delay between cooking and serving meat and poultry products is the usual culprit. Given the right environment, the delay allows *C. perfringens* spores to germinate and multiply. Food must be heavily contaminated for the symptoms of poisoning to manifest. Clinical signs and symptoms are characterized by watery diarrhea and epigastric pain, beginning 24 hours after ingestion. Symptoms usually resolve in 12–24 hours. Fever is uncommon. Diagnosis is confirmed by identifying more than 10^5 organisms/gm of the suspected food, by finding a spore count of more than 10^6/gm in the patient's stool, or by isolating organisms of the same serotype from the stool and suspected food.

Type B poisoning is described later in question 6.

6. What is Pig Bel syndrome?

The Pig Bel syndrome, more officiously known as enteritis necroticans syndrome, was initially observed after World War II in malnourished refugees in Germany and Norway. The disease is caused by consumption of B toxins produced by *C. perfringens* type C in undercooked pork. In a healthy person, the toxin is inactivated by intestinal proteases such as trypsin. However, when patients are either protein-malnourished or ingest protease inhibitors simultaneously with food, the toxin can cause coagulative transmural necrosis of the intestinal wall. The toxin effect may result in perforation, sepsis, and death. The mortality rate is 40%. Pig Bel syndrome may be the most common cause of death among children between age 6–10 years in the highlands of New Guinea. The syndrome persists due to the ritual pig feasting accompanied by the consumption of sweet potatoes, which contain a naturally occurring trypsin inhibitor.

7. What is the leading cause of food poisoning in the United States?

Nontyphoidal salmonellosis is the leading cause. Transmitted via contaminated poultry, eggs, beef, and pork, the syndrome is characterized by nausea, vomiting, and crampy abdominal pain with tenderness, fever, chills, and diarrhea. The patient's stool exam shows a moderate number of white and red blood cells. Blood cultures may be positive in 5–10% of cases and much more frequently in HIV-infected patients.

The treatment in uncomplicated nontyphoidal salmonella is supportive care. Maintenance of intravascular volume is the primary objective. Use of antibiotics is not recommended because of increasing antibiotic resistance and prolongation of *Salmonella* shedding in the stool. However, in neonates, elderly people, people with sickle cell anemia, and immunosuppressed patients, antimicrobial agents should be used without hesitation. In patients without such risk factors, it is preferable to withhold antibiotics if the person appears clinically well.

8. What are risk factors for salmonellosis food poisoning?
- Age under 5 years
- Diminished gastrointestinal motility
- Altered intestinal flora
- Achlorhydria, gastrectomy
- Antacid use
- HIV infection
- Lymphoproliferative disease
- Diabetes mellitus

9. How are botulism and tetanus related?

Botulism and tetanus result from protein neurotoxins generated by two related species of *Clostridium*. The toxins are similar in structure and function but differ markedly in their clinical presentation because they affect different cells in the nervous system. Botulinum neurotoxins affect primarily the peripheral neuromuscular junction and autonomic synapses, with manifestations of weakness. Tetanus toxin can affect the same system, but its manifestations relate to its tropism for inhibitory cells of the central nervous system, with the principal effects of rigidity and spasm.

10. How do you get botulism from food? If you get it, will it kill you?

Food-borne botulism is typically recognized in outbreaks, but some cases are sporadic. Home-canned vegetables, fruits, and fish products are the most common sources. In Alaskans, food preparation involving fish fermentation commonly causes botulism. In China, homemade fermented beans are the leading cause. The pH of the implicated product is usually less than 4.6.

The CDC received reports of 124 cases of food-borne botulism from 1976–1984. The mean number of patients involved in the outbreaks was 2.7. Single cases or small outbreaks were usually related to home-prepared foods. Large outbreaks associated with restaurants accounted for 40% of cases.

Before the advent of critical care units that offer needed respiratory support the case-fatality rate was > 60%. In the early 1970s it was 23%. For 1976–1984, the case-fatality rate fell further to 7.5%. For persons > 60 years old the rate remained high at 30%. Notably the first, or only, case in an outbreak has a 25% risk of death. Subsequent cases, which are diagnosed and treated more quickly, have only a 4% risk of death.

11. How do the toxins of botulism work?

Botulinum toxin consists of a family of seven immunologically distinct molecules. It is among the most potent toxins known with a type A toxin lethal dose of about 1 ng/kg. The toxin prevents the release of acetylcholine at the motor neuron end-plate in neuromuscular junctions, causing weakness and eventually flaccid paralysis if the disease is not recognized and treated.

12. How does one recognize, diagnose, and treat *Clostridium botulinum* food poisoning?

Botulism usually begins at 18–24 hours after ingestion of contaminated food with weakness that frequently intensifies over days or weeks. The presentation is symmetric, descending paralysis with minimal sensory or CNS involvement. Other symptoms often include blurred vision, photophobia, dysphagia, nausea, vomiting, and dysphonia. The differential diagnosis includes Guillain-Barré syndrome, myasthenia gravis (Eaton-Lambert disease), stroke, chemical poisoning, drug reaction, or poliomyelitis. Electromyography is helpful in distinguishing Guillain-Barré syndrome and Eaton-Lambert disease from botulism.

Diagnosis within the first three days of infection is made by identifying the toxin in the patient's stool, serum, or incriminated food. After three days the most sensitive test for *C. botulinum* is a stool culture.

Treatment consists of trivalent antitoxin types A, B, and E to prevent further paralysis. Recovery is gradual over weeks to months.

13. If you eat two salamanders and three colored frogs, why will you probably die?

Most likely because you would eat them if you are lost and starving in the middle of the Amazon jungle and are insane with cerebral malaria. Secondly, people sometimes die during this type of fraternity hazing ritual. Lastly, some of these slimy little critters carry tetrodotoxin, the most lethal seafood toxin known. There are 20 deaths yearly throughout the world via the ingestion of tetrodotoxin in puffer fish liver and roe. Salamanders and colored frogs are carriers of the toxin as well—a fact well known to the indigenous Amazon peoples. Clinical manifestations may begin immediately or several hours after ingestion, including nausea, vomiting, diarrhea, headache, itching and burning of the skin, facial paresthesia, weakness, areflexia, ataxia, convulsions, and respiratory failure.

14. How does the toxin in puffer fish, salamanders, and colored frogs work?

Tetrodotoxin is a heat-stable protein that inhibits nerve conduction through blockade of the neural sodium channels. It is used by Indians in Central and South America as poison for arrows and darts.

15. What is the most common seafood toxin and what are its signs and symptoms?

Ciguatoxin or ciguatera is the most common seafood toxin. It is produced by the dinoflagellate *Gambierdiscus toxicus*. Over 400 species of fish have shown toxicities after ingesting these critters. Because the taste and appearance of poisoned fish are unchanged, identification is nearly impossible. Distribution ranges from Hawaii to Florida. Vomiting and diarrhea begin in the first 8 hours. Headache, myalgia, weakness, reflex loss, perioral dysesthesias, and pruritus occur from 10–24 hours after ingestion. These symptoms evolve into paradoxical sensory disturbances; for example, hot things feel cold. Death is rare.

16. How does ciguatoxin work? What is the recommended treatment?

Ciguatoxin activates the voltage-dependent sodium channels in nerves and muscles. Sodium channels open but do not close. Spontaneous depolarizations occur at resting membrane potential, resulting in an increase in intracellular sodium ions and water. Treatment with mannitol is of some benefit, probably because of its antiedema properties. Mannitol leads to a response in symptomatic patients, resulting in the termination of the illness in 2 days rather than in 1 week with no treatment.

17. What is the second most common cause of seafood poisoning in the United States?

Scombroid fish poisoning ranks second in the United States. This toxin is related to reef fish, including tuna, mackerel, and skipjack. Typical symptoms resemble histamine-like reactions with flushing, pruritus, headache, urticaria, GI hyperactivity and, rarely, bronchospasm. Scombroid poisoning is unlike other illnesses caused by bacterial toxin production. Poorly refrigerated fish undergo bacterial degradation that results in the decarboxylation of histidine to histamine.

18. How do you diagnose and treat scombroid fish poisoning?

Persons consuming contaminated fish experience a bitter or peppery taste with symptoms limited from 3–6 hours after ingestion. Diagnosis is by demonstration of histamine levels greater than 100 mg/gm of fish. The poisoning is treated with H1- and H2-receptor antagonists.

19. Name two complications of the ingestion of foods contaminated with *Escherichia coli* O157:H7.

• Hemolytic uremic syndrome
• Thrombotic thrombocytopenic purpura

20. You didn't think I would end without giving you a table that you can cut out and stick in the back of your "Sanford," did you?

Food Poison	Incubation	Duration	Toxins	Fever	Source
Scombroid	Directly after ingestion	3–6 hr	Histamine-like reaction	Rare	Tuna, mackerel, skipjack
Ciguatoxin	5 min to 30 hr	8.5 days	Open neural sodium channels		Toxin accumulates in tissues of various fish
Tetrodotoxin	Minutes to hours	Not long	Heat-stable; block neural sodium channels		Roe and liver of puffer fish, viscera and skin of salamander and colored frogs
Staphyloccus aureus	1–6 hr	< 24 hr	Enterotoxins	Rare	Food rich in salt, sugar, proteins
Bacillus cereus	1–6 hr	< 24 hr	Heat-stable preformed enterotoxin	Rare	Fried rice from Chinese restaurant
Clostridium perfringens	6–24 hr	24 hr	Heat-labile enterotoxins	Rare	Meat and poultry
Nontyphoidal *Salmonella* spp.	6–48 hr	< 7 days	Enterotoxins that increase cAMP	Yes	Water, contaminated food, poultry, eggs, fish, pork, cheese, vegetables
Clostridium botulinum	12–36 hr	Weeks to months	A through G; inhibit acetylcholine release	Rare	Poorly stored food

cAMP = cyclic adenosine monophosphate.

Note: Other infectious agents such as Norwalk virus, hepatitis A, *Giardia* spp., *Shigella* spp., *Campylobacter* spp., *Vibrio* spp., *Yersinia* sp., *Listeria* sp., and *E. coli* O157:H7 can also be transmitted via food ingestion and present as gastrointestinal problems in outbreaks.

BIBLIOGRAPHY

1. Bishai WR, Sears CL: Food poisoning syndromes. Gastroenterol Clin North Am 22:579–608, 1993.
2. Swift AE, Swift TR: Ciguatera. Clin Toxicol 31(1):1–29, 1993.
3. Watters MR: Organic neurotoxins in seafoods. Clin Neurol Neurosurg 97:119–124, 1995.

42. INFECTIOUS DIARRHEA

James E. Egan, M.D.

1. What is diarrhea?

There is no universal consensus on how to define diarrhea. A clinically useful definition is the passage of three or more loosely formed bowel movements during any 24-hour period. Admittedly, such a definition requires a patient who is an accurate reporter. Other definitions based on 24-hour measurements of stool weight or stool water may be more objective, but such measurements are difficult to obtain and rarely available in the acute setting.

2. What mechanisms of diarrhea are relevant to infections?

The mechanisms of diarrhea can be divided into four large categories: osmotic, secretory, motility-related, and inflammatory. Only two of these, secretory and inflammatory, are involved in infectious diarrhea. **Secretory diarrhea** caused by infectious agents is toxin-mediated and does not involve disruption of the mucosa. *Vibrio cholerae* is the usual prototype for toxigenic diarrhea. This organism adheres to the cells in the upper small intestine and elaborates a toxin that results in loss of intestinal fluid without causing structural damage. **Inflammatory diarrhea** caused by infectious agents involves mucosal invasion as the initial event. *Shigella* species are often considered the prototype for this type of diarrhea.

3. Why should we be concerned with infectious diarrhea?

Infectious diarrhea makes a large contribution to childhood (especially infant and toddler) mortality in the developing world. The publicity associated with outbreaks of *Escherichia coli* O157:H7 from fast-food restaurants in the United States in the past few years reminds us of the universality and potential seriousness of infectious diarrhea. It is estimated that there are over 80 million foodborne illnesses each year in the United States. About 25 million are believed to represent enteric infections that account for over 10,000 deaths. The direct and indirect costs of infectious diarrhea are estimated to be $23 billion per year in the United States alone.

4. How often do bacterial pathogens cause diarrhea?

Bacteria are identified as the cause of infectious diarrhea in 8–15% of cases in the developed world. The most frequently isolated organisms are *Campylobacter* spp., *Salmonella* spp., *E. coli*, and *Shigella* spp. Other bacteria less commonly found as the cause of diarrhea are *Bacillus* spp., *Clostridium* spp., staphylococci, *Vibrio* spp., and *Yersinia* spp.

5. What are fecal leukocytes? How do we use them?

Fecal leukocytes can be found in fecal smears. By convention fecal leukocytes are considered to indicate polymorphonuclear cells (PMNs), although mononuclear cells have been reported with typhoid fever, *Yersinia* spp., and amebiasis. Fecal leukocytes indicate intestinal (usually colonic) inflammation and can be used as a clue in the initial differential diagnosis of diarrheal illness. The presence of fecal leukocytes indicates an inflammatory diarrhea and suggests a certain group of organisms. The absence of fecal leukocytes indicates a noninflammatory or secretory diarrhea and suggests another group of organisms.

6. How are stool specimens tested for fecal leukocytes?

A smear of stool material is placed on a glass slide and diluted with a small volume of saline to create a suspension through which newspaper print can easily be read. A few drops of methylene blue are added to this suspension to stain the leukocytes, and a coverslip is placed over the suspension. After 3–5 minutes the slide is inspected with high-power microscopy (400 × magnification).

If three or more PMNs per high-power field (HPF) are seen in 4 or more fields, the specimen is considered to be positive for fecal leukocytes.

This test presents certain problems for standardization. Obviously the newsprint parameter is difficult to standardize. In addition, although the cutoff value of 3 or more PMNs per HPF is commonly used, cutoff values in the literature range from 1–15 per HPF. The sensitivity and specificity of this test vary widely, depending on the cutoff value as well as the actual dilution factor in specimen preparation. Furthermore, PMNs lyse over time. Examination for fecal leukocytes is best carried out on fresh stool. If a specimen cannot be examined within 1–2 hours, it should be refrigerated. Even with refrigeration lysis continues; as a result, refrigerated specimens should be retained no longer than 24 hours before examination. The detection of lactoferrin, a component of PMN granules, has been developed as a means to circumvent the problem of PMN stability.

7. What is inflammatory diarrhea?

Inflammatory diarrhea can be defined as an acute diarrheal illness accompanied by fever with evidence in the stool, such as pus, mucus, or blood, of an inflammatory process of the GI tract. Some authors do not specifically mention fever in their definitions. Clearly, the more important component of the definition is the presence and degree of inflammatory cells in the stool.

8. What organisms are associated with inflammatory diarrhea?

Shigella spp., enteroinvasive *E. coli*, *Campylobacter* spp., *Salmonella* spp., and *Yersinia* spp. invade the intestinal mucosa and result in inflammatory diarrhea. *Clostridium difficile* and *Vibrio parahaemolyticus* cause this clinical picture primarily as the result of the action of cytotoxins. Inflammatory diarrhea also may be seen with parasites such as *Entamoeba histolytica*, *Balantidium coli*, *Schistosoma mansoni*, and *S. japonicum*. These pathogens, especially early in the course of illness, can manifest without inflammatory changes in the stool. Thus, in the appropriate clinical setting, a negative fecal leukocyte evaluation may need to be repeated.

9. What is dysentery?

Dysentery is used in at least three senses:

1. To refer to a type of diarrheal stool that contains an inflammatory exudate composed of PMNs and blood.

2. To indicate a severe case of inflammatory diarrhea. The qualitative distinction between severe inflammatory diarrhea and dysentery is not clearly defined. Both conditions can be characterized by fever and diarrhea containing inflammatory cells.

3. To indicate specifically the disease process associated with *Shigella dysenteriae*. However, the typical stool of dysentery is present in only about one-third of patients with diarrhea due to *S. dysenteriae*.

BACTERIAL CAUSES

10. Describe the taxonomy of *Campylobacter* spp.

Campylobacter spp. are the most frequently identified bacterial causes of acute infectious diarrhea in the developed world. These gram-negative, spiral, flagellated organisms were first isolated from sheep in 1909. Their contribution to human diarrheal disease was not realized until the mid-1970s when it became possible to culture them readily from stool.

C. jejuni accounts for well over 80% of identified cases of *Campylobacter* enteritis. *C. jejuni* has been further subdivided by molecular techniques into two subspecies, *jejuni* and *doylei*. *C. jejuni* supsp. *doylei* is a much less common cause of *Campylobacter* enteritis and is classified as one of the atypical *Campylobacter* spp.

C. coli is closely related to *C. jejuni* but causes fewer than10% of cases of *Campylobacter* enteritis. Because there is seldom any clinical need to differentiate the two species, the term *C. jejuni* is often used, somewhat loosely, to include both species. There are hundreds of serotypes of *C. jejuni* and *C. coli*.

The phylogenetic group to which *Campylobacter* spp. belong is far removed from the other gram-negative bacteria. *Helicobacter* spp. are in the same phylogenetic group.

11. What are atypical *Campylobacter* organisms?

The growth of atypical *Campylobacter* organisms is not supported by the culture conditions usually employed for *C. jejuni* and *C. coli*, the "typical" organisms. *C. fetus* subsp. *fetus* is a well-known example that causes *Campylobacter* enteritis. More than three-fourths of patients from whom this organism is isolated have a serious medical condition such as atherosclerosis, cirrhosis, diabetes mellitus, or immunodeficiency. Patients with AIDS are becoming the most typical population manifesting this infection.

12. Describe the epidemiology of *Campylobacter* enteritis.

Campylobacter enteritis is primarily a zoonosis. *Cambylobacter* spp. live as commensals in the intestinal tract of a wide variety of birds and mammals. Humans are infected by exposure to foods of animal origin or water contaminated by these animals. The main vehicles of infection are meats, especially poultry, unpasteurized milk, and inadequately chlorinated water. Virtually all surface waters are contaminated with *Campylobacter* spp., even in remote regions, where they are contaminated by wild birds. Although *Giardia* spp. have classically been associated with "backpacker's" diarrhea, *Campylobacter* spp. may be an even more common cause. Major outbreaks of *Campylobacter* enteritis are uncommon. When they occur, they usually result from contaminated water or milk. It is more common to see single sporadic cases or small clusters, such as in a family.

13. Describe the clinical illness and pathology of *Campylobacter* enteritis.

Incubation period ranges from 18 hours to 8 days (mean = 4 days) and depends to some extent on the infecting strain and the load of organisms ingested. Up to one-third of patients have a non-specific flu-like prodrome (fever, headache, myalgias) for as long as a few days. Periumbilical colic is usually the first gastrointestinal symptom and may be sufficiently dramatic that patients come to appendectomy. Diarrhea varies from a few loose movements to profuse watery stools. Fifty percent of patients presenting to an emergency department with *Campylobacter* enteritis report more than 10 stools a day. Although nausea is common, vomiting is not a major feature. Duration of illness is usually only 4–5 days. *Campylobacter* spp. cause acute inflammation in the colon and the small intestine. The predominant site has not been defined. Nonetheless, the colon is affected in most patients, and fecal leukocytes are seen in 66–93% of cases.

14. Should we treat *Campylobacter* enteritis with antibiotics? If we choose to treat, what should we use?

Therapy given to culture-positive patients has not been shown to shorten illness, at least in part because of the interval between onset of illness and diagnosis by culture. Because this interval (4–6 days) is in the same range as the usual duration of illness (4–5 days), failure to shorten illness is easily understood. Some studies that began empiric therapy at presentation, without waiting for culture results, demonstrated a shortened illness. However, illness was shortened by only about 1 day, and in some patients antibiotic resistance developed during treatment. Thus, therapy is generally believed to be indicated only for patients acutely ill at the time of bacteriologic diagnosis or patients with chronic or complicated illness.

Erythromycin continues to be the drug of choice when treatment is undertaken specifically for *Campylobacter* enteritis. Although resistance has been described, it is relatively infrequent and has remained stable for the past 10–15 years. Ciprofloxacin is effective, but resistance rates have been rising since the late 1980s. Resistance is believed to be due, at least in part, to the use of quinolones in poultry. Both gentamicin and imipenem have good activity against *Campylobacter* spp. and may be used in patients with serious systemic infection.

15. Describe the taxonomy of *Salmonella* species.

The technically correct answer to this question, based on DNA studies, is that all *Salmonella* isolates belong to a single species, *S. choleraesuis*. This single species can be divided into seven subgroups based on DNA and host specificity. In this scheme the organism previously known as *Salmonella typhi* is now called *Salmonella choleraesuis* (group I), serotype *typhi*.

Regardless of the correct terminology, the practice is to continue to refer to *Salmonella* organisms by their serotype names as if the serotype names were actually species names. Thus, we continue to encounter the terms *S. enteritidis* and *S. typhimurium*. There are more than 2000 serotypes of *Salmonella* as defined by O (somatic) and H (flagellar) antigens; some serotypes are named for the city in which they were defined or isolated (e.g., *S. heidelberg*).

16. What is the epidemiology of *Salmonella* intestinal infections?

S. typhi and *S. paratyphi* are generally restricted to humans. Transmission usually occurs through ingestion of food or water that has been contaminated by infective feces. Other *Salmonella* serotypes, collectively termed nontyphoidal, are widely disseminated in nature and maintained in animal reservoirs. The source of human infections by nontyphoidal serotypes is usually contaminated food. Poultry has become a major reservoir for the serotype *S. enteritidis* in the United States. Between 1985 and 1992, this one serotype was responsible for 15,162 cases of salmonellosis, 1734 hospitalizations, and 53 deaths. *Salmonella* spp. is the most commonly reported cause of foodborne gastroenteritis outbreaks in the United States.

17. Describe the spectrum of clinical illness and pathology of salmonellosis.

Gastroenteritis is only one of the clinical illnesses produced by *Salmonella* spp. Other clinical illnesses include enteric fever (typhoid and paratyphoid fever); bacteremia; vascular infections, including endocarditis (rare); focal infections, such as osteomyelitis; and a chronic carrier state.

The precise mechanism of *Salmonella* gastroenteritis has not been definitively demonstrated. Although enterotoxins have been demonstrated in *Salmonella* spp., it is believed more likely that diarrhea results from invasion of enterocytes. Nausea, vomiting, and diarrhea usually present within 48 hours of ingestion of contaminated food or water. Usually the diarrhea is of moderate volume with fecal leukocytes but without gross blood or mucus, and self-limited, lasting from 3–7 days.

18. What is enteric fever?

Enteric fever refers to the condition characterized by significant inflammatory reaction in the intestines, especially the lymphoid tissues, associated with prolonged fever and persistent bacteremia. To produce this condition, a pathogen must be able to invade the mucosa and infect cells in Peyer's patches in the distal ileum. *Salmonella* species are the most common causes of enteric fever. *Yersinia enterocolitica* and *Francisella tularensis* are rare causes.

19. What is typhoid fever? What is paratyphoid fever?

Typhoid fever refers to enteric fever caused by *Salmonella typhi*. It occurs rarely in the United States, where its mortality rate is generally less than 1%. Typhoid fever occurs more frequently in developing countries in Africa and Asia, where case fatality rates may be as high as 30%. Diarrhea may result, because organisms make their entry through the enteric mucosa, and has been described in as many as 50% of patients in some series. However, because it usually resolves before the onset of fever, diarrhea is not a necessary component of typhoid fever.

Paratyphoid fever refers to enteric fever caused by serotypes other than *S. typhi* (such as *S. paratyphi*). Paratyphoid fever is usually less severe than typhoid fever.

20. What constitutes the chronic carrier state for *Salmonella* spp.? How often does it occur?

The chronic carrier state is defined as the persistence of *Salmonella* spp. in the stool or urine for longer than 1 year. Chronic carriage develops in 1–4% of *S. typhi* infections and only 0.2–0.6% of nontyphoidal infections. The biliary tract is infected in all chronic enteric carriers; usually 10^6 or more organisms are present in each gram of feces. Urinary tract carriage has been described in countries where *Schistosoma hematobium* is endemic.

21. Who was Typhoid Mary?

Mary Mallon was a chronic carrier of *Salmonella typhi*. She is believed to have been the source of at least 53 cases of typhoid (at least 3 of which were fatal) among the several families for whom she worked as a cook in the New York City area between 1901 and 1915.

22. Should we treat *Salmonella* gastroenteritis?

Antimicrobial therapy should not be used routinely to treat *Salmonella* gastroenteritis, which is usually a self-limited disease lasting 3–7 days. Such therapy has not been reproducibly shown to shorten duration of illness; instead, it has been associated with higher rates of clinical relapse and chronic carriage. Antimicrobial therapy is, however, a consideration to attempt to avoid bacteremia in selected patients. Although bacteremia occurs in less than 5% of patients with *Salmonella* gastroenteritis, certain groups have been identified to be at increased risk. Prophylactic treatment should be considered for: immunocompromised patients, patients with cardiac valvular or mural abnormalities, patients with severe aortic atherosclerosis or aneurysm, and patients with a prosthesis. Prophylaxis is also considered for neonates and patients older than 50 years (although 50 years seems a bit young to me). If prophylaxis is undertaken, the recommended duration of therapy is 48–72 hr or until the patient becomes afebrile. For susceptible organisms, ciprofloxacin, trimethoprim-sulfamethoxazole, or even amoxicillin can be used. Resistance to these drugs is increasing.

23. What should we do to treat chronic carriers of *Salmonella* spp.?

Antibiotic therapy (amoxicillin for 6 weeks or ciprofloxacin or norfloxacin, each for 4 weeks) should be used to attempt to clear the organism. These regimens may be effective in as many as 80% of cases, even in the face of anatomic abnormalities such as biliary or renal stones. Thus, even in patients with an anatomic abnormality, these regimens are recommended as the initial maneuver in attempting to eradicate the carrier state.

24. Describe the taxonomy and epidemiology of *Shigella* spp.

The genus *Shigella* has four species: *S. dysenteriae*, *S. flexneri*, *S. boydii*, and *S. sonnei*. These species are differentiated on the basis of group-specific polysaccharide antigens that compose a portion of the lipopolysaccharide (LPS), biochemical properties, and phage or colicin susceptibility.

Shigella spp. are highly adapted to humans and naturally infect only humans and some non-human primates. The usual mode of transmission is human to human, although food- and water-borne outbreaks have been reported. *Shigella* spp., in contrast to other enteric pathogens, require a small inoculum to cause disease. The infectious dose for *S. dysenteriae* is as few as 10–100 organisms. This dose is easily within the range that can be transmitted by fecal contamination of hands. The expected household transmission rate, when an index case is identified in a family, is about 20%.

Groups at special risk for shigellosis in developed countries are children in day care centers and male homosexuals. *S. sonnei* is the predominant species in the United States, accounting for over 75% of isolates. *S. flexneri*, however, is the most common isolate in male homosexuals.

25. What is the pathology of shigellosis?

The sine qua non of pathogenesis is cellular invasion, which requires the presence of the 220-kb plasmid of *S. flexneri* (or similar plasmids in other species). The molecular basis for the selective invasion by *Shigella* spp. of the colon rather than the small bowel is not understood. Shiga toxin, produced by *Shigella dysenteriae*, type 1, has been purified and studied extensively. It has cytotoxic as well as enterotoxic properties; it also manifests neurotoxic activity (paralysis and death) after experimental administration to animals. Cytotoxins and enterotoxins produced by other species of *Shigella* are also under investigation. Their precise contribution to the pathogenesis of shigellosis remains unclear.

26. What is the Sereny test?

This test was originally described by Sereny in the 1950s to demonstrate the ability of *Shigella* spp. to invade mammalian cells. Organisms are inoculated onto the cornea of a guinea pig or rabbit. If the organism is capable of invasion and replication, purulent keratoconjunctivitis ensues.

27. What is the clinical presentation of shigellosis?

Patients may present with the classic picture of dysentery with frequent, small-volume, bloody stools accompanied by abdominal cramping, fever, and tenesmus. When this picture is accompanied by the presence of sheets of fecal leukocytes, a presumptive diagnosis of *Shigella* spp. or enteroinvasive *E. coli* (EIEC) can be made. However, the classic picture is an uncommon initial manifestation. Up to 90% of patients with shigellosis begin their illness with watery (that is, noninflammatory) diarrhea. Although the stool becomes inflammatory, the process may take as long as a few days. Even with an organism that serves as one of the classic examples of inflammatory diarrhea, the initial diarrheal manifestation is not necessarily inflammatory. The variable initial presentation underscores the great difficulty of attempting to predict the cause of an individual case based on clinical presentation alone.

28. Should antimicrobial therapy be undertaken for shigellosis?

Therapy with antimicrobials to which the organism is sensitive has been shown to shorten the illness and decrease the mortality associated with shigellosis. Virtually all *Shigella* spp. are resistant to tetracycline, many strains are resistant to ampicillin, and resistance to trimethoprim-sulfamethoxazole is increasing. Ciprofloxacin appears to be an effective drug. In the United States and other developed countries, it is possible to use cefixime or even a parenteral drug such as ceftriaxone when necessary. The cost of these drugs prohibits their use in developing countries.

29. What is an enterotoxin? What is an Ussing chamber?

A toxin is classified as an enterotoxin if it stimulates net secretion in ligated rabbit intestinal segments without either histologic or other in vitro assay evidence of tissue damage. A toxin also may be classified as enterotoxin if it stimulates secretion as measured in an Ussing chamber. The Ussing chamber consists of lucite chambers between which either native intestinal epithelium or cultured intestinal monolayers are mounted under conditions of ionic, osmotic, and electrical equilibrium. Anion (usually chloride) secretion and/or sodium chloride absorption can then be measured. An enterotoxin stimulates secretion and inhibits absorption.

30. What is the hemolytic-uremic syndrome (HUS)? What causes it?

The components of HUS are acute renal failure, thrombocytopenia, microangiopathic hemolytic anemia, and central nervous system symptoms. It characteristically presents a few days after an acute diarrheal illness. *E. coli* (serotype O157:H7) and *Shigella dysenteriae* type 1 are the organisms firmly associated with HUS. *E. coli* O157:H7 accounts for 85–95% of cases. The overall rate of HUS in sporadic *E. coli* O157:H7 cases with bloody diarrhea is 5–10%.

Although the precise pathogenesis is unclear, certain toxins appear to be involved. *Shigella dysenteriae* type 1 produces shiga toxin (ST) (see question 25). *E. coli* O157:H7 strains have been found to produce two similar toxins called shiga-like toxin I (SLT I) and SLT II. SLT I is antigenically identical to ST and is neutralized by antisera directed against ST. *E. coli* O157:H7 strains can produce one or both of these toxins. *E. coli* that produce moderate or large amounts of either toxin are called shiga-like toxin-producing *E. coli* (SLTEC). Retrospective studies have shown that patients infected with *E. coli* O157:H7 strains that produce only SLT II are more likely to develop HUS than patients infected with strains that produce both toxins or only SLT I. The precise mechanism of these toxins is unclear.

31. Describe the various subtypes of *E. coli* associated with diarrhea.

Enterotoxigenic *E. coli* (ETEC) causes diarrheal illness in humans and domestic animals via one or more enterotoxins without invading or damaging the intestinal epithelial cells. The incidence of ETEC is equal to or greater than that of rotavirus in the developing world. In many studies ETEC is the most common cause of traveler's diarrhea. The incubation period is 14–50 hours.

Stools are watery and do not contain fecal leukocytes. Illness is self-limited and usually lasts less than 5 days. Antimicrobial therapy has been shown to decrease the duration of diarrhea, but resistant organisms remain a problem.

Enteropathogenic *E. coli* (EPEC) are diarrheagenic *E. coli* that attach to the surface of the enterocyte, leading to the destruction of the microvilli and disruption of the underlying cytoskeleton. They are seen most commonly as a cause of profuse watery diarrhea in infants less than 6 months old in the developing world but also cause outbreaks in the developed world. The diarrhea lasts a mean of 8–18 days but may become chronic in as many as one-fourth of patients and lead to death in a similar portion. Antimicrobial therapy has been shown to be of benefit, but again therapy is complicated by resistance.

Enteroaggregative *E. coli* (EAgg EC) are *E. coli* that adhere to HEp-2 cells in an aggregative pattern (typically described microscopically as "stacked bricks") and do not secrete enterotoxins. EAggEC are classified on the basis of a phenotypic characteristic. No evidence indicates that this phenotype per se is related to the development of diarrhea; therefore, it includes both pathogenic and nonpathogenic organisms. The clinical illness has been described most frequently in the developing world in patients less than 3 years old and appears to generally last longer than 14 days.

Diffusely adherent *E. coli* (DAEC) are *E. coli* again defined on the basis of their behavior with HEp-2 cells. They adhere rather evenly to the entire surface of the cells. DAEC are the least characterized group of *E. coli*. Again there is an association with diarrhea that persists beyond 14 days; the peak age group affected appears to be 4–6 years.

Enterohemorrhagic *E. coli* (EHEC) were first described in 1982 when *E. coli* O157:H7 was found to be the cause of outbreaks of bloody diarrhea. Currently EHEC are defined as SLTECs (see question 30) that can cause diarrhea or HUS. Although over 100 non-O157 SLTECs have been isolated from humans, O157:H7 continues to be the most common cause of human disease.

Cattle (both dairy products and beef) are the main reservoir for EHEC; they generally have no illness associated with the organism. Food products derived from infected cattle or contaminated by their waste products are the main sources of human infection (although contaminated water supplies and infected humans have been described as sources of infection). EHEC have been isolated in 2–3% of ground beef and up to 10% of bulk raw milk samples.

After an incubation period of 3–4 days nonbloody diarrhea (without fecal leukocytes) ensues. In as many as 75% of patients the illness becomes no worse and resolves within 1 week. In the remainder, however, the diarrhea becomes bloody on the second or third day of illness; it is associated with vomiting in about one-half of cases and with fever in less than one-third. Five to ten percent develop HUS.

Antimicrobial therapy has not been shown to shorten the diarrheal illness associated with *E. coli* O157:H7. Furthermore, data about the effect of antimicrobial therapy on the development of HUS are inconclusive. Small studies have variously shown increase, decrease, or no change in the risk for HUS.

Enteroinvasive *E. coli* (EIEC) are *E. coli* that possess a 140-MDa invasion plasmid encoding for virulence genes identical to *Shigella* virulence genes. They were first described in 1973 in an outbreak of bloody diarrhea due to *E. coli* O124, which remains the predominant serogroup. In general, EIEC infection can be seen as a mild culture-negative case of shigellosis. Antibiotic therapy for EIEC has not been studied.

32. Describe the taxonomy and epidemiology of *Vibrio* spp.

The genus *Vibrio* is a member of the family Vibrionaceae and is closely related to members of the Enterobacteriaceae. *Vibrio* spp. are free-living, naturally occurring bacteria in estuarine or marine environments (they are halophilic, i.e., salt-loving). To date approximately 35 species of *Vibrio* have been identified, 12 of which are known human pathogens. *V. cholerae* is the best known species. *V. parahaemolyticus*, *V. hollisae*, *V. fluvialis*, and *V. mimicus* have been described as causes of gastroenteritis in the United States. Gastroenteritis is also the most common manifestation of sporadic non-O1 *V. cholerae* infections. *V. parahaemolyticus* is the most common cause of foodborne illness in Japan.

33. Describe the classification of *V. cholerae*.

V. cholerae is divided into 139 serotypes on the basis of the O antigen of the surface lipopolysaccharide. Serotype O1, until recently, was considered to be the only cause of cholera epidemics. Thus, it was considered separately from all other serotypes. As a result the other serotypes are often referred to as a group of non-O1 or noncholera *Vibrio* serotypes.

V. cholerae serotype O1 (commonly expressed as *V. cholerae* O1) has been divided into two biotypes: the classic and El Tor biotypes. The El Tor biotype is named after the quarantine camp in the Sinai peninsula where it was first isolated in pilgrims returning from Mecca in 1905. The El Tor isolates were noted to produce hemolysins; this is one of the characteristics currently used to differentiate between the two biotypes.

34. What are the *Vibrio* sp. Ogawa, Inaba, and Hikojima serotypes?

Although the term *serotype* is often attached to these names, it probably is more correct to refer to them as subserotypes because they are based on subspecificities of the O1 antigen. To add to the confusion, the term *strain* is also often attached to these names. This system of classification is based on the fact that the O antigen of the *V. cholerae* serotype O1 can be fractionated into A, B, and C antigens. Ogawa, Inaba, and Hikojima are differentiated on the basis of the types and amounts of the three antigens that they express.

35. Describe the major virulence factor for *V. cholerae* O1.

The major virulence factor is cholera toxin (CT), which serves as the model for toxin-mediated diarrhea. CT is a multimeric protein composed of a single A subunit that is surrounded by and noncovalently linked to five B subunits. This B pentamer binds the entire multimer to ganglioside GM1, its receptor on the surface of the enterocyte. The A1 fragment of the A subunit catalyzes the ribosylation of a GTP-binding protein and causes persistent activation of adenylate cyclase and an increase of cyclic adenosine monophosphate (cAMP) in the enterocyte. The increased cAMP stimulates chloride secretion and decreases sodium absorption, leading to the loss of electrolytes and fluid and the production of diarrhea. In addition, some evidence suggests that CT may lead to increased production of prostaglandins, which may independently contribute to loss of water and electrolytes.

36. Is CT production restricted to *V. cholerae* O1?

No. In fact, in Bangladesh as many as 29% of the non-O1 *V. cholerae* strains isolated from patients with gastroenteritis produce CT. The resultant disease may be clinically indistinguishable from disease caused by O1. Why, then, has *V. cholerae* O1 been referred to as the "only" cause of epidemic cholera? The claim is not based on the severity of illness in an individual patient but on whether the illness appears to be part of an epidemic or an isolated case.

37. What is *V. cholerae* O139 Bengal?

V. cholerae O139 Bengal is the designation of the serotype of *V. cholerae* that was found to be the cause of an epidemic of cholera that started in India in October of 1992 and spread to Bangladesh by January of 1993. It is unclear whether this finding will change the traditional association between epidemics and *V. cholerae* O1. Genetic analysis suggests that *V. cholerae* O139 may actually be an El Tor mutant that expresses a variant O antigen.

38. Should we be concerned about cholera in the United States?

Yes. After an absence of nearly 100 years, epidemic cholera (*V. cholerae* O1, biotype El Tor, serotype Inaba) reappeared in the Western Hemisphere in January of 1991. Although the epidemic has not spread to the United States, the same organism was subsequently found in Mobile Bay, Alabama. The presumed source of contamination was the release of ballast water by a vessel that had taken on the water in a port affected by the epidemic.

In addition, an endemic focus of *V. cholerae* along the Gulf of Mexico since at least 1973 has led to sporadic cases of cholera in Texas, Louisiana, Georgia, and Florida. These cases resulted from eating crabs, shrimp, or oysters that had been inadequately cooked or improperly stored or handled after cooking. *V. cholerae* can be recovered from infected crabs boiled up to 8 minutes or steamed up to 25 minutes. The organism responsible for this endemic focus is also biotype El Tor and serotype Inaba; however, it can be distinguished from the epidemic Western Hemisphere strain on the basis of hemolysins, the VcA-3 vibriophage, and chromosomal restriction endonuclease pattern. The organism responsible for the endemic focus in the Gulf of Mexico is sometimes referred to as the "Gulf strain."

Cholera is a cause, albeit uncommonly, of traveler's diarrhea. In the United States it has resulted from ingestion of crabs brought from Ecuador by a tourist and commercially prepared coconut milk imported from Southeast Asia.

39. Who is Cholera Dolores?

Cholera Dolores was a woman from a rural area of the Philippines who was found to excrete *V. cholerae*, biotype El Tor, serotype Ogawa for a period of 42 months from 1962–1966. Duodenal aspiration demonstrated that the source of the organisms was the biliary tree. Because the woman had chronic cholecystitis, her gallbladder was presumed to be the site of chronic carriage. Unlike *Salmonella* spp., chronic carriage is a rare event in cholera. Excretion of organisms rarely lasts longer than 2 weeks.

ANTIBIOTIC-ASSOCIATED COLITIS

40. What is antibiotic-associated diarrhea (AAD)? How does it develop?

AAD is diarrhea that occurs during a course of antibiotic therapy or within 8 weeks (or longer) after its completion and for which no other cause is found. Although the precise mechanism of the diarrhea has not been demonstrated, the common initiating event appears to be disruption of the normal colonic anaerobic flora that are necessary for bowel homeostasis, including protection against enteropathogens. The spectrum of colonic changes associated with AAD ranges from normal mucosa (grossly and histologically) to pseudomembranous colitis. In a minority of cases (15–25% overall) evidence of *Clostridium difficile* is found; this gram-positive, spore-forming anaerobe is the most commonly identified microbial cause. Other organisms that on rare occasions have been associated with AAD are *Salmonella* spp. and *Clostridium perfringens*. *Candida albicans* and *Staphylococcus aureus* are also mentioned as possible causes, but their involvement is more controversial. The overwhelming majority of cases of AAD have no identified microbial cause.

41. What medications cause AAD?

Nearly all agents with antibacterial activity, including antineoplastic compounds such as fluorouracil and methotrexate, have been implicated in AAD. Even the antibiotics used to treat *C. difficile*-related AAD, metronidazole and vancomycin, have been implicated on rare occasions.

42. What is pseudomembranous colitis (PMC)?

PMC refers to colitis characterized by pseudomembranes and is technically a histologic diagnosis. A pseudomembrane is composed of fibrin, mucin, sloughed mucosal epithelial cells, and acute inflammatory cells. On endoscopy, PMC displays multiple, elevated yellowish white plaques that vary in size from a few millimeters to 1–2 cm. PMC is the most severe mucosal change seen in AAD and is virtually always caused by *C. difficile*. In general, as the severity of tissue changes increases, so does the proportion of cases attributable to *C. difficile*. Overall, *C. difficile* accounts for 15–25% of all cases of AAD. When colitis is present, the rate increases to 50–75%, and, when PMC is found, *C. difficile* is found in nearly 100% of cases. Thus, although *C. difficile* may be associated with the full spectrum of changes (including normal colonic mucosa), it is found more readily when pathologic changes are more severe. In the same vein, more severe clinical illness is more likely to be associated with *C. difficile*.

43. What treatment is needed for AAD?

The initial therapy is to discontinue the drug that is believed to have initiated the diarrhea and to restore fluid and electrolytes as needed. Cases of AAD, not related to *C. difficile*, usually respond to this strategy. Even when *C. difficile* is involved, some cases respond to minimal therapy, because what really "cures" *C. difficile* colitis is reconstitution of normal flora. The realization that the antibiotic therapies of *C. difficile* colitis can interfere with this reconstitution argues against antibiotic therapy in mild cases. In addition, the use of antibiotics to treat *C. difficile* is associated with an increased incidence of relapse.

Nonetheless, antibiotic treatment becomes necessary for patients with *C. difficile* diarrhea who fail to respond to discontinuation of the offending drug. Findings on presentation believed to call for antibiotic therapy as a component of the initial management include fever greater than 101° F, white blood cell count > 15,000, bloody diarrhea, severe abdominal pain, and marked dehydration.

Vancomycin, metronidazole, bacitracin, fusidic acid, and teicoplanin have been shown to be effective against *C. difficile*; the first two are the commonly used drugs. Although vancomycin is generally considered to be the gold standard, metronidazole is more frequently chosen because it is much cheaper, is thought to have equivalent efficacy, and does not contribute to the development of vancomycin-resistant enterococci. Both drugs are effective in more than 95% of cases.

Anionic resins, such as cholestyramine and colestipol, also have been used with some success. Anionic resins bind the toxins produced by *C. difficile* and thereby protect mucosal cells. Other methods of treatment intended to reconstitute the colonic flora directly include oral administration of *Saccharomyces boulardii* (a nonpathogenic yeast) or lactobacilli as well as rectal administration of fecal enemas or mixtures of cultured organisms.

44. How does *C. difficile* cause diarrhea?

C. difficile diarrhea is a toxin-mediated disease. Two toxins are produced; toxin A (commonly referred to as the enterotoxin) and toxin B (commonly referred to as the cytotoxin). Toxin A has both enterotoxic and cytotoxic activity and is believed to provide the primary mechanism of diarrhea. Toxin B has only cytotoxic activity, but this activity is several orders of magnitude greater than that associated with toxin A. *C. difficile* strains may be either toxigenic or nontoxigenic. If they are toxigenic, the amount of toxin produced varies widely. Almost all toxigenic strains produce both toxins. Toxin A binds to receptors on the surface of the colonocyte and is internalized. Internalization leads to cell rounding and cell release, which result in tissue damage, erosion of the microvilli, and extravasation of serous fluid into the lumen. Toxin A also appears to be chemotactic for neutrophils, and an inflammatory response is seen. The role of toxin B is less clear; it appears to act in synergy with toxin A.

45. How is *C. difficile* spread?

C. difficile is usually spread from patient to patient via health care personnel. Surveillance studies show that more than one-half of personnel attending patients with *C. difficile* diarrhea have the organism on their hands. Once present in a health care facility, the spores can remain viable for at least several months.

46. Is toxigenic *C. difficile* always associated with diarrhea?

No. The most common example is the widespread presence of toxigenic *C. difficile* in infants and toddlers less than 2 years of age without the presence of diarrhea. In a large survey of adults, 7% were found to be asymptomatic carriers at the time of hospital admission. Twenty-one percent of patients who were culture-negative at admission became infected during hospitalization. Surprisingly, nearly two-thirds of these patients failed to develop diarrhea.

47. How often does a relapse of *C. difficile* diarrhea occur? What causes a clinical relapse? How should a relapse be treated?

Clinical relapse of *C. difficile* diarrhea occurs in 10–25% of successfully treated patients, although some series have reported a relapse rate in as many as 50%. Relapse has been reported as early as 3 days and as late as 5 weeks but usually occurs within 5–10 days after completion of antibiotic therapy directed against *C. difficile*. The relapse generally presents in much the same manner as the initial episode.

The most common mechanism of relapse is believed to be persistence of spores in the gut. (Antibiotics affect only the vegetative form of the organism; they have no effect on the spores.) After the antibiotics have been stopped, the spores may develop into vegetative forms, produce toxin, and again cause diarrhea. Resistance to vancomycin or metronidazole has not been reported for *C. difficile*; thus, relapse does not result from resistant organisms.

If repeat antibiotic therapy is undertaken, the same high response rate is seen. Unfortunately, a second relapse is possible. Multiple relapses have been reported. Various regimens using longer therapy or tapering doses or combinations of the treatment modalities described above have been used to treat multiple recurrences. What is really needed is reconstitution of the usual colonic flora, which ultimately displaces *C. difficile* and stops the illness.

48. What are the methods to diagnose *C. difficile* diarrhea?

The tissue culture toxin assay, the first test developed, is the gold standard by which other tests are measured. The presence of toxin B is indicated if cells in the monolayer round up when exposed to filtered stool supernatant (the cytopathologic effect [CPE]). Although toxin A is the primary cause of diarrhea, toxin A and toxin B production are almost always linked. Thus, the presence of toxin B is a reliable indicator of toxin A. The tissue culture toxin assay is technically difficult and requires at least 2–3 days to complete. Another problem is that the toxin may be destroyed either by proteases or by being frozen and then thawed to be tested in a batch with other specimens.

Enzyme-linked immunosorbent assays (ELISAs) have been developed to detect toxin. All but one measure only toxin A; the remaining assay measures both toxin A and toxin B. In general, the sensitivity and specificity are in the range of 85–90%, and ELISAs offer the advantage of providing an answer within 2–3 hours.

Culturing is probably the most technically difficult method; it is subject to the most variability from lab to lab and is time-consuming. Cultures need to be held for 3 days before they are judged to be negative. In addition, simply growing the organism does not reveal whether it is toxigenic. In some labs up to 25% of the isolates are nontoxigenic. Thus, another step to investigate the toxin status of the organism is required before the isolate is declared a pathogen.

Endoscopy can be used in certain cases and is even considered by some to be a bedside diagnostic test. However, even in PMC, its most severe and characteristic manifestation, histologic diagnosis is recommended. Nonetheless, in a patient with PMC, therapy is often begun on the basis of the endoscopic appearance pending biopsy results. In cases of colitis less severe than PMC, it is increasingly difficult to make such a presumptive diagnosis on the basis of endoscopic appearance alone. Because some series report that 10–30% of cases of PMC have lesions only beyond the reach of the flexible sigmoidoscope, colonoscopy is required to confirm or exclude the diagnosis endoscopically.

Latex agglutination tests detect glutamate dehydrogenase, an enzyme produced by all *C. difficile*. Unfortunately the enzyme is also produced by other anaerobes. Thus, the sensitivity of the test ranges from 70–80% and its specificity from 85–95%. The test does not discriminate between toxigenic and nontoxigenic strains.

DNA probes and polymerase chain reactions (PCRs) are under investigation as diagnostic aids.

None of the above tests is 100% accurate, and test results must be considered in light of the clinical status of the patient. Fully toxigenic strains can be isolated from patients who have no illness.

49. What is nosocomial diarrhea? What causes it?

Nosocomial diarrhea begins more than 72 hours after admission to hospital and persists for at least 2–3 days. The common causes in adults are *C. difficile* (up to about 50%) and *Salmonella* spp. (up to about 10%). *Shigella* sp. also has been reported as a rare cause. Parasitic infections are almost never the cause. Rotavirus and adenovirus are the major causes in pediatric populations. Bacteria (*C. difficile* and *Shigella* spp.) account for a minority of the cases of nosocomial diarrhea described in patients with AIDS. More commonly cytomegalovirus (CMV), *Cryptosporidium* spp., *Microsporidia* spp., and *Candida albicans* are reported in patients with AIDS.

TRAVELER'S DIARRHEA

50. What is traveler's diarrhea?

Traveler's diarrhea refers to the occurrence of 3 or 4 unformed stools in any 24-hour period, along with GI symptoms such as abdominal pain or cramping, in a traveler from a highly industrialized region to a developing tropical region. This definition may be expanded to include any traveler, regardless of point of origin or destination.

Travelers to developing areas (most parts of Latin America, Southern Asia, and Africa) have a high risk of developing diarrhea. Highly industrialized areas (United States, Canada, Northwestern Europe, South Africa, New Zealand, and Australia) constitute a low risk. Other areas are considered to expose the traveler to an intermediate risk. Any large area, however, includes pockets that do not fit the expected pattern for the country or region overall.

The overall risk of diarrhea for travelers from a low-risk area to a high-risk area is about 40%. The risk for a traveler from a low-risk area to an area of intermediate risk is about 10%.

51. What causes traveler's diarrhea?

Bacterial agents are found to be the cause in 80–85% of cases. The accepted bacterial pathogens include ETEC, *Shigella* spp., *C. jejuni*, *Aeromonas* spp., *Plesiomonas shigelloides*, *Salmonella* spp., and noncholera *Vibrio* spp. EAEC and EIEC also have been described as causes. The first three listed are more commonly found, with some geographic and seasonal variation. Rotavirus and Norwalk virus have been shown to be important causes, at least in Mexico. *Giardia lamblia* and *Cryptosporidium* spp. appear to be important causes in the St. Petersburg, Russia area.

52. What measures can we take to avoid traveler's diarrhea?

Travelers generally develop diarrhea from ingestion of contaminated food and/or water. They can exert little control over the manner in which these items are contaminated, but they can control the items that they ingest.

The following high-risk foods and beverages should be avoided: (1) Cooked items served at room temperature; (2) sauces, dressings, and other items in a common open setting, such as a buffet; (3) fruits and vegetables, unpeeled and/or uncooked; (4) tap water or ice, and (5) locally prepared milk.

The following are judged to be low-risk items: (1) cooked food served steaming hot; (2) fruits and vegetables that have been properly washed and prepared by the traveler; (3) breads and crackers (dry foods); (4) peanut butter and items with high sugar content, such as syrups and jellies; (5) bottled carbonated beverages. "Steaming hot" is defined as 59° C. The use of a food thermometer is suggested for the most cautious travelers. The carbonation status of bottled waters is important. Some restaurants prepare "bottled" water by filling bottles from the tap.

53. What are the pros and cons of chemoprophylaxis for traveler's diarrhea? When should we use it?

Because bacteria cause nearly 85% of cases of traveler's diarrhea, prophylaxis with antimicrobial agents can be effective. When the predominant organisms are sensitive to the antimicrobial used, prophylaxis prevents nearly 90% of the expected cases of diarrhea. Thus, prophylaxis may reduce the usual 40% attack rate to 4%. The critical factor is that the predominant organisms need to be sensitive to the antimicrobial used. The extent of resistance to tetracycline and trimethoprim-sulfamethoxazole is sufficiently high that neither can be used for prophylaxis except for areas where they are known to still be effective. Fortunately, both ciprofloxacin and norfloxacin have been shown to be effective prophylactic agents and have not yet met widespread resistance. It should be kept in mind that such prophylaxis is directed against a condition that is usually mild and easily treated, occurs in less than one-half of susceptible people, and may be accompanied by allergic responses in recipients and development of resistance by the pathogens.

Bismuth subsalicylate (BSS) also has been used for prophylaxis. However, it provides only about 65% protection and must be taken with meals and at bedtime to be effective (at least 4 times/day). In contrast, each of the medications described in the preceding paragraph needs to be taken only once a day for protective effect.

The other important factor is the health status of the traveler. Prophylaxis should be considered in any patient who is unusually susceptible or for whom infection may prove unusually deleterious. Examples of such factors and conditions include use of omeprazole or other proton-pump inhibitor, insulin-dependent diabetes mellitus, active inflammatory bowel disease, AIDS, steroid use, heart disease, and cancer.

When prophylaxis is used, it should be started on arrival in the high-risk area and continued for 2 days after return. If the expected duration of the trip exceeds 3 weeks, prophylaxis is not recommended. The use of prophylaxis does not preclude the need for the usual measures to avoid exposure.

54. Is treatment effective after onset of traveler's diarrhea?

Yes. Antimicrobial therapy (trimethoprim-sulfamethoxazole or ciprofloxacin) has been shown to decrease the duration of diarrhea from 60–90 hours (without treatment) to 15–30 hours. BSS (which has antisecretory activity in addition to its antimicrobial effect) also has been shown to be effective. Loperamide (the preferred antimotility agent because of its decreased central effects) also results in symptomatic improvement, sometimes even more quickly than antimicrobial therapy. Antimotility agents, however, should not be used with invasive organisms such as *Salmonella*, *Shigella*, and *Campylobacter* spp. because they increase the contact time of the pathogen with the intestinal mucosa and may lead to more severe disease. If a patient has fever and/or dysentery, antimotility agents should be avoided. In addition, because the antimotility agents do not harm the pathogen, clinical relapses may occur after cessation of therapy.

Because both are effective and have separate modes of action, the combined effect of antimicrobials and an antimotility agent has been investigated. Studies have shown clinical improvement with such combinations; often, however, the benefit has been marginal. More importantly, none of the studies has shown a worsening in the clinical status of the patients.

PARASITIC CAUSES

55. What parasites are reported to cause outbreaks of waterborne gastrointestinal illness in the United States?

The Centers for Disease Control and Prevention (CDC) Surveillance Summary for 1993–1994 lists only two parasites: *Cryptosporidium parvum* and *Giardia lamblia*. *C. parvum* was found in 5 outbreaks associated with drinking water (403,271 cases) and in 6 outbreaks associated with recreational use of lakes and/or swimming pools (693 cases). The numbers for *G. lamblia* are 5 drinking water-associated outbreaks (385 cases) and 4 recreation-associated outbreaks (141 cases). During this period *C. parvum* accounted for the majority of cases documented by the CDC—nearly 100% of cases associated with drinking water and 83% of cases associated with recreational use of water.

56. What are microsporidia?

The term *microsporidia* can actually refer to any member of the phylum Microspora, which contains approximately 100 genera and 1000 species of primitive eukaryotes that are obligate intracellular parasites. These organisms are ubiquitous and infect both vertebrates and invertebrates.

In our context the term *microsporidia* refers to the two species that cause intestinal disease in patients with AIDS: *Enterocytozoon bieneusi* and *Encephalitozoon* (formerly *Septata*) *intestinalis*. *E. bieneusi* has been found in as many as 20% of people infected with HIV and 33% of patients with AIDS. The prevalence of *E. intestinalis* is about one-tenth that of *E. bieneusi*. The latter organism has rarely been described in self-limited diarrhea in immunocompetent individuals. Nonetheless, at this point both organisms are still considered to be pathogens primarily for HIV-infected people. Microsporidia infect and destroy enterocytes, primarily in the distal duodenum and proximal jejunum. This excessive loss of epithelial cells causes clinical illness.

Albendazole has been effective for the relatively few cases of *E. intestinalis* that have been studied. Experience has shown that it is much less effective in the treatment of *E. bieneusi*. A recent report indicates that thalidomide may be effective treatment for *E. bieneusi*. Thalidomide was investigated because one of its actions is to decrease production of tumor necrosing factor alpha (TNF-α), a cytokine found to be increased in patients with *E. bieneusi* diarrhea.

57. Describe briefly the history of *C. parvum*.

The protozoan genus *Cryptosporidium* was originally described in 1907, and initially its species were mainly of interest as agents of bovine and avian diarrheal disease. Between 1976 and 1982 eight human cases of *C. parvum* were reported, six in immunocompromised patients. *C. parvum* has received additional attention since the development of the AIDS epidemic.

58. Describe the epidemiology of *C. parvum*.

C. parvum, although especially prevalent in ruminants, is infectious for most mammals. Dairy farmers and food workers have serologic evidence of significant exposure. Besides cattle, other animals that have been implicated in the transmission of *C. parvum* are rodents, sheep, and household pets (kittens and puppies). In addition to zoonotic transmission, person-to-person transmission occurs from fecal-oral contamination. This mechanism is believed to be responsible for transmission in day care centers, nosocomial outbreaks, and transmission during male homosexual intercourse.

By far, surface water contamination is the source for most cases of cryptosporidiosis. *C. parvum* oocysts have been detected in 65–97% of the surface-water supplies throughout the United States. The municipal water supply in Milwaukee was the source of a large number of cases of cryptosporidiosis in 1994.

59. Do current water treatment practices succeed in removing or inactivating all oocysts of *C. parvum*?

Not always. The water systems implicated in the surface water-associated outbreaks described in the 1993–1994 CDC report met state and federal standards. More stringent Environmental Protection Agency (EPA) standards have become effective since the Milwaukee outbreak. Even when the new standards are met, small numbers of *C. parvum* oocysts can be found in 25–50% of fully treated water samples from municipal treatment plants. The problem is that the oocysts are resistant to chlorine and often are incompletely removed by filtration methods. The public health implications of the persistence of this small number of oocysts even when the new standards are followed is unclear. Obviously immunocompromised patients should be made aware of the potential risk.

60. Briefly describe the course of cryptosporidiosis.

In immunocompetent individuals *C. parvum* is confined to the apical border of enterocytes in the lower jejunum and ileum; it invades the cells but only to the level of the extracytoplasmic compartment beneath the outer limiting membrane of the infected cell. After an incubation period of approximately 1 week, watery, noninflammatory, malodorous diarrhea develops. Severe constitutional symptoms are uncommon, and fever is rarely significant. Spontaneous, complete remission is the rule with the development of protective immunity; thus, no specific antiparasitic therapy is needed. The entire duration of illness is usually about 10–14 days (range = 3–30 days). Shedding of oocysts usually ends within 1–2 weeks after the onset of symptoms but may persist for 2 weeks or more after the end of illness.

In patients with AIDS *C. parvum* appears to be able to infect any portion of the GI tract, including the biliary system and pancreatic duct; increasing evidence also indicates that it can be a pathogen in the respiratory tract as well. In the GI tract, disease is often manifested by a more severe, prolonged, cholera-like illness that may be life-threatening. Symptoms may wax and wane based primarily on the immune status of the patient. Agents such as paromomycin, spiramycin, and azithromycin have been used but with limited effectiveness.

61. Describe the epidemiology of *G. lamblia*.

G. lamblia is the most common protozoan enteropathogen worldwide. (Although *C. parvum* was the most frequently identified pathogen in the CDC report for 1993–1994, *G. lamblia* was the most frequently identified etiologic agent for outbreaks associated with drinking water for 1976–1994 as a whole.) Indirect evidence suggests that giardiasis may be a zoonosis (beavers are most often mentioned); however, the most important well-defined reservoir is infected humans. Most transmission is waterborne. Person-to-person transmission occurs by fecal-oral contact. Inadequate handwashing also may lead to contamination of food items, which then serve as a source of oocysts (the infectious form).

Patients with common variable immunodeficiency or X-linked agammaglobulinemia are at increased risk for giardiasis and generally have more severe disease. Interestingly, *G. lamblia* does not seem to cause more frequent or severe disease in patients with AIDS. Its increased prevalence in male homosexuals is believed to result from increased exposure due to sexual practices.

62. Briefly describe the course of giardiasis.

Excystation of the ingested oocyst occurs in the stomach or possibly the upper small intestine. Although the trophozoite can attach to the surface of the enterocyte, there is no true invasion, and *Giardia* sp. is considered to be basically a luminal pathogen. Diarrhea begins within 3–20 days (mean = 7 days) of exposure and usually resolves spontaneously within 2–4 weeks. Up to 25–30% of patients have persistent diarrhea complicated by malabsorption. Microscopic examination of stool specimens continues to be the mainstay of diagnosis. However, ELISA testing is commercially available, and DNA-based testing is under development. Both metronidazole and tinidazole have > 90% therapeutic efficacy. Furazolidone also may be used, but its efficacy is only in the 80% range.

VIRAL CAUSES

63. Which viruses are believed to be common causes of infectious diarrhea?

Because of the difficulties inherent in developing and performing diagnostic tests for viral pathogens, they are less readily identified than bacteria in patients with diarrhea. Serologic studies provide indirect evidence of infection. Most direct data about viral diarrhea come from pediatric studies.

Rotavirus is usually the most common cause (up to 30–40%) of severe, dehydrating disease that requires inpatient management for children between 6 and 24 months of age. Most older children and adults have little if any disease when infected with rotavirus—presumably the result of immunity from previous infections. In some studies, however, rotavirus has been implicated in as many as 5–10% of diarrheal disease in adults.

Norwalk virus (proposed as the prototype human calicivirus) is a major cause of epidemic gastroenteritis and infects all age groups except infants.

Enteric **adenoviruses** (types 40 and 41) are often considered second in importance only to rotaviruses. Approximately 95% of cases occur before the age of 2 years.

64. Why the geographic names for these viruses, such as Norwalk, Southampton, Hawaii, and Snow Mountain?

Norwalk, Southampton, Hawaii, and Snow Mountain viruses are members of the family Caliciviridae. The initial description was made in 1968 after an outbreak of gastroenteritis in Norwalk, Ohio. Electron microscopy (EM) revealed 27-nm viral particles. The agent was called the Norwalk virus. As additional, similar particles were found in other outbreaks, the geographic naming scheme was continued. This group of viruses, known as the Norwalk-like viruses or small, round structured viruses (SRSVs), were ultimately shown to be human caliciviruses by genomic characterization.

65. What is winter vomiting disease?

Winter vomiting disease is the syndrome of acute nausea and vomiting that is commonly seen during the winter months in temperate climates. Norwalk virus was the first agent identified with this syndrome and for a time was considered to be its principal cause. As it turns out, however, the illness is not restricted to the winter and can be caused by other caliciviruses. Of interest, the original outbreak in Norwalk, Ohio occurred in October (technically not during winter). In addition, although nausea and vomiting are the characteristic manifestations of disease due to Norwalk virus, about one-half of patients in the initial description also had diarrhea. The initial description showed an attack rate of about 50% (by EM of stool); more recent studies have shown an attack rate as high as 80% (by ELISA of stool), with diarrhea occurring 1.5 times as often as vomiting.

DIARRHEA AND HUMAN IMMUNODEFICIENCY VIRUS

66. Review the causes of diarrhea in patients with AIDS. How do we approach their therapy?

Bacterial pathogens such as *Salmonella typhimurium*, *Shigella flexneri*, and *Campylobacter jejuni* may cause recurrent or chronic diarrhea in HIV-infected patients. In fact, chronic salmonellosis is one of the AIDS-defining conditions. The frequency with which pathogens cause diarrhea in patients with AIDS and the difficulty experienced in treating such infections underscore the necessity of immune system activity in eradicating organisms from the body. Because effective immune activity is lacking, therapy directed against the pathogens often becomes chronic or suppressive. Selected pathogens are shown in the table below.

Selected Causes of Diarrhea in Patients with AIDS

PATHOGEN	SITE OF INFECTION	MATERIAL FOR DIAGNOSIS	TREATMENT
Cryptosporidium spp.	Entire GI tract but predominantly small intestine	Stool	Paromomycin? Azithromycin?
Enterocytozoon bieneusi	Small intestine	Stool and/or tissue	Thalidomide? Atovaquone?
Encephalitozoon intestinalis	Small intestine	Stool and/or tissue	Albendazole
Isospora belli	Small intestine	Stool and/or tissue	Trimethoprim-sulfamethoxazole
Cytomegalovirus	Entire GI tract but predominantly colon	Tissue	Ganciclovir, foscarnet
Herpes simplex virus	Rectum, perirectal, esophagus	Tissue	Acyclovir, foscarnet
Adenovirus	Colon	Tissue	None
Mycobacterium avium complex	Small intestine, colon	Stool and/or tissue	Clarithromycin + ethambutol
Histoplasma capsulatum	Colon (disseminated disease)	Tissue	Amphotericin B
Cyclospora spp.	Small intestine	Stool and/or tissue	Trimethoprim-sulfamethoxazole

? Indicates that some data support the use of the listed drug, but it has not been established as the definitive therapy for the infection.

BIBLIOGRAPHY

1. Blaser MJ, Smith PD, Ravdin JI, et al (eds): Infections of the Gastrointestinal Tract. New York, Raven Press, 1995.
2. Fekety R: Guidelines for the diagnosis and management of *Clostridium difficile*-associated diarrhea and colitis. Am J Gastroenterol 92:739–750, 1997.
3. Gianella RA (ed): Acute infectious diarrhea. Gastroenterol Clin North Am 22 (entire volume), 1993.
4. Goodgame RW: Understanding intestinal spore-forming protozoa: *Cryptosporidia, Microsporidia, Isospora,* and *Cyclospora.* Ann Intern Med 124:429–441, 1996.
5. Guerrant RL, Araujo V, Soares E, et al: Measurement of fecal lactoferrin as a marker of fecal leukocytes. J Clin Microbiol 30:1238–1242, 1992.
6. Hamer DH: IDCP Guidelines: Infectious diarrhea: Parts I and II. Infect Dis Clin Pract 6:68–81, 141–152, 1997.
7. Harris JC, Dupont HL, Hornick RB: Fecal leukocytes in diarrheal illness. Ann Intern Med 76:697–703, 1972.
8. LeChevallier MW, Norton WD: *Giardia* and *Cryptosporidium* in raw and finished water. Am Water Works Assoc 87:54–68, 1995.
9. Manabe YC, Vinetz JM, Moore RD, et al: *Clostridium difficile*: An efficient clinical approach to diagnosis. Ann Intern Med 123:835–840, 1995.
10. Sharpstone D, Rowbottom A, Francis N, et al: Thalidomide: A novel therapy for microsporidiosis. Gastroenterology 112:1823–1829, 1997.
11. Soave R: *Cyclospora:* An overview (State-of-the-art Clinical Article). Clin Infect Dis 23:429–437, 1996.

XII. Head and Neck Infections

43. OCULAR INFECTIONS

Timothy J. Zeien, M.D.

Although many eye infections are trivial and self-limiting, each one is potentially dangerous.

1. How does the conjunctiva protect the eye from infection?

The conjunctiva is a thin, translucent mucous membrane that lines the inner surface of the eyelids and covers the anterior sclera. It contributes to the tear film that moistens the eye surface, helps to dilute pathogens, and flushes away foreign substances. In addition, the tear film contains lysozymes, secretory immunoglobulins, and complement components that inhibit bacterial growth and invasion.

2. What are the characteristic findings of conjunctivitis? Why is it important to distinguish conjunctivitis from keratitis?

Characteristic findings of conjunctivitis include a sensation of itching and grittiness in the eye, crusting of the eyelashes with stickiness of the eyelids, conjunctival hyperemia, mucopurulent discharge, and swelling of eyelids in severe cases. It is important to distinguish conjunctivitis from corneal inflammation or keratitis, because keratitis is a vision-threatening condition. Characteristics of keratitis include opacification of the cornea, circumcorneal injection, minimal-to-no discharge, photophobia, pain, and blurred vision that cannot be improved with blinking.

3. What causes conjunctivitis?

Darn near anything—bacteria, viruses, fungi, parasites, allergies, and chemicals.

4. What is the most common cause of bacterial conjunctivitis in the United States? How is it treated?

The most common cause for mucopurulent bacterial conjunctivitis is *Streptococcus pneumoniae*. Other common pathogens include *Staphylococcus aureus*, *Haemophilus influenzae*, and *Moraxella catarrhalis*.

Bacterial conjunctivitis is treated with topical antimicrobial agents, including 10% sulfacetamide, erythromycin, gentamicin, or tobramycin. In addition, warm compresses may be applied to the closed eye for 5–10 minutes 3 times/day. Patients should be told to avoid sharing towels to prevent transmission of infection.

5. What are the clinical manifestations and treatment for purulent bacterial conjunctivitis caused by *Neisseria gonorrhoeae*?

Gonococcal conjunctivitis is an ocular emergency characterized by rapid onset of symptoms, copious purulent discharge, severe chemosis, and extensive lid swelling. Other characteristics may include preauricular lymphadenopathy and concomitant genital discharge.

Treatment must be aggressive because the bacteria can invade the intact cornea, causing keratitis with ulceration and blindness within hours. In contrast to the typical bacterial conjunctivitis described above, treatment of gonococcal conjunctivitis with topical antibiotics alone is inadequate because the ocular finding is a manifestation of systemic disease and thus requires systemic antibiotics. The currently recommended antibiotic treatment is ceftriaxone, 125 mg IV or

IM. For copious ocular secretions, saline irrigation of the eyes can be performed, and topical erythromycin may be used. Lastly, it is important to treat sexual partners; add treatment for chlamydial infection, and promptly consult an ophthalmologist.

6. What is the most common infectious cause of neonatal conjunctivitis in the United States? How is it transmitted?

Neonatal conjunctivitis is most commonly caused by *Chlamydia trachomatis*, serotypes D–K. *C. trachomatis* is transmitted to the neonate during delivery when infected material from the mother's genital tract is transferred to the neonate's eyes. The most common cause of neonatal conjunctivitis overall is silver nitrate.

7. Why is topical antibiotic therapy inadequate for the treatment of neonatal chlamydial conjunctivitis?

There is a strong association between neonatal chlamydial conjunctivitis and neonatal chlamydial pneumonia. After infecting the conjunctivae, chlamydial organisms spread to the nasopharynx and may eventually reach the lungs, causing pneumonia. Because topical erythromycin will not eliminate nasopharyngeal colonization or prevent pneumonia, systemic erythromycin should be used for 2 weeks.

8. What is the leading infectious cause of blindness worldwide?

No, it is not running with a sharp, nonsterilized pencil in your hand. Trachoma is the leading cause of infectious blindness in the world, affecting 500 million people. It is caused by *C. trachomatis*, serotypes A–C. In untreated patients, chronic inflammation leads to corneal scarring and cataract formation, which leads to blindness. If you look at the leading cause of blindness worldwide for all reasons, cataracts lead the list by far.

9. What is the most common infectious cause of blindness in the United States?

Herpes simplex virus (HSV) keratitis. HSV-1 is responsible for most cases. However, HSV-2 may also be a cause when the virus is directly spread from genital lesions to the eye.

10. What are the most common causes of viral conjunctivitis?

Common pathogens include adenovirus, picornavirus, herpesvirus, coxsackie virus, enterovirus, measles, and molluscum contagiosum.

11. How does viral conjunctivitis present compared with bacterial conjunctivitis?

In comparison with bacterial conjunctivitis, viral conjunctivitis classically has a watery rather than purulent discharge and spreads from one eye to the other; conjunctival irritation accompanies constitutional symptoms of fever, sore throat, myalgias, rhinnorhea, and cough consistent with a viral syndrome. Although it is sometimes difficult in clinical practice to distinguish bacterial from viral conjunctivitis, do not make the mistake of blindly (no pun intended) treating everyone with antibiotics (no pus = no antibiotics). More than 90% of conjunctivitis cases are caused by viruses, are self-limited, and resolve in 7–10 days without antibiotic therapy.

12. Which of the seven human herpes viruses have been shown to cause ocular disease?

HSV-1, HSV-2, varicella-zoster virus (VZV), human cytomegalovirus (HCMV), and Epstein-Barr virus (EBV). Human herpes virus (HHV) type 6 and HHV-7 have not been shown to cause ocular disease.

13. What, if anything, is interesting about the pathogenesis of HSV keratitis? What is the typical finding in corneal infection?

The pathogenesis is interesting because most cases of ocular disease are caused by reactivation of latent virus from the trigeminal ganglion rather than from primary infection. When the virus is reactivated, it travels along the ophthalmic division of the trigeminal nerve and infects the eye, causing follicular conjunctivitis, vesicular blepharitis, or epithelial keratitis. When the cornea is involved, slit lamp examination with fluorescein staining often reveals epithelial dendrites, which result from active viral replication in the epithelium.

14. How is herpes keratitis treated?

The affected corneal epithelium should be gently debrided by an ophthalmologist, and topical antiviral drops should be applied 9 times/day for 10 days. The treatment in the absence of corneal involvement is symptomatic, and the disease is often self-limited.

15. What is the most common opportunistic ocular infection in patients with AIDS? What are the classic findings on fundoscopic exam?

HCMV retinitis. The classic finding on fundoscopic exam is a "brushfire" pattern with "flame" hemorrhages. Some also describe the pattern as "cottage cheese and ketchup." Because the lesions are often at the periphery of the retina, it is wise to dilate the eye and use an indirect ophthalmoscope to visualize the entire retina.

16. How is CMV retinitis treated? What are the complications of therapy?

CMV retinitis is usually treated with 2–3 weeks of high-dose induction therapy with intravenous ganciclovir or foscarnet, followed by long-term maintenance therapy. The principal side effect of ganciclovir is myelosuppression, and the primary adverse side effect of foscarnet is nephrotoxicity. Cidofovir is another anti-CMV agent with nephrotoxicity as the dose-limiting adverse event, minimized with probenecid and hydration. Occasionally proteinuria and elevated serum creatinine are seen with cidofovir. The drug has a long half-life, permitting therapy on a weekly or biweekly basis.

Retinal detachment may occur during or after therapy in up to 29% of patients and may be caused by inhibition of scar formation by the anti-CMV treatment, which allows the thin retina to tear easily.

17. What are the ocular manifestations of each stage of Lyme disease? How does treatment differ for each stage?

Lyme disease may involve any portion of the eye, but the ocular manifestations vary depending on the stage of the disease. **Stage 1** consists of conjunctivitis and photophobia, both of which resolve without specific therapy.

In **stage 2**, cranial nerve (CN) palsies develop, including CN-7 (Bell's palsy) and CN-6, which causes diplopia. These manifestations are also self-limiting and require only supportive therapy to prevent complications from exposure keratitis caused by Bell's palsy. Although topical antibiotic therapy is not indicated in the first two stages, it is important to realize that systemic antibiotics are essential for eradication of *Borrelia* sp. in any stage of the disease.

In **stage 3**, severe ocular manifestations involve the anterior segment (keratitis, episcleritis) and posterior segment (iritis, choroiditis, vitritis). Anterior segment disease is treated with topical corticosteroids; optimal treatment of posterior segment disease has not been established, but a 2-week course of intravenous penicillin or ceftriaxone has been used.

18. What is the most serious complication of contact lens wear? Name the two most important pathogens in contact lens-associated corneal infections.

The most serious complication of contact lens wear is infectious keratitis, which may result in permanent visual loss due to corneal scarring. Therefore, a red, painful eye in a contact-lens wearer must be considered to be a result of infectious keratitis until proved otherwise. The most important pathogens are *Pseudomonas aeruginosa* and *Acanthamoeba* species.

19. What are the three major risk factors for the development of acanthamoebic keratitis?

Contact lens wear, corneal trauma, and exposure to contaminated water. *Acanthamoeba* sp., a free-living amoeba, was an infrequent cause of corneal infection before the development of contact lenses and was seen predominantly in cases of penetrating trauma and exposure to polluted water. However, with unhygienic handling of contact lens equipment and improper disinfection regimens, its incidence has increased.

20. What is the treatment for pseudomonal and acanthamoebic keratitis?

Treatment for pseudomonal keratitis is topical fluoroquinolone antibiotics. Current treatment for acanthamoebic keratitis is propamidine isethionate 0.1% (Brolene solution) with neomycin, gramicidin, and polymyxin. Medical and surgical treatments often fail in acanthamoebic keratitis Lastly, **never** patch a contact lens-related abrasion!

21. Compare preseptal cellulitis with orbital cellulitis. Why is the distinction between the two important?

Preseptal cellulitis is an inflammation of the subcutaneous tissues of the eyelid anterior to the orbital septum. Orbital cellulitis is an inflammation of the tissues of the orbit.

Clinical Finding	Preseptal cellulitis	Orbital cellulitis
Fever	Mild to absent	Present
Lid swelling and erythema	Present	Present
Visual acuity	Normal	Reduced
Ocular motility	Normal	Limited
Pain on motion	Absent	Present
Proptosis	Absent	Present
Leukocytosis	Mild to absent	Present
Patient's appearance	Mildly ill	Moderately ill
Conjunctivae/sclera	White	Injected/chemosis

Distinction between the two entities is important because orbital cellulitis has the potential for serious complications. Damage to the optic nerve may result in loss of vision, and extension of infection from the orbit may lead to cavernous sinus thrombosis or meningitis.

22. How does the treatment differ for preseptal and orbital cellulitis?

With preseptal cellulitis, oral antibiotics should be given to cover *S. aureus*, *Streptococcus* spp., and *Haemophilus influenzae*, which are the most frequent causative organisms. With orbital cellulitis, the patient must be hospitalized and treated aggressively with systemic antibiotics. Surgical intervention is sometimes necessary.

ACKNOWLEDGMENT

The assistance of Greg Witkop, M.D., Ophthalmology Service, William Beaumont Army Medical Center, El Paso, Texas, is gratefully acknowledged.

BIBLIOGRAPHY

1. Coston CC, Craven RA: Treating the red eye: Conjunctivitis and its mimics. Emerg Med 26(11):15–29, 1994.
2. Durand M, Adamis A, Baker AS: Infections of the eyelid, lacrimal system, conjunctiva, and cornea. Curr Clin Top Infect Dis 16:125–150, 1996.
3. Martinsen GL: Ocular herpesvirus infections. J Am Optom Assoc 66(4):221–228, 1995.
4. Palmer ML, Hyndiuk RA: Contact lens-related infectious keratitis. Int Ophthalmol Clin 33:23–49, 1993.
5. Podos SM, Yanoff M (eds): Textbook of Ophthalmology, vol 8, St. Louis, Mosby, 1994.
6. Zaidman GW: The ocular manifestations of Lyme disease. Int Ophth Clin 33:922, 1993.

44. OTITIS

Norman Bussell, D.O., and Donald R. Skillman, M.D., FACP

1. What is the annual incidence of otitis media in children and adults?

In children less than 2 years old, the annual incidence may be as high as 50%. By age 7 years it has decreased to around 10%. In adults the annual incidence has decreased to approximately 0.25%.

2. What are the common pathogens in acute otitis media in adults?

Most studies show *Haemophilus influenzae*, *Streptococcus pneumoniae*, and *Moraxella catarrhalis* to be most common pathogens, isolated in about 50% of cases. Other isolated organisms include other streptococcal species (6%) and *Staphylococcus aureus* (3%). The *H. influenzae* are usually all non-typeable.

3. Name seven risk factors for recurrent and severe otitis media in children.

1. The age of the child at the first episode of otitis media is inversely associated with recurrent risks. This "early and often" risk is believed to be due to increased respiratory infections, decreased immunocompetence, and/or eustachian tube angles.

2. Males are at greater risk than females.

3. There is a higher prevalence among American Indian and Eskimo children compared with Caucasian children, who have a higher prevalence than black children.

4. Seasonal variation is correlated with winter months and upper respiratory infection seasons.

5. Children who were breastfed for at least 4 months have a decreased incidence.

6. Group day care center attendees have an increased incidence.

7. Parental tobacco use also increases the risk.

4. What are some of the complications of untreated otitis media?

The spontaneous clinical recovery rate for otitis media is 50–60% for all causes. However, the consequences of untreated infection can be grim. Hearing loss with its associated impact on language skills, cognitive development, and emotional development is the most serious. Tympanic membrane rupture, formation of retraction pockets and cholesteatoma, structural damage to the ossicles, acute labyrinthitis, and facial paralysis are other potential outcomes. More serious and rare complications are meningitis, extradural abscess, subdural empyema, brain abscess, and lateral sinus thrombosis.

5. What are the differences between acute, recurrent, and chronic otitis media?

Acute otitis media is defined as the presence of middle ear effusion in association with the signs and symptoms of an acute infection, such as fever, irritability, and otalgia. An asymptomatic middle ear effusion is defined simply as otitis media with effusion. Recurrent otitis media is defined as three or more episodes of acute otitis media within 6 months or four or more episodes in 1 year. Chronic otitis media occurs when the effusion has been present for at least 12 weeks.

6. What is the first line of treatment for routine acute otitis media?

Amoxicillin, even in the era of penicillin-resistant *S. pneumoniae* (see the next question). Many alternative agents are available as single drugs and sometimes as combinations in the same bottle, including erythromycin, sulfisoxazole, trimethoprim-sulfamethoxazole, azithromycin, clindamycin, and a wide variety of oral cephalosporins. Mothers prefer single daily doses of pleasant-tasting liquids for their children. Pharmaceutical budget analysts have different ideas about the best choice.

Otitis media during the first 6 weeks of life may be caused by gram-negative bacteria, including *Pseudomonas* spp. It also may present atypically with rhinorrhea, irritability, feeding difficulty, cough, and diarrhea. Most patients are afebrile. A routine 10-day course of antibiotic treatment may not result in cure, and pseudomonal organisms are often recovered from the ears of treatment failures (whether or not it was the organism initially isolated). An antipseudomonal antibiotic, therefore, should be included in the initial treatment of children under 6 weeks of age with otitis media; therapy should be continued for more than 10 days.

7. How do you treat otitis media that has failed to respond to routine treatment?

Because otitis media is not typically a life-threatening infection, a stepwise approach to management may be followed. Amoxicillin frequently will not eradicate resistant pneumococci, especially highly-resistant strains, from middle ear fluid. Assume that for every 100 patients treated for otitis media about one-fourth of cases (25 patients) are caused by pneumococci. Of these 25 patients, about one-fifth (5 patients) will be infected with penicillin-resistant strains. About 50% of patients will be cured regardless of therapy; thus only about 2–3 patients per 100 will fail amoxicillin because of penicillin resistance. Myringotomy or tympanocentesis is appropriate in patients who fail to respond to therapy. Either procedure should clarify the nature of the causative bacteria and permit sensitivity testing.

Beta-lactamase-producing *Haemophilus* or *Moraxella* sp. also may cause failure of amoxicillin treatment. Several oral cephalosporins are effective against amoxicillin-resistant strains, but none is more active than amoxicillin against penicillin (PCN)-resistant pneumococci or PCN-susceptible pneumococci. All beta-lactam antibiotics (penicillins and cephalosporins) given at standard oral doses are ineffective against otitis media caused by highly PCN-resistant strains of pneumococci.

PCN-resistant pneumococci isolated from middle ear fluid of children in some parts of the United States have been resistant to both erythromycin and trimethoprim-sulfamethoxazole. Clindamycin has excellent in vitro activity against most PCN-resistant strains and has been used successfully (sometimes in combination with rifampin) in children with PCN-resistant pneumococcal otitis media that failed to respond to beta-lactam therapy.

In patients who do not respond to oral antibiotics, parenteral therapy with ceftriaxone (once daily for 3 days) or myringotomy may be needed.

8. What organism can produce hemorrhagic bullous myringitis?

Mycoplasma pneumoniae. Bullous myringitis has been associated with experimentally induced *M. pneumoniae* infection in about 20% of volunteers. However, true bullous myringitis in naturally occurring mycoplasma disease is rare. Middle ear fluid of 771 patients was studied, and *M. pneumoniae* was isolated in only one case. Mycoplasmas do not appear to play a significant role in acute otitis media, yet some patients with lower respiratory tract disease due to *M. pneumoniae* may have concomitant otitis media. The absence of myringitis, bullous or otherwise, should not dissuade you from a diagnosis of mycoplasma pneumonia.

9. Into what categories can otitis externa be divided?

- Acute diffuse (bacterial)
- Acute localized
- Chronic
- Eczematous
- Fungal
- Malignant (sometimes called necrotizing)

10. What are the normal flora in the external ear canal? What are the common pathogens isolated from infected canals?

Staphylococcus epidermidis and *Corynebacteria* species are the normal residents. The usual suspect pathogens are *Pseudomonas aeruginosa* and *S. aureus.*

11. Do anaerobic organisms play a significant role in otitis externa?

In one study designed to isolate all types of bacteria, aerobes were isolated in 67% of infections, and anaerobic bacteria were isolated in 17%. Mixed aerobic and anaerobic cultures were found in 9%. Predominant anaerobic organisms were *Peptostreptococcus* sp. and *Bacteroides* sp.

12. What is swimmer's ear?

Swimmer's ear is acute diffuse otitis externa. It usually occurs during hot humid weather. Gram-negative bacilli play a significant role, with *P. aeruginosa* as the major pathogen.

13. What is malignant otitis externa?

Malignant otitis externa is an invasive infection of the skin of the external ear canal that spreads via the fissures of Santorini to the subcutaneous tissues, then erodes through the junction of the cartilaginous and osseous canals. The primary organism involved in this beastly process is *P. aeruginosa*.

14. What disease has a strong association with malignant otitis externa?

Most studies report that 90–100% of patients with malignant otitis externa have diabetes mellitus.

15. Does cerumen play a good, bad, or ugly role in otitis externa?

All of the above: it is good for you, bad for germs, and revoltingly ugly. It tastes awful, too. Cerumen serves an antimicrobial role by establishing a low pH environment that is inhospitable to pathogens. It also contains lysozyme and immunoglobulins.

16. How significant is otomycosis?

Fungi have been identified in about 9% of otitis externa cases. The most common organisms are *Candida* and *Aspergillus* species. Rarely does otomycosis represent invasive disease, but it may be potentially lethal. Most often the fungus grows on desquamated debris and cerumen and contributes little or nothing to the pathology.

17. If a patient with HIV reports otorrhea, what type of otitis would be of concern?

Malignant otitis externa is the worry, regardless of HIV status. Presenting symptoms include otalgia and otorrhea. A facial nerve palsy may be present initially; involvement of other cranial nerves may appear later. Some report decreased hearing. The pinna may be tender, and the presence of trismus indicates involvement of the temporomandibular area. Systemic symptoms occur in a small minority of patients. The external auditory canal is abnormal in almost all patients. It is inflamed, swollen, or erythematous, and a purulent discharge is present. The tympanic membrane may be intact or perforated. Lymphadenopathy and parotid swelling may be seen.

P. aeruginosa is isolated in virtually all patients with malignant external otitis. Although other organisms may be isolated, for practical purposes this may be considered a specific pseudomonal disease.

18. How do you treat malignant otitis externa?

With aggressive persistence, using both surgery and antibiotics. Surgeons are needed to drain pus and debride granulation tissue and necrotic material (bone and cartilage). The extent of surgery is defined by sites and severity of infection. The patient may need canal debridement, bone or cartilage debridement, mastoidectomy, or facial nerve decompression. A suboccipital approach may be required to drain and debride the floor of the skull. Relatively minor surgery usually suffices, in combination with aggressive antibiotics.

Historically, antibiotic therapy consisted of an aminoglycoside in combination with a beta-lactam agent with good antipseudomonal activity. Therapy is ordinarily continued for at least 4 weeks for relatively limited disease and 6–8 weeks or longer if extensive disease is present. Oral fluoroquinolone therapy for 6 weeks, as a single agent, may be effective.

Good follow-up and observation are necessary to ensure adequacy of treatment (and avoid litigation). Treatment failures occur despite optimal therapy, and relapses may occur as long as 4–12 months, but usually within 3 months, after termination of antibiotics.

19. What organism tends to cause chronic suppurative otitis media? How is it treated?

The most common pathogen isolated from the middle and external ear of children and adults with suppurative otitis media is *P. aeruginosa* (as high as 72%). The microbiology of chronic middle ear infections is complex, but *P. aeruginosa* has been identified in 67% of specimens obtained directly from the middle ear of children with chronic suppurative otitis media and in one study was the only organism grown in 31%.

Tympanomastoid surgery was considered standard management for chronic suppurative otitis media unresponsive to topical and oral antimicrobial therapy. However, medical management with parenteral antibiotics and daily aural toilet resulted in resolution of most chronic suppurative otitis media, without cholesteatoma. Approximately 2–3 weeks of therapy (with mezlocillin, ceftazidime, or ciprofloxacin) produced good responses in most patients.

BIBLIOGRAPHY

1. Bojrab DI, Bruderley T, Abdulrazzak Y: Otitis externa. Otolaryngol Clin North Am 29:761–782, 1996.
2. Brook I, Frazier EH, Thompson DH: Aerobic and anaerobic microbiology of external otitis. Clin Infect Dis 15:955–958, 1992.
3. Lucente FE: Fungal infections of the external ear. Otolaryngol Clin North Am 26:995–1006, 1993.
4. Mandell GL, Bennet JE, Dolin R (eds): Principles and Practice of Infectious Disease, 4th ed. New York, Churchill Livingstone, 1995.
5. Schwartz LE, Brown RB: Purulent otitis media in adults. Arch Intern Med 152:2301–2304, 1992.
6. Teele DW, Klein JO, Rosner B, et al: Epidemiology of otitis media during the first seven years of life in children in greater Boston: A prospective, cohort study. J Infect Dis 160:83–94, 1989.

45. PHARYNGITIS

Paul J. Carson, M.D.

1. What infectious agents cause pharyngitis? Which are the most common?

Viruses, by far, cause most cases of pharyngitis in both adults and children. The most common viruses are those causing the common cold, rhinovirus and coronavirus. Among bacterial agents, group A β-hemolytic streptococci (GABHS) account for up to 15% of infections. Major causes of pharyngitis are listed below.

Infectious syndromes

Bacterial	Fungal	Viral
Streptococcus pyogenes	*Candida albicans*	Rhinovirus
Chlamydia trachomatis	(moniliasis)	Coronavirus
Mycoplasma pneumoniae		Adenovirus (pharyngo-
Haemophilus influenzae		conjunctival fever)
Treponema pallidum (syphilis)		Coxsackie A (herpangina)
Neisseria gonorrhoeae		Herpes simplex virus
Mycobacterium tuberculosis		Aphthous stomatitis
Borrelia vincentii (Vincent's angina)		Parainfluenza
Corynebacterium diphtheriae		Influenza
Arcanobacterium haemolyticum		

Systemic (noninfectious) syndromes

Pemphigus vulgaris	Neutropenia	Chemotherapy
Erythema multiforme	Allergy	

2. Can any of the infectious causes of pharyngitis be distinguished by clinical features?

Most cases of pharyngitis—viral and bacterial—cannot be distinguished on clinical grounds. However, there are a few notable exceptions. Adenovirus typically causes a more severe form of pharyngitis associated with conjunctivitis in up to one-half of cases (pharyngoconjunctival fever). Some strains of Coxsackie virus may cause herpangina, which is characterized by 1–2-mm vesicles on the soft palate, uvula, and tonsillar pillars. The lesions eventually rupture to become small white ulcers. Coxsackie A16 infection may cause typical vesicles on the tongue, buccal mucosa, and peripheral extremities that suggest classic hand, foot, and mouth disease. *Arcanobacterium hemolyticum* has been increasingly recognized as a cause of pharyngitis in adolescents and young adults. It may be associated with a diffuse, pruritic, maculopapular rash on the extremities and trunk, similar to scarlet fever.

3. What causes of pharyngitis are most common in adolescents and college-aged patients?

Although routine viruses and GABHS are common in all populations, adolescents and young adults are prone to several other organisms. Epstein-Barr virus and primary herpes simplex virus infections are common causes of pharyngitis. Although not routinely checked, mycoplasmal, chlamydial, and arcanobacterial infections have also been frequently seen in studies of this population when carefully looked for.

4. Should any medical emergencies be considered in the evaluation of a patient presenting with sore throat?

Yes. Patients with parapharyngeal space infection, tonsillar or peritonsillar abscess, and epiglottitis may present with the initial complaint of sore throat. Clinical suspicion should be raised when patients appear toxic or septic, cannot swallow their own secretions, are stridorous, or have significant trismus. These are medical emergencies that may require rapid control of the airway and possible surgical intervention. Diphtheria, although rare, is another potential medical emergency that should be considered in the patient with pharyngitis. The diagnosis should be contemplated in patients without an immunization history who appear toxic and have a tough, gray, adherent pharyngeal exudate. Complications include airway obstruction, cranial and peripheral nerve paralysis, and myocarditis. Timely therapy with antitoxin may significantly decrease morbidity. Special media are required for culture, and the laboratory should be notified that diphtheria is a possibility.

5. What is meant by group A and β-hemolytic streptococci?

Streptococci are differentiated by a number of microbiologic techniques in the laboratory. One method is to describe how they grow on a blood-agar plate. The growing colonies may lyse the hemoglobin in the surrounding blood cells to varying degrees. Gamma-hemolysis involves no visible breakdown; alpha-hemolysis is an incomplete hemolysis that gives a greenish hue to the zone surrounding the colony; and beta-hemolysis is due to complete breakdown of the hemoglobin, which results in a clear zone surrounding the colony. The numerous streptococci that cause β-hemolysis are further classified by the Lancefield system, in which bacteria are grouped serologically by whether they bear certain carbohydrates on their surface (A, B, C, D, or G). Although groups B, C, and G have been associated with pharyngitis, GABHS (or *Streptococcus pyogenes*) is the most common bacterial cause of acute pharyngitis.

6. What clinical features characterize GABHS pharyngitis?

Unfortunately, clinical criteria cannot distinguish streptococcal pharyngitis from other causes; however, some features are suggestive. Streptococcal infections are more common in 5–15 year olds, especially in the winter and spring. Temperature elevation may be higher than with viral infections ($\geq 38.5°$ C in up to 74% of cases). Tender anterior cervical adenopathy is seen in 50% of cases. A pharyngeal exudate is seen in 45% of cases but also may be seen in many other bacterial and viral infections. "Doughnut lesions" (red, raised, or hemorrhagic lesions with a yellow center) are highly diagnostic of GABHS but occur in only 10% of cases. Cough and rhinorrhea favor a viral etiology and are negative predictors for GABHS, especially in adults.

7. Describe the different laboratory methods used for diagnosing GABHS pharyngitis.

The gold standard is a culture on blood agar taken from a swab of the tonsillar area and posterior pharynx. Many laboratories add trimethoprim-sulfamethoxazole to the media and incubate under anaerobic conditions to suppress growth of normal flora and promote growth of GABHS. Growth is usually apparent within 18–24 hours but may take up to 48 hours. Newer, more rapid screening tests detect group A carbohydrate directly from the swab within minutes by either a latex agglutination assay or enzyme-linked immunoabsorbent assay (ELISA).

8. Does a negative rapid streptococcal screen rule out GABHS pharyngitis?

No. Although these tests are fairly specific for GABHS, sensitivity varies widely. Depending on the assay and adequacy of the specimen, sensitivity may range from 40–90%. If streptococcal pharyngitis is clinically suspected and the rapid screen is negative, a formal throat culture should be performed.

9. What other laboratory tests may be useful in evaluating the patient with pharyngitis?

An elevated white blood cell (WBC) count > 15,000, especially with a left shift, suggests streptococcal pharyngitis over nonbacterial causes. When clinical or epidemiologic factors suggest the possibility of an atypical organism (diphtheria, gonorrhea, herpes simplex, *Arcanobacterium*), the laboratory should be notified so that the most appropriate culture medium is used rather than the standard medium selective for GABHS.

An atypical lymphocytosis noted on the WBC differential may be particularly helpful in suggesting Epstein-Barr virus (EBV) infection, although other viral infections may cause the same reaction. A rapid "spot" test (e.g., monospot) for heterophil antibodies may be done when EBV infection is suspected. These tests may not turn positive until the second or third week of illness, and false-positive reactions may occur. IgM antibodies to EBV capsid antigen may be seen early in infection and are specific for EBV when the diagnosis remains in question.

10. What complications may follow infection with GABHS?

Complications may be described as suppurative or nonsuppurative. Suppurative complications are primarily tonsillar and peritonsillar abscess. The most significant nonsuppurative sequela is rheumatic fever, which has an endemic incidence of 0.3% and an epidemic incidence up to 3%. Rheumatic fever follows only streptococcal infections of the pharynx and occurs an average of 19 days after onset of infection. Poststreptococcal glomerulonephritis may follow either pharyngitis or pyoderma in up to 10–15% of cases that involve a "nephritogenic strain."

11. What are the goals of therapy for GABHS pharyngitis?

1. To eliminate streptococci from the pharynx and to prevent further spread of infection
2. To prevent suppurative and nonsuppurative complications of therapy
3. To hasten clinical recovery. (Symptoms from untreated streptococcal pharyngitis are usually limited to 3–5 days; treatment shortens the duration by about 24 hours.)

12. Does delay in therapy while waiting for a culture result increase the risk of complications from GABHS infection?

No. The decreased risk for rheumatic fever associated with treatment may still be seen even if treatment occurs up to 9 days after onset of symptoms.

13. What is the standard therapy for GABHS pharyngitis?

Penicillin is still the drug of choice in the nonallergic patient. Benzathine PCN G, 1.2 million units in a single intramuscular dose for adults or 600,000 units for children less than 60 pounds, is quite effective and eliminates the problem of patient compliance. Penicillin V in a twice-daily regimen for 10 days also has been shown to be effective. Doses of 500 mg twice daily for adults and 250 mg twice daily for children younger than 12 are recommended. In penicillin-allergic patients, erythromycin and clindamycin are acceptable alternatives. If the allergy is not immediate hypersensitivity, cephalosporins are also acceptable.

14. Has antibiotic resistance become a problem with GABHS?

Despite reports of microbiologic failure after treatment with penicillin, clinical failure is rare, and no true in vitro resistance to penicillin has yet been reported. Reports of erythromycin resistance are increasing, particularly in Europe. Sulfonamides and tetracyclines should not be used because resistance is common.

15. What do Vincent's angina and Ludwig's angina have to do with pharyngitis?

Vincent's angina and Ludwig's angina are old terms applied to two characteristic syndromes that may present as "sore throat." Vincent's angina (also called trench mouth) is a necrotizing, exudative gingivostomatitis caused by a mixed infection with *Fusobacterium necrophorum*, oral spirochetes, and other anaerobes. It typically occurs in the debilitated elderly or people with poor oral hygiene. Symptoms include putrid breath, odynophagia, and gingival-buccal ulceration. Vincent's angina responds to treatment with penicillin. Ludwig's angina refers to odontogenic infection that spreads to the floor of the mouth and submandibular space. It presents as a rapidly spreading sublingual and submandibular cellulitis. Treatment includes parenteral antibiotics and close airway monitoring.

16. Which sexually transmitted diseases may present with pharyngitis?

Gonorrhea, chlamydia, and herpes simplex may cause pharyngitis after orogenital contact. Gonorrhea typically causes a purulent exudative pharyngitis, whereas herpes leads to its typical painful vesicles followed by shallow ulceration. Secondary syphilis may cause a patchy enanthema or shallow ulceration involving the oropharynx. Acute primary infection with HIV causes a mononucleosis-like syndrome 2–4 weeks after infection. Recognizing this syndrome in high-risk patients may be especially important, because early intervention may alter the natural history of the disease.

CONTROVERSIES

17. Should antibiotics be given empirically to patients presenting with pharyngitis without making a laboratory diagnosis?

For: This practice is commonly done by many physicians for several reasons: (1) patients expect some kind of treatment when they come to a physician; (2) it may cost less to treat anyone suspected of GABHS and then proceed with a culture to prove the diagnosis; (3) treatment is greatly expedited; and (4) recent studies suggest that even people without proven GABHS or culture may benefit slightly (symptomatically) from antibiotics.

Against: Physicians in fact have a poor record in judging clinically who is likely to have GABHS. Widespread overtreatment with antibiotics for mostly viral upper respiratory tract infections is probably a major reason for the burgeoning epidemic of antimicrobial resistance. Furthermore, in most patients symptoms resolve with or without antibiotics in almost the same amount of time, and delay of therapy does not increase the risk of complications. Most experts strongly discourage the routine use of empiric antibiotics for upper respiratory tract infections.

18. What is the significance of recurrent pharyngitis with throat cultures repeatedly positive for GABHS? How should it be managed?

Clinicians frequenlty face this complex issue. Do throat cultures repeatedly positive for GABHS represent true infection or repeated viral pharyngitis in a patient who is a carrier for GABHS? Treatment failure, as defined by a positive culture at the end of therapy for GABHS pharyngitis, occurs in up to 20% of patients. Speculative explanations include possible antibiotic tolerance, inactivation of the antibiotic by other pharyngeal flora that produce β-lactamase, and noncompliance with the medication. Further compounding this problem is the fact that up to 15–20% of healthy school-age children at times may be carriers for GABHS. In practice, persistent carriage of GABHS at the end of appropriate therapy does not seem to cause clinical problems, possibly because the bacteria become attenuated by treatment. Cultures after a course of therapy should not be done routinely. It is harder to ignore the recurrently symptomatic patient with a positive culture. Treatment with rifampin for the last 4 days of a 10 day course of penicillin therapy or treatment with clindamycin may eradicate the carrier state. Differentiating the carrier state from true recurrent infection may be aided by several clinical and laboratory features:

Streptococcal Carrier	*Repeated Episodes of GABHS Pharyngitis*
Signs and symptoms of viral infection	Signs and symptoms consistent with GABHS
Wrong season	Seasonal clustering
Little clinical response to antibiotics	Marked clinical response to antibiotics
GABHS present between episodes	No GABHS between episodes
No response to antistreptolysin 0 or antideoxyribonuclease-B	Response to antistreptolysin 0 or antideoxyribonuclease-B
Same serotype of GABHS	Different serotypes of GABHS

From Berger MA: Treatment failures and carriers: Perception or problem? Pediatr Infect Dis J 13:576, 1994, with permission.

BIBLIOGRAPHY

1. Berger MA: Treatment failures and carriers: Perception or problem? Pediatr Infect Dis J 13:576, 1994.
2. Bisno AL: Acute pharyngitis: Etiology and diagnosis. Pediatrics 97:949–954, 1996.
3. Mandell GL, Bennett JE, Dolin R (eds): Principles and Practice of Infectious Diseases, 4th ed. New York, Churchill Livingstone, 1995.
4. Stollerman GH: Penicillin for streptococcal pharyngitis: Has anything changed? Hosp Pract 30:80–83, 1995.
5. Vuknir RB: Adult and pediatric pharyngitis: A review. J Emerg Med 10:607–616, 1992.

XIII. Cardiac Infections

46. INFECTIVE ENDOCARDITIS

Robert R. Tight, M.D.

1. What is infective endocarditis?

Infective endocarditis (IE) is a microbial infection of the endothelial lining of the heart. The characteristic lesion of IE is the vegetation, an infected platelet-fibrin clot that typically also contains white blood cells and a few erythrocytes. Vegetation may be located at any endothelial site but most often occurs on cardiac valvular endothelial surfaces.

2. What infectious agents cause IE?

Although many different microorganisms may cause IE, the majority are caused by streptococci, particularly *Streptococcus viridans*. In one large series, streptococci (including enterococci) caused 56% of episodes of IE. The second most common cause of IE is staphylococci. Approximately 20% of cases of IE are caused by *Staphylococcus aureus*, and another 5–6% are caused by coagulase-negative staphylococci. Gram-negative bacteria, including the HACEK group of microorganisms, cause a smaller number of cases of IE. Other bacteria, as well as fungi, cause 2–3% of cases of IE, and some cases are apparently culture-negative. The percentage of culture-negative IE ranges from 2–10%.

Microbiologic Etiology in 2345 Episodes of IE

ORGANISM	%
Streptococci (mostly *S. viridans*)	56
Enterococci	6
Pneumococci	3
Staphylococci	25
S. aureus	19
Coagulase-negative	6
Gram-negative bacteria	6
Fungi	1
Other	3
Culture-negative	9

Modified from Kaye D (ed): Infective Endocarditis, 2nd ed. Philadelphia, Lippincott-Raven, 1992, with permission.

3. What is the HACEK group of microorganisms?

The HACEK group of microorganisms consists of a group of slow-growing, fastidious, gram-negative bacilli that are part of the normal oral flora. They include ***H**aemophilus parainfluenzae*, *H. aphrophilus*, ***A**ctinobacillus actinomycetemcomitans*, ***C**ardiobacterium hominis*, ***E**ikenella corrodens*, and ***K**ingella kingae*. Treatment for IE caused by each of the HACEK microorganisms is the same: a 4-week course of ceftriaxone or combination ampicillin/gentamicin.

4. What cardiac conditions are associated with an increased risk of IE?

Cardiac conditions in the highest risk category include prosthetic cardiac valves (bioprosthetic and homograft valves); previous bacterial endocarditis; and complex cyanotic congenital heart disease, such as tetralogy of Fallot. Other cardiac conditions that confer an increased risk of IE include acquired valvular dysfunction, such as rheumatic heart disease, hypertrophic cardiomyopathy, and mitral valve prolapse with valvular regurgitation. A few cardiac conditions *not* associated with an increased risk of IE include isolated secundum atrial septal defect, previous coronary artery bypass graft surgery, and a cardiac pacemaker or implanted defibrillator.

Cardiac Conditions Associated with Endocarditis

Endocarditis prophylaxis recommended	Endocarditis prophylaxis not recommended
Prosthetic cardiac valves	(negligible risk)
Previous IE	Isolated secundum atrial septal defect
Complex cyanotic congenital heart disease	Previous coronary artery bypass graft surgery
Acquired valvular dysfunction	Cardiac pacemakers and implanted
(e.g., rheumatic heart disease)	defibrillators
Hypertrophic cardiomyopathy	
Mitral valve prolapse with valvular regurgitation	

Dajani AS, Taubert KA, Wilson W, et al: Prevention of bacterial endocarditis: Recommendations of the American Heart Association. JAMA 277:1794–1801, 1997, with permission.

5. What clinical findings suggest a diagnosis of IE?

A wide variety of nonspecific symptoms and physical findings occur in patients with IE. A history of night sweats, fatigue, myalgias, arthralgias, and weight loss is common. Mucocutaneous abnormalities on physical examination often include petechiae, splinter hemorrhages, Osler's nodes (small, raised, tender nodules, red to purple in color, that are located in the pulp spaces of the terminal phalanges of the fingers and toes), and Janeway lesions (painless macules, 1–4 mm in diameter, on the palmar and plantar surfaces). Other nonspecific physical examination findings include Roth spots (retinal hemorrhages with central clearing), clubbing, and splenomegaly. Toxic encephalopathy and various neurologic abnormalities due to septic emboli to the central nervous system may dominate the clinical presentation. Although no clinical findings are diagnostic of endocarditis, **fever** associated with a cardiac **murmur**, particularly if the murmur is a new regurgitant murmur or a changing murmur, are most suggestive of the diagnosis.

6. How is the diagnosis of IE established?

IE may be definitively diagnosed by histologic and microbiologic studies of vegetation obtained at surgery or autopsy. Because it is desirable to diagnose IE noninvasively, recently published diagnostic criteria, sometimes designated the Duke criteria (after studies done by the Duke University Endocarditis Service) are promising. These criteria place diagnostic prominence on distinctive echocardiographic findings. In brief, two major criteria are required for definitive diagnosis. The first is multiple positive blood cultures that grow *Streptococcus viridans, S. bovis,* HACEK microorganisms, or *Staphylococcus aureus* or enterococci acquired in the community and in the absence of a primary focus. The second major criterion consists of typical echocardiographic findings, particularly findings on transesophageal echocardiography (TEE): oscillating intracardiac mass on valve or supporting structures or in the path of a jet stream; valve ring abscess; new dehiscence of a prosthetic valve; or new valvular regurgitation. Recent studies have documented that the noninvasive diagnosis of IE with TEE approaches the pathologic/microbiologic diagnosis in sensitivity and specificity.

7. What is the natural history of untreated IE?

The natural history of IE is invariably clinical deterioration and eventual death from some complication. In some cases, this course of events is acute, lasting just a few days up to a few weeks. Acute bacterial endocarditis (ABE) usually is caused by organisms such as *Staphylococcus aureus, Streptococcus* (group A) *pyogenes,* and *Streptococcus pneumoniae.* In the preantibiotic era, ABE caused by *Neisseria gonorrhoeae* was well-recognized, although currently gonococcal ABE is rare. Although these organisms often cause ABE in patients with underlying valvular heart disease, at least 25% of cases of ABE occur in patients with no underlying valvular disease. In brief, ABE is caused by highly virulent bacteria capable of infecting even normal heart valves.

More often the course of IE lasts 3–12 months or longer. Patients experiencing the subacute form of IE typically have disease caused by *Streptococcus viridans*, *Enterococcus faecalis*, or one of the HACEK microorganisms. IE caused by these organisms usually occurs in patients with underlying valvular or other cardiac disease. A few well-documented cases from before the antibiotic era document survival for over 2 years before development of the inevitable fatal complications.

8. List at least five life-threatening complications of IE.

Five life-threatening complications of IE include intractable congestive heart failure due to valvular insufficiency; chronic renal failure; central nervous system hemorrhage or embolic infarction; ruptured mycotic (infective) aneurysm; and pulmonary emboli arising from right-sided IE, as is typically seen in intravenous drug users. The term *mycotic aneurysm* is a misnomer and does not imply a fungal etiology. A mycotic aneurysm is merely an infected aneurysm.

9. What are the most common sites of septic embolization in patients with IE?

Although infrequently detected clinically, the spleen is the most common site of embolization in IE. In one study, splenic arterial emboli (usually clinically silent) with infarction occurred in nearly 50% of patients with endocarditis. Left upper quadrant abdominal pain radiating to the shoulder, perhaps with an associated left pleural effusion or friction rub, should suggest this diagnosis. Less often, splenic abscess may develop and cause persistent fever despite appropriate antibiotic treatment. Renal emboli are the second most common site of embolization in IE. Many renal emboli are silent; microscopic hematuria is the only clue.

Cerebral embolism is a common, often disastrous, complication of IE. On occasion, the initial presentation of IE is dominated by an acute cerebrovascular hemorrhage or infarct or "aseptic" meningitis. This complication may confuse the clinical picture and delay diagnosis of IE.

Other less common sites of embolic phenomena include central retinal artery occlusion with resultant sudden monocular blindness and mesenteric emboli with associated abdominal pain, ischemic colitis, diarrhea, and melena. Coronary artery emboli may lead to myocardial infarction, myocardial abscess, and arrhythmias. Finally, emboli to bone may result in osteomyelitis.

10. What is the goal of therapy of IE?

The goal of therapy of IE is neither clearance of bacteremia nor symptomatic improvement, which may occur after only a few days of antibiotic therapy. The goal of antimicrobial therapy is sterilization of all vegetations, which typically requires that proper antibiotics, sometimes in combination, be given for an appropriate duration so that relapse does not occur after completion of therapy.

11. What are the basic principles of antimicrobial therapy of IE?

Effective antimicrobial therapy of IE requires the use of a bactericidal antibiotic given for a prolonged duration (usually 2–6 weeks). In some cases, combination antimicrobial therapy is mandatory for cure. Finally, recent emphasis has been placed on cost-effective antimicrobial therapy, resulting in outpatient treatment in selected cases once clinical stability has been achieved.

12. Describe three treatment regimens for IE caused by penicillin-sensitive (minimal inhibitory concentration of penicillin G ≤ 0.1 μg/ml) *S. viridans* with cure rates of at least 90%.

1. **Penicillin G**, 20,000,000 U/day IV for 4 weeks, has been used for many years. This regimen is preferred for patients over the age of 65 and for patients with preexisting renal disease or decreased auditory acuity.

2. **Penicillin G plus streptomycin**, given for a total duration of 2 weeks, has been found to be quite effective in recent years. This regimen has the obvious advantage of shortening the duration of therapy from 4 weeks to 2 weeks.

3. **Ceftriaxone**, 2 gm/day in a single dose for 4 weeks, has been associated with very high cure rates in recent studies. This regimen is suitable for outpatient therapy and thus can provide more cost-effective therapy than hospital-based regimens.

13. How is IE different in intravenous drug users?

IE in intravenous drug users is more likely to be a right-sided infection, whereas in other patients IE is usually left-sided. In intravenous drug users, IE is most commonly staphylococcal in etiology, whereas in other patients the etiology is most commonly streptococcal. IE in intravenous drug users may be easier to cure than in other patients. For instance, right-sided IE caused by *S. aureus* in an intravenous drug user can usually be cured with a 2-week course of bactericidal combination antistaphylococcal therapy, whereas a minimum of 4 weeks of therapy is generally required to cure left-sided IE caused by *S. aureus*.

14. What are two types of IE in which combination antibiotic therapy is required for cure?

Effective therapy for **enterococcal endocarditis** requires a combination of a cell-wall active antibiotic, usually penicillin G, ampicillin, or vancomycin, and an aminoglycoside, generally streptomycin or gentamicin. In the absence of gentamicin or streptomycin the cell-wall active agents are only bacteriostatic for the enterococci, and bacteremia and clinical symptoms promptly recur once therapy with penicillin G, ampicillin, or vancomycin is discontinued. In the presence of the aminoglycoside a synergistic bactericidal effect is achieved.

The overall mortality rate in **prosthetic valve IE** approximates 40%. Thus, even with the most effective medical treatment regimens, prognosis is not good. Prosthetic valve IE requires combination therapy for a prolonged duration, usually 6 weeks. Staphylococcal prosthetic valve IE is commonly caused by nafcillin-resistant strains that require a 6-week course of combination vancomycin and rifampin, with gentamicin added for the first 2 weeks.

The choice of antimicrobial therapy for streptococcal prosthetic valve IE is based on precise susceptibility studies. In brief, penicillin or ampicillin is generally given for at least 6 weeks with gentamicin or streptomycin for at least the first 2 weeks and sometimes for the entire duration of treatment.

15. Has antibiotic resistance become a problem in therapy of IE?

In recent years, antibiotic-resistant staphylococci and enterococci have become an increasing problem in IE management. IE caused by methicillin-resistant *S. aureus* (MRSA) requires treatment with vancomycin. Recent studies indicate that vancomycin is less rapidly bactericidal against *S. aureus* than is nafcillin for methicillin-sensitive *S. aureus* (MSSA). Patients treated for MRSA IE with vancomycin tend to be febrile and bacteremic longer than patients treated with nafcillin for MSSA endocarditis.

The most ominous form of antibiotic resistance in IE has been the recent emergence of enterococci resistant to penicillin/ampicillin, gentamicin/streptomycin, and vancomycin. Patients infected with penicillin/ampicillin-resistant enterococci can still be effectively treated with combination vancomycin/aminoglycoside, although this regimen is associated with higher toxicity. Patients with enterococcal IE caused by a streptomycin-resistant enterococci can be effectively treated with combination penicillin/ampicillin-gentamicin therapy or with vancomycin/gentamicin therapy. Most, but not all, gentamicin-resistant enterococci are also streptomycin-resistant. Those which are streptomycin-sensitive can be treated with penicillin/ampicillin-streptomycin. However, enterococci resistant to both gentamicin and streptomycin cannot be effectively treated with a combination regimen that is reliably bactericidal. Recently, enterococcal strains, usually *E. faecium*, that are resistant to penicillin/ampicillin, aminoglycosides, and vancomycin have emerged. Although investigational antibiotics (teicoplanin, streptogramin combination) have been effective in some patients, many have been resistant to all attempts at therapy with a subsequently high mortality rate.

16. What is the role of surgery in the management of IE?

Surgical excision of an infected native cardiac valve and implantation of a valve prosthesis must be seriously considered in patients with **repeated embolic events**. Once effective antimicrobial therapy has been given for at least 1 week, the risk of embolic events decreases. Thus, a single embolic event, especially before diagnosis or in the first few days of therapy, need not be an indication for valve surgery. A second embolic event, however, may be the predecessor of disastrous complications that are potentially avoidable with appropriate surgical management.

Uncontrollable infection is another indication for surgery. This complication is fairly infrequent now that effective therapy is available for many types of IE. Fungal endocarditis and unusual types of endocarditis, such as Q-fever endocarditis, often cannot be effectively controlled and may require surgery.

Finally, **intractable congestive heart failure** may occur despite bacteriologic cure of IE. In such cases, prosthetic valve implantation can be life-saving.

17. How is adequacy of therapy monitored? How is relapse recognized? How is cure established?

These questions are commonly asked by patients and family members. Cure of IE can be verified only after antimicrobial therapy is stopped and 2 months have subsequently elapsed without recurrence of bacteremia. Some authorities insist on a 6-month interval. A common practice is to obtain blood cultures on several occasions after completion of therapy, such as 1, 2, 4, and 8 weeks after therapy. If all blood cultures are negative for the previously cultured infectious agent, the patient may be assured that the infection has been cured.

Meticulous, frequent clinical re-evaluation is the most important aspect of monitoring adequacy of therapy. Persistent or recurrent fever may be a sign of treatment failure or may be due to drug-related hypersensitivity, thrombophlebitis with or without pulmonary embolism, or sterile embolism to other organs. Positive posttherapy blood culture for the infecting organism establishes relapse and mandates prompt reevaluation and retreatment. Patients whose symptoms have been present for more than 3 months before initiation of therapy tend to have a somewhat higher relapse rate.

18. State the rationale for IE prophylaxis.

Patients with certain structural abnormalities of the heart or great vessels are at increased risk for development of IE. About 15–25% of cases of IE occur in temporal association with invasive dental or surgical procedures. The microorganisms most likely to cause endocarditis after a given procedure are fairly predictable, as are their antimicrobial susceptibilities. IE prophylaxis thus is recommended for certain dental, respiratory tract, gastrointestinal tract, and genitourinary tract procedures.

19. How has the epidemiology of IE changed since the preantibiotic era?

Two factors have changed: the age of the patients and their underlying cardiac diseases. In the preantibiotic era, most cases of IE occurred in patients younger than 30 years. Today most IE occurs between the ages of 30 and 60 years. Roughly 25% of cases recur in patients older than 60 years.

Rheumatic heart disease accounts for much less of the underlying cardiac disease today than in the preantibiotic era. Congenital heart disease, degenerative valvular heart disease, and mitral valve prolapse with valvular regurgitation now represent the majority of underlying cardiac disease in patients with IE.

CONTROVERSY

20. Must all patients with *Staphylococcus aureus* bacteremia be treated as if they have IE?

For: S. *aureus* is a virulent pathogen that, when bacteremic, may invade even normal heart valves. The result often is a rapidly progressive form of acute bacterial endocarditis. In one small series over 30% of episodes of S. *aureus* bacteremia associated with a readily removable focus of infection, usually an intravenous line, nevertheless resulted in IE. Distinguishing between patients with S. *aureus* bacteremia and IE and patients with S. *aureus* bacteremia without IE is difficult. Thus, it may be best to treat all patients with S. *aureus* bacteremia as if they have S. *aureus*

IE—namely, with intravenous antistaphylococcal therapy (such as nafcillin, vancomycin, or cefazolin) for at least 4 weeks.

Against: In certain settings, *S. aureus* bacteremia is associated with a low risk of severe complications, such as IE. Examples include *S. aureus* bacteremia associated with an intravascular catheter that is promptly removed, patients who rapidly become afebrile, and patients without underlying heart disease and cardiac murmurs. The great majority of such patients (> 90% in several series) can be effectively treated with a 2-week course of intravenous antistaphylococcal therapy. Thus, treating all patients as if they have IE results in treating a majority of patients for an unnecessarily prolonged duration.

BIBLIOGRAPHY

1. Dajani AS, Taubert KA, Wilson W, et al: Prevention of bacterial endocarditis: Recommendations of the American Heart Association. JAMA 277:1794–1801, 1997.
2. Durack DT, Lukes AS, Bright DK, et al: New criteria for diagnosis of IE: Utilization of specific echocardiographic findings. Am J Med 96:200–207, 1994.
3. Kaye D (ed): Infective Endocarditis, 2nd ed. New York, Raven Press, 1992.
4. Raad I, Sabbagh MF: Optimal duration of therapy for catheter-related *Staphylococcus aureus* bacteremia—a study of 55 cases and review. Clin Infect Dis 14:75–81, 1992.
5. Sekeres MA, Abrutyn E, Berlin JA, et al: An assessment of the usefulness of the Duke criteria for diagnosing active infective endocarditis. Clin Infect Dis 24:1185–1190, 1997.
6. Wilson WR, Karchner AW, Dajani AS, et al: Antibiotic treatment of adults with infective endocarditis due to streptococci, enterococci, staphylococci, and HACEK microorganisms. JAMA 274:1706–1713, 1995.

XIV. Respiratory Syndromes

47. SINUSITIS

Karen Fagin, M.D., and David R. Haburchak, M.D.

1. Define sinusitis. How is it classified?

Sinusitis is inflammation of paranasal sinus cavities and surrounding tissues. Acute sinusitis is of recent onset, chronic sinusitis of more than 1 month's duration. Sinusitis is qualitatively distinctive in immunocompromised and normal hosts and may be caused by community or nosocomial organisms as well as noninfectious causes. Infectious types of sinusitis include viral, mixed viral/bacterial, bacterial, and fungal.

2. What are the important anatomic and histologic characteristics of the paranasal sinuses?

The maxillary, frontal, ethmoid, and sphenoid sinuses are bony chambers lined with ciliated respiratory epithelium and covered with a thin layer of mucus. Cilia transport mucus through the sinus ostia toward the nares regardless of gravity orientation, thereby maintaining normal sterility.

3. What are the pathologic manifestations of sinusitis?

Most cases of sinusitis occur in the context of increased viscous material in sinus cavities after viral, allergic, or physical exposure. Parasympathetic and inflammatory mediators provoke goblet cell mucus deposition on walls of sinuses, which is visualized radiographically as "mucosal thickening." Cilia appear unable to transport this thick mucus, resulting in fluid collection. Simultaneous ostial-meatal and maxillary-infundibular occlusion are common and may contribute to delayed clearance and failure to maintain bacterial or fungal sterility of the sinus. These secondary pathogens may be invasive. Chronic sinusitis is associated with damage to the mucosa and squamous metaplasia.

4. What are the risk factors for sinusitis?

Risk factors include any condition that impedes mucociliary clearance of secretions: viral or allergic upper airway disease; nasal polyps, tumors, foreign bodies, or septal deviation; cystic fibrosis; ciliary defects; and cigarette smoke. Maxillary dental abscesses and immunodeficiency enhance risk of infection.

5. What is the incidence of viral and bacterial sinusitis?

It is estimated that 90% of common colds are associated with viral sinusitis. Between 0.5% and 2% of colds are complicated by bacterial sinusitis. There are approximately 2 million patient visits yearly for presumed bacterial sinusitis in the United States.

6. How can the causative organism be identified?

Quantitative cultures of sinus puncture aspirates are the gold standard. Nasal cultures or samples obtained from sinus endoscopy are usually contaminated by nasopharyngeal flora and are of little diagnostic significance.

7. What are the most prominent bacterial causes of acute and chronic sinusitis?

Acute sinusitis: *Streptococcus pneumoniae, Hemophilus influenzae, Moraxella catarrhalis,* and *Chlamydia pneumoniae.*

Chronic sinusitis: anaerobes, staphylococci, gram-negative rods.

8. What clinical findings separate bacterial from viral sinusitis?

Individual clinical findings may have limited sensitivity and specificity. However, history of purulent nasal secretions, cough, and sneezing each have sensitivity greater than 70%. Maxillary toothache, fever, poor response to decongestants, and sinus tenderness each have specificity greater than 65% for bacterial disease. Air-fluid level with flat meniscus on limited sinus computed tomography (CT) and elevated erythrocyte sedimentation rate (ESR) or C-reactive protein also appear helpful to confirm bacterial disease. Finally, symptoms persisting longer than 7 days after viral infection suggest secondary bacterial sinusitis.

9. When are radiographic and endoscopic procedures indicated?

Patients suspected of intracranial or orbital extension or fungal etiology should have limited sinus CT and sinus endoscopy for precise anatomic and microbiologic diagnoses. Failure to respond to therapy and frequently relapsing disease are also indications for evaluation.

10. What are the management imperatives of acute sinusitis?

Critical disease (signs suggestive of intracranial or orbital involvement)
  • Obtain head CT, lumbar puncture, and surgery consultation
  • Start intravenous empiric broad-spectrum antibiotics (vancomycin plus ceftriaxone)
Serious disease (fever, facial pain, edema, erythema, toothache, air-fluid level on radiograph or CT)
  • Prescribe amoxicillin/clavulanate or cefuroxime axetil, adjunctive decongestants, and guaifenesin
  • Close follow-up for complications
Routine disease (symptoms of cold with no improvement after 7 days)
  • Antibiotics and adjunctive therapy as above

11. How long should antibiotics be given?

Usually 10 days of therapy is sufficient in the absence of complications. Chronic sinusitis may require therapy for 6 weeks or longer.

12. Which hospitalized patients are at risk for nosocomial sinusitis?

Patients with nasal packing or prolonged nasal intubation are at increased risk.

13. What are the common bacterial causes of nosocomial sinusitis?

Staphylococcus aureus, Pseudomonas aeruginosa, Klebsiella pneumoniae, Enterobacter sp., and *Proteus mirabilis* are reported most commonly.

14. When and how is fungal sinusitis manifest?

Fungal sinusitis is much less common than bacterial sinusitis and is seen most often in the immunocompromised or allergic host. **Chronic indolent fungal sinusitis** may occur in normal hosts and is characterized by granulomatous inflammation of sinus cavities with isolation of *Aspergillus* sp., usually after heavy exposure. **Mycetoma** or fungus ball may occur in normal or allergic hosts. **Allergic fungal sinusitis** is associated with mucinous material containing fungal hyphae, eosinophils, and cellular debris in asthmatics. **Invasive fungal sinusitis** occurs most commonly in acidotic diabetics, patients on dialysis, leukemics, and patients with AIDS after environmental exposure to *Aspergillus* or *Rhizopus* sp.

15. What is the therapy for fungal sinusitis?

Therapy is directed at reversal of predisposing acidosis or immunodeficiency, control of allergy with steroids, and surgical debridement of infected tissue. Systemic amphotericin B is helpful to limit spread of infection.

16. What are the complications of sinusitis?

- Meningitis
- Cranial osteomyelitis
- Brain abscess
- Orbital cellulitis
- Venous thrombophlebitis

Complications should be suspected in the presence of high fever, severe headache, or ocular symptoms such as chemosis, proptosis, or abnormal extraocular movement.

17. When is sinus surgery indicated?

Surgery is indicated for chronic sinusitis refractory to medical management, fungal sinusitis, or complications of acute sinusitis. CT findings direct surgical correction of anatomic abnormalities. Endoscopic surgery is performed to enlarge sinus ostia. Traditional surgery may be used to produce drainage windows, debride diseased mucosa, or remove osteomyelitic bone.

18. When is referral indicated in sinus disease?

If there is no response to two courses of antibiotics in conjunction with decongestive and steroid therapy, an ear-nose-throat surgeon should be consulted. If immune deficiency is suspected, IgA and IgG subset immunoglobulin levels should be evaluated and an infectious disease specialist should be consulted. Referral to an allergist may be indicated if symptoms or laboratory signs suggest allergic etiology.

CONTROVERSY

19. Which adjunctive therapies are better—systemic decongestants or nasal sprays?

Topical therapies may be effective in decreasing nasal edema and providing some relief of airflow obstruction and rhinorrhea. They do little to promote flow of viscous mucus but may provoke rhinitis medicamentosa and rebound vasodilatation. Intranasal steroids are not effective in experimental rhinovirus infections but are useful in patients with nasal polyps. Systemic decongestants are helpful but slower in action and may provoke hypertension. Patients on antihypertensive therapy should be monitored closely.

BIBLIOGRAPHY

1. Dolan RW, Chowdhury K: Diagnosis and treatment of intracranial complications of paranasal sinus infections. J Oral Maxillofac Surg 53:1080–1087, 1995.
2. Guarderas JC: Rhinitis and sinusitis: Office management. Mayo Clin Proc 71:882–888, 1996.
3. Gwaltney JM: Acute community-acquired sinusitis. Clin Infect Dis 23:1209–1225, 1996.
4. Morpeth JF, Rupp NT, Dolen WK, et al: Fungal sinusitis: An update. Ann Allergy Asthma Immunol 76:128–140, 1996.
5. Newman U, Platts-Mills TAAE, Phillips CD, et al: Chronic sinusitis: Relationship of computed tomographic findings to allergy, asthma, and eosinophilia. JAMA 271:363–367, 1994.
6. Sethi DS, Winkelstein JA, Lederman H, et al: Immunologic defects in patients with chronic recurrent sinusitis: Diagnosis and management. Otolaryngol Head Neck Surg 112:242–247, 1995.
7. Singh B, Van Dellen J, Ramjettan S, et al: Sinogenic intracranial complications. J Laryngol Otol 109:945–950, 1995.
8. Willett LR, Carson JL, Williams JW: Current diagnosis and management of sinusitis. J Gen Intern Med 9:38–45, 1994.
9. Williams JW, Simel DL: Does this patient have sinusitis? JAMA 270:1242–1246, 1993.
10. Iwen PC, Rupp ME, Hinrichs SH: Invasive mold sinusitis: 17 cases in immunocompromised patients and review of the literature. Clin Infect Dis 24:1178–1184, 1997.

48. COMMUNITY-ACQUIRED PNEUMONIA: PUBLIC ENEMY NO. 1

Lisa L. Zacher, M.D., FCCP

1. Why is community-acquired pneumonia (CAP) public enemy no. 1?

Pneumonia is the leading cause of death due to infectious disease and the sixth leading cause of death in the United States. Nearly one-half of the deaths from infection were caused by respiratory infections, mostly in persons older than 65 years. Between 1980–1992 mortality due to respiratory tract infections increased 20%—from 25 to 30 deaths per 100,000. In the outpatient setting the mortality rate is low (1–5%) but approaches 30% if the patient requires admission to the intensive care unit.

2. What is the most common organism associated with CAP in children? In adults younger than 65? In the elderly?

Streptococcus pneumoniae is still the most common single pathogen in all age groups (except newborns).

3. Name the major route of acquisition of CAP.

Aspiration from a previously colonized upper airway. Other routes include inhalation, hematogenous spread, and direct inoculation from contiguous infected sites.

4. What organisms are always pathogenic (i.e., not colonizers) when isolated from the respiratory tract?

Legionella sp.	*Mycobacterium tuberculosis*	*Histoplasma capsulatum*
Mycoplasma pneumoniae	*Pneumocystis carinii*	*Coccidioides immitis*
Influenza virus	*Toxoplasma gondii*	*Blastomyces dermatitidis*
Respiratory syncytial virus	*Strongyloides* sp.	

5. Name the most common pathogens in outpatients younger than age 60 who have no coexisting illnesses.

Streptococcus pneumoniae, Mycoplasma pneumoniae, respiratory viruses, *Chlamydia pneumoniae,* and *Haemophilus influenzae.*

6. Can "typical" and "atypical" presentations reliably predict microbial causes?

No. Advanced age and coexisting illnesses are important factors in the clinical presentation of pneumonia. Pneumococcal pneumonia occurs with increased incidence in elderly, immunocompromised, and alcoholic patients; the "typical" presentation (abrupt onset, single shaking chill, pleuritic chest pain, rusty sputum, lobar consolidation) is rarely seen except in an otherwise healthy person. Atypical pneumonias were historically associated with *Mycoplasma pneumoniae* and viruses. Extrapulmonary symptoms are prominent (headache, myalgias, nausea, diarrhea, nonproductive cough, ill-defined pulmonary infiltrates). A prospective study of 359 cases of CAP found no distinctive clinical features diagnostic for any of the etiologic agents, although high fever occurred more often in Legionnaire's disease.

7. What makes CAP in the elderly different?

Pneumonia in the elderly is commonly "atypical" in presentation; patients are often afebrile or hypothermic. Frequently, the only finding is an altered mental status. The pulmonary inflammatory response may be delayed, and it is common for the chest radiograph to progress despite appropriate antibiotic therapy. Underlying illnesses (e.g, chronic obstructive pulmonary disease

[COPD], heart disease) may influence radiographic features. Large-volume aspiration and poor nutrition were independent risk factors for development of pneumonia. The main pathogens causing pneumonia in hospitalized patients over age 65 years are *Streptococcus pneumoniae* and *Chlamydia pneumoniae*. Gram-negative bacilli are uncommon (5%). The elderly also are more likely to require hospitalization and to die from CAP.

8. What organisms are associated with CAP that requires hospitalization?

Causative Organisms in 359 Cases of Community-acquired Pneumonia

ORGANISM	DEFINITIVE	PRESUMPTIVE	TOTAL	%
Streptococcus pneumoniae	16	39	55	15.3
Haemophilus influenzae	1	38	39	10.9
Legionella sp.*	17	7	24	6.7
Chlamydia pneumoniae	19	3	22	6.1
Aerobic gram-negative organisms[†]	2	19	21	5.9
Staphylococcus aureus	4	8	12	3.3
Streptococcus sp.[‡]	2	8	10	2.8
Pneumocystis carinii	9	0	9	2.5
Mycoplasma pneumoniae	5	2	7	2.0
Miscellaneous[§]	4	6	10	2.8
Virus (varicella zoster)	0	1	1	0.3
Postobstructive	0	19	19	5.3
Aspiration	0	12	12	3.3
Unknown	0	0	118	32.9
Total	79	162	359	100

* *L. pneumophilia* (22 patients), *L. micdadei* (2).
[†] *Pseudomonas aeruginosa* (7), *E. coli* (4), *Klebsiella* sp. (3), *Enterobacter cloacae* (2), *Acinetobacter* sp. (1), *Proteus* sp. (1), *Providencia* sp. (1), *Pasteurella* spp. (1), *Acinetobacter/Serratia* spp (1).
[‡] *S. sanguis* (1), group B (4), group C (1), group F (1), *Enterococcus* sp. (1), other (2).
[§] *M. tuberculosis* (4), *M. catarrhalis* (3), *B. fragilis* (1), *Actinomyces israelii* (1), multiple anaerobes (1).
From Fang GD, et al: New and emerging etiologies for community-acquired pneumonia with implications for therapy: A prospective multicenter trial of 359 cases. Medicine 69:309, 1990, with permission.

The causative organism of nearly 40–50% of pneumonia cases remains unknown despite multiple diagnostic tests, including use of convalescent serology. Gram-negative bacilli are uncommon causes of CAP.

9. List the organisms that have been associated with pneumonia in the following clinical settings.

Smokers	*Haemophilus influenzae*
Alcoholics	*Klebsiella pneumoniae*
Splenectomy	Encapsulated organisms (*S. pneumoniae, H. influenzae*)
Leukemia	Aspergillus and other fungus (especially if neutropenic)
Cystic fibrosis	*Pseudomonas* sp.
Bird exposure	*Chlamydia psittaci*
Milk/postparturition products	*Coxiella burnetii* (Q fever)
Rabbit exposure	*Francisella tularensis* (tularemia)
Rats	Plague, Leptospirosis
Deer mouse	Hantavirus
Travel to Southeast Asia	*Pseudomonas pseudomallei*
Travel to Asia, Africa, or Central and South America	Paragonimiasis

10. What factors predict mortality in CAP?

Male sex	Neoplastic disease
Pleuritic chest pain	Neurologic disease
Hypothermia	Bacteremia
Systolic hypotension	Leukopenia
Tachypnea	Multilobar radiographic pulmonary infiltrate
Diabetes mellitus	

11. What antibiotics should be chosen empirically?

The American Thoracic Society (ATS) guidelines define four patient categories based on age, comorbid factors, and severity of illness. These categories are believed to relate not only to microbial etiology but also to prognosis and outcome.

1. Outpatient pneumonia without comorbidity in patients 60 years old or younger: macrolide (erythromycin) or tetracycline (in macrolide-allergic or intolerant patients). Consider newer macrolides (azithromycin or clarithromycin) in smokers with *H. influenzae* pneumonia and in erythromycin-intolerant patients.

2. Outpatient pneumonia with comorbidity and/or age ≥ 60 years: second-generation cephalosporin or trimethoprim/sulfamethoxazole or beta lactam/beta lactamase inhibitor. If infection with *Legionella* sp. is a concern, a macrolide should be added.

3. Hospitalized patients with CAP: second- or third-generation cephalosporin or beta-lactam/beta lactamase inhibitor. Add macrolide if infection with *Legionella* sp. is a concern. Rifampin may be added if *Legionella* sp. is documented.

4. Hospitalized patients with severe CAP: macrolide plus third-generation cephalosporin with antipseudomonal activity or other antipseudomonal agents (imipenem/cilastatin, ciprofloxacin). Because of the high mortality of *P. aeruginosa* pneumonia, an aminoglycoside should be added to the first few days of treatment. If *Legionella* sp. is documented, consider addition of rifampin.

5. The newest fluoroquinolones, levofloxacin and sparfloxacin, are promising therapeutic options for CAP. These drugs have a convenient once-daily dosing schedule and are active against the major respiratory pathogens. Both have enhanced activity against *S. pneumoniae*, including penicillin-resistant strains. However, judicious use because of their broad activity is recommended to avoid further antibiotic resistance patterns.

12. How long should the pneumonia be treated?

In general, *S. pneumoniae* should be treated for 7–10 days. Longer courses of therapy (10–14 days) may be required for *M. pneumoniae, C. pneumoniae,* and *Legionella* sp. Immunocompromised patients with Legionnaire's disease may require up to 21 days of therapy. Shorter treatment courses may be possible with the introduction of the new macrolide azithromycin (5 days). However, at current doses, azithromycin does not achieve high serum levels and should not be used in patients with suspected bacteremia or in moderately to severely ill patients.

13. When can antibiotics be switched from parental to oral therapy?

Two randomized, controlled studies reported good clinical response with switching from parental to oral therapy on day 3 and day 6. A more practical approach, although not based on solid evidence, is to switch to oral therapy when the clinical condition has stabilized and fever has resolved.

14. Which oral antimicrobials achieve serum levels comparable to parental therapy?

Doxycycline, minocycline, chloramphenicol, trimethoprim/sulfamethoxazole, and most fluoroquinolones.

15. When should pneumonia resolve on chest radiograph?

Complete radiographic clearance of CAP in an inpatient and outpatient setting occurred in 50% of patients at 2 weeks, 64% at 4 weeks, and 73% at 6 weeks. If the patient is older, has bacteremic pneumonia, COPD, alcoholism, or underlying chronic illness, radiographic clearing is only 25% at 4 weeks. Clearance was faster in outpatients and nonsmokers.

16. When should a physician be concerned about penicillin-resistant pneumococci?

Levels of penicillin-resistant *S. pneumoniae* are greater than 25% in some areas of the United States and exceed 40% in parts of Europe. The emergence of resistant organisms has important implications for the selection of empiric regimens. Most strains have intermediate resistance and can be treated with high doses of penicillin or certain third-generation cephalosporins. Vancomycin or imipenem/cilastatin is recommended for high-level penicillin-resistant pneumococci. Of note, the mortality rate is similar for resistant and sensitive strains. The newer fluoroquinolones may have a role in therapy.

17. Who should get the influenza vaccine?

1. All persons older than 65.
2. Patients with underlying chronic illnesses such as COPD, heart failure, and diabetes mellitus
3. Residents of chronic care facilities
4. Persons who transmit to high-risk persons, such as health care workers, nursing home employees, and household members

18. What bacterial superinfection is most frequently seen with influenza?

Streptococcus pneumoniae is the most common bacterial pathogen complicating influenza. The incidence of pneumonia caused by *Staphylococcus aureus*, however, increases significantly during influenza periods and accounts for 25% or more of secondary bacterial infections in some series.

19. To whom, when, why, and how often should a physician give the pneumococcal vaccine?

To whom: Good candidates include patients with chronic cardiopulmonary disease, asplenia, liver disease, alcoholism, or diabetes and persons older than 65 years. Poor responders include patients with renal failure, malignancy (especially chronic lymphocytic leukemia or myeloma), or HIV.

When: Efficacy decreases with age. Thus, physicians should screen for candidates at age 50.

Why: Each year pneumococcal disease kills about 32,000 people in the United States. The overall case-fatality rate is approximately 5%. Many of these deaths can be prevented with a single injection of pneumococcal polysaccharide vaccine.

How often: Revaccination is not routine. The vaccine offers 10-year protection despite early antibody drop. Consider revaccination in high-risk patients after 6 years or in patients who received the 14-valent vaccine. (The current vaccine is effective against 23 serotypes, which account for 90% of clinical infections.)

20. Describe the potential complications of pneumonia.

Because of concern about development of a complicated parapneumonic effusion or empyema, a repeat chest radiograph with sampling of pleural fluid should be obtained if clinical response to therapy is inadequate. Chest tube drainage with or without installation of lytic agents, thoracoscopy, or thoracotomy may be needed for definitive treatment. Hematogenously spread infections include meningitis, arthritis, endocarditis, pericarditis, and peritonitis. Progression to adult respiratory distress syndrome, sepsis, or multiorgan dysfunction syndrome may further complicate pneumonia.

21. Which patients with pneumonia should be tested for *Legionella* sp.?

Legionnaire's disease is more common in the elderly, cigarette smokers, diabetics, immunosuppressed people, and patients with chronic lung, heart, or kidney disease. Especially high-risk populations include transplant recipients, patients taking corticosteroids, and patients with hairy cell leukemia. Testing should be reserved for patients who are immunosuppressed, do not respond to beta-lactam antibiotics, or have a classic presentation. Avoid testing in areas with a low incidence of *Legionella* (< 5%).

22. What is TWAR?

An unusual strain of *Chlamydia* was first reported in 1985 and designated TWAR because of its similarity to a conjunctival chlamydial isolate recovered in Taiwan (TW-183) and a pharyngeal isolate from the United States (AR-39). TWAR is distinct from other forms of *Chlamydia* and has been given the species designation *Chlamydia pneumoniae*. Approximately 50% of adults worldwide have significant titers to *C. pneumoniae* with few geographic variations. Immunity, however, is short lived. Infections are markedly underdiagnosed because many patients are asymptomatic and accurate tests are not generally available. The drugs of choice are macrolides or tetracyclines.

CONTROVERSIES

23. Should antibiotic regimens be based on sputum Gram stain and culture results?

For: (1) Sensitivity and specificity are higher with attention to collection and processing. (2) Finding pneumococci on Gram stain allows directed therapy. No organisms but many leukocytes suggest possibility of *Legionella* sp., *C. pneumoniae*, *Mycoplasma* sp., or viral etiology. Direct staining of sputum may be diagnostic for some pulmonary infections (*Mycobacterium* sp., *Nocardia* sp., endemic fungi, *Legionella* sp., and *P. carinii*). (3) Recovery of organisms not part of normal respiratory flora or demonstration of a resistant organism in patients already receiving antibiotics can direct therapy. If isolation of penicillin-resistant pneumococci is anticipated, cultures should be obtained. (4) Emergence of resistant organisms is an increasing concern when empiric regimens are used.

Against: (1) Patients often have nonproductive cough. (2) Prior use of antibiotics ruins yield. (3) Sensitivity and specificity of Gram stains are poor (gram-negative oragnisms are often missed, whereas gram-positive organisms are overcalled). (4) Routine cultures often demonstrate pathogens, but sensitivity and specificity are low. (5) Early empiric therapy directed at likely pathogens can improve the outcome, whereas identification of the pathogen is not associated with improved survival rates.

24. Are serologic tests useful?

For: Useful in epidemiologic surveys. Serologic tests for *Legionella* sp., *Mycoplasma* sp. (including cold agglutinins), viral agents, endemic fungi, and other unusual pathogens should be considered in nonresponding patients.

Against: Serologic methods based on demonstrating antibody response between acute and convalescent serum samples are not rapid diagnostic tools and are not useful in the initial evaluation of patients with CAP. Convalescent titers are often not done, negating even the epidemiologic value.

BIBLIOGRAPHY

1. Bartlett JG, Mundy LH: Community-acquired pneumonia. N Engl J Med 333:1618–1624, 1995.
2. Fang GD, Fine M, Orloff J, et al: New and emerging etiologies for community-acquired pneumonia with implications for therapy: A prospective multicenter trial of 359 cases. Medicine 69:307–316, 1990.
3. Fine MJ, Smith MA, Carson CA, et al: Prognosis and outcomes of patients with community-acquired pneumonia: A meta-analysis. JAMA 275:134–141, 1995.
4. Niederman MS, Bass JB, Campbell GD, et al: Guidelines for the initial management of adults with community-acquired pneumonia: Diagnosis, assessment of severity, and initial antimicrobial therapy. Am Rev Respir Dis 148:1418–1426, 1993.
5. Centers for Disease Control and Prevention. Pneumonia and Influenza Death Rates - United States, 1979-1994. MMWR 44:535-537, 1995.
6. Mittle RL, Schwab RJ, Duchin JS, et al: Radiographic resolution of community-acquired pneumonia. Am J Respir Crit Care Med 149:630–635, 1994.
7. Pinner RW, Teutsch SM, Simonsen L, et al: Trends in infectious diseases mortality in the United States. JAMA 275:189–193, 1996.
8. Riquelme R, Torres A, El-Ebiary M, et al: Community-acquired pneumonia in the elderly: A multi-variate analysis of risk and prognostic factors. Am J Respir Crit Care Med 154:1450–1455, 1996.

49. NOSOCOMIAL PNEUMONIA IN NONINTUBATED PATIENTS

Benjamin W. Berg, M.D.

1. Nosocomial pneumonia is the most common hospital-acquired infection in the United States. True or false?

False. Nosocomial pneumonia is the *second* most common hospital-acquired infection after urinary infection. However, nosocomial pneumonia is the most common *lethal* infection acquired by hospitalized patients. Nosocomial pneumonia accounts for approximately 15% of all hospital-acquired infections. Mortality in patients with nosocomial pneumonia ranges from 8–40%. Higher mortality rates are seen in patients in the intensive care unit (ICU). Attributable mortality rates of 30–33% are reported.

2. What is the most common source of infecting organisms in bacterial nosocomial pneumonia?

Aspiration of organisms colonizing the oropharynx or upper gastrointestinal tract is the most common source for bacterial nosocomial pneumonia. After hospitalization the oropharynx becomes rapidly colonized with aerobic gram-negative bacilli. Colonization occurs in 30–40% of moderately ill patients and in 60–75% of ICU patients. Aspiration is present in 45% of normal subjects during sleep, and many hospitalized patients have a predisposition to aspiration.

3. Risk factors for nosocomial pneumonia have been identified. True or false?

True. Patients with the following risk factors are at increased risk for nosocomial bacterial pneumonia:

Definite risks	Probable risks
Age > 60 years	24-hour ventilator circuit changes
Intubated patients (surgery included)	Hospitalization in fall or winter
Depressed level of consciousness	Stress bleeding prophylaxis with H_2 blockers
Chronic lung disease	Supine position
Prior administration of antibiotics	Presence of nasogastric tube
Large volume aspiration	

Individual risk can be further evaluated by the following scheme, which allows consideration of multiple risks that have been identified inconsistently in different patient study populations:

- Host factors: extremes of age, immune status, specific disease processes (e.g., diabetes, cystic fibrosis, malignancy).
- Factors that enhance colonization of the oropharynx and GI tract: admission to ICU, antimicrobial therapy.
- Aspiration-promoting conditions: supine position, nasogastric tube, gastroesophageal reflux disease, neurologic disorders, swallowing dysfunction.
- Exposure to respiratory therapy devices or other contaminated hospital equipment: intubation, lung disease, surgery, poor handwashing practices.
- Impaired respiratory clearance mechanisms: diminished mental status, decreased cough reflex, immobilization, head and neck or thoracic surgical procedures, underlying lung disease.

4. How is nosocomial pneumonia transmitted?

- Aspiration of oropharyngeal flora (most common mechanism).
- Inhalation of aerosols containing pathogenic organisms from respiratory therapy equipment or person-to-person transmission.

- Hematogenous spread of infection from a distant body site (uncommon). Translocation of gastrointestinal flora is hypothesized to occur in some patients.
- Cross-contamination from gloves, hands, or devices.
- Contaminated hospital water supply (associated with *Legionella* spp. infection).

5. Match the mode(s) of transmission for the following organisms which have been described in nosocomial pneumonia.

Organism	Mode(s) of transmission
1. *Legionella* species	a. Person-to-person respiratory droplets
2. *Mycobacterium tuberculosis*	b. Fomite or hand contamination
3. Respiratory syncytial virus (RSV)	c. Hospital water supply
4. Aspergillosis	d. Inhalation of environmental organisms
5. *Pseudomonas* species	

Answers:

1—c. Person-to-person transmission has not been described. Aerosolized hospital water supply in showers, medical devices, and hospital cooling towers have been implicated as sources in nosocomial legionellosis.

2—a. *M. tuberculosis* survives well outside the body but is not infectious unless aerosolized.

3—a, b. Primarily in pediatric settings. Portal of entry is nasal or conjunctival mucosa.

4—d. Inhalation of spores in immunocompromised patients is the most common portal of entry.

5—b, c. Contaminated respiratory therapy equipment and health care workers' cross-contamination are modes of transmission for gram-negative nosocomial infection in addition to the more common aspiration mechanism.

6. *Aspergillus* spp. cause nosocomial pneumonia in immunocompromised patients. Name three specific conditions that predispose to nosocomial invasive pulmonary aspergillosis.

1. Neutropenia (absolute neutrophil count < 500/mm^3) from any cause
2. Bone marrow transplantation
3. Solid organ transplantation

Invasive aspergillosis is a severe respiratory infection with a mortality rate of over 90% in neutropenic patients. It is most often encountered in patients with absolute neutrophil counts of < 500/mm^3 from leukemia or chemotherapy. Patients undergoing bone marrow transplantation are susceptible to a greater extent than patients with heart, kidney, or liver transplants.

7. In what proportion of patients with hospital-acquired pneumonia is a definitive pathogen identified?

No specific pathogen is identified in up to 50% of patients with nosocomial pneumonia. This finding is similar to the data for community-acquired pneumonia. In patients who undergo invasive procedures for diagnosis, including bronchoscopy with quantitative cultures of brush or bronchoalveolar lavage samples and transthoracic needle aspiration, specific diagnoses are made more often.

8. Do viruses cause nosocomial pneumonia?

Yes. Influenza and respiratory syncytial virus (RSV) are the most common causes of viral nosocomial pneumonia. Hospital outbreaks of viral pneumonia are most commonly encountered in the setting of concurrent community outbreaks. Most commonly influenza affects elderly persons, whereas RSV occurs on pediatric wards. Immunocompromised patients and patients with chronic medical conditions are most susceptible. Respiratory droplet transmission and transmission by hands and fomites has been documented. Infectivity is greatest during the first three days of illness. Diagnosis can be made by culture for both RSV and influenza.

9. Is respiratory isolation required for patients with nosocomial pneumonia or other hospitalized patients with pneumonia?

Some patients with pneumonia should be placed in respiratory isolation to prevent nosocomial spread of infection by respiratory droplets. *M. tuberculosis* is the most commonly recognized organism for which respiratory isolation is advised. Other organisms for which respiratory isolation is advised include influenza, and possibly *Pneumocystis carinii*, which may be transmissible to immunocompromised and elderly patients. Handwashing remains the most effective method of preventing person-to-person transmission of nosocomial pneumonia agents. During RSV and influenza outbreaks all persons contacting an infected patient should wear masks and follow strict handwashing protocols.

10. Name four preventive strategies for nosocomial pneumonia.

1. Administer amantadine or rimantadine to all patients and staff without contraindications during an influenza outbreak.

2. Administer pneumococcal polysaccharide and influenza vaccines to patients at high risk for complications of pneumococcal pneumonia. Included in this category are patients over 65 years of age and patients with chronic cardiopulmonary disease, diabetes, alcoholism, cirrhosis, or cerebrospinal fluid leaks. Immunosupressed children and adults and patients with functional or anatomic asplenia also should be vaccinated. In some studies 20% of early nosocomial pneumonia is caused by *Streptococcus pneumoniae*.

3. Elevate the head of the bed 30–45°. This strategy is particularly important in patients at risk for aspiration, including patients with nasogastric tubes or endotracheal tubes.

4. Wear gloves for handling respiratory secretions or objects contaminated with respiratory secretions of any patient. Wash hands after removing gloves.

11. Which organisms predominate in nosocomial pneumonia?

Bacterial infection accounts for over 90% of reported cases of nosocomial pneumonia. Viruses, protozoans, parasites, and fungi are much less commonly reported. Data from a variety of sources regarding the frequency of bacterial species in nosocomial infection are presented in the following table.

Frequency of Bacterial Species in Nosocomial Infection

GRAM-NEGATIVE AEROBES	FREQUENCY	GRAM-POSITIVE AEROBES	FREQUENCY	ANAEROBIC BACTERIA	FREQUENCY
50–75% OF ALL INFECTIONS	(%)	17–56% OF ALL INFECTIONS	(%)	7–35% OF ALL INFECTIONS	(%)
Pseudomonas aeruginosa	17–25	*Staphylococcus aureus*	15–30	*Peptostreptococcus* spp.	14
Klebsiella spp.	7–23	*Streptococcus* spp.	1–31	*Peptococcus* spp.	11
Escherichia coli	6–14			*Fusobacterium* spp.	10
Enterobacter spp.	4–11			*Bacteroides fragilis*	8
Proteus spp.	3–11			*Prevotella* spp.	9

Polymicrobial infections are present in up to 40% of cases of nosocomial bacterial pneumonia. Anaerobic infections are frequently polymicrobial and may be more likely in patients with aspiration.

12. Are any organisms associated with proportionally higher mortality rates in nosocomial pneumonia?

Yes. Pseudomonal infections are associated with higher mortality rates than infections caused by other organisms. The mortality attributable to pseudomonal nosocomial pneumonia increased from 27 to 43% in one study of ventilator-associated pneumonia. Mortality rates of up to 70% have been reported in patients with *P. aeruginosa* nosocomial pneumonia. Bacteremia is present in 2–6% of patients with nosocomial pneumonia and is also associated with an increased mortality (up to 58%).

13. Which patients with nosocomial pneumonia require ICU management?

Patients with nosocomial pneumonia who are at risk for respiratory failure from hypoxemia or hypoventilation or who have signs of sepsis should be monitored in an ICU setting. The following criteria may be used as guidelines for ICU admission:

1. **Oxygenation:** progressive hypoxia. Arterial oxygen saturation < 90% on FiO_2 of 35% or more.

2. **Ventilation:** progressive respiratory acidosis with arterial blood pH < 7.3.

3. **Metabolic status:** progressive metabolic acidosis with arterial blood pH < 7.3.

4. **Hypotension:** requirement for vasopressor agents or failure to respond to IV volume infusion.

5. **Respiratory therapy:** frequent suctioning or chest physiotherapy requirements, especially in patients with underlying lung disease.

These criteria are minimal guidelines to integrate into the total clinical evaluation of an individual patient. ICU admission should be based on the capabilities of individual institutions and individual patient's physiologic and other clinical parameters.

14. What are the diagnostic criteria for nosocomial pneumonia?

Nosocomial pneumonia is by definition a process that is acquired after admission to the hospital. This definition is complicated by the fact that patients who are admitted from long-term care facilities or skilled nursing facilities with pneumonia share the epidemiologic and microbiologic characteristics of patients with pneumonia acquired in the hospital. Thus nosocomial pneumonia can be diagnosed in patients who acquired infection outside the acute hospital setting. The following criteria are used to diagnose nosocomial pneumonia:

- New pulmonary infiltrate
- Respiratory symptoms—cough, sputum production, dyspnea
- Fever
- Elevated white blood cell count
- Positive Gram stain or culture of respiratory secretions

15. What is the specificity of the clinical diagnostic criteria for nosocomial pneumonia?

The clinical criteria for diagnosis of nosocomial pneumonia are highly nonspecific, especially in ventilated patients. Many patients are treated empirically based on clinical criteria. When strict pathologic and quantitative microbiologic criteria are applied, nosocomial pneumonia rates in ICU patients have fallen from 26% (using clinical criteria) to 9% (using strict microbiologic criteria). Similar studies have not been conducted in nonventilated and non-ICU patients. Accurate diagnostic criteria with high sensitivity and specificity depend on accurate microbiologic diagnosis, usually requiring bronchoscopy with quantitative culture of bronchoalveolar lavage fluid or a protected specimen brushing of the distal airways. These techniques increase diagnostic specificity to 70–100% but may cause complications.

16. Match the organism with the specific risk factor(s) for nosocomial pneumonia.

Organism	Risk factor
Legionella spp.	Aspiration
P. aeruginosa	Head trauma or coma
Aspergillus spp.	Corticosteroid therapy
S. aureus	Diabetes and/or renal failure
Anaerobic organisms	Prolonged hospitalization
	Neutropenia
	Underlying structural lung disease (e.g., emphysema, bronchiectasis)
	Prior antibiotic therapy

Answers:

Legionella spp.—corticosteroids, prolonged hospitalization, prior antibiotics.

P. aeruginosa—underlying structural lung disease, prolonged hospitalization, prior antibiotics.

Aspergillus spp.—neutropenia.

S. aureus—head trauma, diabetes, renal failure, IV drug abuse, coma.

Anaerobic organisms—aspiration.

17. List three conditions that can clinically mimic nosocomial pneumonia.

1. Pulmonary embolism
2. Cardiogenic or noncardiogenic pulmonary edema
3. Chemical aspiration pneumonitis

These conditions, in addition to alveolar hemorrhage, bronchoalveolar carcinoma, pulmonary infarction, pulmonary lymphoma, amiodarone toxicity, and others, may cause failure to respond to therapy. Failure to follow the expected clinical course after initiation of empiric therapy for nosocomial pneumonia should prompt reevaluation for alternative diagnoses or a specific microbiologic diagnosis.

18. When can a hospitalized patient with active pulmonary tuberculosis be taken out of respiratory isolation?

Controlled data regarding the transmissibility of tuberculosis after initiation of therapy are sparse. A large body of anecdotal, inferential, and accidental data allows a practical approach to the problem of a potentially infected person who is in the hospital. Sputum smears correlate well with infectivity. For patients with negative sputum smears on three occasions, respiratory isolation is not required. After initiation of therapy for tuberculosis, sputum smears may remain positive for a prolonged interval, especially in patients with cavitary disease. An interval of two weeks of effective therapy (with attention to resistance patterns) has been traditionally used to define noninfectivity, regardless of sputum smear status. Discharge to the home environment after this interval is also most likely to be safe, because virtually all household contact purified protein derivative (PPD) skin test conversions are due to exposure before diagnosis.

Many hospitals maintain respiratory isolation until the sputum smear is negative in patients who continue to require hospitalization for treatment of tuberculosis or other reasons. This prudent strategy prevents nosocomial outbreaks. Nosocomial transmission of tuberculosis by smear-negative index cases has been described.

19. What are the major complications of nosocomial pneumonia?

The major complications of nosocomial pneumonia relate to the underlying host status, infecting organism, and efficacy of therapy. Pleural effusion is commonly found and mandates evaluation. Progression from a simple parapneumonic effusion to a complicated effusion can be predicted by a pH < 7.2 and lactate dehydrogenase level > 1000 IU/L. The presence of pus defines empyema, and tube thoracostomy is usually indicated. A complicated parapneumonic effusion defined by low pH (< 7.2), positive Gram stain, positive culture, glucose < 40 mg/dl, or exudative characteristics requires serial evaluation with repeat thoracentesis or placement of a thoracostomy tube to minimize the risk of empyema. Other complications include bacteremia and sepsis, hemoptysis, bronchopleural fistula formation, cavitation, adult respiratory distress syndrome, and pleuritic pain.

CONTROVERSY

20. Does selective decontamination of the GI tract prevent nosocomial pneumonia?

Selective decontamination of the gastrointestinal tract (SDD) has been hypothesized to remove or diminish the endogenous reservoir of gram-negative anaerobic organisms, which are associated with the majority of nosocomial pneumonia infections. This strategy was first used in leukemic patients and later in mechanically ventilated patients in efforts to decrease the incidence of nosocomial pneumonia.

Results of studies reveal that application of nonabsorbable antibiotic pastes and IV antibiotics clearly diminish pharyngeal and respiratory colonization with gram-negative organisms. In some studies gram-negative pneumonia was also decreased; however, an increase in pneumonia caused by gram-positive organisms offset the decrease in gram-negative infections. In other studies the overall rate of nosocomial pneumonia decreased. In 12 of 13 controlled trials SDD was associated with decreased rates of infection in SDD (8–52%) vs. control (27–81%) groups.

Analyses of overall mortality rates and length of hospital stay have failed to reveal any consistent benefit. Concerns about increased cost and emergence of resistant bacteria combined with the lack of definitive demonstrated benefit have caused some to question the potential benefit of SDD. Nonetheless, the potential benefit remains significant, and studies to evaluate appropriate populations for application of SDD are ongoing.

BIBLIOGRAPHY

1. American Thoracic Society. Hospital-acquired pneumonia in adults: Diagnosis, assessment of severity; initial antimicrobial therapy and preventive strategies. A consensus statement. Am Rev Respir Crit Care Med 153:1711–1725, 1996.
2. Bergogne-Berezin E: Therapy and prevention of nosocomial pneumonia. Chest 108:26s–34s, 1995.
3. Centers for Disease Control and Prevention: Guidelines for prevention of nosocomial pneumonia. MMWR 46(No. RR-01), 1997.
4. Craven DE, Steger KA: Epidemiology of nosocomial pneumonia: New perspectives on an old disease. Chest 108:1s–15s, 1995.
5. Mandell LA, Marrie TJ, Niederman MS: Initial antimicrobial treatment of hospital-acquired pneumonia in adults: A conference report. Can J Infect Dis 4:317–321, 1993.
6. Selective Decontamination of the Digestive Tract Trailists Collaborative Group: Meta-analysis of randomized controlled trials of selective decontamination of the digestive tract. BMJ 307:525–532, 1993.
7. Sepkowitz KA: How contagious is tuberculosis? Clin Infect Dis 23:954–962, 1996.

50. VENTILATOR-ASSOCIATED PNEUMONIA

Joseph M. Parker, M.D.

1. What is the incidence of nosocomial pneumonia in mechanically ventilated patients?

The risk of developing ventilator-associated pneumonia (VAP) has been estimated at approximately 1–3% per patient day of mechanical ventilation.

2. What are the consequences of VAP?

Nosocomial pneumonia is the second most common cause of nosocomial infection; however, it is the most common cause of mortality due to a hospital-acquired infection. The attributable mortality of VAP in various studies ranges from 27–33%. Mortality is even higher in patients infected with virulent organisms (*Pseudomonas aeruginosa* and *Acinetobacter* sp.).

3. What are the most common pathogens isolated from patients with VAP?

Based on the National Nosocomial Infection Study (NNIS) data from 1986–1989, *P. aeruginosa* (17%), *Staphylococcus aureus* (16%), *Enterobacter* sp. (11%), *Klebsiella pneumoniae* (7%), and *Escherichia coli* (6%) were the most commonly isolated organisms. *P. aeruginosa* and *S. aureus* appear to be increasing in incidence over the past decade.

4. Aspiration is believed to be the most common mechanism for developing VAP. Where are the primary reservoirs colonized by pathogenic organisms?

The oropharynx, endotracheal tube, stomach, respiratory therapy equipment, paranasal sinuses, and trachea have been implicated as reservoirs for aspiration of infected secretions into the distal airways and for development of VAP.

5. What are recognized risk factors for the development of VAP?

1. **Host factors.** Acute and chronic illnesses lead to rapid oropharyngeal colonization with gram-negative organisms. Immunosuppression prevents an adequate host response to a bacterial challenge.

2. **Surgery.** Postoperative atelectasis, mucus plugging, and decreased clearance of lower airway secretions contribute to the development of VAP.

3. **Medications**. Broad-spectrum antibiotics abolish normal flora and lead to colonization with more virulent and frequently antibiotic-resistant organisms.

4. **Invasive devices.** The endotracheal tube prevents normal lower airway clearance of organisms by coughing and ciliary transport and provides a conduit for the introduction of bacteria. Nasogastric or orogastric tubes interrupt the normal function of the lower esophageal sphincter, leading to greater incidence of gastric reflux and aspiration.

5. **Respiratory therapy devices.** The ventilator tubing condensate quickly becomes colonized with large amounts of bacteria. If the patient is turned or the bed rail is raised carelessly, the patient is placed at risk.

6. How does the lower airway defend itself from a bacterial challenge?

The alveolar macrophage (AM) is the primary cell that serves to maintain the sterility of the gas-exchanging airways. The AM is capable of eliminating a challenge of 10^5 or fewer *S. aureus*. Higher numbers of organisms or more virulent organisms (*Pseudomonas*) cause the AM to initiate an inflammatory response manifested by the release of cytokines (tumor necrosis factor in particular) and the recruitment of polymorphonuclear leukocytes in an attempt to contain the infection.

7. List diagnoses other than pneumonia that may produce fever and radiographic infiltrates.

The mnemonic is **TPA = 123**: T (1), P (2), and A (3).

Tumor: lymphoma (leukemia in particular)

Pulmonary infarction or embolism

Pulmonary hemorrhage

Aspiration

Atelectasis

Adult respiratory distress syndrome (ARDS; fibroproliferative phase)

8. Clinicians frequently rely on the portable anteroposterior (AP) chest radiograph in establishing the presence of infiltrates suggestive of VAP. How effective are AP chest radiographs in demonstrating infiltrates?

AP chest radiographs are relatively insensitive for detecting infiltrates in the lower lung fields. A study comparing AP films with CT scans of the chest found that 26% of infiltrates were not seen on AP films, particularly in the lower lung fields. ARDS in particular lowers the sensitivity and specificity of this technique.

9. What are the usual clinical criteria for VAP? How sensitive and specific are they?

Fever (temperature > 38° C), leukocytosis, new or worsening radiographic infiltrate, purulent sputum, and sputum or tracheal aspirate Gram stain with > 25 polymorphonucleocytes and < 10 squamous epithelial cells per low power field are the usual clinical criteria. They have moderate-to-high sensitivity (60–90%) but relatively low specificity (< 50%).

10. It is common clinical practice to treat the organism cultured from the endotracheal secretions. What may be the true clinical utility of the endotracheal tube aspirate Gram stain and culture?

Studies using tissue culture and other invasive techniques have found the concordance of the etiologic organism with endotracheal cultures to be as low as 40%. The true value in the endotracheal culture and Gram stain may be in excluding VAP. When bacteria are not seen on the Gram stain, pneumonia is present in less than 5% of cases.

11. Sampling of lower respiratory secretions in the involved area of the lung is used to establish the causative organism or to exclude the presence of VAP. What methods are currently available? What are their respective sensitivity and specificity?

1. **Bronchoscopic protected specimen brush** (PSB) uses a telescoping catheter that is protected from upper airway contamination to obtain lower airway secretions. This methods collects a small amount of fluid (0.1 ml) for quantitative cultures. It has a high specificity (approximately 90%) and a moderate-to-high sensitivity (80%).

2. **Bronchoscopic bronchoalveolar lavage** (BAL) is the technique of instilling 100–200 ml of saline into a distal airway to sample what is believed to be approximately one million alveoli. This method has a higher sensitivity (90%) but somewhat lower specificity by some studies than PSB (80–90%). More recently, the use of protected BAL catheters has duplicated PSB's specificity while retaining the sensitivity of the BAL.

3. **Other available methods** for obtaining lower respiratory secretions include blind BAL with a specially designed catheter, transthoracic needle aspiration, and lung biopsy.

12. What are the respective thresholds for distinguishing positive from negative results of PSB and BAL to establish the presence and causative organism of suspected VAP?

Quantitative cultures with $\geq 10^3$ colony-forming units (CFU) for PSB and $\geq 10^4$ CFU for BAL are considered to be consistent with the diagnosis of VAP. Cultures with one log growth below these thresholds should be interpreted with caution. Serial studies and/or the clinical course should dictate the clinician's response.

13. Which mechanically ventilated patients are at risk for complications of invasive bronchoscopic techniques for suspected VAP?

High risk	Moderate risk
$PaO_2 < 70$ with $FiO_2 > 70\%$	PEEP > 10 cm H_2O
Positive end-expiratory pressure (PEEP) > 15 cm H_2O	Auto-PEEP > 15 cm H_2O
Active bronchospasm	Prothrombin time (PT) >
Recent myocardial infarction	1.5 × control
Unstable arrhythmia	Increased intracranial pressure
Mean arterial pressure < 65 mm on vasopressors	
Platelet count < 20,000	

14. How commonly are patients with VAP infected at another site? What are the most common sites of infection?

A recent study by Meduri et al. found concomitant infection in 14 of 19 patients with well-documented VAP, some of whom had more than one additional site. Catheter-related infections, sinusitis, and urinary tract infections were the most common. Organisms other than the causative agent identified in the patient's VAP were found in approximately 50% of cases.

15. What interventions are available and effective for preventing VAP?

1. Infection control and surveillance
2. Hand washing
3. Isolation of patients with resistant organisms
4. Nutritional support with enteral feeding
5. Semierect positioning (> 30°)
6. Use of sucralfate for gastrointestinal bleeding prophylaxis
7. Careful handling of respiratory therapy equipment, changing ventilator circuits > 48 hr
8. Continuous lateral bed rotation

16. Most cases of VAP represent endemic infection; however, some (< 5%) cases of VAP are epidemic. What are the common routes of epidemic transmission of VAP?

1. **Contact transmission** by direct physical contact, indirect contact with contaminated inanimate objects, and droplet contact.

2. **Airborne transmission** by aerosolized particles over a distance.

Epidemic VAP pathogens include many of the same organisms as endemic VAP; additional pathogens include viral (influenza, respiratory syncytial virus), fungal (*Aspergillus* sp.), and atypical organisms (*Legionella* sp., mycobacteria).

17. What are potential reasons for antibiotic failure in VAP?

1. Misdiagnosis of the original pneumonia—a noninfectious cause of fever and infiltrate or an alternate infectious process.

2. Misdiagnosis of the causative agent—lack of sensitivity or specificity of the diagnostic technique or an opportunistic or unusual organism.

3. Inadequate antibiotic coverage—drug resistance, polymicrobial infection, or antibiotic inappropriate for the organism.

18. What are the potential patterns of response in antibiotic failure?

Pattern	Cause
Rapid deterioration (< 72 hr)	Misdiagnosis—not pneumonia, wrong organism, or resistant organism
Nonresolving pneumonia	Misdiagnosis
	Persistent organism due to resistance, wrong regimen, superinfection
Improvement followed by deterioration	Acquired resistance, superinfection, polymicrobial infection

19. How should a clinician respond to suspected antibiotic failure in VAP?

In general, an additional diagnostic test (PSB or BAL) should be performed with the following changes:

1. **Sterile culture** ($< 10^2$ CFU)—continue use of antibiotics if used less than 72 hr; discontinue and consider another cause of fever and infiltrate if antibiotics used more than 72 hr.

2. **Indeterminate culture** (PSB 10^2 or BAL $10^2–10^3$ CFU) **and stable patient**—continue current medications.

3. **Positive culture** (PSB $\geq 10^3$ or BAL $\geq 10^4$ CFU) **or unstable patient**—add or change coverage.

CONTROVERSY

20. Is selective gut decontamination an effective means of preventing VAP?

For: Oropharyngeal and gastric colonization occurs early in mechanically ventilated patients at risk for VAP. Aspiration of oropharyngeal or gastric contents is the most common means for the development of VAP; therefore, suppression of bacterial pathogens with antibiotics, usually topical nonsystemically applied antibiotics, may decrease the bacterial load and allow lower respiratory defense mechanisms to clear the challenge effectively. Studies using selective gut decontamination have demonstrated a decreased incidence of VAP and reduced rates of colonization with pathogenic organisms.

Against: Suppression of bacterial colonization may result in development of resistant organisms or colonization by more virulent organisms. Some pathogens (notably *P. aeruginosa*) may directly colonize the trachea, thus bypassing the treated areas. Although studies have demonstrated that the incidence of VAP may be reduced by this method, no studies have demonstrated a substantial decrease in mortality or morbidity. Selective gut decontamination, therefore, increases the cost of medical care without demonstrable benefits.

BIBLIOGRAPHY

1. Fagon JY, Chastre J, Hance AJ, et al: Nosocomial pneumonia in ventilated patients: A cohort study evaluating attributable mortality and hospital stay. Am J Med 94:281–288, 1993.
2. Kollef MH: Ventilator-associated pneumonia: A multivariate analysis. JAMA 270:1965–1970, 1993.
3. Meduri GU, Mauldin OL, Wunderink RG, et al: Causes of fever and pulmonary densities in patients with clinical manifestations of ventilator-associated pneumonia. Chest 106:221–235, 1994.
4. Wunderink RG: The diagnosis of nosocomial pneumonia. Pulmon Crit Care Update 10(2):1–10, 1994.
5. Wunderink RG (ed): Pneumonia in the intensive care unit. Clin Chest Med 16:1–227, 1994.

XV. Cerebrospinal Infections

51. MENINGITIS

R. Scott Miller, M.D.

1. How does classification by syndromes of central nervous system infection help in the initial approach to a patient?

Clinical manifestations of central nervous system (CNS) infections depend on the anatomic site involved, acuteness of presentation, and underlying disease processes. Although not always present, fever, headache, nuchal rigidity, altered mental status, ataxia, and/or seizures should alert the clinician to the possibility of a CNS infection.

Acute meningitis syndrome is the most common CNS infection and represents a true medical emergency. Dominant features include onset of fever, headache, photophobia, and meningismus over hours to days. Acute meningitis syndromes are classified into bacterial and aseptic (viral, culture-negative bacterial, fungal, mycobacterial, and noninfectious) causes.

Subacute meningitis is defined by duration of symptoms longer than 1 week. It is caused by slow-growing agents such as *Mycobacterium tuberculosis* or *Borrelia burgdorferi* as well as by fungi such as *Cryptococcus neoformans*.

Chronic meningitis is defined by duration of months or years, often with intermittent symptoms. Common causes include tuberculosis and neurosyphilis.

Meningoencephalitis refers to infections involving both the leptomeninges and cerebrospinal fluid (CSF) as well as brain parenchyma. Symptoms include altered mental status (often earlier in the illness than meningitis) and localizing neurologic signs.

Parameningeal infections, including subdural empyema and epidural abscess or brain abscess, are space-occupying lesions that may mimic symptoms of acute meningitis.

2. What are the portals of entry into the CNS?

Most infectious agents gain access to the CNS via the bloodstream and choroid plexus, although exact mechanisms are poorly understood. For example, enteroviruses invade across the brain microvasculature after a generalized viremic phase. Contiguous spread from adjacent sites (otitis media or sinusitis), retrograde intraneuronal transportation (as in polio or herpes simplex virus [HSV]), post-operative infection or trauma, and infection through indwelling devices (CSF shunts) are the other mechanisms of access to the CNS.

3. Why do certain organisms show neurotropism (i.e., have the potential to cause bacterial meningitis)?

Many organisms are capable of causing bacteremia, but relatively few are able to seed the meninges. Certain strains of bacteria possess specific virulence factors that allow successful invasion into the CNS. Recently these processes have been described for neonatal *Escherichia coli* meningitis. The initial step is adherence to epithelial cells, which involves specific pili or the bacterial capsule. Encapsulated K1 *E. coli* strains evade complement-mediated phagocytosis in the bloodstream and are able to sustain bacteremia. Specific S-fimbria on the organism's surface contain a sugar, which facilitates adherence to CNS microvasculature. An outer membrane protein (OmpA) contributes to invasion ability in vitro and allows translocation via intracellular vacuoles.

4. Why is the CSF considered an area of impaired host resistance?

In the absence of inflammation, the CSF is markedly impaired in its intrinsic ability to fight infections; hence, high bacterial loads may exist in this compartment (up to 10 million colony-forming units/ml of CSF). The impaired resistance is due to the following factors:

- Absence of measurable complement and specific antibody and hence inefficient opsonization and phagocytosis
- Initial paucity of phagocytic cells
- Poor antibiotic penetration (typically 10% or less of serum levels)

Therefore, optimal antibiotic therapy requires a drug with bactericidal effect to sterilize the CSF.

5. What are the common pathogens in acute bacterial meningitis?

Two factors have affected the epidemiology of acute bacterial meningitis in the past decade: development and implementation of the *Haemophilus influenzae* type B vaccines and emergence of penicillin-resistant strains of *Streptococcus pneumoniae*. Overall, pneumococcal meningitis is now the most common cause of bacterial meningitis in the United States. The relative frequency (shown top to bottom) with which each of the various bacterial pathogens causes meningitis is age-related:

Bacterial Pathogens Causing Meningitis

NEONATES (AGE < 1 MO)	CHILDREN (1 MO TO 18 YR)	ADULTS (OVER 18 YR)
Group B streptococci	*Neisseria meningitidis*	*S. pneumoniae*
E. coli (principally K1)	*Streptococcus pneumoniae*	*N. meningitidis*
Listeria monocytogenes	*H. influenzae* type B	Gram-negative bacilli
		L. monocytogenes

6. How has the *H. influenzae* type B conjugate vaccine (Hib) affected the epidemiology of bacterial meningitis?

The development and use of the *H. influenzae* type B (Hib) conjugate vaccines in the mid 1980s dramatically changed the epidemiology of bacterial meningitis. The incidence of meningitis secondary to *H. influenzae* type B fell 82% in U.S. children under the age of 5 yr between 1985 and 1991. No other organisms have filled the void, leading to an overall reduction in bacterial meningitis.

7. What are common causes of acute aseptic meningitis?

Bacterial causes include parameningeal infections, partially treated bacterial meningitis, and difficult-to-culture organisms such as *Mycoplasma* or *Rickettsia* spp. More common are viral etiologies, most of which may overlap in clinical involvement and cause encephalitis. Enteroviruses are the most common, occurring during the summer and fall in temperate climates and year-round in the tropics. Arboviruses are transported by various arthropod vectors; therefore, their prevalence can be assessed by seasonal activity and geographic distribution of the vector. Herpes viruses may cause many clinical syndromes, including encephalitis, meningitis, transverse myelitis, or localized neuritis. HIV can cause acute meningoencephalitis as part of its acute viremia, which may be associated with a flu-like or mononucleosis-like syndrome.

8. What are signs and symptoms of acute meningitis?

The typical presentation of headache, fever, and meningismus with or without mental status changes is noted eventually in about 85% of patients. In many cases, particularly young children and infants, however, the clinical manifestations of meningitis are nonspecific. Clinicians should keep a high index of suspicion for meningitis and exclude it with a lumbar puncture if meningitis is considered.

In neonates, the symptoms are often subtle and more suggestive of a sepsis syndrome. Fever, lethargy, gastrointestinal dysfunction with vomiting and/or anorexia, and seizures are most commonly seen. The bulging fontanelle is seen rarely (20%) in full-term infants and less often in premature infants because the open skull sutures at birth can expand head size in response to increased intracranial pressure.

Children and adults typically present with fever, nuchal rigidity, headache and neck pain, lethargy, irritability, nausea and vomiting, and photophobia. Seizures occur in 30–40% of children with meningitis. In adults as in children, lethargy or altered mental status is the strongest predictor of acute bacterial meningitis.

9. What are Brudzinski's and Kernig's signs?

Brudzinski described several signs of meningeal irritation. The best known, nape-of-the-neck sign, is now regarded as Brudzinski's sign. The sign is considered positive when passive flexion of the neck results in flexion of the hips and knees.

The modified Kernig's test is performed with the patient lying supine. The hip is flexed onto the abdomen with knee flexed. A positive sign is signified by resistance with passive extension of the knee in this position. Both are seen rarely in neonates and only in about 50% of children and adults with meningitis.

10. Are there certain clues to aseptic meningitis? Parameningeal disease?

There is significant overlap in the clinical presentation of bacterial and aseptic meningitis as well as in early laboratory CSF parameters. Enteroviral meningitis in neonates is associated with a greater risk of multiorgan involvement and increased mortality, similar to that of overwhelming bacterial sepsis. In children and adults, enteroviral meningitis typically runs a benign course; abnormal neurologic findings are rarely reported. A typical pattern includes insidious onset of symptoms over one to several days during summertime and rapid relief of headache after lumbar puncture due to the drop in intracranial pressure.

Intracranial suppuration (brain abscess, subdural or epidural abscess) should be considered in the presence of focal neurologic signs or multiple cranial nerve palsies. If symptoms are subacute, CNS imaging should be the first step in the evaluation. If acute onset is suggestive of meningitis, blood cultures should be obtained and antimicrobials started without a delay for imaging. Spinal epidural abscess presents as acute or progressive back pain and localized tenderness associated with fever, and should prompt an early evaluation with magnetic resonance imaging (MRI) or computed tomographic (CT) myelography. Chronic epidural abscess more commonly is associated with abnormalities on plain spinal radiographs.

11. When does a CT scan need to be done before a lumbar puncture?

Once acute meningitis syndrome is entertained on the basis of history and physical examination, a lumbar puncture should be promptly obtained for diagnosis, and antibiotics then should be initiated pending results. Most experts agree that CT scans are overused in the initial management of meningitis and result in unnecessary delays in diagnosis and treatment.

Mild elevations in intracranial pressure are to be expected with meningitis and should not delay lumbar puncture. Markedly increased intracranial pressure is manifested by significant papilledema, a dilated, nonreactive pupil, ocular motion abnormalities, drowsiness or stupor, bradycardia, and hypertension. These findings warrant delay of lumbar puncture for CT scan to exclude patients at high risk for brain herniation. In such cases, blood cultures should be obtained and empiric antibiotics should be started before CT scan.

Persons with late-stage AIDS (CD4 count below 100 cells/ml) have increased likelihood of CNS mass lesions without localizing signs. Although controversial, CNS imaging probably is warranted before lumbar puncture.

12. Should I wear a mask in addition to gloves when performing an lumbar puncture?

For: Easily performed and anecdotal reports of possible contamination of cultures with oral flora support use. Inexpensive.

Against: No randomized study supports wearing of a mask, and it is not widely practiced.

13. Discuss the complications of diagnostic lumbar puncture.

Brain herniation is the most serious complication and can best be avoided by foregoing lumbar puncture in high-risk patients and removing a minimum of fluid. Lumbar puncture through a local site of suppuration is contraindicated because it may cause bacteremia and secondary meningitis.

Postdural puncture headache (PDPH) occurs in 12–38% of persons. It is characterized by an upright postural headache with usual onset 6–48 hours after lumbar puncture and may be associated with tinnitus and hearing loss. Evidence supports CSF hypotension due to ongoing CSF leak at dural puncture and resultant stretching of cranial contents upon assuming an upright position. Incidence of PDPH can be reduced by using the smallest needle practical and aligning the plane of the bevel parallel to the longitudinal axis of the spinal cord to separate, not cut, dural fibers. Bed rest after lumbar puncture shows no benefit over early ambulation in several trials. If a PDPH occurs, a trial of IV hydration with or without caffeine may be tried. If PDPH does not resolve in 24 hours, an epidural blood patch is highly effective.

14. When should antibiotics be started? What if lumbar puncture is delayed for an imaging study?

Given the potential of neurologic morbidity and mortality from bacterial meningitis, potent bactericidal antibiotics should be started promptly after presentation, ideally within 30 minutes of presentation. Clinical data to support this notion are inconclusive, but in animal data progressive bacterial endotoxin release was noted by *E. coli* not exposed promptly to antibiotics. Endotoxin release leads to more inflammation and risk of sequelae.

The majority of delay in administration of antibiotics in the emergency department is avoidable. If the patient with suspected meningitis presents with stupor, focal neurologic signs, or marked papilledema, a CT scan is warranted. In this case, blood cultures should be obtained and antibiotics started before imaging. Lumbar puncture should be performed promptly after CT scan if no mass lesion is detected. Although CSF cultures are usually rendered sterile by 24 hours of parenteral antibiotics, CSF white blood cell count and chemistry panels are not significantly altered for 48–72 hours.

15. How do CSF studies help to distinguish bacterial from aseptic meningitis?

Despite overlap between these groups, history, physical examination, and CSF results can distinguish many differing causes of meningitis.

	Normal	*Bacterial*	*Viral*
Opening pressure (mmH$_2$0)	< 180	> 180	< 180–220
White blood cells (per µl)	0–5	100–10,000	50–1000
Glucose (mg/dl)	45–65	< 40	> 45
CSF/serum glucose ratio	0.6	< 0.4	0.6
Protein (mg/dl)	20–45	> 150	50–100

Cell differential is often a confusing CSF parameter and should be considered in context with values listed above. As a rule, bacterial meningitis has neutrophilic predominance, although 10% of bacterial meningitis are initially mononuclear especially if white blood cells are < 1000/mm^3. Likewise, 25–75% of viral meningitides begin with a polymorphonuclear leukocyte predominance before eventually showing lymphocyte predominance.

16. What role do CSF bacterial antigen studies play in the diagnosis of meningitis?

Latex particle agglutination tests for soluble bacterial capsular antigens (*H. influenzae* type B, *S. pneumoniae*, *N. meningitidis*, *Streptococcus agalactiae* and *E. coli* K1) add little to the Gram stain and culture of bacterial meningitis in patients who have not been pretreated with antibiotics. Sensitivity ranges from 44–100% (mean = 80%) and is slightly less than Gram stain.

In persons pretreated with antibiotics, antigen studies may play a more important role, but Gram stain and culture may still be positive up to and occasionally after 48 hours. Furthermore, if blood cultures were obtained prior to antibiotics, they may yield the pathogen. Overall, antigen testing may yield a specific diagnosis for smear-negative, culture-negative bacterial meningitis in 5–7% of cases. Maxson offers a rational, cost-effective approach:

1. 1 ml of CSF is saved and refrigerated or frozen
2. If Gram stain is negative and cultures reveal no growth at 48 hours, antigen testing can then be performed.

Given changes in empiric therapy for resistant pneumococci, immediate *S. pneumoniae* antigen testing for gram stain-negative acute meningitis is warranted (see question 19).

17. What tests best exclude fungal and mycobacterial meningitis?

Fungal meningitis can occasionally be detected on Gram or silver stain of concentrated CSF, although often the burden of organisms is too low to detect by microscopy. Cryptococcal antigen by latex agglutination is a reliable, rapid diagnostic test. Likewise, acid-fast stain has a low yield (< 1%) unless large volumes (20 ml of CSF) are concentrated (sensitivity 10–25% in experienced hands).

A common mistake is obtaining insufficient CSF for culture of fungi or mycobacteria. If fungi or mycobacteria are considered in the differential diagnosis, at least 20 ml of CSF should be concentrated and cultured, if not contraindicated by mass lesion or hydrocephalus. Often the CSF is obtained by a second lumbar puncture after initial tests fail to reveal alternate causes. Polymerase chain reaction may prove to be a useful rapid diagnostic test in the future.

18. What recommendations are made for empiric therapy based on initial clinical and laboratory data?

When antibiotics are to be initiated with unavailable or inconclusive Gram stain results, therapy should be based on patient's age and risk factors. In general, a third-generation cephalosporin (ceftriaxone or cefotaxime) should be initiated. Ampicillin should be added in patients less than 3 months or more than 50 years of age to provide additional coverage for *Listeria* sp. or *S. agalactiae*. Immunocompromised patients (chemotherapy, underlying leukemia/lymphoma, or long-term steroids) warrant additional gram-negative coverage of ceftazidime in addition to ampicillin. Patients with wounds or CSF shunts should include staphylococcal coverage with vancomycin. Corticosteroid therapy should be considered simultaneously according to criteria outlined below.

Gram stain or antigen studies should narrow coverage toward the presumptive pathogen, and in the case of gram-negative rods an aminoglycoside should be added. Further modification should be based on return of culture and sensitivity data.

19. How have rising rates of penicillin-resistant pneumococci affected empiric therapy?

Emergence of penicillin-binding protein alterations in *S. pneumoniae* has led to increasing resistance to penicillin worldwide. Fifteen percent of *S. pneumoniae* isolates from New York City in 1995 were nonsusceptible to penicillin, defined as a minimal inhibitory concentration (MIC) ≥ 0.1 µg/ml. Twenty-two percent of strains at Children's Medical Center in Dallas in 1994 were resistant to penicillin, and 7% were also resistant to cefotaxime/ceftriaxone. Vancomycin (15 mg/kg IV every 6 hr up to 2 gm/day) should be added to the third-generation cephalosporin if pneumococci appear to be likely pathogens by Gram stain or antigen studies. Adjunctive glucocorticoids should be considered carefully in this setting because steroids diminish vancomycin levels in the CSF in animal models. Children appear to be less affected than adults. In suspected cephalosporin-resistant pneumococcal meningitis, repeat lumbar puncture should be considered 24–36 hours after the start of therapy to ensure eradication of the pathogen.

20. What is the role of corticosteroids in adjunctive therapy?

Although cell-wall active antimicrobials rapidly sterilize the CSF, the release of cell-wall products (lipopolysaccharide, peptidoglycan, and teichoic acid) that increase the inflammatory response may contribute to a degree of neurologic sequelae. Dexamethasone, given at or before the first dose of antibiotic (at 0.15 mg/kg every 6 hr for 4 days), has been found to ameliorate this inflammation in animal and some human studies. Routine use is still controversial, but most authors agree that the benefit is limited to steroids started within 4 hours of initial antibiotic therapy.

In children?

For: Four trials in children older than 2 months showed decreased audiologic and neurologic sequelae. A trial in pneumococcal meningitis in Turkey showed a similar trend in benefit that did not achieve statistical significance.

Against: The four trials showing benefit contained primarily *H. influenzae* meningitis, now a rare pathogen due to the Hib vaccine.

In adults?

For: One prospective, randomized trial in patients with advanced disease at presentation showed benefit; only in the *S. pneumoniae* group. Quagliarello, therefore, recommends corticosteroids for patients with positive Gram stain of CSF and evidence of increased intracranial pressure.

Against: No placebo-controlled or blinded studies support use of corticosteroids. Moreover, rising penicillin resistance in the only subgroup to show benefit, *S. pneumoniae*, may require vancomycin, whose poor penetration into the CSF is further impaired by corticosteroids.

21. What are recommended lengths of therapy for common pathogens?

Few controlled trials address this issue. Meningococcal meningitis is effectively treated with 7 days and perhaps less of penicillin or ceftriaxone. Lin showed that a 7-day course of ceftriaxone was as effective as a 10-day course in children with nonmeningococcal meningitis, although most cases were due to *H. influenzae*. Gram-negative bacilli (excluding *H. influenzae*) probably warrant longer treatment courses of 3–4 weeks. It is important to remember that the most important criteria for discontinuation are clinical response and improved laboratory parameters; length of therapy should be individualized according to these criteria.

22. What complications of meningitis should the treating physician look out for?

Early complications of increased intracranial pressure, cranial nerve palsies, and seizures have already been discussed. Both children and adults can develop infectious vasculitis and cerebral infarction. Children may develop subdural effusion due to increased vascular permeability in the subdural space from the adjacent infection, and the effusion may produce mass effect or become infected, leading to prolonged fever. Hyponatremia and syndrome of inappropriate antidiuretic hormone secretion are common features of childhood bacterial meningitis, occurring in about 50% of cases due to *H. influenzae*. Hearing loss is the most common long-term neurologic sequelae (10% overall), followed by mental retardation, spasticity or paresis, and seizures.

BIBLIOGRAPHY

1. Adams WG, Deaver KA, Cochi SL, et al: Decline of childhood *Haemophilus influenzae* type B (Hib) disease in the Hib vaccine era. JAMA 269:221–226, 1993.
2. Centers for Disease Control and Prevention: Surveillance for penicillin-nonsusceptible *Streptococcus pneumoniae*—New York City 1995. MMWR 46(14):297–299, 1997.
3. Friedland IR, Jafari H, Ehrett S, et al: Comparison of endotoxin release by different antimicrobial agents and the effect upon inflammation in experimental *Escherichia coli* meningitis. J Infect Dis 168:657–662, 1993.
4. Geisler PJ, Nelson KE, Levin S, et al: Community-acquired purulent meningitis: a review of 1,316 cases during the antibiotic era, 1954–1976. Rev Infect Dis 2:725–745, 1980.
5. Kuntz KM, Kokmen E, Stevens JC, et al: Post-lumbar puncture headaches: Experience in 501 consecutive patients. Neurology 42:1884–1887, 1992.
6. Lin TY, Chrane DF, Nelson JD, et al: Seven days of ceftriaxone is as effective as ten days treatment for bacterial meningitis. JAMA 253:3559–3563, 1985.
7. Maxson S, Lewno MJ, Schutze GE: Clinical usefulness of cerebrospinal fluid antigen studies. J Pediatr 125:235–238, 1994.

8. Meier C, Oelschlager TA, Merkert H, et al: Ability of *Escherichia coli* isolates that cause meningitis in newborns to invade epithelial and endothelial cells. Infect Immun 64:2391–2399, 1996.

9. Paris MM, Ramilo O, McCracken GH: Management of meningitis caused by penicillin-resistant *Streptococcus pneumoniae*. Antimicrob Agents Chemother 39:2171–2175, 1995.

10. Quagliarello VJ, Scheld WM: Treatment of bacterial meningitis. N Engl J Med 336:708–716, 1997.

11. Radetsky M: Duration of symptoms and outcome in bacterial meningitis: An analysis of causation and the implications of a delay in diagnosis. Pediatr Infect Dis J 11:694–698, 1992.

12. Scheld WM, Whitely RJ, Durack DT (eds.): Infections of the Central Nervous System, 2nd ed. New York, Raven Press, 1997.

13. Schuchat A, Robinson K, Wenger JD, et al: Bacterial meningitis in the United States in 1995. N Engl J Med 337:970–976, 1997.

14. Tunkel AR, Scheld WM: Acute meningitis. In Mandell GL, Bennett JE, Dolan E (eds): Principles and Practice of Infectious Diseases, 4th ed. New York, Churchill Livingstone, 1995, pp 831–865.

15. Verghese A, Gallemore G: Kernig's and Brudzinski's signs revisited. Rev Infect Dis 9:1187–1192, 1987.

XVI. Skin and Soft Tissue Infections

52. ECTOPARASITES

W. Michael Botkin, M.D.

1. What is scabies?

Scabies is a disease caused by an infestation with the itch mite, *Sarcoptes scabiei* var. *hominis*. This organism is introduced to the new host primarily by close contact, but it has been reported to be transmitted by fomites or casual contact on rare occasions. It has masqueraded under the terms seven-year itch and army itch; people in Wisconsin have called it the Michigan itch. Crowded conditions, poor hygiene, and malnutrition facilitate its spread from person to person.

2. How does scabies cause disease in humans?

The scabies organisms are barely visible. The adult female measures 0.4 ¥ 0.3 mm, and the male is half this size. After fertilization on the skin surface the male dies and the female starts burrowing to lay her eggs. The female burrows between 2–4 mm per day and lays 2–3 eggs per day for a total of 10–25 eggs before dying in the distal end of the burrow. In a typical infestation the host has only 10–15 organisms, but there may be thousands in immunosuppressed patients.

3. How do I diagnose scabies?

During the first month there are usually no signs or symptoms of infestation. With continued exposure, however, the host mounts an immunologic reaction that gives rise to the clinical picture. The typical case presents with pruritus that is particularly severe at night and may occur on any part of the body, although it is most commonly seen in finger webs, genitalia, wrists, waist, axillae, buttocks, and umbilical areas. On examination papules and often burrows are noted in the involved areas. The intense pruritus often leads to secondary excoriations and superimposed pyodermas.

4. Do any laboratory tests aid in the diagnosis of scabies?

Yes. The scabies prep is performed by carefully observing the involved areas for a burrow— under good lighting and with magnification. The best area to test is the end of the burrow where the mature female is located. When this area is identified, a drop of mineral oil is placed on the skin, and the burrow is unroofed, placed on a glass slide, and examined with a microscope. A positive preparation may reveal the adult mite with its 4 pairs of short legs; the posterior legs are associated with long, protruding spines. The diagnosis also may be made by observing the eggs (see figure, top of next page), immature larvae, or scybala (feces). This last item is best left to experienced microscopists who know their scybala.

5. How do I treat scabies?

The drug of choice is permethrin. It is applied in a thin coat from the neck down in adults and older children and includes the head in young children. Areas to emphasize are the areas of clinical involvement as noted above and the nails. It is particularly important to trim the nails and clean their undersurfaces well with a brush before applying the medication. The medication is left on the patient for 8–12 hours and then washed off. A single application cures 90% of patients, but because of the 10% failure rate many clinicians treat again in 1 week. Alternative drugs include lindane, 6–10 % sulfur ointment, and crotamiton. It is recommended that others in the household and close contacts be treated to prevent reinfestation. It is important to tell the patient

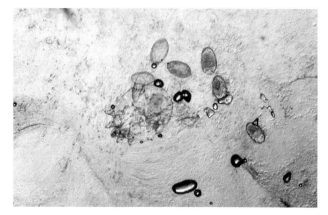

Eggs of scabies. (Slide courtesy of Cary Dunn, M.D., Dermatology Service, Tripler Army Medical Center, Honolulu.)

up front that symptoms are caused by an allergic reaction to the organisms and that they can expect to remain itchy for several days up to 4 weeks after treatment has killed the organisms and eggs but before they are totally shed from the skin surface. After completion of the treatment, all articles of clothing, sheets, towels, and gloves should be washed in a machine on the hot cycle for 10–20 minutes. Articles not washable can be put in a dryer at the same temperature or simply bagged for 1–2 weeks because the mites are reported to die within 4 days off the human host. The itching can be treated with your favorite antipruritic (I prefer hydroxyzine); secondary infection, if present, should be treated like any other pyoderma.

6. Should I know about any variants of the disease?

The most serious of the variants is the crusted variant, also called **Norwegian scabies**. This condition is often seen in immunosuppressed patients and has been responsible for hundreds of infections in institutions—particularly nursing homes, hospitals, homeless shelters, and hospices. Norwegian scabies often occurs on the face, scalp, palms, soles, and extensor surfaces; sometimes it is mistaken for psoriasis, eczematous dermatitis, or seborrhea. Patients teem with thousands of organisms and are a great source of institutional epidemics. Treatment of staff, patients, and visitors and prevention of nosocomial spread are discussed by Estes and Estes.[4] Scabies should be suspected in any immunosuppressed patient with itching or atypical rash. Norwegian scabies is not always associated with pruritus because the immunosuppressed patient does not react to the organism.

Another type of scabies is the exaggerated form, which is often mistaken for a drug reaction because of its widespread nature. Scabies is often missed completely if prior treatment has been given with systemic or potent topical steroids; this condition is termed **scabies incognito**. Immunosuppressed patients sometimes need to be treated with alternating agents, such as lindane and permethrin, to eradicate heavy infestations and possibly resistant organisms. Ivermectin, in a single oral dose, has been used in veterinary practice and in epidemics in other parts of the world. It may be available for human use in the United States in the not too distant future.

7. What variants may be seen in children?

Infants and young children often have involvement of the scalp and face as well as typical areas. Vesicles and pustules are also frequently seen, particularly on the hands and feet.

8. I treated my patient twice, but he still has nodules without burrows or papules. Should I treat him a third time?

The patient probably has a condition called **nodular scabies**, but you should repeat the scraping to confirm the absence of organisms. Nodular scabies occurs most frequently in the axilla, genitalia, and trunk. The histologic picture is a marked lymphohistiocytic reaction pattern without apparent retained organisms. Nodules may be treated with injected steroids or potent topical steroids, but they clear spontaneously and do not require further scabicidal therapy.

9. My patient was exposed to a nursing home patient with scabies, and lesions appeared in only 2 weeks. Doesn't it take a month to manifest scabies?

Several cases with short incubation periods have been noted and may be due to acquisition of excessive organisms. In addition, atopic patients may react earlier because of cross-reactivity to house dust mites.

10. My dog has mange and the veterinarian asked me if I itched. Can I catch it?

You will not get mange, but after contact with the dog you may have animal scabies. The *Sarcoptes* organism has been identified on at least 40 different mammalian hosts. Because it is mostly species-specific, full-fledged disease is seen only in the primary host. The animal owner may note symptoms of pruritus in areas contacting the infected animal—usually the thighs, anterior trunk, and forearms. Studies have noted this condition in up to one-third of owners. In addition to pruritus, objective lesions include erythematous papules, vesicles, urticarial lesions (some with a central puncta), and pustules. Burrows are not seen in nonhuman forms, and in most cases it is nearly impossible to identify the organism on the surface of human skin.

11. How do I treat patients exposed to mange?

You don't. Most authors recommend only symptomatic treatment of humans, with isolation of the owner from the animal until it is clear of disease.

12. The veterinarian told me that my cat has *Cheyletiella*. Will this affect my family?

Cheyletiella spp. is a mite that infests pets. Humans may develop an eruption from contact with affected animals. The lesions are small papules, urticarial papules, or frank wheals; occasionally, small vesicles or pustules may appear, particularly in children. The lesions are located on the same areas involved in patients with animal scabies. The disease is usually acquired from a puppy but also may be acquired from cats, rabbits, and guinea pigs. The organisms belong to several discrete species and are sometimes referred to as "walking dandruff" because they are observed to move under microscopic examination of animal skin scrapings. Lesions are not positive on human scrapings. The management strategy is to treat the animal definitively and the human symptomatically.

13. What should I know about chiggers?

Chiggers are baby mites of over 3000 species, only a few of which are important to humans. The most common in the United States is the harvest mite, *Eutrombicula* sp. The larvae are seen in the southern two-thirds of the United States, and the incidence peaks from June to early August, depending on latitude and numbers of larvae. The larvae migrate to the tip of vegetation and jump onto a passing host after being alerted by the host's carbon dioxide aura. They then migrate rapidly and frequently set up housekeeping at a point of clothing constriction, such as the top of socks or waistbands. They secrete a small amount of protein-digesting enzymes in their saliva and begin to digest the host's tissue. The organism then drops off the host, and symptoms appear hours later—the exact time depends on prior exposure to the antigens of the organism. On a few virgin hosts, organisms may be viewed with a magnifying lens after engorgement, but an experienced host will scratch the organism off so that usually they are missed. Pruritus begins and increases over about 24 hours. As the immunologic reaction develops, urticaria, papules, vesicles, and even frank bullae may appear. Treatment is symptomatic with the proviso that any clothing worn and not washed may be a source of reinfestation. Remember what mom told you: wear clean clothes, and keep your room clean.

14. I have seven parakeets and canaries. They appear sick, and I itch. Is there a connection?

You may be infested with bird mites. The presentation is the same as with other nonscabies infestations. The birds are treated for mites, and exposed humans are treated with systemic antipruritics and topical lotions containing menthol and camphor. The same condition may be seen in people who come into contact with wild birds nests, such as children, window washers, and roofers.

15. What other mite infestations should I know about?

In taking the history of a patient with pruritus and clinical suggestions of bites, you should consider the diagnosis of the *Acariformes* group of mites. Specific diseases are named after the product to which patients are exposed. Baker's itch is due to stored grains; other examples include copra itch, onion mites, tea or coolie itch, and grocer's itch (from all of the above plus fruits, cheese, and other produce).

16. My patient has severe pubic itching and a few blue macules. Is this scabies?

Probably not. The patient most likely is infested with the pubic louse, *Phthirus pubis*. Both scabies and pubic lice are sexually transmitted. Infestation with pubic lice is associated with severe itching, and the blue macules are called maculae cerulae. They are believed to be caused by the breakdown of bilirubin to biliverdin by enzymes secreted by the mite after biting the host. If you look closely in the pubic area, you can often see the organisms and their eggs (nits). The male is about 1.25 mm, and the female is 1.75 mm. On examination the pubic louse resembles a crab with short muscular limbs; hence its common name. The organism has 6 legs with well-developed claws that grasp hairs in the involved area.

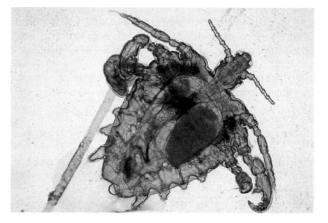

Pubic louse. (Slide courtesy of Cary Dunn, M.D., Dermatology Service, Tripler Army Medical Center, Honolulu.)

17. How is infestation with pubic lice treated?

Patients often treat infestation with pubic lice with over-the-counter pyrethrins such as RID. Effective prescription agents include permethrins and lindane. I prefer lindane shampoo of the entire body for 4 minutes, repeated in 1 week. It is necessary to remove the nits with a comb. The comb should be soaked in a pediculicide for at least 1 hour before it is used again.

18. The sexual partner of my patient with pubic lice has blepharitis. Is this related?

Probably. Pubic lice easily infest eyelashes and eyebrows. They are readily visible with good light and magnification. Treatment consists of application of petrolatum to the area 3 times/day for 3 days. This condition has become more common with the increasing variety of sexual activity (scalp involvement has been reported in rare cases).

19. What else should I worry about in patients with pubic lice?

Patients with pubic lice often have other associated venereal diseases. As many as one-third have been reported to have a second sexually transmitted disease. Pubic lice may be seen in up to 5% of patients in STD clinics. Do not forget to treat the patient's sexual partner.

20. How do patients with head lice present?

Patients with head lice (*Pediculus humanus* var. *capitis*) present with scalp itching, often with an associated impetigo or eczematization of the scalp, neck, or upper back. Lice and nits can be visualized with good lighting and simple magnification. Hairs can be plucked and examined for nits that are cemented to the hairs. The lice themselves are rarely seen; they are $\frac{1}{10}$–$\frac{1}{6}$ of an inch long, wingless, and gray to creamy white.

21. What is the treatment for head lice?

Treatment is with several nonprescription agents. Pyrethrins such as RID are the most commonly used agents. They require two applications 1 week apart because they are not ovicidal. Permethrin agents such as Nix theoretically require only a single application because they kill both eggs and adult lice. The old standby lindane may be used, but it is available only by prescription and is considered more toxic than the other agents. Another point about treatment is the necessity to get rid of the nits attached to the hairs; in many districts, children are not admitted to school until they are nit-free. The nits are removed by combing the hair, but they are often quite resistant to the comb and are more easily removed after soaking the comb or hair in a white vinegar solution or after using an 8% formic acid rinse sold as a commercial preparation called Step 2 Nit Removal System.

22. How do body lice present?

Body lice (*Pediculus humanus* var. *corporis*) are not residents of the body surface. They live in the seams of clothing and go onto the skin surface only to feed. Patients are usually homeless or victims of war or overcrowding. Most present with red macules, papules, urticarial lesions, and excoriations. Lesions are often noted in the axilla or upper back. Pyoderma secondary to scratching of the intensely itching lesions is a common finding. In endemic settings many clinicians treat the patient with a hot shower and clean clothes. For heavy infestations some treat the patient with one of the drugs used for head lice, such as a permethrin or pyrethrin, and the clothing with insecticide powders. Body lice may carry rickettsial and borrelial diseases.

23. What is cutaneous larva migrans?

Cutaneous larva migrans, also known as creeping eruption, is most often caused by larvae of roundworms that infest dogs or cats (usually *Ancylostoma braziliense*, but others may be involved). It is frequently seen in the southern United States and other subtropical and tropical areas. Humans are accidently exposed when they contact animal feces, usually in a sandy area frequented by animals. As the larvae penetrate the skin, they form a papule that over time begins to move in a long serpiginous track that is slightly elevated and may manifest vesiculation. Lesions are usually seen on the feet, buttocks, and thighs. The rate of migration is usually about 2 cm/day. Treatment consists of topical thiabendazole, applied 2–4 times/day for 1 week. Oral Ivermectin may be used as a single dose; oral thiabendazole also may be used, but it has a greater number of gastrointestinal side effects.

24. What is swimmer's itch?

Swimmer's itch is a skin condition caused by penetration of human skin by a cercarial form of a bird schistosome. It is seen most commonly in the flyways of the north central United States. The victim may note itching within 10 minutes of exposure; itching may be associated with urticaria and red macules and papules. The eruption occurs usually on the exposed areas of the body. Symptoms peak in a few days and resolve in about 1–2 weeks. The condition is usually acquired close to shore where the cercaria are released from the involved snails. Swimmer's itch may be seen in salt water and confused with seabather's eruption. Treatment consists of oral and topical antipruritics; organisms do not persist for more than a few days.

25. What is seabather's eruption?

Seabather's eruption is believed to be caused by the larval form of the thimble jellyfish (*Linuchi unguiculata*). Itching may begin while the victim is in the water but more commonly develops after water exposure. The involved area is under the swimsuit in contrast to swimmer's itch. Lesions are small red papules or urticarial lesions. They localize about follicles and may result in residual pigmentation. Lesions resolve spontaneously in 1–2 weeks. On rare occasions the condition is associated with fever, particularly in children. The patient should shower immediately on becoming symptomatic, and the swimwear should be thoroughly washed. Symptomatic control of itching and treatment of any associated infection are the only required therapy.

26. What is myiasis?

Myiasis results from tissue invasion by any of a number of fly larvae (maggots). The larvae may inhabit an open wound surface, extending the ulceration but also debriding the surface. Some species, particularly screwworms, may cause sinuses and widespread destruction of surrounding healthy tissue. The other variety of myiasis leads to a furuncle-type lesion after direct skin invasion by certain larvae. The most common example in this hemisphere is *Dermatobia hominis*. Lesions are typically symptomatic, with patient complaints of pain or burning. Some patients report the sensation that the boil is "moving." Close examination often reveals a central puncta, which is the larval breathing tube. Treatment is to open the furuncle and extract the larvae. In patients with destruction of surrounding tissue, treatment includes irrigation and careful debridement of the lesion.

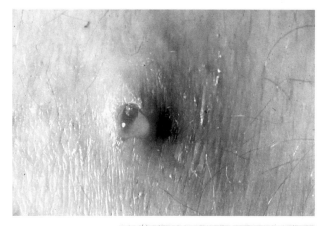

Boil of myasis. (Slide courtesy of Cary Dunn, M.D., Dermatology Service, Tripler Army Medical Center, Honolulu.)

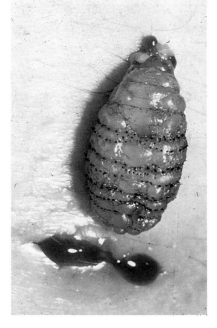

Fly larva removed after incision of boil. (Slide courtesy of Cary Dunn, M.D., Dermatology Service, Tripler Army Medical Center, Honolulu.)

BIBLIOGRAPHY

1. Cabrera R, et al: The immunology of scabies. Semin Dermatol 12:15–21, 1993.
2. Demis DJ (ed): Clinical Dermatology, 24th ed. Philadelphia, Lippincott-Raven, 1997.
3. Elston DM: Bugs and bites. Del Med J 68:445–450, 1996.
4. Estes SA, Estes J: Therapy of scabies: Nursing homes, hospitals and the homeless. Semin Dermatol 12:26–33, 1993.
5. Kalter DC, et al: Parasitic diseases. In Arndt KA, et al (eds): Cutaneous Medicine and Surgery. Philadelphia, W.B. Saunders, 1996, pp 1172–1189.
6. Knutson RM: Furtive Fauna. New York, Penguin Books, 1992.
7. Levisohn DR: Injurious effects in humans induced by arthropods. In Demis DJ (ed): Clinical Dermatology, 24th ed. Philadelphia, Lippincott-Raven, 1997, pp 1–39.
8. Millikan LE: Mite infestations other than scabies. Semin Dermatol 12:46–52, 1993.
9. Orkin M: Scabies in AIDS. Semin Dermatol 12:9–14, 1993.
10. Paller AS: Scabies in infants and small children. Semin Dermatol 12:3–8, 1993.
11. Parish LC, Schwartzman RM: Zoonoses of dermatological interest. Semin Dermatol 12:57–64, 1993.
12. Rasmussen JE: Body lice, head lice, pubic lice and scabies. In Arndt KA, et al (eds): Cutaneous Medicine and Surgery. Philadelphia, W.B. Saunders, 1996, pp 1190–1199.

53. SECRETS LURKING UNDER THE SKIN: FASCIITIS

Joel D. Brown, M.D., DTMH, FACP

1. Why should I read this chapter?

What you know and do not know about skin and soft tissue infections can make the difference between life and death. Think of the cross-sectional anatomy of the affected area:

- Is the infection limited to the skin (impetigo or erysipelas)?
- Does it extend to the underlying soft tissues (cellulitis), the fascia (fasciitis), the muscle (myositis), the periosteum (periostitis—often due to an overlying inflammation), the bone and bone marrow (osteomyelitis), or internal organs (intraabdominal abscess or empyema necessitans)?
- Does the history suggest that the infection began in the skin or in a deeper organ such as the bone? Special imaging may help in some patients, but it also may delay therapy; surgical exploration may be quicker and treats as well as defines the anatomy of the infection.
- Is the onset rapid or slow?

Soft tissue infections are often divided into confusing groups that are hard to remember. It is more important to judge the clinical acuity and urgency of therapy—particularly the need for early surgical consultation. Below are typical questions that should run through your mind.

2. What may cause abnormal gas in the soft tissues?

1. Infections with gas-forming organisms, particularly anaerobic bacteria. Gram-negative facultative aerobes (e.g., *Escherichia coli*) also may liberate gas, particularly in diabetics.
2. Spread of atmospheric air through breaks in skin may have a ball valve effect (e.g., walking on a lacerated foot may lead to subcutaneous crepitus).
3. Spread of gas from a gas-containing organ (e.g., bowel or lung)
4. Hydrogen peroxide wound irrigations
5. Compressed air procedures or accidents (dental drills or goosing with pneumatic air equipment—not funny)

3. Discuss the cause and significance of skin anesthesia in a patient with acute "cellulitis".

The skin changes from acutely tender to anesthetic as the fasciitis damages the cutaneous nerves that perforate through the fascia.

4. How can you differentiate erysipelas from acute fasciitis?

It is not always easy. Erysipelas usually has a subtle palpable border, is sharply demarcated, and is often associated with regional adenopathy. Fasciitis spreads rapidly and has no palpable border. Both conditions may be associated with superficial skin necrosis and blebs or bullae, but this process is slower in erysipelas. Acute streptococcal fasciitis almost always causes severe toxicity, which is less likely in erysipelas. Ask for consultation in difficult cases.

5. What can be done, short of major surgical exploration, to help diagnose fasciitis?

Ask a surgical colleague to make a small incision and pass a probe to the fascia; if the fascia layer separates easily, it is necrotic and infected. (For this simple procedure, the surgeon will be paid twice what you are paid). A frozen biopsy of the fascia may indicate fascial infection. Sometimes the surgeon may not have much experience with necrotizing fasciitis and may settle for a less disfiguring diagnostic procedure than extensive surgical exploration when the diagnosis is unclear.

6. What forms of treatment should be used when one suspects or has proved the diagnosis of fasciitis?

Appropriate antimicrobials and early surgical consultation with a low threshold for surgical exploration. Extensive, often disfiguring debridement—perhaps repetitive—is required. Patients with pure clostridial cellulitis, nonclostridial anaerobic cellulitis, or infected vascular gangrene may not be acutely ill, but patients with clostridial myonecrosis or streptococcal necrotizing fasciitis may be severely ill and require intensive care.

7. Fasciitis should be suspected in which of the following settings?
a. Chickenpox with sudden appearance of spreading cellulitis
b. Cellulitis at the site of illicit intravenous drug injection
c. Early-onset (within 1–2 days) infection of traumatic or surgical wound
d. Facial cellulitis after onset of dental infection
e. All of the above

Answer: e. Chickenpox lesions may become secondarily infected with *Streptococcus pyogenes*. Wound infections with *S. pyogenes* typically have an incubation period of 1–3 days and should be suspected in early-onset infections; most other wound infections are not manifest until 3–5 days later. (Our surgical colleagues have an oral tradition that simplifies the typical later onset of wound infections: "wind, water, wound . . . whatever." Works for them!) Dental infections due to mixed anaerobic/aerobic bacterial infections may spread to the fascia of the face and chest.

8. How do you distinguish clostridial myonecrosis from clostridial cellulitis by the gas pattern seen on radiographs?

Radiographs of clostridial myonecrosis often show gas outlining the muscle fibers in a feathery pattern, whereas in cellulitis the gas is confined to bubbles in the subcutaneous tissues only. (The radiologist gets paid lots for this simple interpretation).

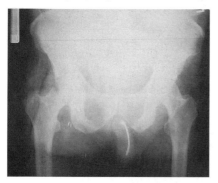

Radiograph of the pelvis in a patient with myonecrosis due to *Clostridium septicum*. Note the gas outlining the muscle fibers of the right thigh.

9. What organism is most likely to cause cellulitis, fasciitis, myositis, or all three in a patient with erythema of the body and palms, shock, and multiorgan failure?

Group A beta-hemolytic streptococci (*Streptococcus pyogenes*). Such a clinical picture helps to define the toxic shocklike syndrome due to the streptococcal exotoxin A that causes scarlet fever. It acts as a superantigen, i.e., an antigen that does not require processing by the host macrophage system, which rapidly stimulates production of inflammatory cytokines. The mortality rate approaches 30%.

10. What is Fournier's gangrene?

Necrotizing fasciitis of the genitals and perineum in males due to mixed aerobic/anaerobic bacterial infection. It is more common in diabetics and often follows perineal or genital infection (e.g., perirectal abscess, infected circumcision, complications of urethral procedures). Patients with Fournier's gangrene require aggressive surgical debridement; however, the separate blood supply of the testes allows these organs to be spared.

11. What is the appropriate empiric antimicrobial therapy to supplement surgical debridement for suspected necrotizing fasciitis?

Gram stains of tissues or fluids may offer a clue to monobacterial infections such as pure clostridial (large gram-positive rods) or streptococcal (gram-positive cocci in chains) infections, which may be treated with specific narrow-spectrum agents. Otherwise, one should use agents effective against anaerobes (e.g., ampicillin/sulbactam, metronidazole, or clindamycin) and gram-negative aerobes (e.g., gentamicin) or broad-spectrum agents effective against both (e.g., piperacillin/ tazobactam, or meropenem). Experimental animal models of group A streptococcal fasciitis suggest that clindamycin is much more effective. In fact, penicillin was not much more effective than placebo, perhaps because large numbers of bacteria may be in a stationary growth phase, during which cell wall-active agents such as penicillin may be ineffective (the Eagle effect). Cell wall-active agents require actively dividing cells to kill microbes. For this reason many clinicians add clindamycin when treating such infections.

BIBLIOGRAPHY

1. Mathieu D, Neviere R, Teillon C, et al: Cervical necrotizing fasciitis: Clinical manifestations and management. Clin Infect Dis 21:51–56, 1995.
2. Nickle JC, Morales A: Necrotizing fasciitis of the male genitalia. Can Med Assoc J 129:445, 1983.
3. Stamenkovic I, Lew PD: Early recognition of potentially fatal necrotizing fasciitis: The use of frozen-section biopsy. N Engl J Med 310:1689–1693, 1984.
4. Stevens DL, Tanner MH, Winship J, et al: Severe group A streptococcal infections associated with a toxic shock-like syndrome and scarlet fever toxin A. N Engl J Med 321:1–7, 1989.
5. Wilson GJ, Talkington DF, Gruber W, et al: Group A streptococcal necrotizing fasciitis following varicella in children: Case reports and review. Clin Infect Dis 20:1333–1338, 1995.

54. FEVER WITH DERMATITIS

Joseph C. English III, M.D., and T. Keith Vaughan, M.D.

1. Define exanthem and enanthem.

An **exanthem** is defined as any generalized cutaneous dermatitis (inflammation of the skin) that appears rapidly. The term literally means to burst forth. The rash may be composed of macules, papules, vesicles, pustules, petechiae, or polymorphous lesions. An **enanthem** is any sudden eruption on mucosal surfaces. Both processes often occur in association with a febrile illness.

2. Name the five classical exanthems of childhood and the etiologic agent of each.

- Measles (rubeola)—paramyxovirus
- Rubella (German measles)—togavirus
- Scarlet fever (scarlatina)—group A beta-hemolytic streptococcus
- Erythema infectiosum (fifth disease)—parvovirus B19
- Exanthem subitum (roseola infantum)—human herpesvirus 6 and 7

3. Describe the clinical presentation of measles.

Measles occurs in the age range from infants to young adults during the winter and spring-time. The infection is acquired through respiratory transmission. The incubation period is approximately 10 days. The prodromal symptoms consist of a miserable patient with high fever, coryza (profuse nasal discharge), conjunctivitis, and **Koplik spots** on the buccal mucosa (the pathognomonic enanthem of measles). A dusky red maculopapular (also referred to as morbilliform) eruption develops initially (1–2 days after prodromal symptoms) behind the ears and in the scalp line. The term *maculopapular* describes a dermatitis in rapid transition from macules to papules. The dermatitis eventually spreads to the entire torso and extremities, persisting for up to 7 days. A secondary change of brawny desquamation follows. There are three forms of measles:

    1. Typical—in an unimmunized individual

    2. Modified measles—in partially immune hosts (prodrome and rash less severe)

    3. Atypical measles—in patients given killed measles virus vaccine, which was used until 1967. Treatment is supportive, and prevention is obtained by receiving the live attenuated MMR (measles, mumps, rubella) vaccine in infancy.

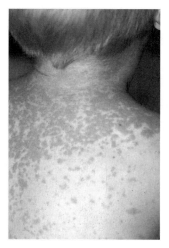

The classic cephalad-to-caudal progression of early measles.

4. Describe rubella. When is an infection with rubella extremely hazardous?

Rubella is also a virus acquired through respiratory transmission, mainly in the springtime. Its incubation period is up to 21 days before a mild prodrome of low-grade fever and malaise develops. Within 24–48 hours a generalized maculopapular eruption develops along with characteristic suboccipital and postauricular adenopathy. Petechiae may develop on the soft palate and are referred to as **Forchheimer's sign**, the enanthem of rubella. Treatment is supportive, and prevention is obtained by receiving the MMR vaccine in infancy.

A rubella infection during pregnancy can be devastating to the fetus in the first trimester. Congenital rubella syndrome causes dysorganogenesis in the cardiopulmonary, gastrointestinal, nervous, and hematopoietic systems. Affected infants are referred to as **blueberry muffin babies** because of multiple purplish-blue cutaneous lesions that represent dermatoerythropoiesis. Prevention is by ensuring that all females are immunized during infancy.

5. Describe the enanthem and exanthem of scarlet fever.

Scarlet fever is caused by a group A beta-hemolytic streptococcal bacteria that produce the pyrogenic exotoxin A, B, or C. The disease presents with acute onset of fever, malaise, and pharyngitis. The characteristic enanthem may precede the exanthem. The tongue is initially coated, and protruding erythematous papillae (**white strawberry tongue**) eventually develop into the **red strawberry tongue** as the coating dissipates. The cutaneous eruption develops shortly after the initial fever and is a gritty or sandpaper-like micropapular eruption. In flexural junctions of the extremities, petechiae may develop and are referred to as **Pastia lines**. The diagnosis of scarlet fever is sometimes made when the patient presents with the classical end-stage aspect of the exanthem: marked desquamation of large scales on the hands, feet, and flexural areas. The treatment of scarlatina is antistreptococcal antibiotics given orally.

6. What do scarlet fever and rheumatic fever have in common?

Both are initiated by group A beta-hemolytic streptococcal infections. Rheumatic fever, however, is a nonsuppurative acute inflammatory response of the host to the bacterium that causes secondary arthritis, chorea, carditis, subcutaneous nodules, and a classic skin finding called **erythema marginatum**, which consists of erythematous annular lesions on the torso with a slightly elevated border. These lesions may spread rapidly and have a tendency to be transient in nature.

7. What are the clinical findings and characteristic skin changes associated with erythema infectiosum?

Parvovirus B19 virus is transmitted via the respiratory route, multiplies in red blood cell precursors, and then results in classic cutaneous findings. A mild low-grade fever and malaise often precede a bright red, slapped-cheek appearance. After the initial facial eruption appears, a characteristic reticulated erythema develops on the extremities and occasionally on the buttocks. By the time the rash presents, the child is no longer infectious. Treatment is supportive.

Pregnant patients may not realize that they have been exposed to the virus until it is too late to avoid contact. On rare occasions, contact during pregnancy may lead to hydrops fetalis or stillbirth.

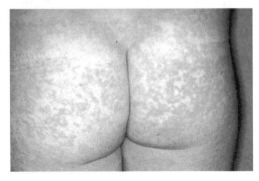

Reticulated erythema on the buttock in erythema infectiosum. (Photo from U.S. military dermatology teaching slides.)

8. What other diseases are associated with parvovirus B19 infection?

1. Papular-purpuric gloves-and-socks syndrome: sudden onset of confluent erythema and papules that become petechial and purpuric, and are localized to the hands and feet with a distinctive cut-off at the wrist and ankle; often associated with fever and oral ulcers.

2. Pruritus and arthritis in adults: occurs only in women; after infection, a symmetric polyarthritis associated with pruritus develops for up to 4 years' duration.

3. Aplastic crisis in sickle cell anemia: infection causes red blood cell precursor hemolysis, which may compromise the patient with an underlying hemolytic process, inducing a transient aplastic state that results in a severe anemia.

9. What presents first in exanthem subitum (roseola infantum): fever or dermatitis?

Exanthem subitum is a common cause of sudden, otherwise symptomless, high fever in children primarily from 6–36 months of age. Convulsions (febrile) and lymphadenopathy may accompany the high-grade fever, which lasts for approximately 3–4 days before the dermatitis of exanthem subitum appears. The defervescence also occurs suddenly; infants feel well by the time the dermatitis develops. Discrete rose-colored macules appear on the neck, trunk, and buttocks (less commonly on the face and extremities) and last only 1–2 days. There is no enanthem, and treatment is supportive.

10. Describe varicella zoster infection and its effect during pregnancy.

Varicella (chickenpox) is an exanthem caused by the varicella zoster virus, which has an incubation period of up to 21 days, is spread via respiratory route, and is highly contagious. The rash is pruritic and consists of vesicles on an erythematous base. Secondary changes (crusting) occur as new lesions continue to develop, and polymorphic lesions may aid in the clinical diagnosis. Lesions also may occur on mucosal membranes.

The diagnosis also may be aided by performing a Tzanck preparation (or, less commonly, a skin biopsy) and demonstrating multinucleated giant cells. More recently, direct immunofluorescence of a smear from the floor of an unroofed vesicle also has been used to confirm the diagnosis. Treatment is supportive; acyclovir may be used in cases complicated by pneumonia or encephalitis.

Varicella only should occur in a pregnant patient with no history of varicella or negative varicella serology. If the infection occurs during the first and/or second trimester, the severe congenital varicella syndrome (CVS) consisting of limb hypoplasia, chorioretinitis, and cutaneous scarring may occur. The incidence rate for CVS is 0.4% in the first trimester and 2% in the second trimester. A more common result is the mostly asymptomatic intrauterine fetal varicella infection with potential for subsequent development of early childhood herpes zoster. During the third trimester, maternal infection 5 days before or 2 days after delivery may cause a severe neonatal varicella infection (mortality rate: 20%) due to the lack of maternal antibodies to protect the neonate. The exposed/infected mother or neonate is treated with varicella zoster immunoglobulin and acyclovir.

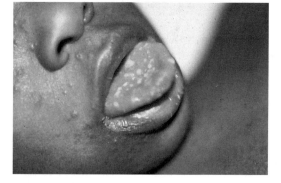

Multiple vesicles of varicella on the face and tongue.

11. What other viral infections may cause exanthems?

The nonpolio enteroviruses may cause a wide spectrum of cutaneous eruptions that are associated with fever. Examples include the coxsackievirus, echovirus, and enterovirus. In addition, adenovirus and Epstein-Barr virus may produce fever and dermatitis. The dermatitis of these viral infections may be polymorphous.

12. Several different viruses may cause one recognizable reactive process called Gianotti-Crosti syndrome. What are its characteristics?

Gianotti-Crosti syndrome is an acute, transient papular dermatitis of children and is accompanied by fever and malaise. A characteristic monomorphic eruption of nonpruritic, erythematous 1–5-mm papules appears suddenly over the face, limbs, and buttocks. The papules tend to coalesce on the cheeks, remaining more discrete on the limbs. The lesions are somewhat firm, continue to develop over a few days' time, and fade slowly with desquamation. There is no enanthem; inguinal or axillary adenopathy may be present.

Gianotti-Crosti syndrome may be caused by a number of viruses, including coxsackie A, respiratory syncytial virus, Epstein-Barr virus, rotavirus, and hepatitis A virus. A similar reactive process (Gianotti disease), associated with infection with certain hepatitis B subtypes, may cause liver enzyme elevations and, less commonly, a symptomatic anicteric hepatitis. Treatment of Gianotti-Crosti syndrome is supportive; the disease is nonscarring and self-limited.

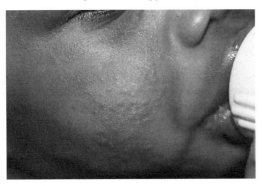

The classic papular eruption on the face in a patient with Gianotti-Crosti syndrome. (Photo from U.S. military dermatology teaching slides.)

13. Name two newly recognized exanthems associated with asymmetry.

Unilateral laterothoracic exanthem (ULE) and **asymmetric periflexural exanthem of childhood** (APEC). ULE presents in young children as erythematous papules in the axilla and unilateral chest wall that spontaneously resolve in 4 weeks. Mild prodromal symptoms and fever also may occur. APEC begins as cutaneous erythematous papules predominant in the axilla or inguinal folds. No etiologic agents have been found for either disease, and some authors believe that they may be variations of the same condition.

14. List the diagnostic criteria for Kawasaki syndrome.

1. Fever lasting longer than 5 days with no identifiable cause and no response to antibiotics or antipyretics
2. At least four of the following:
    (1) Bilateral, nonpurulent conjunctivitis
    (2) Mucous membrane involvement (red fissured lips, strawberry tongue)
    (3) Edema and erythema of hands and feet
    (4) Polymorphous truncal exanthem, followed by acral and perineal desquamation
    (5) Cervical lymphadenopathy > 1.5 cm

15. Specify the etiologic agent, treatment, and major complications of Kawasaki syndrome.

The **etiology** is unknown but may represent a host immune response to a bacterial superantigen. **Treatment** consists of intravenous immunoglobulin and high-dose aspirin. The **major**

complications are thrombocytosis and cardiac disease. In the acute phase, arrhythmias from inflamed cardiac tissue may develop. Arrhythmias may be followed by coronary artery aneurysms and platelet thrombi resulting in heart failure during the subacute phase. The resulting fibrosis and scarring of the myocardium and arteries may lead to ischemic heart disease and death. Male children under the age of 1 year are at greatest risk.

16. What are bacterial superantigens? How do they activate the immune system?

Superantigens are most often bacterial toxins; staphylococcal enterotoxins and streptococcal exotoxins are the most commonly studied. An important difference between superantigens and standard antigens is that the superantigen can independently elicit a strong primary immune response. The superantigen can stimulate T cells solely through the activation of the variable beta portion of the T-cell receptor. In addition, the superantigen can bind to major histocompatibility complex (MHC) class II proteins to activate accessory cells without prior antigen processing. Therefore, the process is not restricted to MHC class II proteins. Superantigens also cause massive release of cytokines (interleukin-1, tissue necrosis factor) and activation of B-cell antibody production. The toxins also may have a direct effect on targeted tissue and play a role in psoriasis, atopic dermatitis, toxic shock syndrome (TSS), staphylococcal scalded skin syndrome (SSSS), and a newly described, recurrent, toxin-mediated perineal erythema.

17. List the diagnostic criteria for staphylococcal toxic shock syndrome.

1. Major criteria (4 must be present)
   (1) Fever
   (2) Diffuse macular erythroderma with late desquamation of palms and soles
   (3) Conjunctival, oropharyngeal, or vaginal hyperemia
   (4) Hypotension (systolic blood pressure < 90 mmHg)
2. Minor criteria (three or more must be present)
   (1) Elevated creatine phosphokinase
   (2) Elevated liver functions
   (3) Elevated renal functions
   (4) Thrombocytopenia
   (5) Hypocalcemia and hypophosphatemia
   (6) Change in mental status
   (7) History of diarrhea or vomiting
   (8) Cardiopulmonary disease (myocarditis, adult respiratory distress syndrome)
3. All cultures and serologic studies must be negative for other diseases.

18. Is toxic shock syndrome caused only by *Staphylococcus aureus* enterotoxins or improper tampon use?

No. Currently improper use of tampons accounts for the minority of TSS cases. The incidence of streptococcal toxic shock-like syndrome is now increasing.

19. Describe the differences between staphylococcal and streptococcal TSS.

The systemic signs and symptoms of TSS, regardless of the etiologic agent, are identical. However, the cutaneous findings vary. Streptococcal TSS is associated with desquamative macular erythroderma and possible bullae formation; 80% of cases are associated with a necrotizing fascitis or myositis. Blood cultures are positive in more than 50% of cases, and antistreptolysin O titers are elevated. The mortality rate of staphylococcal TSS is < 5%, whereas the fatality rate of streptococcal TSS is 30%. Staphylococcal TSS is treated with beta-lactamase–resistant antistaphylococcal antibiotics, whereas streptococcal TSS is treated with antistreptococcal antibiotics.

20. What is staphylococcal scalded skin syndrome (SSSS)?

SSSS is a toxin-mediated disease caused by *Staphylococcus aureus*. The disease presents with acute onset of fever and cutaneous tenderness. The epidermolytic toxin causes cleavage of the skin above the granular layer, with characteristic flaccid blisters and subsequent denudation. Culturing of the skin is negative because the bacteria are located at distant foci, often in the nasopharynx. The disease most often affects children but may affect adults with renal insufficiency who cannot adequately excrete the epidermolytic toxin. SSSS is treated with antistaphylococcal antibiotics.

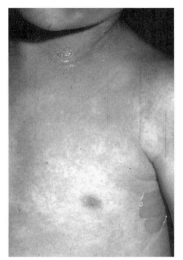

Erythematous, tender skin with an area of denudation of the skin characteristic of SSSS.

21. Define petechia, purpura and ecchymosis.

Petechia is a circumscribed deposit of blood in the skin (outside the blood vessel) less than 2 mm in diameter. **Purpura** is a circumscribed deposit of blood in the skin from 2 mm–1.0 cm in diameter. **Ecchymosis** is a deposit of blood greater than 1 cm.

22. Name four diseases that may present with fever and petechia/purpura and their respective causative agent.

1. Rocky Mountain spotted fever—*Rickettsia rickettsii* (tick-borne)
2. Meningococcemia—*Neisseria meningitidis*
3. Disseminated gonorrhea—*Neisseria gonorrhoeae*
4. Subacute bacterial endocarditis—*Streptococcus viridans*

23. Give an example of a disease that is transmitted by a mosquito and may cause an exanthem.

Dengue fever is an acute flavivirus infection that presents with fever and myalgia; it is commonly known as **breakbone fever**. Defervescence is followed by generalized maculopapular dermatitis. A hemorrhagic variant with a bleeding dyscrasia presents with petechial dermatitis. It is most commonly encountered in Southeast Asia and Africa but now has been reported in South America and Texas. The disease is transmitted by the mosquito, *Aedes aegypti*.

24. What may be associated with fever and dermatitis other than an underlying infectious agent?

1. Drug reactions
   (1) Maculopapular eruptions (e.g., sulfa drugs, thiazide diuretics, amoxicillin—in association with infectious mononucleosis)
   (2) Erythema multiforme and toxic epidermal necrosis (e.g., allopurinol, sulfa drugs, phenytoin)
   (3) Hypersensitivity reactions (e.g., phenytoin, minocycline)
   (4) Serum sickness-like reaction (e.g., cephalosporins)

2. Generalized erythroderma
   (1) Exacerbation of underlying dermatitis (e.g., psoriasis, atopic dermatitis)
   (2) Leukemic phase of cutaneous T-cell lymphoma
   (3) Underlying malignancy
   (4) Idiopathic

DISCLAIMER

The opinions and assertions contained herein are the private views of the authors and are not to be construed as official or reflecting the policies of the Department of Defense or Department of the Army.

BIBLIOGRAPHY

1. Arnold HL, Odom RB, James WD: Andrew's Diseases of the Skin, 8th ed. W.B. Saunders, Philadelphia, 1990, pp 436–485.
2. Baselga E, Drolet BA, Esterly NB: Purpura in infants and children. J Am Acad Dermatol 37:673–705, 1997.
3. Benenson A: Control of Communicable Diseases in Man, 15th ed. Washington, DC, American Public Health Association, 1990, pp 117–122.
4. Bialecki C, Feder HM, Grant-Kels JM: The six classic childhood exanthems: A review and update. J Am Acad Dermatol 21:891–903, 1989.
5. Cherry JD: Contemporary infectious exanthems. Clin Infect Dis 16:199–207, 1993.
6. Frieden IJ: Childhood exanthems. Curr Opin Pediatr 7:411–414, 1995.
7. Frieden IJ, Resnick SD: Childhood exanthems old and new. Pediatr Clin North Am 38:859–887, 1991.
8. Habif TP: Clinical Dermatology: A Color Guide to Diagnosis and Therapy, 3rd ed. St. Louis, Mosby, 1996, pp 409–444.
9. Kellner B, Kiati I, Krafchik B: Congenital varicella syndrome. Pediatr Dermatol 13:341–344, 1996.
10. Leung DYM, Meissner HC, Fulton D, et al: The potential role of bacterial superantigens in the pathogenesis of Kawasaki syndrome. J Clin Immunol 15:11S–17S, 1995.
11. Leung DYM, Norris DA: The role of bacterial superantigens in psoriasis and atopic dermatitis. Prog Dermatol 31:1–14, 1997.
12. Manders SM, Heymann WR, Atillasoy E, et al: Recurrent toxin-mediated perineal erythema. Arch Dermatol 132:57–60, 1996.
13. McCuiag CC, Russo P, Powell J, et al: Unilateral laterothoracic exanthem: A clinicopathologic study of forty-eight patients. J Am Acad Dermatol 34:979–984, 1996.
14. Meissner HC, Leung DYM: Kawasaki syndrome. Curr Opin Rheumatol 7:455–458, 1995.
15. Resnick SD: Staphylococcal toxin-mediated syndromes in childhood. Semin Dermatol 11:11–18, 1992.
16. Trofa AF, DeFraites RF, Smoak BL, et al: Dengue fever in US military personnel in Haiti. JAMA 277:1546–1548, 1997.
17. Wolf JE, Rabinowitz LG: Streptococcal toxic shock-like syndrome. Arch Dermatol 131:73–77, 1995.

55. PYODERMAS

Bonnie Cary Freitas, M.D.

1. What is pyoderma?

Pyoderma is defined broadly as any purulent disease of the skin. The term is used by some to describe impetigo.

2. List and describe the different forms of purulent skin infection, including the most common etiologic agent.

Lesion	Etiologic Agent	Description
Impetigo	*Staphylococcus aureus*, Group A streptococci (GAS)	Honey-colored crusts
Ecthyma	GAS	Deep, punched-out ulcer with yellow crust
Folliculitis	*S. aureus*, *Pseudomonas* sp.	Multiple small pustules around hair follicles
Furuncle	*S. aureus*	Superficial inflammatory abscess
Carbuncle	*S. aureus*	Multiple draining abscesses
Erysipelas	GAS	Edematous erythema with distinct leading edge
Cellulitis	GAS, *S. aureus*, polymicrobial (diabetics)	Tender, erythematous, warm area without distinct borders
Paronychia	GAS, *S. aureus*, gram-negative organisms	Swelling, pain, and erythema surrounding nail bed

3. One way to classify pyoderma is by the anatomic location within the skin that is affected. Match the lesion with the portion of the skin anatomy involved.

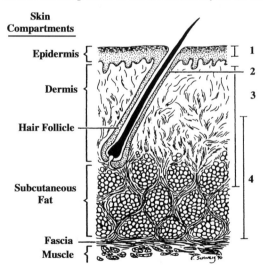

Answers: 1, Impetigo; 2, Folliculitis; 3, Erysipelas; 4, Cellulitis. (From Feingold DS: Staphylococcal pyodermas. Semin Dermatol 12:332, 1993, with permission.)

4. How do primary and secondary pyoderma differ in pathogenic mechanism?

Primary—normal skin is colonized with bacteria that are introduced intradermally after a minor abrasion, scratch, or insect bite.

Secondary—skin that has been previously damaged by burns, dermatoses, or trauma is secondarily colonized and infected by bacteria.

5. Describe the typical clinical findings of classic impetigo, and identify the population primarily affected.

Lesions affect exposed areas of skin, with most cases occurring in the lower extremities. Facial involvement may follow a previous nasopharyngeal infection with GAS. The lesions begin as small vesicles, which quickly transform into pruritic, pustular lesions covered with a thick yellow crust. Regional lymphadenopathy may be present. Healing is slow but generally does not lead to scarring.

Most cases of impetigo occur in children and are caused by GAS and *S. aureus*. Impetigo is highly infectious with outbreaks in hot, humid climates where children are in close contact with one another.

6. What is bullous impetigo? How does its pathogenesis differ from the nonbullous form?

Bullous impetigo accounts for 10% of cases of impetigo and is caused by *S. aureus*. Seen primarily in children, the bullous form begins as vesicles and progresses to flaccid bullae. The bullae rupture, leaving a shiny "varnished" appearance.

The pathogenesis differs because the lesions form as response to toxins produced by *S. aureus*, whereas the lesions of classic impetigo are produced by neutrophil invasion and pus formation.

7. In GAS, what is M protein? What role does it play in the pyodermal disease process?

M protein is the primary virulence factor in GAS with more than 80 recognized serotypes. The protein prevents phagocytosis of the bacteria by interfering with complement activation via the alternative pathway. Specific M serotypes have been associated with the subsequent development of glomerulonephritis.

8. Describe the serious sequelae that can result from classic (nonbullous) impetigo.

Acute glomerulonephritis (AGN). The latent period from infection with GAS to AGN is approximately 21 days. Children are affected more commonly but have a better prognosis than adults. AGN affects 2–15% of patients with streptococcal skin infections. Certain nephritogenic strains of GAS (M type 49, 55, 57, 60) are implicated in outbreaks. Treatment of the initial skin infection with antibiotics does not alter the subsequent risk of developing AGN. Anti-DNase B and antihyaluronidase are more useful markers of disease in post-pyoderma AGN. Anti-streptolysin O (ASO) titers are used for this purpose in post-pharyngitis AGN. Although GAS pharyngitis may lead to rheumatic fever, GAS pyoderma does not. Differing M serotypes of the streptococci are believed to account for the difference in rheumatogenicity.

Cellulitis. Impetigo may spread to involve deeper dermal and subcutaneous tissues. Prompt recognition is required with institution of systemic antibiotics.

9. What is the treatment of impetigo?

A few small lesions may be soaked with antiseptic soap and water until the crusts are removed. A topical antibiotic such as mupirocin or bacitracin is then applied to the clean base 2–3 times/day, for 1 week. More extensive lesions benefit from the addition of an oral antibiotic, which covers the potential pathogens. Options include cephalexin, dicloxacillin, or azithromycin. Unresponsive or serious infections may require an intravenous antibiotic, such as nafcillin.

10. What is ecthyma?

Although similar to impetigo, ecthyma is a deeper infection usually caused by GAS and characterized by a deep, punched-out ulcer with yellow-green crust. Ecthyma occurs on the lower legs, predominantly the shins and dorsum of the feet, and may result in scar formation. Ecthyma gangrenosum, a lesion seen in immunocompromised patients, is caused by *Pseudomonas aeruginosa* and is distinct from ecthyma.

11. Which organism is uniquely associated with folliculitis after swimming pool or hot tub exposure?

Folliculitis after exposure to inadequately chlorinated water is frequently caused by *Pseudomonas aeruginosa*. Development of pruritic lesions occurs approximately 48 hours after exposure. Otitis externa caused by the same organism may accompany the folliculitis and is best treated with polymyxin B-neomycin-hydrocortisone ear drops 4 times/day. The folliculitis typically heals spontaneously within 5 days.

Note: Do not confuse uncomplicated otitis externa ("swimmer's ear") with malignant otitis externa. Diabetics may be affected by an acute, invasive pseudomonal otitis externa, which requires more aggressive therapy with outpatient fluoroquinolones or inpatient intravenous antibiotics.

12. What is the difference between a furuncle and carbuncle? What is the best treatment for each?

A furuncle is a deep inflammatory nodule caused by *S. aureus*. A furuncle develops from a previous follicular infection and is best treated by incision and drainage.

A carbuncle is a collection of furuncles in the dermis and subcutaneous tissues generally underlying thick skin (nape of neck and back) with multiple draining sinuses along hair follicles. Fever, malaise, and bacteremia may accompany the lesion. Treatment is best accomplished with antibiotics such as dicloxacillin, clindamycin, or a macrolide. Surgical drainage may be necessary if the lesion is sufficiently fluctuant.

13. Is recurrent furunculosis a sign of an underlying immune deficit?

Most cases of recurrent furunculosis are not associated with a disorder of immune or cellular function. Obesity, diabetes mellitus, drug abuse, chronic hemodialysis, and corticosteroid treatment may act as predisposing factors.

14. What measures may be used for prophylaxis against recurrent furunculosis?

Treating patients with recurrent furunculosis is a challenging task. Good skin hygiene with frequent handwashing and cleansing with chlorhexidine, an antimicrobial wash, may decrease colonization and subsequent attacks. Clothes and bed linens should be washed in hot water daily to prevent recurrent autoinoculation. Eradication of nasal carriage of *S. aureus* may be achieved with 2% topical mupirocin applied 3 times/day to the nares for 5 days or by therapy with oral rifampin. Unfortunately, treatment with either modality has led to the development of resistance.

15. What is hydradenitis suppurativa?

Hydradenitis suppurativa is caused by keratin plugging of the apocrine glands in the axilla and groin. It is frequently complicated by secondary infection with *S. aureus*, leading to recurrent abscesses, draining sinuses, and scar formation.

16. Describe the clinical presentation of erysipelas and the known risk factors.

Erysipelas is a superficial skin infection that involves the lymphatics and is characterized by a painful, edematous erythematous lesion with a raised leading edge. It is caused by infection with GAS, although cultures of the skin or leading edge rarely yield the responsible organism.

Areas of compromised lymphatic drainage are at highest risk of involvement. Radical mastectomy, chronic lymphedema, and venous insufficiency are predisposing risk factors. Erysipelas also may result in lymphatic obstruction, making it more likely to recur in previously affected sites.

17. How does cellulitis differ from erysipelas by location within the skin?

Cellulitis involves the deep dermis and subcutaneous fat, whereas erysipelas affects the superficial dermis, leading to lymphatic obstruction.

18. What factors predispose a person to developing cellulitis?

Any patient with a chronic debilitating disease or immunosuppression is at increased risk of cellulitis. Specific factors include diabetes, chronic renal failure, chronic lymphedema, venous stasis, cirrhosis, cancer, or immunosuppression from disease or drugs (corticosteroids).

19. What bacterial agents are frequently implicated in cellulitis?

GAS and *S. aureus* are the most commonly implicated organisms. However, in certain populations other organisms may be isolated:

Diabetics: a polymicrobial infection may be present secondary to GAS, *S. aureus*, anaerobes, enterobacteriaceae, and enterococci.

Head and neck cellulitis in children: *Haemophilus influenzae.*

Fish, meat, and poultry handlers: *Erysipelothrix rhusiopathiae* (erythematous lesion resembling erysipelas at a portal of entry [e.g., the hands]).

Ingestion of raw seafood in cirrhotics and diabetics: *Vibrio vulnificus* (bacteremia from ingestion seeds the skin with resulting cellulitis and bullae).

20. Describe the typical clinical presentation of cellulitis.

Cellulitis begins as an area of warm, tender erythema with swelling. Frequently there is an obvious portal of entry for infection. Fever, leukocytosis, and regional tender lymphadenopathy often develop.

21. What is the treatment for cellulitis?

A limited area of involvement in patients without predisposing risk factors may be treated with oral first-generation cephalosporins or the newer macrolides. However, patients with predisposing risk factors and patients with more severe or extensive involvement should be treated with intravenous antibiotics such as nafcillin, cefazolin, vancomycin, or clindamycin.

If the patient is diabetic or immunocompromised, broader coverage is needed to include gram-negative pathogens. Among the many choices are second- or third-generation cephalosporins, ampicillin/sulbactam, and meropenem.

22. Name the causes of cellulitis associated with blebs.

- *Vibrio vulnificus*
- *Aeromonas hydrophilia*
- *Staphylococcus aureus*
- Severe group A streptococci
- Necrotizing fasciitis (not strictly a cellulitis, but must be considered in the differential diagnosis; caused by clostridia, mixed aerobic and anaerobic bacteria, and GAS)
- Pemphigus (also not a cellulitis but must be considered in the differential diagnosis)
- Rarely *Campylobacter* spp. (and case reports of other gram-negative bacteria)
- *Pseudomonas aeruginosa* (in ecthyma gangrenosum)
- *Pyoderma gangrenosum* (not an infection but may be confused with ecthyma)

BIBLIOGRAPHY

1. Ayoub EM, Ferrieri P: Infectious Disease, 5th ed. Philadelphia, J.B. Lippincott, 1994.
2. Bass JW: Treatment of skin and skin structure infections. Pediatr Infect Dis J 11:152–155, 1992.
3. Bisno AL: Group A streptococcal infections and acute rheumatic fever. N Engl J Med 325:783–793, 1991.
4. Feingold DS: Staphylococcal and streptococcal pyodermas. Semin Dermatol 12:331–335, 1993.
5. Swartz MN: Principles and Practice of Infectious Diseases, 4th ed. New York, Churchill Livingstone, 1995.

56. WOUND INFECTIONS

Steve Granada, M.D.

1. What kind of fool would put maggots into an open wound?

Ambroise Paré, the French surgeon who gave up using boiling oil to treat wounds, noted the value of maggots after the Battle of St. Quentin in 1557. Napoleon's military surgeon noted that maggots attack only rotting substances, not living tissues. A Confederate Army surgeon, J. F. Zacharia, used maggots during the American Civil War (sometimes known as the War of Northern Aggression) and reported "eminent satisfaction. . . . I am sure I saved many lives by their use, escaped septicemia, and had rapid recoveries." A Union Army physician, W. W. Keen, observed that maggots were "disgusting" but did no apparent harm.

William S. Baer, clinical professor of orthopedics at Johns Hopkins, observed beneficial effects of maggots during World War I in France. In 1928 he treated four children with seemingly incurable osteomyelitis with maggots obtained from a local blowfly. After 6 weeks, all were completely healed. His success heralded the golden age of maggot therapy (1928–1948), and, as judged by numerous case reports, they still seem to be very helpful.

2. What are the classic signs of an infected wound?

The classic signs of infection are erythema, pain or tenderness, swelling, heat, and pus. The classic signs of inflammation include all of the above except pus. Some amount of inflammation is required for wound healing. A clear "yes" or "no" answer regarding the presence of infection is difficult in wounds with no pus and/or negative cultures.

3. What types of wound infections may benefit from hyperbaric oxygen?

The current use of hyperbaric oxygen as an adjunct therapy in wounds can be divided into three main categories:

1. Diseases for which the weight of evidence supports hyperbaric oxygen as effective therapy:
   • Clostridial myonecrosis
   • Compromised skin grafts and flaps
2. Diseases for which the weight of evidence suggests that hyperbaric oxygen may be helpful:
   • Refractory osteomyelitis
   • Selected problem wounds (i.e., diabetic foot infections and leg ulcers due to arterial insufficiency)
3. Diseases for which the weight of evidence does not support the use of hyperbaric oxygen, but for which it may be helpful:
   • Necrotizing fasciitis
   • Thermal burns

4. What are the most common complications from infected wounds?

The most common complications are cellulitis, fasciitis, tenosynovitis, sepsis, septic arthritis, osteochondritis, and osteomyelitis.

5. Louis Pasteur once said, "The germ is nothing. It is the terrain in which it is found that is everything." How does his statement apply to predicting wound infection and/ or sepsis?

Wound monitoring by swab cultures or biopsies allows identification and quantification of an organism. Quantitative microbiology alone cannot predict the risk of sepsis. If > 100,000 organisms/gram of tissue are present in a wound, an infection may or may not exist. However, the nature of the organism is still important. For instance, gram-negative organisms are not always equal to gram-positive organisms in extent of pathogenicity. Attempts to use other systemic microbial indicators have not been successful (e.g., endotoxins, tissue necrosis factor, or other cytokines). There is no single perfect predictor of wound infections or systemic sepsis. The risk of complications depends on risk factors that affect the tissue in which the wound is found: (1) host status, (2) amount of contamination, (3) mechanism and depth of injury, and (4) time of injury before treatment started.

6. Why is the medical history of the host important in wound evaluation?

Many diseases and conditions can affect the number and function of polymorphonuclear cells and macrophages, including diabetes mellitus, malnutrition, alcohol abuse, hepatic or renal insufficiency, asplenia, malignancies, and extremes of age.

Conditions that result in impaired delivery of nutrients, oxygen, and white blood cells due to decreases in cutaneous blood flow include diabetes mellitus, atherosclerotic peripheral vascular disease, collagen vascular diseases, and severe congestive heart failure.

Medications that are immunosuppressive or impede blood clotting should be sought, especially glucocorticoids. Cancer chemotherapy or radiation therapy also suppress the immune response.

7. What factors related to the wound are most important in considering the risk of infection?

1. Age of the wound. The earlier a wound is closed, the less likely it will become infected. A wound left untreated for > 3 hours has a potential bacterial proliferation of > 1,000,000 organisms/gram of tissue.

2. Mechanism of injury. Injury may be secondary to shearing forces (i.e., sharp injury) or due to impact (i.e., blunt injury). Large or deep wounds are more prone to infection. Blunt injuries sustain larger amounts of kinetic energy, which result in microvascular disruption, edema, and devitalized tissue; thus, they are more prone to infection.

8. How do you describe a wound?

Anatomic location, measured size, depth, (what types of tissue are involved), and appearance of tissue along the edges of the wound are important to document. Close inspection for arterial bleeding, gross particulate matter (e.g., feces, saliva), foreign bodies (e.g., glass), devitalized tissue, and level of tissue/structure involvement should be performed.

9. What are the most common organisms found in simple wounds?

For traumatic wounds during initial presentation to the emergency department, culture biopsies found pure aerobic cultures in 66.5% of wounds and mixed aerobic/anaerobic cultures in 32%. Two or more pathogens were usually isolated. The most common included *Staphylococcus aureus* (52%), streptococci (52%), clostridia (23%), enterobacteria (23%), and anaerobic gram-negative bacilli (1.5%). Studies involving infected (as opposed to contaminated) wounds in which purulent material was cultured confirm that staphylococci and streptococci are the most common pathogens associated with wound infections.

10. If indicated, what empiric antibiotic treatment should be started in patients with a simple wound?

The initial selection of antimicrobial agents may be guided by Gram stain. Most wound infections are due to staphylococci and streptococci which are sensitive to first-generation cephalosporins and penicillinase-resistant penicillins. Wounds contaminated with feces or manure often develop obligate anaerobes and coliforms, thus requiring second- and third-generation cephalosporins, a penicillin/beta-lactamase combination, or the combination of clindamycin and an aminoglycoside. Levofloxacin as single agent may provide adequate and inexpensive coverage for wounds infected by multiple bacteria, but it has limited anaerobic activity.

11. Should antibiotics be given as prophylaxis in nonsurgical wounds?

About 90–95% of wounds treated in the emergency department heal when given appropriate wound care, such as irrigation, debridement, and foreign body removal. The routine use of antibiotics for simple wounds is therefore not indicated.

12. When should antibiotics be used in early wound management before clinical evidence of infection?
Antibiotics are appropriate if:
1. The wound is heavily contaminated with feces or saliva
2. The wound was caused by an animal or human bite
3. The patient is prone to development of infective endocarditis
4. The patient has an orthopedic prosthesis
5. The patient presents with wounds involving lymphedematous regions
6. The patient has extensive intraoral wounds
7. A high risk wound is found in a compromised patient: contaminated wound, old wound, or devitalized tissue in a diabetic person.

13. Describe the two types of diabetic ulcers.
Neuropathy is the most common underlying cause of wounds in diabetic patients, followed by vascular occlusive etiologies. Most neuropathic ulcers occur under the foot, particularly at the metatarsal heads, and soft tissue of the toes. Clinically, if ankle pulses are present with signs of good arterial perfusion, the ulcer is probably neuropathic. In addition, when compared with ischemic ulcers, neuropathic ulcers have marked marginal thickening and keratosis.

14. What is the Wagner classification?
The Wagner classification of diabetic foot ulcers captures the range of possible presentations:
Grade 0:   Skin intact, but bony deformities or keratosis present
Grade I: Ulceration down to dermis only
Grade II: Ulceration involving tendons and/or joint capsule
Grade III: Ulceration down to the bone
Grade IV: Localized gangrene
Grade V: Gangrene involving a major portion of the foot

15. How useful are standard and nuclear imaging techniques in the assessment of diabetic foot ulcers?
Infected foot ulcers in diabetic patients require rapid diagnosis. The presence of an abscess or cellulitis may be determined by a good physical exam; computed tomography (CT) and magnetic resonance imaging (MRI) are useful in detecting deep infections, abscesses, and bony involvement (MRI is especially adept at this). Bone scans and plain films are poor techniques for finding deep infections. Osteomyelitis may be difficult to differentiate from diabetic osteodystrophy by technetium[99] bone scan. Bone scans combined with radiologically labeled white blood cells can give a diagnostic accuracy of 90%.

16. What are the most common causes of cellulitis in the adult?
Group A streptococci and *Staphylococcus aureus* are the most common causes of cellulitis. The infection may spread rapidly, involving the subcutaneous tissues. Previous trauma (lacerations, puncture wounds) or underlying skin lesions (ulcer, furuncle) predispose to the development of cellulitis.

17. What are the four major threats to life and limb that should be considered in every initial evaluation of a chronic skin ulcer?
1. Venous thrombosis
2. Acute arterial occlusion
3. Severe systemic or regional infections
4. Metabolic abnormalities
Patients with venous stasis ulcers are at risk for deep venous thrombosis and extensive secondary cellulitis. Arterial ulcers may culminate in acute thrombotic occlusion. Patients with pressure ulcers are at risk for deep tissue infection and sepsis. Diabetic patients have the additional risk of developing diabetic ketoacidosis and/or hyperosmolar coma.

18. Name the five most common pathogens isolated from dog bite wounds.

Pathogens are usually components of the normal oral flora of dogs and include alpha-hemo-lytic streptococci, *Staphylococcus aureus*, EF-4, *Capnocytophaga canimorsus*, and *Haemophilus* species. EF-4 is one of the gram-negative bacilli without a genus and species name. It is called EF-4 because of the letter and number designation, based on growth characteristics, assigned by the Centers for Disease Control and Prevention. EF means *eugonic fermenter*; the organism grows well through fermentation of glucose. In addition, 25–30% of cases grow anaerobic bacteria. *Pasteurella multocida* is isolated from 20–30% of dog bite wounds (and over 90% of cat bites).

19. What are the five main classifications of chronic skin ulcers?

1. **Pressure ulcers:** often located in the ischium, sacrum, and hip trochanter. Bed-ridden patients are predisposed to pressure ulcers.

2. **Venous stasis ulcers:** often occur in the setting of chronic venous insufficiency manifest clinically by lower extremity edema, stasis dermatitis, and hyperpigmentation. Venous stasis ulcers are shallow, tender, pliable (they move with skin), and usually located along the long saphenous system.

3. **Arterial ulcers:** occur in the lateral ankle, toes, heel and ball of the foot, fifth metatarsal, and head of the first metatarsal. Resting pain is the clinical hallmark. A history of claudication is also common.

4. **Diabetic ulcers:** classified as either neuropathic or ischemic in etiology (see question 13).

5. **Self-induced (factitious) ulcers**

20. Do crepitations on physical exam or gas on plain films indicate gas gangrene?

True gas gangrene is a rare cause of gas in tissues. Gas gangrene does not always present with gas, but when it does, the radiographs are pathognomonic. The gas is located within, not between, the muscle groups, resulting in a " feathering " appearance. The most common cause of gas in a wound is due to air entering when the wound was inspected. The second most common cause is an infection with aerobic gas-producing gram-negative bacilli.

21. Can seaweed help wounds to heal?

Kelp is the source of complex polysaccharide biosynthetic dressings called alginates. Alginates are derived from salts of alginic acid, and the material is best classified as a gel. Exudate from the wound is required to transform the gel into a therapeutic gel matrix. The alginate dressing has been shown to be effective in treating ulcers, pressure sores, and full-thickness surgical defects. The underlying requirement is that the wound is exudative.

BIBLIOGRAPHY

1. Arndt K: Types of Topical Medications: Manual of Dermatologic Therapeutics with Essentials of Diagnosis, 4th ed. Boston, Little, Brown, 1989.
2. Baer WS: The treatment of chronic osteomyelitis with the maggot (larva of the blowfly). J Bone Joint Surg 13:478, 1931.
3. Chisholm CD: Wound evaluation and cleansing. Emerg Med Clin North Am 10: 665–670, 1992.
4. Kahn RM, Goldstein EJC: Common bacterial skin infections. Postgrad Med 93:175–182, 1993.
5. Laing P: Diabetic foot ulcers. Am J Surg 167(Suppl):31S–36S, 1994.
6. Lindsey D: Soft tissue infections. Emerg Med Clin North Am 10:737–748, 1992.
7. Lindsey D, Quenzer RW: Infection Following Bites, Wounds, and Burns: Infectious Disease in Emergency Medicine. Boston, Little, Brown, 1992.
8. Piacquadio D: Alginates: A "new" dressing alternative. J Dermatol Surg Oncol 18:990–998, 1992.
9. Rodgers KG: The rational use of antimicrobial agents in simple wounds. Emerg Med Clin North Am 10:753–763, 1992.
10. Thomson PD, Smith DJ: What is infection? Am J Surg 167(Suppl):7S–11S, 1994.
11. Tibbles PM, Edelsberg JS: Hyperbaric-oxygen therapy. N Engl J Med 275:1642–1647, 1996.
12. Trott A: Chronic skin ulcers. Emerg Med Clin North Am 10:823–841, 1992.
13. Wijetunge DB: Management of acute and traumatic wounds: Main aspects of care in adults and children. Am J Surg 167(Suppl):56S–60S, 1994.

XVII. Urinary Tract Infections

57. URINARY TRACT INFECTIONS

William Salzer, M.D.

1. What is the pathogenesis of bacterial cystitis in otherwise healthy women?

Sticky question. The periurethral epithelium becomes colonized with enteric bacterial flora. Strains of gram-negative rods that cause cystitis tend to express type 1 fimbriae (pili), which bind to mannose residues on the surface glycoproteins of uroepithelial cells. Upon entering the bladder, these strains are more likely to adhere to the epithelium and produce infection.

2. What are the risk factors for cystitis in women?

Remember, most things that taste good or feel good are bad for you. Unfortunately in healthy young women it is often sex. Onset of or increased frequency of intercourse (honeymoon cystitis) is a risk factor. Also use of a diaphragm with spermicide markedly increases the risk of cystitis, probably through alteration of vaginal bacterial flora by the spermicide. In older women estrogen deficiency may enhance colonization of the periurethral area with uropathogens, or incomplete emptying of the bladder due to prolapse may predispose to urinary tract infection (UTI).

3. What are the signs and symptoms of acute cystitis?

Dysuria, frequency, urgency, suprapubic pain, often with pyuria, sometimes gross hematuria. Fever is usually absent unless pyelonephritis is present.

4. What is the differential diagnosis of a woman with acute cystitis?

Vaginitis due to *Candida* or *Trichomonas* spp.
Urethritis due to *Chlamydia trachomatis* or *Neisseria gonorrhoeae*
Genital herpes simplex
Allergic reactions or irritation
Trauma

5. How should one diagnose acute cystitis?

In a woman with typical symptoms, without fever or flank pain, a simple urine leukocyte esterase dipstick or microscopic urinalysis showing pyuria is quite sensitive and moderately specific; it is also the most cost-effective means (in this age of managed care) of diagnosis. Urine culture and sensitivity should be performed in all patients who fail or relapse after empirical antibiotic therapy.

6. True or false: urine cultures must grow > 100,000 colony-forming units (CFU)/ml to diagnose UTI.

Partly true, partly false. A urine culture growing this many colonies of a single uropathogen indicates true infection (highly specific) but may occur in patients without symptoms (see question 22). On the other hand, studies using suprapubic bladder aspiration have shown that some women with clinical cystitis may have only 100–1000 CFU of bacteria, indicating that counts as low as 100 CFU may be significant in patients with typical symptoms and signs.

7. What are the antibiotics of choice for empirical treatment of cystitis?

Unfortunately, amoxicillin, sulfa alone, or nitrofurantoin will fail in 30% of cases because of antibiotic resistance in community bacterial isolates. The current drug of choice is trimethoprim/sulfamethoxazole (TMP/SMX) one double strength dose 2 times/day. In sulfa-allergic patients, trimethoprim, 100 mg 2 times/day, works as well. Fluoroquinolones may be used but are more expensive.

8. How long should uncomplicated cystitis be treated?

Three days of antibiotic therapy is more effective than single-dose therapy and is as effective as 7 days. If the patient fails or relapses soon after 3-day therapy, urine culture and sensitivity tests should be obtained. Antibiotic resistance, pyelonephritis, or an alternate diagnosis should be suspected.

9. In a healthy woman with frequent recurrences of cystitis, what can be done?

Abstaining from sexual intercourse would help, but unfortunately (or fortunately) abstinence is not acceptable to most patients. Women who use diaphragm and spermicide should be advised to use a different form of contraception. Voiding after intercourse and cranberry juice are *not* effective. Daily antibiotic prophylaxis or postcoital dosing with one-half single-strength dose of TMP/SMX, trimethoprim, or nitrofurantoin is effective in reducing recurrences. Another cost-effective strategy is patient-initiated antibiotic therapy at the onset of symptoms, which saves the patient the time and expense of a physician visit.

10. What makes TMP/SMX, TMP, nitrofurantoin, and fluoroquinolones so special in the treatment of UTIs?

Because their spectrum of antibiotic activity is restricted to aerobic gram-negative enteric bacteria, they markedly reduce the numbers of these bacteria in the stool and rarely select antibiotic-resistant strains. Penicillins, cephalosporins, tetracyclines, or sulfa alone alters the normal vaginal and stool flora, enhancing the risk for vaginal candidiasis and selecting antibiotic-resistant gram-negative bacteria in the stool, which may subsequently cause UTI.

11. When should you obtain imaging studies or refer a woman with recurrent cystitis to a urologist?

Not often. Imaging studies are performed to detect structural abnormalities of the urinary tract that are amenable to treatment. Women with onset of cystitis after puberty rarely have significant structural abnormalities unless frequent relapses with the identical bacterial strain occur.

12. What about cystitis in men?

In older men cystitis occurs most often in association with prostatic enlargement; frequent relapses are seen with chronic bacterial prostatitis. Cystitis occurs in younger men much less frequently than in women and is associated with insertive anal intercourse (another compelling reason for condom use) and colonization of the glans with gram-negative enteric bacteria in uncircumcised men. Men with cystitis should be treated with a 7-day course of antibiotics and do not need further work-up unless the infection recurs.

13. What are the etiologic agents of infectious epididymitis?

In young men, causative agents are sexually transmitted pathogens—*Chlamydia trachomatis* and gonococci. In older men, the etiology is usually gram-negative enteric bacteria, often in association with bladder catheters or bacterial prostatitis.

14. What is the pathogenesis of pyelonephritis?

Bacteria enter the bladder and ascend to the kidneys. Strains of gram-negative bacteria that cause pyelonephritis tend to express P-fimbriae, which bind to gal-gal residues of glycolipids that are abundant on the surface of epithelial cells of the upper urinary tract.

15. What are the signs and symptoms of pyelonephritis?

Sometimes none (especially in elderly and immunosuppressed patients), sometimes only symptoms of cystitis (silent pyelonephritis). Most patients with pyelonephritis have fever, chills, and leukocytosis; some will have flank pain and tenderness of the costovertebral angle.

16. Must every patient with pyelonephritis be hospitalized for treatment?

Patients with no signs of sepsis and no nausea or vomiting that interferes with oral therapy may be treated on an outpatient basis if close follow-up is available. Oral TMP/SMX or a fluoro-quinolone should be used.

17. What is an appropriate IV antibiotic regimen for hospitalized patients with uncomplicated pyelonephritis?

Many regimens are available: TMP/SMX, third-generation cephalosporins, ampicillin and gentamicin, or fluoroquinolones. When the patient becomes afebrile (usually in 2–3 days), switch to oral therapy based on culture results to complete 14 days of therapy.

18. What do you do if the temperature does not go down promptly?

First, be patient. In most patients with pyelonephritis the temperature will decrease gradually over 2–3 days. In the patient whose fever and white blood cell count increase or do not decrease after 3 days of therapy, suspect a complication and consider ultrasound or computed tomography to exclude perinephric abscess, stones, or other causes of obstruction.

19. What is meant by complicated UTI? Why does it matter?

Complicated means a structural or functional abnormality of the urinary tract: neurogenic bladder, catheters, urinary diverting procedures, stones, vesiculoureteral reflux, or anatomic obstruction. Affected patients are more difficult to treat because they often have antibiotic-resistant bacteria, which because of the structural problems are more difficult to eradicate.

20. What about UTIs in patients with renal transplants?

Cystitis in patients with renal transplants often proceeds to pyelonephritis because of the short, denervated ureter. Unless a perinephric abscess has ensued, pain over the graft is absent because the transplanted kidney is not innervated. Treatment should be continued for at least 2 weeks unless pyelonephritis can be ruled out, which is usually not possible.

21. Why do nephrologists dislike TMP/SMX or, more specifically, TMP?

1. TMP causes hyperkalemia. It is structurally similar to amiloride and inhibits the distal tubular sodium absorption and potassium secretion.

2. TMP causes elevation of serum creatinine. It inhibits the proximal tubular secretion of creatinine so that serum creatinine rises but glomerular filtration rate has not decreased.

22. What is asymptomatic bacteruria?

Surgical colleagues can answer this one: > 100,000 CFU of bacteria in a urine culture in a patient with no symptoms of UTI. Asymptomatic bacteruria is present in 1–2% of healthy, non-pregnant women, 10–20% of ambulatory elderly people, and up to 40% of debilitated elderly men and women.

23. Do all people with > 100,000 CFU in the urine require treatment?

Only if they have symptoms or signs of UTI or if they are pregnant. Treatment of asymptomatic bacteruria in elderly populations and other groups is of no benefit (remember, it is hard to make an asymptomatic patient feel better) in terms of long-term morbidity from UTI or mortality. Treatment also may be harmful, resulting in side effects and encouraging the appearance and spread of antibiotic-resistant bacteria.

24. What antibiotics are safe and effective in pregnant women with UTI?

Amoxicillin, first-generation cephalosporins, or nitrofurantoin is recommended. Sulfa, TMP, and aminoglycosides have some risk to the fetus. Tetracyclines or quinolones should not be used because of major effects on fetal bones.

25. When should urine cultures be performed in patients with long-term bladder catheters?

Only in the presence of signs or symptoms suggesting local or systemic bacterial infection. In this population urine cultures are never sterile (asymptomatic bacteriuria).

26. When do you treat a positive urine culture in patients with a chronic bladder catheter?

Only if they have local symptoms of UTI or signs suggesting urosepsis. I repeat, urine cultures are always positive. Antibiotic treatment does not sterilize the urine; it merely selects bacteria or fungi resistant to therapy. Treat only if you have to!

27. Does chronic suppressive or prophylactic therapy have any benefit for chronically catheterized patients?

No. Antibiotics select more resistant pathogens, which complicate treatment of symptomatic infections when they do develop.

28. Who gets candiduria?

Generally patients with catheters, stents, conduits, or other structural abnormalities who have received broad-spectrum antibiotics.

29. How should candiduria be managed?

First, remove catheters or other hardware whenever possible. In patients with catheter-related infections, amphotericin B bladder washes will eradicate the yeast, but recurrences are common if the catheter remains. Oral fluconazole has shown some promise, but chronic therapy in patients with persistent structural defects often selects azole-resistant strains such as *Candida krusei* and *C. glabrata*.

BIBLIOGRAPHY

1. Alappan R, Perazella MA, Buller GK: Hyperkalemia in hospitalized patients treated with trimethoprim-sulfamethoxazole. Ann Intern Med 124:316–320, 1996.
2. Boscia JA, Kobasa WD, Knight RA, et al: Epidemiology of bacteriuria in an elderly ambulatory population. Am J Med 80:208–214, 1986.
3. Gugliemo BJ, Stoller ML, Jacobs RA: Management of candiduria. Int J Antimicrob Agents 4:135–139, 1994.
4. Hooton TM, Scholes D, Hughes JP, et al: A prospective study of risk factors for symptomatic UTI in young women. N Engl J Med 335:468–474, 1996.
5. Nicolle LE: Prevention and treatment of catheter-related infections in older patients. Drugs Aging 4:379–391, 1994.
6. Stamm WE, Hooton TM: Management of urinary tract infections in adults. N Engl J Med 329:1328–1334, 1993.
7. Medical Clinics of North America 75(2):whole issue on UTI, 1991.

XVIII. Maternal and Pediatric Infections

58. INFECTIONS IN PREGNANCY

Cecilia Del Moral, M.D., and Donald R. Skillman, M.D., FACP

1. What is parvovirus B19? Why should pregnant women fear it?

Parvovirus B19 is the smallest single-stranded DNA virus. It grows in erythroid precursor cells and is the cause of erythema infectiosum (fifth disease), prolonged arthralgia and arthritis (in adults), and transient aplastic crisis in patients with chronic hemolytic anemia (e.g., sickle cell disease). Immunosuppressed people may develop severe chronic anemia. It is highly contagious, with transmission via respiratory secretions. Intrauterine infection can result in fetal anemia with hydrops fetalis and fetal death. Fortunately, intrauterine infection occurs in less than 10% of infections acquired in the first half of pregnancy.

2. Does pregnancy have anything to do with human papillomavirus (HPV)?

HPV is a DNA virus of great interest not only because of a dramatic increase in incidence but also because of its potential role in genital tract malignancy. HPV is associated with condyloma acuminata, cervical intraepithelial neoplasia, and invasive carcinoma. Flat warts are seen on the external genitalia and cervix. In unusual circumstances, the lesions may become so large that they mechanically obstruct the birth of the child. Viral replication is enhanced during pregnancy, possibly because of the associated mild immunologic suppression. The most common types are 6 and 11. Treatment for small condylomas includes electrocautery, cryocautery, and laser; for large lesions surgical removal may be necessary. Podophyllin should definitely *not* be used during pregnancy.

3. What do you know about herpes simplex virus during pregnancy?

Herpes simplex, a DNA virus of type I and type II, is transmitted via physical contact through skin or mucosa. In pregnant women infected for the first time, the risk of herpetic outbreak at delivery is 36%. A mother in whom genital herpes was diagnosed before pregnancy with a history of less than 6 outbreaks per year has a 13% risk of outbreak at delivery. On the other hand, in the same mother with more than 6 outbreaks per year, the risk increases to 25%. In 1988, the American College of Obstetrics and Gynecology recommended that at the time of delivery, women need to be examined for the presence of active herpetic lesions. If identifiable genital lesions are found or prodromal symptoms of a herpes recrudescence are described, she should be delivered abdominally, regardless of how long her membranes have been ruptured. If there are no visible lesions and no prodromal symptoms, a vaginal delivery is indicated. Acyclovir, valacyclovir, and famciclovir decrease the duration of herpes attacks and the frequency of recurrent attacks. In pregnancy, these drugs should be reserved for life-threatening maternal illness and not used for routine recurrent herpetic eruptions.

4. How is cell-mediated immunity (CMI) affected during pregnancy?

Investigations of the immunocompetency of pregnant women indicate selective depression of CMI of variable clinical significance. As this chapter illustrates, many infections are much more serious when acquired by pregnant women.

5. Why are urinary tract infections more common during pregnancy? What are the most common pathogens isolated in asymptomatic bacteriuria?

Relative obstruction of the ureters during pregnancy is due to the enlarging uterus, which compresses or blocks the ureters. Progesterone also enhances relaxation of the smooth muscle in the ureters and bladder. Pregnancy-induced glycosuria and aminoaciduria provide an excellent medium for bacteria to proliferate. The most common pathogens are the usual suspects: *Escherichia coli*, *Klebsiella pneumoniae*, *Proteus mirabilis*, *Enterobacter* spp., *Staphylococcus saprophyticus*, and group B streptococci.

6. What does cytomegalovirus (CMV) do during pregnancy?

CMV is another double-stranded DNA virus. It may remain latent after a primary infection and is the most common cause of congenital viral infection. Fifty percent of pregnant women are positive for CMV antibodies, usually indicating past infection. Transmission is via close or intimate contact, and the fetus can be infected transplacentally during the viremic phase of the mother's infection. Severe sequelae are seen in children whose mothers had a primary infection: microcephaly with periventricular calcification, hepatosplenomegaly with jaundice, and thrombocytopenic purpura. Survivors may have chorioretinitis with general cerebral degeneration. The lungs, eyes, kidneys, or pancreas also may be affected. CMV replicates in the kidney, and viruria is a consistent finding in infected neonates. Amniotic fluid culture appears to be a promising method for diagnosis. There is no effective and safe treatment for CMV infection in pregnancy. Prevention is the ideal solution. A live attenuated vaccine appears to be protective.

7. Is rubella a concern during pregnancy?

Rubella, an RNA togavirus, is transmitted by droplet infection and has an incubation period of 14–21 days. Maternal infection in the first 8 weeks of pregnancy leads to fetal infection in over 90% of cases. First-trimester rubella produces serious defects in 25–50% of fetuses and "minor" defects in even more. Infection acquired during the third and seventh week of gestation usually leads to death from serious anomalies. Congenital deafness is the primary concern for infants who acquire infection between the ninth and thirteenth weeks of gestation. Fetuses who acquire rubella during this time of organogenesis also may develop heart disease, cataracts, and cerebral and somatic retardation. Rubella-related problems present even after organogenesis is complete and sometimes are not recognized until the child reaches school age. Hearing defects, diabetes, growth retardation, and eye and heart abnormalities have been found.

8. What advice is appropriate for a woman who is not immune to rubella and wants to get pregnant?

Prepubertal or nonpregnant women without documented antirubella antibodies should be immunized and wait at least 3 months after vaccination before trying to get pregnant. In the authors' opinion, women also should wait until they are finished with school, have a reasonable job with good health care coverage, or are happily married to someone with a satisfactory income. Uncannily, it's easier to get pregnant than to buy cigarettes. (In the editor's opinion, the same may be said for men.)

9. What should a pregnant women do if she is exposed to measles and is not already immune?

She should receive gammaglobulin (0.5 ml/kg) within 6 days after exposure. With measles infections, spontaneous abortions and premature deliveries are common. Measles virus crosses the placenta, and newborns develop typical exanthematous lesions. Pregnant women with active measles should receive gammaglobulin (0.25 ml/kg). Women who have never had measles or documented immunity should receive two doses of live virus vaccine 1 month apart at least 30 days before becoming pregnant.

10. What is toxoplasmosis? What are its risks if acquired during pregnancy?

Toxoplasma gondii is an intracellular protozoan parasite. Acute infections in adults go unrecognized in up to 90% of the cases. The risk of fetal infection is estimated to be 1 in 8,000 in the United States. Disease is transmitted to the fetus in about one-half of women who acquire the infection while pregnant. Risk to the fetus is not uniform throughout pregnancy but is directly related to the gestational age at the time of maternal acquisition; infection early in gestation has the worst consequences. Potential problems include micro- or macrocephaly, hydrocephalus, carditis, hepatitis, splenomegaly, retinochoroiditis, dermatitis, and lesions in almost any organ. Ninety percent of neonates are asymptomatic at birth, but many who are left undiagnosed and untreated may subsequently develop chorioretinitis and/or learning disabilities. In a recent study of mothers who acquired toxoplasmosis during the first 16 weeks of pregnancy, spiramycin treatment limited infection of fetuses to only 3.7%.

11. How can *T. gondii* be diagnosed during pregnancy?

Prenatal diagnosis with a detailed sonogram is used to search for evidence of in utero infection: hydrocephalus, microcephaly, intracranial or hepatic calcifications, ascites, hydrops, or placental thickening. Fetal blood acquired by cordocentesis can be tested for fetal toxoplasma-specific IgM, IgA, and IgE (which do not cross the placenta), and *T. gondii* may be isolated in culture. Nonspecific indicators are white blood cell count and differential, platelet count, and liver enzyme levels. Using this combined approach, investigators in France have successfully identified approximately 90% of congenitally infected neonates before birth. Spiramycin, 1 gm orally every 8 hr, should be started immediately in women with possible acute infection by toxoplasma and continued for the remainder of the pregnancy. Spiramycin is currently not approved by the Food and Drug Administration but is available on a case-by-case basis.

12. What happens if a woman gets hepatitis E during pregnancy?

Hepatitis E virus (HEV) is transmitted via the oral-fecal route, most commonly through contaminated drinking water. Usually infection is self-limited; as with hepatitis A, no progression to chronic hepatitis, no late hepatic sequelae, and no evidence for persistent HEV infection have been found. HEV is endemic in developing countries, where the attack rates for pregnant women appear to be higher. During pregnancy, fulminant hepatitis and disseminated intravascular coagulation are common, particularly during the third trimester. For infected pregnant women, the case fatality rate is as high as 20%. Mortality does not appear to be related to poor nutrition or a general susceptibility of pregnant women to develop fulminant hepatitis; pregnancy does not increase the risk of fulminant disease and death in women who acquire acute hepatitis A infection. Currently there is no vaccine against HEV, and immunoglobulin has not proved effective in preventing infection. Pregnant women who plan travel to areas endemic for HEV should be counseled about the risks of acquiring hepatitis E during pregnancy.

13. What factors increase the risk of transmission of hepatitis B to neonates?

• High titers of Dane particles (complete virions)
• Hepatitis B surface antigen, presence of e antigen
• High hepatitis B virus DNA levels

Ninety percent of cases of hepatitis B acquired in infants during the neonatal period result in chronic infection. Although hepatitis B surface antigen can be found in breast milk, no evidence indicates that breast feeding increases the risk of transmission. Cesarean delivery is not currently recommended for reduction of vertical transmission of viral hepatitis.

14. What can you do for an infant born to a mother with positive hepatitis B surface antigen?

Hepatitis B vaccine and hepatitis B immunoglobulin should be administered to seropositive neonates within 12 hours of delivery. This protocol prevents transmission of the virus in more than 90% of cases. The hepatitis B vaccine series is currently recommended for all infants, regardless of the hepatitis B status of their mothers.

15. What is Lyme disease? How do you treat it during pregnancy?

Lyme disease is caused by the spirochete *Borrelia burgdorferi*, which is transmitted by ticks. Because of problems seen with syphilis (which is also a spirochete), initial concern about possible fetal infection and teratogenicity if Lyme disease was contracted during pregnancy was great. A survey conducted in 1994 by 162 neurologists raised doubts about the existence of prenatally acquired neuroborreliosis. Acute Lyme disease is treated with oral antibiotics (see chapter on tickborne disease for discussion of treatment). No evidence indicates that more aggressive intravenous therapy is warranted for Lyme disease in pregnant women, except for the usual indications of severe acute disease, neurologic complications, and chronic disease.

16. What is the effect of *Treponema pallidum* on children who acquire it in utero?

Fetal infection before the fourth month of gestation is rare because the placenta provides a protective barrier until later in gestation. Treatment of a luetic mother during the first 4 months of pregnancy usually ensures that the fetus will not be infected. A virtually pathognomonic sign of congenital syphilis is necrotizing funisitis. This inflammatory process involves the matrix of the umbilical cord, with typical syphilitic perivascular inflammation and obliterative endarteritis. It should be suspected when the umbilical cord is swollen and discolored red, white, and blue to resemble a barber's pole.

Congenital syphilis may present with rhinitis (snuffles), followed by a diffuse maculopapular desquamative rash with extensive sloughing. A vesicular rash with bullae may develop. The lesions are teeming with spirochetes. Generalized osteochondritis and perichondritis may alter the architecture of bones, most prominently the nose (saddle nose) and metaphyses of the lower extremities (anterior bowing or "saber shin"). The liver is often heavily infected; associated signs are splenomegaly, anemia, thrombocytopenia, and jaundice. Neonatal death can be caused by liver failure, pneumonia, or pulmonary hemorrhage. An immune-complex glomerulonephritis may develop, usually about the fourth month of life.

Other common findings are recurrent arthropathy and bilateral knee effusions (Clutton's joints); widely spread, peg-shaped upper central incisors with central notching (Hutchinson's teeth); frontal bossing; and poorly developed maxillas. Penicillin is virtually risk-free for neonates, and all neonates born to syphilitic mothers should be treated.

17. *Chlamydia trachomatis* is responsible for what disease?

C. trachomatis is the most common sexually transmitted disease in the United States. The prevalence in pregnant patients is 2–31%. It may cause acute urethritis, cervicitis, and acute pelvic inflammatory disease. Chlamydial infection may present clinically as urethritis or pyuria with a negative urine culture. Diagnosis is made by a direct immunofluorescence test using monoclonal antibodies against *C. trachomatis*. Chronic inflammation and scarring with either recurrent or persistent infection may lead to tubal occlusion, infertility, and increased risk of ectopic pregnancy. Sexual partners of women diagnosed with chlamydial infection require treatment.

18. What bacteria cause most perinatal infections?

Group A streptococci were once responsible for most puerperal fevers. Group B streptococci are part of the normal flora of the genital tract in 25–55% of pregnant women. Streptococci are the most common cause of neonatal sepsis and meningitis in the United States, accounting for approximately 6,200 cases per year. Streptococcal infection should be suspected in patients with prematurely ruptured membranes, septic abortion, endometritis, chorioamnionitis, or pelvic peritonitis. Group A streptococci are transmitted by person-to-person contact. The modern use of aseptic techniques and early recognition and treatment have significantly reduced the incidence of streptococcal infections.

19. What is so special about coccidioidomycosis and pregnancy?

When infection occurs during pregnancy or is active when conception occurs, coccidioidomycosis can be especially dangerous. Dissemination is 40–100 times more common than in the general population, and only one in eight affected pregnant women survives. Rates of dissemination and mortality are higher the later in pregnancy that infection is acquired. Only 60% of pregnant patients with active infection produce offspring who survive beyond the neonatal period, and one-third of these are delivered prematurely.

Coccidioidomycosis should be suspected in pregnant residents or travelers to endemic areas when a febrile illness develops. If the *Coccidioides immitis* complement fixation test is elevated, a diagnostic work-up is urgent. If active infection is present, consider abortion or early delivery. The same regimen of amphotericin B should be given as for nonpregnant patients. Treatment appears to enhance survival and is safe for the fetus if the pregnancy is continued.

The parasitic phase of *C. immitis* and specific binding proteins for mammalian hormones are stimulated by female sex hormones, which may help to explain the danger of this disease for pregnant women.

20. What two diseases can *Listeria monocytogenes* cause in fetuses or newborns?

Pregnant women may harbor *L. monocytogenes* asymptomatically in their genital tract and rectum and transmit the infection to their infants. But overall colonization rates are low. Perinatal listeriosis may take two forms: the early form, which results from an intrauterine infection producing granulomatosis infantisepticum, a devastating illness; and the late form, presumably acquired during or immediately after birth, presenting as meningitis in the second or third week of life.

BIBLIOGRAPHY

1. Creasy RK, Resnik R: Maternal Fetal Medicine: Principles and Practice, 3rd ed. Philadelphia, W.B. Saunders, 1994.
2. Mandell GL, Bennett JE, Dolin R (eds): Principles and Practice of Infectious Disease, 4th ed. New York, Churchill Livingstone, 1995.
3. Niswander KR, Evans AT: Manual of Obstetrics, 5th ed. Boston, Little, Brown, 1996.
4. Levinson WE, Jawetz E: Medical Microbiology and Immunology, 3rd ed. Norwalk, CT, Appleton & Lange, 1995.
5. Tuomala R, Cox SM (eds): Infections in obstetrics. Infect Dis Clin North Am 11(1) [entire issue], 1997.

59. NEONATAL INFECTIONS

Carmen D. Cetrone, D.O., and Denise M. Demers, M.D.

1. When does vertical transmission of human immunodeficiency virus (HIV) take place?

Transmission of HIV from mother to child may occur in utero as early as the eighth week of gestation, at delivery, and after birth through breastfeeding. The risk of transmission is reduced from approximately 25% to 8% when zidovudine (AZT) is given according to the AIDS Clinical Trial Group (ACTG) Protocol 076. Although this protocol involved the use of AZT before, during, and after delivery, treatment can begin at any stage, including infants less than 12 hours old born to untreated HIV-positive women. Recent research suggests that high-dose AZT fed to newborn experimental animals may incite cancers at a later age. Although all mothers must be counseled about the unknown long-term risks of AZT, the reduced risk of transmitting HIV must be emphasized. Clinical trials to evaluate combination antiretroviral therapy in this setting are currently underway.

2. What is the ACTG Protocol 076 regimen?

Pregnant women (beginning at 14–34 weeks' gestation): AZT, 100 mg orally 5 times/day.

Pregnant women in labor: AZT, 2 mg/kg loading dose intravenously over 1 hour, followed by continuous intravenous infusion of 1 mg/kg/hr until delivery.

Neonate: AZT syrup, 2 mg/kg/dose every 6 hours beginning within 8–12 hours after birth and continuing for 6 weeks.

3. Why are HIV-positive mothers in the United States told not to breast feed their infants, whereas mothers in developing countries are not restricted?

The risk of HIV transmission from breastfeeding is estimated at 10–20%. In the U.S. and other nations where formula and water supplies can be assumed to be uncontaminated, this risk is unnecessary. For children in developing countries where infectious diarrhea and subsequent dehydration accounts for the majority of deaths, the risk of formula feeding is greater than the estimated risk of HIV transmission from breastfeeding.

4. What infectious agents cause ophthalmia neonatorum?

Infectious causes listed from most to least common include *Chlamydia trachomatis, Staphylococcus aureus, Haemophilus* spp., *Streptococcus pneumoniae,* enterococci, herpes simplex virus (HSV)-2, HSV-1, and *Neisseria gonorrhoeae.* In addition, various chemical agents, including those put into the eye to prevent infection, are the most common cause in the first day of life.

5. What are reasonable guidelines for the management of a neonate born to a mother who received intrapartum antimicrobial prophylaxis for prevention of early-onset group B streptococcal disease?

If signs or symptoms of sepsis are present in the neonate, a full diagnostic evaluation is performed and empiric antimicrobial therapy is initiated. A full diagnostic evaluation includes complete blood count and differential, blood culture, and chest radiograph if respiratory symptoms are present. Lumbar puncture is performed at the discretion of the physician. If no signs or symptoms of sepsis are present but the estimated gestational age of the neonate is less than 35 weeks, a full diagnostic evaluation should be performed and empiric antimicrobial therapy initiated. If no signs or symptoms of sepsis are present and the estimated gestational age of the neonate is 35 weeks or older, the duration of maternal intrapartum antimicrobial prophylaxis (IAP) before delivery must be considered. If the duration is 4 hours or less, the asymptomatic neonate should receive a limited evaluation (complete blood count with differential and blood culture) and be observed for 48 hours. If sepsis is suspected after the limited evaluation, the neonate should receive a full diagnostic evaluation and empiric antimicrobial therapy should be initiated. If the duration of IAP is more than 4 hours, the asymptomatic neonate requires no evaluation or empiric therapy but should be observed for 48 hours.

6. What immunoprophylaxis is indicated in the neonate born to a hepatitis B surface antigen-positive mother?

Neonates born to HBsAg-positive mothers should receive hepatitis B immune globulin (HBIG) within 12 hours of birth. The initial dose of hepatitis B vaccine should be given concurrently at a different site.

7. What are the common acute clinical manifestations of symptomatic congenital cytomegalovirus infection?

Ninety percent of cytomegalovirus (CMV) infection is asymptomatic. Clinically apparent infection classically involves multiple organ systems, notably the reticuloendothelial system and central nervous system.

Hepatomegaly. Enlargement of the liver accompanied by splenomegaly is perhaps the most common manifestation of congenital CMV infection. Although marked elevation of hepatocellular enzymes is rare, mild elevation is common.

Splenomegaly. Enlargement of the spleen is common. In some congenital CMV infections, splenomegaly and petechiae may be the only recognized abnormalities at birth.

Jaundice. Jaundice that persists beyond the time of physiologic jaundice is common. The direct fraction of bilirubin typically rises late in the first week of life and may reach 50% of the total bilirubin.

Petechiae. Thrombocytopenia secondary to CMV-mediated megakaryocytic bone marrow suppression is a common manifestation. Petechiae frequently present several hours after birth and may disappear within 48 hours or persist for weeks after birth. Although most neonates have platelet counts of 20,000–60,000, some have petechial rashes without associated thrombocytopenia.

Microcephaly. A head circumference less than the fifth percentile may be seen in about one-half of all surviving patients who were born with symptomatic CMV infection. Occasionally hydrocephalus may result from obstruction of the fourth ventricle.

Ocular abnormalities. Chorioretinitis is the most common ocular defect. Other abnormalities, such as cataracts, microphthalmos, blindness, retinal necrosis, and optic disc malformations, have been reported.

Fetal growth retardation. Intrauterine growth retardation has been reported in up to one-half of all cases of symptomatic CMV infection.

Dental defects. An apparent enamel defect in the primary dentition has been reported in cases of symptomatic CMV infection and to a lesser degree in asymptomatic infection. The enamel has been described as opaque and moderately soft, with yellowish discoloration.

Sensorineural deafness. Sensorineural hearing loss is probably the most common neurologic deficit caused by congenital CMV infection and appears to be the leading cause of deafness in children. It may be present in both symptomatic and subclinical congenital CMV infection.

8. What is the appropriate management of asymptomatic neonates born to mothers with genital HSV infection?

A neonate born to a mother with a history of genital herpes but no active lesions is at a low risk for acquiring HSV infection—whether the infant is born via vaginal delivery or cesarean section when membranes are intact. No special evaluation is necessary during the neonatal period. An asymptomatic neonate born to a mother with active genital herpes or positive perinatal HSV cultures should be isolated from other neonates for up to 4 weeks of age. Before discharge of asymptomatic neonates, parents and other caregivers should receive information about HSV infection and early signs and symptoms of disease. The neonate should be cultured for HSV after 24–48 hours of age. Possible recovery sites include the eye, oropharynx, nasopharynx, rectum, and suspicious skin lesions. Some data support the use of weekly surveillance cultures from the above sites for 4–6 weeks after birth. If at any time a culture is positive, cultures should be repeated, a lumbar puncture should be performed, and therapy with acyclovir or vidarabine should be initiated.

9. A neonate is exposed to *Chlamydia trachomatis* during vaginal delivery. What are the two most common clinical manifestations of exposure? When would you anticipate their occurrence?

Conjunctivitis. *C. trachomatis* is the most common infectious cause of conjunctivitis in the neonatal period and occurs in 25–50% of exposed infants. Most cases present after the fifth day of life and before 2 weeks of age. Typically a watery discharge becomes purulent over 1–2 days. Erythema of the bulbar conjunctiva is common and is usually accompanied by markedly swollen eyelids. Cell culture, direct fluorescent antibody (DFA) testing, and electroimmunoassay (EIA) of conjunctival scrapings are highly sensitive and specific.

Pneumonia. Chlamydial pneumonia typically presents between the fourth and eleventh weeks of life. Infants usually are afebrile but may exhibit low-grade fever. Respiratory findings include tachypnea, cough, and inspiratory rales. Wheezing is uncommon. Chest radiographs reveal bilateral interstitial infiltrates and hyperexpansion of the lungs. Blood studies often reveal eosinophilia and elevated immunoglobulins.

10. How are neonatal chlamydial infections treated?

Conjunctivitis and pneumonia must be treated with oral erythromycin, 50 mg/kg/day for 14 days. Topical ophthalmic ointment is not recommended because it has no effect on the nasopharyngeal carriage of *C. trachomatis*. The mother and her sexual partner should be referred for evaluation and treatment.

11. A mother and newborn are ready to be discharged from the hospital. A sibling at home has active chickenpox. The mother and newborn have no varicella skin lesions. What preventive measures should be considered before discharge?

If the mother has a history of varicella infection, the mother and newborn may be discharged home. If the mother does not have a history of varicella infection, she should be tested for varicella antibodies. If the antibody test is positive, the mother and newborn may be discharged home. If the antibody test is negative, varicella zoster immunoglobulin (VZIG) should be given to the mother and newborn before discharge.

12. A 32-year-old woman with a history of systemic lupus erythematosus and no prenatal care delivers a well-appearing term infant. Laboratory samples drawn shortly before delivery reveal a positive VDRL/RPR. What further evaluation is indicated in the newborn?

A nontreponemal antibody test, such as the rapid plasma reagin (RPR) or Veneral Disease Research Laboratory (VDRL) test, should be performed on the newborn. Antiphospholipid antibodies typically present in patients with systemic lupus erythematosus (SLE) cross-react with a phospholipid antigen used in nontreponemal antibody tests. This phenomenon produces a false-positive nontreponemal antibody test for syphilis. The IgG antibodies freely cross the placenta, causing a false-positive result in the newborn. Although maternal history of SLE strongly suggests a false-positive result, syphilis cannot be ruled out without further testing. The mother and newborn should receive a treponemal antibody test such as the fluorescent treponemal antibody, absorbed (FTA-ABS) or microhemagglutination–*Treponema pallidum* (MHA–TP) test. If the RPR is positive secondary to a cross-reacting antibody in the mother's serum, the FTA-ABS and MHA-TP will be negative. If the treponemal tests in the mother and newborn are positive, a presumptive diagnosis of maternal syphilis with possible infant infection should be considered, and further evaluation is warranted. Treponemal tests are not 100% specific for syphilis. Positive reactions occur in patients with other spirochetal diseases such as yaws, pinta, leptospirosis, rat-bite fever, and Lyme disease.

13. What are the clinical manifestations of congenital toxoplasmosis?

Most cases of congenital toxoplasmosis are asymptomatic in the neonatal period. At birth, only 1 in 10 infants has severe generalized disease. Generalized disease is often indistinguishable from other causes of congenital infection. Although congenital toxoplasmosis may present with various signs and symptoms, it is often immediately considered when the classic triad of chorioretinitis, hydrocephalus, and intracerebral calcifications is present. This triad was found in the first proven case of congenital toxoplasmosis described in 1939. Toxoplasmosis must be considered in all infants with signs or symptoms of congenital infection, even when signs consistent with the classic triad are absent. In neonates with generalized infection, neurologic signs are universally present and may appear as abnormal spinal fluid, convulsions, intracranial calcifications, chorioretinitis, or hydrocephalus. Any or all of these findings may be accompanied by fever, anemia, jaundice, intrauterine growth retardation, hepatosplenomegaly, lymphadenopathy, and petechial rash.

14. What are the common permanent manifestations of congenital rubella infection?

Classically, congenital rubella syndrome is characterized by the combination of eye defects (e.g., microphthalmia, glaucoma, chorioretinitis, cataracts), sensorineural hearing loss, congenital heart disease, and neurologic abnormality. This definition dates back to 1941, when Gregg described these defects in a neonate with congenital rubella infection. It has since become apparent that congenital rubella infection may produce a wide spectrum of abnormalities, infecting one or all fetal organs. In utero infection with rubella may result in asymptomatic disease, subtle defects recognized after infancy, severe multiple anomalies recognizable at birth, or fetal wastage. Many of the permanent manifestations of congenital rubella infection result from aberrant organogenesis and scarring secondary to tissue destruction. Cardiac anomalies occur in almost one-half of all neonates infected during the first 8 weeks of gestation. Patent ductus arteriosus is the most common lesion, followed by peripheral pulmonary artery stenosis and pulmonary valvular stenosis. Sensorineural hearing loss is by far the most common consequence of congenital rubella infection and is often the only recognizable defect. Some studies have reported an 80% incidence of hearing loss in infected infants. Other neurologic manifestations include microcephaly, meningoencephalitis, developmental delays, and behavior disorders. Congenital rubella infection disrupts the growth of the pigmentary layer of the retina, producing a "salt-and-pepper" retinopathy. Cataracts are present in about 30% of all cases, with half of these cases exhibiting unilateral involvement.

15. What are the typical clinical manifestations and outcomes of perinatal HSV infection limited to the skin, eye, and mouth?

Characteristic vesicular lesions of HSV usually appear between 1 and 2 weeks of age. These lesions may cluster at former scalp lead sites or on the presenting part of the body that was in direct contact with the virus during birth. Distant vesicular lesions may occur on any part of the body, and cases of vesicular lesions limited to the oropharynx have been reported. Recurrences during the first 6–12 months of life are common, regardless of whether the neonate receives appropriate antiviral therapy at initial presentation. Infection of the eye with HSV may lead to keratoconjunctivitis, chorioretinitis, cataracts, and retinal detachment even if appropriate antiviral therapy is initiated. The incidence of mortality from localized disease is extremely low, but significant morbidity has been reported. It is estimated that 20–30% of children with skin, eye, and mouth disease will develop neurologic impairment; some experts recommend suppressive oral acyclovir to reduce sequelae.

16. What are the possible modes of transmission for congenital and neonatal tuberculosis?

Congenital tuberculosis is defined as infection that occurs in utero. It may be acquired via passage from the infected placenta or by inhalation or ingestion of infected amniotic fluid. Neonatal tuberculosis is defined as infection acquired after birth from infected mothers, family members, or caregivers. It may be acquired by inhalation or ingestion of infected droplets, ingestion of infected breast milk, or contamination of traumatized skin or mucous membranes.

17. What are the common clinical manifestations of early congenital syphilis?

Liver. Hepatomegaly, with or without splenomegaly, occurs in nearly all neonates with congenital syphilis. Jaundice secondary to syphilitic hepatitis or hemolysis may be the only sign of disease. Elevation of hepatocellular enzymes is common and may worsen after penicillin therapy is initiated.

Lymph nodes. Nontender lymphadenopathy may occur in about 50% of neonates with congenital syphilis. It commonly is associated with hepatosplenomegaly. Enlargement of the epitrochlear nodes, a rare sign in other diseases, warrants a high index of suspicion for congenital syphilis.

Hematologic abnormalities. Coombs-negative hemolytic anemia is a common finding early in the neonatal period in infants with congenital syphilis. A hydropic infant with such an anemia strongly suggests the diagnosis of congenital syphilis. White blood cell counts are usually within normal limits, but leukopenia and leukocytosis have been reported. Thrombocytopenia secondary to decreased platelet life span may be present.

Skin and mucous membranes. A pink or red maculopapular rash that gradually becomes coppery-brown is the most common skin manifestation of congenital syphilis, but petechiae and a vesiculobullous eruption (pemphigus syphiliticus) also may occur. All three frequently involve the palms and soles. Mucous membrane manifestations, such as a highly infectious mucoid nasal discharge (snuffles) and mucosal erosions, may develop.

Skeletal involvement. Osteochondritis, osteomyelitis, and periostitis are common manifestations of untreated congenital syphilis. The lesions tend to be multiple and symmetric and most often involve the metaphyses and diaphyses. Although not pathognomonic for syphilis, destruction of the tibial tubercle (Wimberger's sign) is suggestive of congenital disease. Physical exam findings may be subtle. Subjective observation of decreased movement of one or more extremities may be the only sign of disease.

Kidney. Easily recognizable signs and symptoms of nephrotic syndrome may appear between 2–3 months of age. The most common finding is generalized edema with ascites.

18. Which infectious diseases must be considered in a neonate with nonimmune hydrops fetalis?
Chagas disease, cytomegalovirus, leptospirosis, parvovirus B19, syphilis, and toxoplasmosis.

19. Candidal infection is frequently acquired by an infant from the infected vagina during birth. What are possible clinical manifestations?
In term infants, localized infection of the mucous membranes (thrush) is by far the most common manifestation of candidal infection acquired during birth. Lesions are typically whitish-gray and may be found on the tongue, soft palate, buccal mucosa, gums, or tonsils. Another benign condition in the term infant is vesicular or pustular dermatitis around the umbilicus, perineum, axillae, or intertriginous areas. These conditions may be treated with appropriate topical antifungal medications. In premature infants, cutaneous findings may be associated with severe systemic disease, including early-onset respiratory distress, leukocytosis, and spreading dermatitis resembling streptococcal or staphylococcal infection. Systemic antifungal therapy is essential.

20. What is the pathogenesis of osteomyelitis in neonates?
The bony skeleton of the neonate may be infected by several different mechanisms. Seeding of the skeletal system during the course of neonatal sepsis is by far the most common route of entry for microorganisms. Direct inoculation of bacteria after radial artery catheterization, femoral venipuncture, multiple lumbar puncture, fetal scalp monitor placement, or capillary heel sampling has been implicated in some cases. Soft tissue infections, such as an infected cephalhematoma, may migrate into underlying bony structures and cause parietal osteomyelitis. Finally, infection may be transmitted through the placenta, as seen (almost exclusively) in congenital syphilis.

21. What are the most common causes of neonatal sepsis and meningitis in the United States?
Classically, physicians have taught that the three most common causes of sepsis in the neonate are, in descending order, group B streptococci, *Escherichia coli*, and *Listeria monocytogenes*. This "pearl" is useful but limited because it neglects the emergence of an important pathogen in the modern nursery: *Staphylococcus epidermidis*. The increased isolation of *S. epidermidis* has coincided with the use of multiple broad-spectrum antibiotics and invasive monitors and vascular access devices in low-birth-weight infants with immature immune systems. *S. epidermidis* can adhere to and grow on the synthetic surfaces used to manufacture common intravascular catheters, which may serve as a persistent source of bacteremia. Removal is often necessary. Finally, most strains of *S. epidermidis* produce beta-lactamase, rendering them resistant to penicillins and requiring treatment with vancomycin.

22. Which enterovirus is most commonly associated with neonatal myocarditis?
Enteroviral myocarditis in the neonate is often a devastating disease associated with coxsackie B1–5. It is usually seen in infants less than 10 days old. Nonspecific manifestations, such

as poor feeding, lethargy, mild respiratory distress, and fever, may precede the abrupt onset of cardiac failure and shock. The mortality rate is reported at 30–50% but may be higher in infants with concomitant meningoencephalitis, pneumonia, or hepatitis.

CONTROVERSIES

23. What is the vertical transmission rate of hepatitis C?

Currently it is thought that perinatal HCV transmission is rare unless the mother is concomitantly infected with HIV. Newer polymerase chain reaction (PCR) studies may reveal higher rates of transmission than previously predicted by serologic studies. Virus has been identified in the breast milk of 0–29% of seropositive women. Therefore, formula feeding is recommended for infants of hepatitis C-positive women.

24. Which neonates should be considered for prophylaxis against respiratory syncytial virus (RSV) with high-dose RSV immune globulin?

RSV immune globulin (RSVIG) should be considered in all preterm infants of less than 32 weeks' gestation who will be less than 6 months of age at the onset of RSV season. Infants with a gestational age less than 28 weeks may benefit from prophylaxis for up to 12 months of age. RSVIG also should be considered for children less than 2 years of age with bronchopulmonary dysplasia who require or have required oxygen within 6 months of the onset of RSV season. At present, RSVIG is not approved by the Food and Drug Administration for children with congenital heart disease and is contraindicated in neonates with cyanotic congestive heart disease. Prophylaxis should be initiated before the onset of RSV season and terminated at the end of RSV season.

25. What are the current recommendations for the use of ribavirin in patients at risk for infection with RSV?

There are no definitive indications for use of ribavirin because of concerns about cost, safety, and efficacy. Use of ribavirin may be considered in infants at high risk for severe or complicated infection. This group includes infants with bronchopulmonary dysplasia, cystic fibrosis, or other chronic lung disease; congenital heart disease, including pulmonary hypertension; gestational age less than 37 weeks; and immunosuppressive diseases as well as infants receiving immunosuppressant therapy. Severely ill infants hospitalized with RSV disease also should be considered (e.g., oxygen saturation consistently < 93% on room air by pulse oximetry, PaO_2 < 65 mmHg, or increasing $PaCO_2$ by arterial blood gas determination). Ribavirin therapy should be considered in infants with RSV disease that is not initially severe but may be associated with increased risk of progressing to a more complicated course. This group includes infants less than 6 weeks of age and infants with multiple congenital anomalies, metabolic disease, or neurologic disease.

BIBLIOGRAPHY

1. AIDS Clinical Trial Group Protocol 076. MMWR 43(RR-11), 1994.
2. Annunziato PW, Gershon AG: Herpes simplex virus infections. Pediatr Rev 17(12):415–423, 1996.
3. Committee on Infectious Diseases, American Academy of Pediatrics: Reassessment of the indications for ribavirin therapy in respiratory syncytial virus infections. Pediatrics 97:137–139, 1996.
4. Committee on Infectious Diseases, American Academy of Pediatrics: Red Book. American Academy of Pediatrics, 1997.
5. American Academy of Pediatrics and American College of Obstetricians and Gynecologists: Guidelines for Perinatal Care, 3rd ed. American Academy of Pediatrics, 1992.
6. Long SS, Pickering LK, Prober CG (eds): Principles and Practice of Pediatric Infectious Diseases. New York, Churchill Livingstone, 1997.
7. PREVENT Study Group: Reduction of hospitalization by respiratory syncytial virus immune globulin. Pediatrics 99:93–99, 1997.
8. Remington JS, Klein JO (eds): Infectious Diseases of the Fetus and Newborn Infant, 4th ed. Philadelphia, W.B. Saunders, 1995.
9. Schuchat A, et al: Prevention of perinatal group B streptococcal disease: A public health perspective. MMWR 45 (RR-7), 1996.

XIX. Emporiatrics

60. TRAVEL MEDICINE: EMPORIATRICS

Larry K. Miller, M.D.

1. What recommendations do you have for travelers looking for medical advice?

They should be evaluated by their physician or travel clinic at least 4 and preferably 6 weeks before departure. They should bring their complete itinerary, list of previous immunizations, medical history, list of current medications, and summary of any special recommendations from their travel agent. This schedule should allow sufficient time for necessary immunizations and to start antimalarial prophylaxis if required.

2. What is the essential first step in preparation of the departing traveler and in evaluation of the returning traveler with illness?

An accurate travel itinerary must be obtained to prepare the traveler for potential illness exposures and to form a comprehensive differential diagnosis in the case of the ill returning traveler. Key elements are:

1. Travel destinations (including intermediate stops) along with accurate arrival/departure dates

2. Purpose of the travel (pleasure or business)

3. Travel in urban versus rural areas

4. Extent of contact with local inhabitants (health care work or sexual contacts)

5. Unusual exposures

6. Vaccination history/requirements

7. Malaria prophylaxis (presence of resistant *Plasmodium falciparum*, which drug used, compliance)

3. Of all the perils facing the international traveler, which is the most likely to result in injury or death?

Approximately 25,000 injuries and 750 deaths are estimated to occur in travelers each year as a result of motor vehicle accidents.

4. List the immunizations commonly recommended for adult travelers.

Immunization	Type	Schedule	Booster	Comments
Cholera	Inactivated bacterial	Two 0.5 ml doses > 1 week apart (SQ or IM)	6 mo	Low efficacy, no longer required by WHO
Hepatitis A	Inactivated viral	Two 1 ml doses at 0 and 6–12 months (IM)	6–12 mo	Largely replaced immune globulin
Hepatitis B	Recombinant viral	Three 1 ml doses at 0, 1, 6 months (IM)	Unknown	For travelers at risk of blood exposure or sexual contact

(Continued on following page)

Immunization	Type	Schedule	Booster	Comments
Immune serum globulin	Immunoglobulins	0.02 ml/kg for < 3 months' protection; 0.06 ml/kg for up to 5 months' protection (IM)	Every 3–5 mo as long as risk remains	Difficult to acquire in U.S., largely replaced by hepatitis A vaccine
Influenza	Inactivated viral	One 0.5 ml dose (IM)	Annual	Same as current ACP recommendations Consider for all travelers to the tropics
Japanese encephalitis	Inactivated viral	Three 1 ml doses at 0, 7, and 30 days (SQ)	3 yr	Delayed anaphylaxis Consider for > 30 days' travel to SE Asia, especially rural areas
Measles	Live viral	One 0.5 ml dose SQ (monovalent or MMR)	None	Give > 2 weeks before or > 3 months after immunoglobulin
Meningococcus	Inactivated bacterial	One 0.5 ml dose (SQ)	None	Travel to areas of high endemicity; required for Hajj
Pneumococcus	Polysaccharide	One 0.5 ml dose (SQ)	6 yr	Same as current ACP recommendations
Poliomyelitis	eIPV: enhanced potency inactivated virus	Three 0.5 ml doses at 0, 1–2, and 6–12 months (SQ) if no childhood series	Once as adult	Polio eradicated in Western hemisphere
Rabies	Inactivated viral	Three 1 ml IM doses at 0, 7, and 21–28 days	3 yr	Complete series 3 weeks before starting chloroquine
Tetanus–diphtheria	Bacterial toxoid	Three 0.5 ml doses at 0, 1, and 6–12 months (SQ or IM)	5 yr	5-year booster precludes need for TIG/booster for tetanus-prone wounds
Typhoid	Ty21a:live attenuated bacterial	Four doses at 0, 2, 4, and 6 days (PO)	5 yr	Start mefloquine 1 week after series completed
Typhoid	VI CPS	One 0.5 ml dose (IM)	2 yr	Fewer side effects and best choice in pregnancy
Typhoid	Heat-phenol inactivated	Two 0.5 ml doses > 4 weeks apart (SQ)	3 yr	High incidence of side effects
Yellow fever	Live attenuated virus	One 0.5 ml dose (SQ)	10 yr	Avoid in travelers with egg allergy and in immunocompromised. Only vaccine still mandated by WHO

SQ = subcutaneously, IM = intramuscularly, PO = orally, WHO = World Health Organization, ACP = American College of Physicians, MMR = measles-mumps-rubella vaccine, TIG = tetanus immunoglobulin.

5. Since cholera vaccine has only about a 50% efficacy, should it be recommended?

No countries have officially required proof of cholera vaccination for travelers coming directly from the United States since 1988. Some African countries require vaccination for travelers coming from areas where cholera is present. In this case a single documented injection is usually adequate for entrance and can spare the traveler the risks of an injection at the point of entry. Other travelers with peptic ulcer disease treated with H_2-receptor blockers or proton-pump inhibitors, prior gastric resection, or achlorhydria should be offered cholera immunization because gastric acidity is the primary defense against cholera.

6. Who should receive yellow fever vaccination?

Yellow fever is a flaviviral disease spread by the bite of *Aedes* mosquitoes. It is currently restricted to areas of Africa, South America, and Panama. Epidemics still occur, with mortality rates up to 50%. As of December, 1996, 17 countries require yellow fever immunization for direct travel from the United States, and many countries require an international certificate of immunization if the traveler is coming from (even passing through) a high-risk area. The certificate technically becomes valid 10 days after the vaccination is received. It is a safe, attenuated live viral vaccine requiring only one injection with boosters every 10 years. Because of rare reports of encephalitis in infants, it should never be given to children < 6 months of age. As the vaccine is prepared from virus grown in eggs, it is contraindicated in people with life-threatening egg allergies. Because it is a live virus vaccine, it should be avoided in pregnant and immunosuppressed travelers, unless the risk of the disease outweighs the risk of the vaccine. Concomitant administration of cholera vaccine with yellow fever vaccine can decrease immune response to both vaccines; therefore, these vaccines should be separated by 3 weeks.

7. Is Japanese encephalitis a real risk to the traveler? What is the risk of the vaccine?

Japanese encephalitis, another flaviviral disease, is found in Asia and spread by infected *Culex* mosquitoes. Although most infections remain asymptomatic, case fatality rates rise to 20–30% in clinical illness, with frequent persistent neurologic sequelae. The risk to travelers has been estimated at about 1:1,000,000 per 1 week of urban travel but increases to 1:20,000 per 1 week in rural rice-growing or pig-farming areas. (Pigs serve as amplification hosts.) The vaccine is currently recommended for travelers staying longer than 30 days in rural Southeast Asia. The vaccine has a reported efficacy of about 90%. Side effects are frequent: local pain and erythema, 20%; fever and constitutional symptoms, 10%; urticaria, angioedema, anaphylaxis, 15–62/10,000 doses. The more severe allergic reactions may be delayed up to 2 weeks after the last injection, resulting in current recommendations that travelers complete their series 2 weeks before departure.

8. What should be used for the prevention of hepatitis A in frequent travelers—immune serum globulin or one of the hepatitis A vaccines?

In the United States, immune serum globulin has been difficult to obtain because of recent reports that the intravenous preparation (not the intramuscular preparation) had been linked to cases of hepatitis C. There also have been concerns that pooled gamma globulin from the USA may have lower titers of antihepatitis A because of the relative infrequency of hepatitis A in the population. The two licensed formalin-inactivated, whole-virus hepatitis A vaccines, VAQTA and Havrix, are available for travelers 2 years of age and older. Both are about 90% effective 10 days after receipt of the initial dose; efficacy increases to 90–100% after 4 weeks. Cost is about $30 for 3–5 months' protection with immune globulin compared with $125 for up to 20 years' protection with vaccines. If cost were not a problem, one of the vaccines would be best for the frequent traveler.

9. Should travelers routinely receive pre-exposure antibiotic prophylaxis for diarrhea?

Most travelers should not. The exception is the traveler making a brief trip for a specific purpose who cannot afford even brief inconvenience from diarrhea. In this case, a once-daily dose of a fluoroquinolone is probably the regimen of choice. Recent studies have shown that the combination of a single dose of a fluoroquinolone and loperamide is safe and even more efficacious than more prolonged therapy with antibiotic alone and that 63% of the patients had no further diarrheal stools after the start of therapy.

10. What are the current drugs of choice for malaria prophylaxis in travelers?

Although malaria is caused by four species of Plasmodium (*P. falciparum, P. vivax, P. ovale,* and *P. malariae*), almost all mortality in nonimmune travelers is due to *P. falciparum.* Mefloquine, 250 mg once weekly, remains the drug of choice for travel to all parts of the world with chloroquine-resistant *P. falciparum,* except the border regions between Thailand, Cambodia, and Burma, where doxycycline, 100 mg/day, is recommended because of frequent mefloquine resistance. Both regimens are reported to be approximately 90% efficacious. Mefloquine is now believed to be safe for use in pregnancy, whereas doxycycline remains contraindicated. Chloroquine base, 300 mg once weekly, is the drug of choice for most of the Middle East, Central America west of the Panama Canal Zone, Mexico, Haiti, and the Dominican Republic, where only chloroquine-sensitive *P. falciparum* is found. Mefloquine and chloroquine should be started at least 2 weeks before entering a malarious area to allow for adequate serum levels, whereas doxycycline may be started just 1–2 days before entry. All drugs should be continued until 4 weeks after the last possible malarial exposure. At present, terminal prophylaxis with primaquine to eradicate the hypnozoite stages of *P. vivax* and *P. ovale* is offered only to travelers with more intense, prolonged rural exposures.

11. What adjuncts to drug prophylaxis are available to help decrease the risk of malaria?
Malaria is transmitted by the bite of female *Anopheles* mosquitoes, which are predominantly night feeders. Any tactic that decreases night-time exposure also decreases the risk of infection:
- Remain indoors after dark
- Stay in hotels with window screens
- Use pyrethrin room spray
- Treat clothing with permethrin
- Wear long pants and long sleeved clothing
- Use permethrin-impregnated mosquito nets
- Use insect repellents with up to 35% diethyltoluamide

12. Does the traveler who cannot take mefloquine or doxycycline have any alternative when traveling to areas with chloroquine-resistant malaria?
Chloroquine alone and chloroquine plus proguanil (when traveling to Africa) are currently the only alternatives recommended by the Centers for Disease Control and Prevention. Because these regimens are not as effective as mefloquine or doxycycline, travelers who are not sulfa-allergic should carry a self-treatment dose of Fansidar (3 tablets of pyrimethamine/sulfadoxine), to be taken if they develop symptoms consistent with malaria and are not within 24 hours of medical care. Mefloquine should not be used for empiric self-treatment because of the risk of CNS side effects; halofantrine should not be used because of possible cardiotoxicity.

13. What activities, immunizations, and medications are best avoided by pregnant travelers?
Pregnant women beyond 36 weeks' gestation and those with sickle cell disease, anemia with Hgb < 8.5 gm, or a history of recurrent deep venous thrombosis should not fly. Activities that subject the patient to extremes of pressure, such as scuba diving with possible risk of decompression illness and high-altitude trekking with risk of resultant low-birth-weight infants, should be avoided. First-trimester exposure to high temperatures that raise maternal core temperatures (e.g., saunas, hot tubs) can result in fetal neural tube defects. Most vaccines, including live yellow fever vaccine, can be used during pregnancy if the benefit outweighs the risk, although the measles-mumps-rubella (MMR), live attenuated oral typhoid (Ty21a), and bacille Calmette-Guérin (BCG) vaccines should be avoided. Current data are insufficient to allow use of live varicella vaccine or inactivated hepatitis A vaccine in pregnancy. Mefloquine and chloroquine are considered safe in pregnancy, but primaquine should not be used until after delivery because of the risk of severe hemolysis in a G6PD-deficient fetus. Doxycycline has been associated with abnormal tooth and bone development; sulfa medications may displace bilirubin from binding sites, causing severe jaundice at the time of delivery; and fluoroquinolones may or may not be associated with joint abnormalities. All are contraindicated in pregnancy.

14. What are the symptoms of acute mountain sickness (AMS)? How can it be prevented? How can it be treated?
Acute mountain sickness is characterized by headache, nausea, vomiting, tinnitus, insomnia, decreased appetite, sleep disorder, and dulled level of consciousness, usually 6–24 hours after rapid ascents to altitudes > 2500 meters. AMS should be differentiated from exhaustion, dehydration, hypothermia, and infection. It is usually self-limited, resolving in 24–72 hours unless it progresses to more severe altitude illnesses such as high-altitude cerebral edema (HACE) or high-altitude

pulmonary edema (HAPE). Gradual acclimatization by following a graded assent can prevent AMS. AMS can be treated by descent or low-flow oxygen therapy. Acetazolamide, 125–250 mg twice daily for 24–48 hours before ascent and continued for 24–48 hours at altitude, can hasten acclimatization, and analgesics and antiemetics can ameliorate both headache and nausea. Dexamethasone, 4 mg orally every 6 hours, can be used in place of the acetazolamide if the traveler cannot take sulfa-based medications. HACE and HAPE are potentially life-threatening and should be treated with emergency descent along with the short-term use of oxygen, dexamethasone (HACE), nifedipine (HAPE), and hyperbaric therapy.

15. What are the most common causes of fever in a traveler returning from a tropical vacation? What is the initial approach to evaluation?

The most common tropical infections are malaria, arboviral diseases such as dengue, hepatitis, enteric fever, rickettsial diseases, and leptospirosis. Malaria should be considered in anyone who has traveled to or even just passed though a malarious region in the 12 months before presentation. A differential diagnosis can be developed from the history, including travel history, physical examination, and knowledge of which diseases are present in the region visited. Initial lab tests should include thick and thin malaria smears, complete blood count, liver function tests, urinalysis, blood, urine, and stool cultures, and arboviral and other serologies as indicated.

16. What are the common causes of prolonged diarrhea in a returned traveler? How should they be treated?

Although most travelers' diarrhea is caused by enterotoxigenic *Escherichia coli* (ETEC), *Shigella* spp., *Salmonella* spp., or *Campylobacter* spp., persistence of diarrhea longer than 10–14 days should suggest the presence of *Giardia* sp., *Cryptosporidium* sp., *Cyclosporum* sp., and *Microsporidium* sp. Cryptosporidia, cyclospora, and microsporidia may result in prolonged and/or relapsing disease in HIV-infected patients.

Organism	Drug of Choice
Giardia sp.	Metronidazole
Cryptosporidia	Paromomycin
Cyclospora	Cotrimoxazole
Microsporidia	Albendazole

17. List the parasitic causes of hypereosinophilia that may be seen in the returning traveler.

Parasitic Causes of Eosinophilia

Angiostrongyliasis	Loiasis
Ascariasis	Onchocerciasis
Filariasis (*Wuchereria* sp., *Brugia* sp., *Mansonella* sp.)	Schistosomiasis
	Strongyloidiasis
Gnathostomiasis	Trichinellosis
Hookworm (*Ancylostoma* sp., *Necator* sp.)	Tropical pulmonary eosinophilia
Liver flukes (*Clonorchis* sp., *Opisthorchis* sp., *Fasciola* sp.)	Visceral larva migrans

Adapted from Wilson ME: A World Guide to Infections. New York, Oxford University Press, 1991.

18. Are sexually transmitted diseases (STDs) a cause for concern among travelers?

Gonorrhea, syphilis, chancroid, lymphogranuloma venereum, herpes, and HIV as well as hepatitis B and cytomegalovirus are well reported among travelers. A whole industry has grown up to promote sexual tourism. Low rates of condom use have been reported. Travelers should be counseled as to the increased risk of STDs and HIV in many parts of the world, and condom use should be encouraged. The World Health Organization (WHO) estimates that 75% of HIV infections are transmitted sexually with an efficacy of 0.1–1.0% per contact. This transmission rate is frequently enhanced in the developing world because the presence of genital ulcer disease results in much greater risk from even a single exposure. Hepatitis B vaccination should be considered for frequent travelers or travelers anticipating sexual contact with the indigenous population. A history of sexual exposure should be sought during the evaluation of returning travelers with unexplained fevers.

19. With regard to rabies, what advice would you give an asymptomatic patient who in the process of his pre-travel screen reveals that he had sustained a nonprovoked dog bite 6 months previously while hiking in rural India?

Although the incubation period for clinical rabies usually ranges from 20–90 days, rabies has been reported to develop as rapidly as 4 days after exposure and to have been delayed as long as 19 years. Clinical disease is preventable only if immunotherapy is initiated before the virus gains access to the CNS. Because no reliable test can exclude the diagnosis of rabies, the patient should receive postexposure prophylaxis with both rabies immune globulin (RIG), 20 IU/kg body weight with one-half the dose infiltrated around the previous bite site and the other half administered intragluteally, and either human diploid cell vaccine (HDCV) or rabies vaccine adsorbed (RVA), given as 1-ml intradeltoid injections on days 0, 3, 7, 14, and 28.

20. What are the concerns about immunization and increased risk of infection in the HIV-infected traveler?

The patient's level of immunosuppression is initially evaluated by determining the CD4 lymphocyte level. In general, patients whose CD4 count ranges from 200–500 cells or better do fairly well with travel. Live viral and bacterial vaccines such as MMR, polio, typhoid Ty21a, and BCG are avoided. Enhanced inactivated polio virus vaccine and the Vi intramuscular typhoid vaccine can provide equivalent coverage if required. Yellow fever vaccine does not seem to impart an increased risk if the CD4 count is > 200 cells. Highly compromised patients with < 200 cells may be at risk for measles pneumonia with the vaccine strain and disseminated infection with BCG. Other nonlive vaccines are fairly well tolerated, although the patient's ability to mount an immune response decreases with progressive HIV disease. Concern that immunization may transiently worsen the patient's HIV disease seems to be fading with the availability of aggressive antiretroviral treatment regimens.

The HIV-infected patient is at risk of developing more severe gastrointestinal disease (e.g., salmonellosis, shigellosis, campylobacterial or giardial infection, amebiasis, infection with cryptosporidia, microsporidia, cyclospora, or isospora). Reports of increased risks of visceral leishmaniasis, Chagas disease, and progressive primary disease with *Mycobacterium tuberculosis* as well as the potential need for more advanced medical care should be taken into account when the HIV-infected patient is selecting a travel destination.

ACKNOWLEDGMENT

The Chief, Bureau of Medicine and Surgery, Navy Department, Washington, DC, Clinical Investigation Program, sponsored this report, no. 84-16-1968-647, as required by HSETCINST 6000.41A. The views expressed in this article are those of the authors and do not reflect the official policy or position of the Department of the Navy, Department of Defense, or the United States Government.

BIBLIOGRAPHY

1. Auerbach PS (ed): Wilderness Medicine, 3rd ed. Mosby, St. Louis, 1995.
2. Centers for Disease Control and Prevention: Health Information for International Travel, 1996–1997. Atlanta, U.S. Department of Health and Human Services, 1996.
3. DuPont HL, Steffen R: Textbook of Travel Medicine and Health. Philadelphia, B.C. Decker, 1997.
4. Ericsson CD, DuPont HL, Mathewson JJ: Single dose ofloxacin plus loperamide compared with single dose or three days of ofloxacin in the treatment of traveler's diarrhea. Trav Med 4:3–7, 1997.
5. Humar A, Keystone J: Evaluating fevers in travelers returning from tropical countries. BMJ 312:953–356, 1996.
6. Jong EC, McMullen R: The Travel and Tropical Medicine Manual. Philadelphia, W.B Saunders, 1995.
7. Shoff WH, Shepherd SM (eds): Travel-related Emergencies. Emerg Med Clin North Am 15(1):1997.
8. Wilson ME: A World Guide to Infections. New York, Oxford University Press, 1991.

61. MALARIA

H. James Beecham III, M.D.

1. Name the four species of the protozoa genus *Plasmodium* that cause human malaria.

1. *P. falciparum:* the species responsible for most malaria fatalities worldwide; does not produce relapsing malaria.

2. *P. vivax:* the most common form of relapsing malaria; rarely fatal.

3. *P. ovale:* a much less common form of relapsing, nonfatal malaria.

4. *P. malariae:* a less common and sometimes milder form of malaria. Capable of low-grade, chronic infections that may be transmitted through blood transfusions from donors with subclinical infections.

2. What species of malaria cause most human disease worldwide?

P. falciparum and *P. vivax* are responsible for most cases of malaria worldwide. *P. falciparum* causes most malaria fatalities. *P. vivax* (along with *P. ovale*) has a potentially dormant liver stage capable of evading treatments for acute blood stage disease and may produce clinical malarial relapses weeks or months after infection.

3. Who should be suspected of having acute malaria?

Any patient or traveler evaluated for fever within or recently returning from a country known to be endemic for malaria. Most acute cases present with fever, chills, headache, and myalgias. Up to 50% of cases also have gastrointestinal symptoms such as diarrhea, nausea, and vomiting. Gastrointestinal symptoms may be pronounced and have been known to cause the primary physician to exclude malaria from the differential diagnosis. In one reported series this mistake resulted in delayed treatment for malaria and fatal outcomes. The clinical presentation may be delayed, less dramatic, and somewhat attenuated in a patient who is taking malaria chemoprophylaxis.

4. Once malaria is diagnosed, what are the most important considerations in choosing the appropriate treatment?

1. Severity of illness and whether the infection is due to *P. falciparum* and thus potentially life-threatening.

2. Whether the infection was acquired in an area with known chloroquine-resistant *P. falciparum*. If so, a drug other than chloroquine must be used.

3. Whether the infection is associated with a relapsing form of malaria—*P. vivax* or *P. ovale*. If so, treatment with primaquine to kill the dormant liver stage is also indicated.

5. What are the major features of severe or complicated malaria?

Altered mental status	Shock
Coma	Parasitemia > 3%
Respiratory distress	Severe anemia (< 21%)
Convulsions	Renal failure (creatinine > 3mg/dl)
Hypoglycemia (< 40 mg/dl)	Elevated hepatic transaminases (> 3 times normal)

For treatment purposes, complicated malaria should be assumed to be due to chloroquine-resistant *P. falciparum*, and intravenous antimalarials should be initiated.

6. When should exchange transfusions be considered as adjuvant therapy in treating malaria?

Exchange transfusions are controversial but may be considered in seriously ill patients with complicated malaria who have parasitemia in the range of 5–15%.

7. What is the drug of choice for patients who present with uncomplicated *P. falciparum* malaria after returning from travel in a country (such as Haiti or the Dominican Republic) that is still free of chloroquine-resistant *P. falciparum*?

Such patients should be treated with chloroquine orally. Chloroquine is well tolerated, and years of usage have proved that it is also safe in pregnant women.

8. What is the drug of choice for patients who present with severe, complicated, life-threatening malaria?

In the United States parenteral quinidine gluconate is recommended for severe malaria infection. Complicated malaria is most commonly associated with *P. falciparum* infection. Before 1991, the Centers for Disease Control (CDC) provided parenteral quinine for severe malaria because quinine was not commercially available in the United States. In April 1991, after reviewing data about the clinical efficacy of intravenous quinidine gluconate (the dextrorotatory diastereoisomer of quinine), which is more widely available in American hospitals, the CDC recommended the use of parenteral quinidine gluconate as the drug of choice for persons with complicated malaria. Guidelines for its use are detailed in the *Morbidity and Mortality Weekly Report*, April 19, 1991, Vol. 40, No. RR-4. Since this recommendation, there have been isolated reports of difficulty in obtaining quinidine gluconate in some hospitals because of changes in the frequencies of its usage.

9. Why may hypoglycemia be seen in malaria cases?

1. *Plasmodium*-infected red blood cells utilize glucose at a rate 75 times greater than normal red blood cells.

2. Quinidine and quinine may stimulate insulin secretion, resulting in hyperinsulinemia and thus significant hypoglycemia.

3. In acute malaria hepatic gluconeogenesis is impaired and may contribute to hypoglycemia.

Clinically, hypoglycemia is most often associated with cerebral malaria and tends to be more common in younger children and pregnant women.

10. How may infection with *P. vivax* cause serious disease?

P. vivax infection is not usually associated with fatal disease, but deaths have been reported after spontaneous or traumatic ruptures of an enlarged spleen.

11. Name two precautions with the use of primaquine in treating the liver stages of *P. vivax* or *P. ovale* infection.

1. Primaquine is a potent oxidant and may cause hemolysis in some patients with glucose-6-phosphate dehydrogenase (G-6-PD) deficiency.

2. Use of primaquine is contraindicated in pregnant women.

12. A 45-year-old man presents with fever and myalgia. He is an air cargo pilot whose recent travel history includes a flight to Haiti 5 days ago. He remained overnight in Port-au-Prince and noted bites by mosquitoes. He took no malaria chemoprophylaxis. What is the likelihood that his acute illness is due to malaria?

Highly unlikely. The incubation period for malaria ranges from as early as 8–9 days up to 40 or more days after the bite of the infected mosquito. If related to exposure in Haiti only 5 days ago, the illness may be due to one of the shorter incubating diseases of the Caribbean region, such as classic dengue fever, but not to malaria.

13. You are consulted by a traveler about to embark on a 21-day tour of African game parks. What standard reference publication provides guidance about medical recommendations for international travel?

The Centers for Disease Control and Prevention's *Health Information for International Travel*, which is published annually by the CDC. It is available through the Superintendent of

Documents, U.S. Government Printing Office, Washington, DC 20402, (202) 512-1800. The Traveler's Health Section of the CDC maintains a Fax Information Service at (404) 332-4565; on the Internet, the World Wide Web address is http://www.cdc.gov.

14. What are two of the most common causes of sudden clinical deterioration in patients with severe, complicated malaria ?

Hypoglycemia and bacterial sepsis.

15. Malaria transmission occurs in areas of Central and South America, Haiti and the Dominican Republic, Africa, the Indian subcontinent, Southeast Asia, parts of the Middle East, and Oceania. From what region of the world are most U.S. cases acquired?

According to the CDC, 800–1000 cases of malaria are reported each year in the United States. Over 80% of U.S. cases of malaria are acquired in sub-Saharan countries of Africa. In addition, over 80% of the fatal cases of malaria reported in the United States are acquired in sub-Saharan Africa.

16. What personal preventive advice should be given to travelers about to embark to a high-risk malaria endemic area?

1. Malaria mosquitoes (*Anopheles* sp.) bite primarily between dusk and dawn.

2. Travelers should wear clothes that cover most of the body and remain in well-screened areas.

3. Travelers should purchase insect repellent that contains between 30–35% DEET (N,N diethylmethyltoluamide) for use on exposed skin.

4. If they are living in more primitive conditions, travelers should use mosquito nets and a pyrethroid-containing flying insect spray in living and sleeping areas during evening and night-time hours.

5. Bed nets are more effective when sprayed with permethrin spray.

6. Malaria may occur despite preventive efforts as early as 8–9 days after initial exposure in an endemic area or several months (sometimes delayed for several months past the usual presentation) after departing the area. Therefore, at the onset of any malarial symptoms such as fevers, the traveler should seek immediate medical evaluation.

17. Name the four most commonly prescribed antimalarial drugs in chemoprophylactic regimens for travelers to endemic areas.

Mefloquine, doxycycline, chloroquine, and primaquine. Each drug has specific indications, adverse reactions, and contraindications that should be reviewed before prescribing. For more detailed information about malaria chemoprophylaxis (country-specific because of the presence or absence of chloroquine-resistant *P. falciparum* and other factors such as mefloquine resistance) see the CDC's *Health Information for International Travel*.

18. What two mechanisms of action may account for the lethality of *P. falciparum*?

1. The extent of red blood cell invasion by the parasite. *P. vivax* and *P. ovale* tend to invade only young red blood cells (reticulocytes), whereas *P. malariae* invades only aging erythrocytes. *P. falciparum* invades erythrocytes of all ages, producing much higher levels of parasitemia.

2. *P. falciparum* causes rosetting, which is the clumping or binding of uninfected erythrocytes to microscopic "knobs" on the surface of infected erythrocytes. This, along with enhanced endothelial cytoadherence, causes obstruction and plugging of the microvasculature, with impairment of local blood flow and cell death.

19. Are corticosteroids beneficial as ancillary treatment in severe malaria ?

No. High-dose corticosteroids, aspirin, hyperimmune serum, cyclosporine, and heparin have been shown to confer no benefit and may be harmful.

20. How many hours after the initiation of antimalarial treatment should a drop in parasitemia be seen?

Failure to see a reduction in parasitemia within 24–48 hours of oral antimalarial treatment may be an indication for initiation of intravenous antimalarial therapy. This finding may suggest the presence of a resistant strain. Peripheral blood smears should be monitored daily until no parasites have been seen for 2–3 days.

21. What are the most common errors in the treatment of malaria ?

Delay in starting treatment, which is usually due to one or more of the following factors:

1. Initial blood smear is negative and not repeated.

2. Drug of choice is not readily available.

3. Lack of high index of suspicion of malaria due to (1) presentation with fever and gastrointestinal symptoms, (2) failure to take an adequate travel history, or (3) lack of knowledge about the incubation period of malaria.

BIBLIOGRAPHY

1. Berg SW (ed): Navy Medical Department Guide to Malaria Prevention and Control, "Malaria Blue Book." Norfolk, VA, Navy Environmental Health Center, 1995.
2. Centers for Disease Control: Health Information for International Travel. Centers for Disease Control and Prevention, National Center for Infectious Diseases, Division of Quarantine, 1996.
3. Kean BH, Reilly PC: Malaria—the mime: Recent lessons from a group of civilian travelers. Am J Med 6:159–164, 1976.
4. White NJ: The treatment of malaria. N Engl J Med 335:800–806, 1996.
5. Wyler DJ: Malaria: Overview and update. Clin Infect Dis 16:449–456, 1993.
6. Wyler DJ: Malaria chemoprophylaxis for the traveler. N Engl J Med 329:31–37, 1993.

62. LEPTOSPIROSIS

Eric A. Crawley, M.D.

1. Describe the organism responsible for leptospirosis.

Leptospirosis refers to the illness caused by infection with a pathogenic serovar of the spirochete species, *Leptospira interrogans*. It is an aerobic, tightly coiled, motile organism with a terminal hook. It stains gram-negative but is best visualized with dark field microscopy. Over 200 different serovars have been identified, many of which cause disease in humans. Leptospirosis is a zoonosis; humans are accidental hosts.

2. What are the most common symptoms encountered?

By far the three most common symptoms, in descending order of prevalence, are fever, headache, and myalgia, each occurring in approximately 90% of patients. The headache is often bifrontal and severe and may mimic the headache seen in rickettsial disease. Photophobia, and nuchal rigidity are not uncommon. Myalgia, often profound, is typically more severe in the lower extremities. Other symptoms include cough, dyspnea, nausea, vomiting, pharyngalgia, hemoptysis, and hematemesis. Any constellation of the above may be encountered; the typical presentation suggests a nonspecific infectious entity.

3. What are the common risk factors for development of leptospirosis?

Leptospirosis is acquired through exposure to water, urine, or animal tissues containing the organism. Historically, occupational exposures were most commonly associated with infection; in the industrial world, however, recreational exposures have become more prevalent. Specific implicated exposures include swimming or wading in mud or water, ingestion of surface or catchment water, and contamination of cuts or abrasions with rodent urine. Specific occupations at risk include sewer, aquaculture, and farm workers, veterinarians, butchers, and military personnel.

4. How is the diagnosis established?

Culture of leptospires from blood, cerebrospinal fluid (CSF), or urine is diagnostic. A serologic diagnosis remains the more common means of making the diagnosis. Blood and CSF cultures are positive at initial presentation, whereas urine becomes positive in 1–2 weeks in untreated individuals. The microscopic agglutination test is most commonly performed and is considered positive when a fourfold rise is seen from acute and convalescent titers. Compatible clinical cases are described as presumptive when the acute titer is > 1:200 but fails to show a fourfold increase. An enzyme-linked immunosorbent assay (ELISA) is also available commercially. Leptospires also can be demonstrated in tissue specimens via direct fluorescent antibody staining. Physicians should maintain a high clinical suspicion in patients with a compatible history; most cases go undiagnosed.

5. Is antibiotic therapy effective?

Treatment with penicillin G, 6 million U/day, was shown to be effective in severe leptospirosis even when given late in the course. Duration of fever, renal insufficiency, and total days hospitalized were markedly reduced, and leptospiruria was prevented. Doxycycline, 100 mg two times/day orally, also was shown to be effective in mild leptospirosis, with reduction in fever and overall symptoms and prevention of leptospiruria. Other agents believed to be effective include amoxicillin, 500 mg every 6 hr, and ampicillin, 500–750 mg every 6 hr.

6. Is there a means of preventing infection in persons at risk?

Yes. It has been demonstrated that 200 mg of doxycycline weekly was effective prophylaxis among soldiers at risk. This regimen was 95% effective, with an attack rate of 4.2% in the placebo group compared with 0.2% in the treated group. The indications for prophylaxis are not clear, but if a limited, high-risk exposure is expected, prophylaxis seems reasonable.

7. What control measures are effective in reducing risk of infection?

Control of animal reservoirs, particularly rodents, may reduce the risk of infection. Other approaches include treatment of water supplies at risk, avoidance of water exposure, and use of protective clothing. Effective animal vaccines have been used in cattle, sheep, and domestic dogs.

8. What is the most effective means of culturing the organism?

The organism is readily cultured with appropriate specimen handling and culture techniques. The organism can be isolated from the blood or CSF early in the course of illness. Urine cultures become positive in untreated people 1–2 weeks into the illness. The organism should be cultured in Fletcher's medium, and the laboratory should be alerted to the possibility of leptospirosis so that sufficient culture time may be allotted. Cultures may take several weeks to become positive.

9. What are the typical laboratory and radiographic features of leptospirosis?

It is useful to think of anicteric and icteric leptospirosis as opposite ends of the spectrum of disease because the laboratory abnormalities found in each are significantly different.

Anicteric leptospirosis is associated with less marked derangement in laboratory values. The typical anicteric patient demonstrates a mild leukocytosis with left shift. Renal insufficiency is sometimes seen, but otherwise normal laboratory values are the rule. CSF studies are usually unremarkable in both spectrums of disease.

In icteric or severe illness, multiple laboratory abnormalities are the norm, including leukocytosis or leukopenia, anemia that usually is mild, and thrombocytopenia, which may be in the 20–50,000 range. Elevation in serum creatinine with preserved electrolytes is seen in most patients. Liver-associated enzyme testing demonstrates elevations in bilirubin, which may be quite marked, as well as liver enzyme elevations 2–5 times normal values. Creatinine kinase may be elevated. Significant derangement in prothrombin time or activated partial thromboplastin time is uncommon. Arterial blood gas analysis may demonstrate hypoxemia and respiratory alkalosis.

The chest radiograph often demonstrates abnormalities, including a pattern of diffuse alveolar filling, either from alveolar hemorrhage or noncardiogenic pulmonary edema, or localized infiltrates similar to bronchopneumonia. Pleural effusions also have been described.

10. Describe the clinical features of Weil syndrome.

Weil syndrome is a fulminant variant of leptospirosis associated with icterus and multiorgan dysfunction. Although the syndrome was initially described by Adolph Weil in 1881, the causative organism was not identified until 1915 by Inada and Ido. The syndrome is typically marked by the development of icterus, oliguric renal failure, and evidence of systemic vasculitis in a patient with febrile illness. Vasculitis may lead to hemorrhagic complications, most notably pulmonary hemorrhage resulting in hypoxemic respiratory failure. The development of the adult respiratory distress syndrome has been described. Although uncommon, severe illness with multiorgan dysfunction may occur in the absence of icterus. Classically described as a biphasic illness, Weil syndrome may well present as one acute infection.

11. What is the prognosis of severe leptospirosis (Weil syndrome)?

Mortality is most closely related to age and presence of icterus. The mortality rate on average is 5–10%. Traditionally, the most common cause of death is renal failure. With the availability of dialysis and hemofiltration, death due to respiratory failure has become more common. Respiratory failure usually results from hemorrhagic pneumonitis with massive hemoptysis and asphyxiation or from development of adult respiratory distress syndrome. With antibiotic therapy and supportive care, patients who survive the initial insult can expect a full recovery, including normalization of renal function.

12. Is there any particular geographic distribution of leptospirosis?

Leptospires are ubiquitous and found on all inhabited continents. Cases of leptospirosis have been reported globally, but the disease is more prevalent in tropical regions. There appears to be a tendency toward more severe illness among cases reported from the tropics, especially the Far East.

13. What seasonal or environmental factors affect the incidence of disease?

For poorly understood reasons, the illness is more common during summer months or the rainy season in the tropics. Mass outbreaks have been associated with natural disasters such as flooding. The disease also has a 4–5 year periodicity. Conditions that increase the number of persons coming in contact with water, such as summer months or flooding, are believed to play a role in the seasonal pattern. The theory that leptospires deposited by animals at the edge of bodies of water enter the water as levels rise also may help to explain the seasonal pattern.

14. What is the role of vaccination?

Leptospirosis vaccines are most commonly used in veterinary medicine and animal husbandry. Leptospirosis among cattle and sheep is a major cause of fetal wastage and has significant economic impact. Vaccination of cattle has been shown to reduce infection and consequently fetal wastage. Preliminary evidence suggests that in regions where farm animals represent the major reservoir for leptospirosis, vaccination has decreased the incidence of human disease.

Human immunization is not widely utilized and the efficacy is controversial. Natural immunity is highly protective but is serovar-specific. Immunization is feasible but hampered by the large number of immunologically distinct pathogenic serovars, which makes the development of a widely protective vaccine difficult.

BIBLIOGRAPHY

1. De Brito T, Bohm GM, Yasuda PH: Vascular damage in acute experimental leptospirosis of the guinea-pig. J Pathol 128:177–181, 1979.
2. Farr RW: Leptospirosis. Clin Infect Dis 21:1–8, 1995.
3. Heath CW, Alexander AD, Galton MM: Leptospirosis in the United States: Analysis of 483 cases in man,1949–1961. N Engl J Med 273:915–922, 1965.
4. Im J, Yeon KM, Han MC, et al: Leptospirosis of the lung: Radiographic findings in 58 patients. Am J Roentgenol 152:955–959, 1989.
5. McClain JBL, Ballou WR, Harrison SM, et al: Doxycycline therapy of leptospirosis. Ann Intern Med 100:696, 1984.
6. Sasaki DM, Pang L, Minette HP, et al: Active surveillance and risk factors for leptospirosis in Hawaii. Am J Trop Med Hygiene 48:35–43, 1993.
7. Takafuji ET, Kirkpatrick JW, Miller RN, et al: An efficacy trial of doxycycline chemoprophylaxis against leptospirosis. N Engl J Med 310:497–500, 1984.
8. Watt G, Padre LP, Tuazon L, et al: Placebo-controlled trial of intravenous penicillin for severe and late leptospirosis. Lancet 1:433–435, 1988.
9. Watt G, Alquiza LM, Padre LP, et al: The rapid diagnosis of leptospirosis: A prospective comparison of the dot enzyme-linked immunosorbent assay and the genus-specific microscopic agglutination test at different stages of illness. J Infect Dis 157:840–842, 1988.

XX. Emerging Pathogens

63. HANTAVIRUSES

Chun Ho So, M.D., and Donald R. Skillman, M.D., FACP

> I hope we never lose sight of one fact, that this was all started by a mouse.
> *Walt Disney*

1. What are hantaviruses?

Hantaviruses are single-stranded, enveloped viruses related to members of the family Bunyaviridae. Their genome consists of three negative-sense RNA segments cleverly termed the L (large), M (medium), and S (small) segments. The L-segment encodes for a viral transcriptase, the M-segment encodes for the envelope glycoproteins (G1 and G2), and the S-segment encodes for the nucleocapsid protein. Each envelope contains three nucleocapsids. Intact hantavirus particles are pleomorphic, varying from spherical to oval, with an average diameter of 80–110 nm. Many different hantaviruses are found in different geographic locations worldwide. New ones are still being identified.

2. How are hantaviruses transmitted?

Hantaviruses are pure zoonotic infections. Whereas the primary vectors for other members of the Bunyaviradae family are arthropods, no study to date has implicated transmission of hantaviruses by arthropod vectors. Hantavirus vectors are mostly rodents: field mice, voles, and rats. Each particular hantavirus appears to favor a specific rodent endemic to a particular region. Infected rodents shed infectious virions in their urine, feces, and saliva. The primary route of infection is via inhalation of the shed virions from aerosolized urine or feces. There have also been reports of infection arising from direct contact with contaminated secretions and from rodent bites. Human-to-human transmission has not been documented.

3. Do rodent vectors infected with hantaviruses exhibit symptoms of illness?

No. The key to hantavirus survival and transmission is asymptomatic infection of rodent vectors. Infection begins with a viremic phase lasting about 1 week, during which the virus is disseminated throughout the host's blood and organs. Antigens can be detected in blood, lungs, spleen, parotid glands, kidneys, saliva, feces, and urine throughout the life of the host.

An immune response with production of neutralizing IgM and IgG antibodies occurs after the viremic phase. Despite these antibodies, infected rodents shed infectious virions in their saliva, urine, and feces. The duration and mechanism of shedding are yet to be fully determined.

4. How did the term hantavirus originate?

It came from the prototype hantavirus, Hantaan virus, which causes hemorrhagic fever with renal syndrome (HFRS) in Asia. This syndrome is not new and it is recognized in other parts of the world. Epidemics fitting the syndrome of HFRS were described as early as 960 A.D. Sporadic cases were noted in the American Civil War, in the USSR in 1913 and again in the 1920s and 1930s, and in Manchuria in the 1940s.

HFRS came to the attention of the western world in the 1950s during the Korean conflict. Over 3000 cases were diagnosed among the United Nations Forces, which mounted an intensive search for the etiologic agent. Finally, in 1976 convalescent sera from patients with HFRS was found to react with an undefined antigen in the lungs of *Apodemus agrarius* mice trapped along the banks of the Hantaan river near the border between North and South Korea. The virus responsible for HFRS was isolated in 1978, and the name *Hantaan virus* was coined. Antigenically distinct types of the hantavirus have been subsequently characterized in other parts of the world.

5. Describe some of the hantaviruses that cause human disease, along with their hosts, geographic location, and associated clinical syndromes.

Hantaviruses are ubiquitous (one is probably in the room with you right now). More hantaviruses that affect humans are being characterized throughout the world. Different viruses cause different clinical symptoms, but overlap is substantial. Each hantavirus appears to be associated with a unique rodent host. Some hantaviruses, such as the Prospect Hill virus, have not been associated with a clinical syndrome.

Hantavirus	Rodent Host	Geographic Locale	Clinical Syndrome
Hantaan	*Apodemus agrarius* (striped field mouse)	Korea, China, Russia, Siberia, central Asia, Europe	Severe HFRS
Dobrava/Belgrade	*Apodemus flavicollis* (yellow field mouse)	Most of Europe, Asia Minor	HFRS
Seoul	*Rattus norvegicus* (Norway rat)	Worldwide—related to shipping	Mild HFRS
Puumala	*Clethrionomys glareolus* (bank vole)	Mostly Europe	NE
Four Corners or Sin Nombre	*Peromyscus maniculatus* (deer mouse)	Southwest United States	HPS
Black Creek Canal	*Sigmodon hispidus* (cotton rat)	South Florida	HPS/more renal involvement
Bayou	*Orysomys palustis* (rice rat)	Louisiana	HPS/more renal involvement
New York-1	*Peromyscus leucopus* (white-footed mouse)	Eastern U.S., Canada	HPS
Prospect Hill	*Microtus pennsylvanicus* (meadow vole)	United States, Canada	No known human disease

HFRS = hemorrhagic fever with renal syndrome, HPS = hantavirus pulmonary syndrome, NE = nephropathica epidemica.

6. Where and when was a hantavirus first detected and isolated in the United States?

On May 14, 1993, several unexplained deaths were recognized in the Four Corners area (where Utah, Arizona, New Mexico, and Colorado meet). The first to die were a young Native American couple who were struck suddenly with a viral-like prodrome, developed rapidly progressive respiratory failure, and died within 5 days of each other. Dr. Bruce Tempest of the Indian Health Service noted reports of comparable deaths within the same time frame. A hantavirus was considered because of clinical similarity to hemorrhagic fever with renal syndrome, but without renal involvement. Antibody screening and polymerase chain reaction techniques eventually revealed a novel hantavirus as the cause. This hantavirus has had various names, but sin nombre virus (SNV) seems to be the one that stuck.

SNV has been present in North America for many years. Cases in New Mexico (1975) and Idaho (1978) were diagnosed retrospectively using the case definition of hantavirus pulmonary syndrome (HPS) developed in 1993 by the Centers for Disease Control and Prevention. In 1994, a man who had the clinical syndrome of HPS in Utah in 1959 was found to have IgG antibodies to SNV. Navajo elders noted that twice in this century after a heavy rainfall season, with prosperous growth of the piñon nut crop, there were many unexplained deaths among healthy young

Navajos. With the exuberant piñon nut crop the deer mouse population booms. The Four Corners outbreak in 1993 also followed a season of heavy rains, with a robust piñon nut crop and a 10-fold increase in the deer mouse population.

7. How many cases of hantavirus infection have been confirmed in the United States as of December 18, 1996?

Since its initial isolation in 1993 through December 18, 1996, 155 cases of hantavirus infection have been confirmed. The cases come from 26 states, with the majority clustered west of the Mississippi River, mainly in New Mexico (29), Arizona (22) and California (14). Most cases in the U.S. are caused by SNV through the vector *Peromyscus maniculatus* (the wily deer mouse).

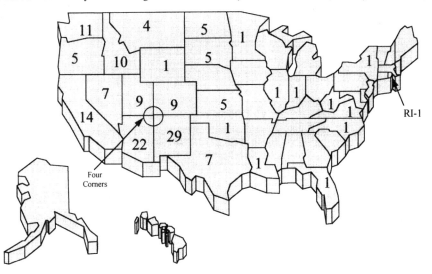

State-by-state number of hantavirus cases as of December 18, 1996.

8. What clinical syndromes have been attributed to hantavirus infection?

Although some hantavirus infections are asymptomatic (e.g., the Prospect Hill virus; see question 3), three disease syndromes have been frequently observed:

1. Hemorrhagic fever with renal syndrome (HFRS). Most of these viruses come from Old World rodents (i.e., Far East).

2. Hantavirus pulmonary syndrome (HPS). Viruses often come from Western Hemisphere rodents.

3. Nephropathia epidemica (NE). This syndrome is seen most often in western Europe and is caused primarily by the Puumala virus.

9. What are the five clinical phases of HFRS?

1. **Prodromal febrile phase:** general flulike symptoms, with back and abdominal pain. It may mimic anything from pyelonephritis to a surgical abdomen. Facial flushing, petechiae, and conjunctival bleeding may be observed as result of endothelial injury and vascular leakage. Marked leukocytosis appears.

2. **Hypotensive phase:** septic shock picture, often requiring vasopressors and copious intravenous fluids. Thrombocytopenia is marked, and abnormalities in the coagulation cascade may occur with prominent capillary hemorrhage and bleeding.

3. **Oliguric phase:** decreased urinary output, uremia, and multiple laboratory abnormalities (e.g., increased blood urea nitrogen and creatinine, electrolyte problems, proteinuria). This phase usually starts during the hypotensive phase because of decreased renal perfusion and

renal vascular injury. Increased bleeding is due to uremia, which interferes with platelet function; the degree of hemorrhagic complications varies (epistaxis, dermal purpura, gastrointestinal bleeding, hematuria, strokes). Fifty percent of deaths occur during the oliguric phase.

4. **Diuretic phase:** high volume diuresis, 3–6 L/day, with gradual improvement in renal function. This phase is the beginning of clinical recovery, if the patient survives.

5. **Convalescent phase:** a gradual return to the usual state of health. Complete recovery is the usual course, assuming no major organs were permanently damaged (e.g., stroke).

10. What are the clinical manifestations of HPS?

HPS has the typical prodromal phase of HFRS, but the major organ system involved is the lungs. Once a patient develops dyspnea, the interval to development of shock and noncardiac pulmonary edema requiring intubation and mechanical ventilation is as short as 4 hours. HPS is usually not associated with severe renal or hematologic complications, but both are sometimes observed. HPS carries a high mortality rate due to respiratory compromise.

11. What are the clinical manifestations of NE?

NE is considered a benign disease (although the patient may not agree) because the overall mortality rate is less than 1%. Typically the onset of symptoms is similar to HFRS. Some degree of hypotension may be observed, but the septic shock state is not seen. The main features are interstitial nephritis and renal hemorrhage, which cause acute renal failure. Other features are severe central nervous system symptoms manifest by severely ill appearance (e.g., confusion, lethargy) and meningeal signs that may be mistaken for meningitis (cerebrospinal fluid is usually normal). Full recovery is the expected outcome. Fewer than 1% of patients may require dialysis.

12. What is the underlying pathophysiology of hantavirus infection?

For each of the three clinical syndromes caused by hantaviruses, the pathophysiology involves damage to the vasculature and vascular beds of multiple organ systems. Each syndrome involves specific organs, but overlap is common. The destructive process involves direct and indirect destruction of vascular beds. Direct damage results from viral invasion of endothelial cells, with subsequent replication and cellular injury. Damage to the endothelium leads to increased capillary permeability. Indirect vascular damage results from circulating immune complex deposition as well as activation of both arms of the complement cascade. Activation of the kallikrein, kinin, and renin systems also has been described. Immune complement deposition on platelets causes thrombocytopenia, platelet dysfunction, and prolonged bleeding time. Depressed coagulation factors leading to prolonged prothrombin time (PT) and partial thromboplastin time (PTT) also have been seen.

13. What is the overall case-fatality rate from hantavirus infection?

Of the cases confirmed in the U.S. to date, the overall case-fatality rate as of Dec. 18, 1996, is 47.7%. No effective therapy has been developed. The overall mortality rate for HFRS ranges from 5–10%. Up to 100,000 cases are reported each year in China alone, resulting in 5,000–10,000 deaths. The overall mortality rate for NE is < 1%, and many people are asymptomatic after acquiring the infection, as evidenced by positive antibody titers.

14. In which body compartments can hantaviruses be isolated from infected humans?

Hantaviruses have been found in plasma, cerebospinal fluid, and cells, particularly peripheral blood monocytes. Viruses have been detected for up to 7 days in plasma and up to 2 weeks in monocytes. Hantaviruses have not been isolated from saliva, breast milk, urine, or semen of infected humans.

15. Are vaccines available for hantaviruses?

In China, where the annual incidence of HFRS is 50,000–100,000 cases, a recombinant protein vaccine has been developed that elicits a neutralizing antibody response. Neutralizing antibody is also present in serum of patients who recover from disease and offers the potential for prophylactic treatment in certain circumstances. Apparently some people parenterally exposed to hantavirus in laboratory accidents did not develop illness after receiving convalescent plasma. However, the risk of immune complex formation with the rapid appearance of antibodies in natural infections (which do not appear to reduce disease) argues against therapy with immune plasma. No vaccine of proven benefit is yet available. Human trials with inactivated mouse and rat brain preparations were listed as "underway" in a 1991 textbook of virology.

16. What tests are available for diagnosis of hantavirus infection?

1. Serum can be tested for IgM and IgG antibodies against a panel of heterologous hantaviral antigens with an enzyme-linked immunosorbent assay (ELISA).

2. Polymerase chain reaction (PCR) can be done on RNA extracted from body fluids and frozen tissue specimens using hantavirus-specific oligonucleotide primers.

3. Immunohistochemical assays for viral antigens can be done on formalin-fixed specimens using monoclonal or polyclonal antibodies.

17. Where and how do you report suspected hantavirus infections?

Notify your local public health or preventive medicine officials, the Infection Control Service, and your friendly infectious disease specialist. The CDC has a hotline for reporting suspected hantavirus cases and obtaining more information: 1-800-532-9929.

18. What drug therapies are available for hantavirus infections?

From 1985–1987 a trial using intravenous ribavirin was conducted in 242 patients with serologically confirmed HFRS in mainland China. A fourfold decrease in mortality was noted in the treated group (2% of 125 ribavirin-treated patients vs. 8% of 117 placebo-treated patients). A significant decrease in progression to oliguria and bleeding complications was also noted in the ribavirin group. The only adverse effect from ribavirin was development of reversible anemia.

Although a few sporadic case reports have shown some decrease in case fatality rates after treatment of HPS with ribavirin, the overall mortality rate did not appear to change. Subsequent analysis revealed no clear positive influence on outcome. To date, no specific effective pharmacologic therapy is indicated for the treatment of hantavirus infection.

19. What preventive measures can be taken to avoid hantavirus infection?

Rodent control in and around the home is the best prevention strategy. Keep food, water, and garbage in rodent-proof containers. Do not leave pet food and water out overnight. Three inches of gravel under mobile homes prevent burrowing. Metal roof flashing can be placed around the base of wooden, earthen, or adobe buildings. Use traps or rodenticides (approved by the Environmental Protection Agency) regularly. Relocate woodpiles, animal feed, trash cans, and vegetable gardens at least 100 feet from dwellings.

When cleaning areas with small numbers of rodents, wear Latex or rubber gloves and wet down the area with a general household disinfectant such as Lysol, bleach and water, or ammonia. In areas with large numbers of rodents, add goggles and a high-efficiency particulate air (HEPA) filter mask to the protective ensemble. Wash gloved hands in soap and water, and wash again after removing gloves.

Laboratory work with hantaviruses should be conducted under BL-3 or higher-level containment conditions.

20. Who in the United States is at greatest risk of hantavirus infection?

Hantavirus does not appear to be limited to any age, ethnic group, or geographic region. Although over 50% of HPS cases have been reported from the Four Corners states, this finding reflects the large proportion of cases from the outbreak in the spring of 1993 and the disproportionately active surveillance for HPS in Four Corners compared with elsewhere. In contrast to HFRS, HPS does not appear to affect males more often than females.

Exposure to hantavirus is greatest in people who work, play, or live in closed areas with active rodent infestation. Beware of crawl spaces, opening of air conditioning equipment after winter storage, and cleaning of barns and sheds. Travel is safe in areas where hantavirus has been reported. The risk of exposure to hikers, campers, and tourists is small. Rodents and their dens should be avoided. Infested shelters should not be used until cleaned and disinfected.

21. Does the incidence of hantavirus infection follow a seasonal pattern?

Both HPS and HFRS have a spring-summer seasonality. In contrast to HFRS, HPS is not associated with a high incidence of cases in the fall.

22. How should rodents potentially infected with hantavirus be collected and handled?

A smart person will leave this job to trained experts. If you are elected or volunteered as the trained expert, get the *Guidelines for Removing Organs or Obtaining Blood from Rodents Potentially Infected with Hantavirus*, which is available from the Centers for Disease Control and Prevention by calling 404-639-1510. The supplement contains many details and outlines many mandatory safety procedures.

23. How is HPS diagnosed?

First, you must be smart enough to suspect the infection. The current CDC definition for a suspected case of HPS is twofold: (1) febrile illness (temperature $\geq 38.3°$ C) in a previously healthy person, characterized by adult respiratory distress syndrome or bilateral interstitial pulmonary infiltrates that develop within 1 week of hospitalization and respiratory compromise that requires supplemental oxygen, or (2) unexplained respiratory illness resulting in death, with an autopsy examination demonstrating noncardiogenic pulmonary edema with no identifiable specific cause of death. Excluding criteria include: (1) predisposing underlying medical condition (e.g., cancer, AIDS, steroid therapy) and (2) acute illness that provides a likely explanation for the respiratory illness. In addition to the compatible clinical syndrome, confirmed cases must have positive serology, positive PCR, or positive immunohistochemical assay results for hantavirus.

24. Discuss the medical management of HFRS.

Management is phase-specific and must be individualized. Close observation and supportive care are vital. Hospital admission and trauma avoidance are important to avoid exacerbation of vascular injury. Patient transport should be minimized. Bed rest is essential, especially early in the course. Sedation and narcotics may be needed for restlessness and pain due to vascular extravasation. Fluid balance and volume status require vigilant management to avoid overload in early phases and to cover losses during polyuric later phases. Hypotension requires intravascular volume expanders such as albumin rather than dextrose, saline, or electrolyte solutions. Pressors may be needed.

Electrolytes must be managed carefully; beware of hyperkalemia, an occasional cause of death. Hemodialysis may be necessary for acute renal failure. Secondary infection is a concern, but avoid the salt load associated with some antibiotics. The efficacy of heparin for control of bleeding due to disseminated intravascular coagulation is unproven in clinical trials.

Intravenous ribavirin reduced mortality and improved many aspects of disease manifestation in trials conducted in mainland China. The loading dose was 30 mg/kg IV, followed by 16 mg/kg IV every 6 hours for 4 days, then 8 mg/kg IV for 3 days. The principal adverse effect was reversible anemia.

BIBLIOGRAPHY

1. Centers for Disease Control and Prevention: Hantavirus pulmonary syndrome—United States, 1995 and 1996. MMWR 45:291–295, 1996.
2. Khan AS, Khabbaz, Armstrong LR, et al: Hantavirus pulmonary syndrome: The first 100 US cases. J Infect Dis 173:1296–1303, 1996.
3. McKee KT Jr, LeDuck JW, Peters CJ: Hantaviruses. In Belshe RB (ed): Textbook of Human Virology, 2nd ed. St. Louis, Mosby, 1991, pp 615–632.
4. Warner SG: Hantavirus illness in humans: Review and update. South Med J 89:264–270, 1996.
5. Yao ZQ, Yang WS, Zhang WB, et al: The distribution and duration of Hantaan virus in the body fluids in patients with hemorrhagic fever with renal syndrome. J Infect Dis 160:218–224, 1989.

64. CAT SCRATCH DISEASE

Judy M. Vincent, M.D.

1. What is the causative organism of cat scratch disease (CSD)?

The causative organism of CSD is *Bartonella henselae*, which was formerly known as *Rochalimaea henselae*. The current name was adopted in 1995.

2. What is the pathogenesis of CSD?

B. henselae causes bacteremia in flea-infested, well-appearing cats that are usually less than 1 year old. The organism is transmitted among cats by the cat flea; it is transmitted to humans by a cat scratch, bite, or other intimate contact. The scratch heals quickly and usually does not appear inflamed. About 2 weeks after the scratch, a 3–4-mm solid, verrucous papule may develop in the line of the scratch. About 4 weeks after the scratch, the regional lymph node proximal to the scratch begins to enlarge. At the onset of lymphadenopathy the scratch is completely healed and may be detectable only as a thin, white, fibrous scar.

3. What is the typical clinical presentation of CSD?

The typical patient presents with a lymph node that has enlarged slowly over 10–14 days. Typical CSD has one of the most predictable courses of all diseases: 2 weeks coming, 2 weeks staying, 4–8 weeks going. The lymph node takes about 2 weeks to reach its maximal size. It stays the same size for another 2 weeks and then resolves slowly over the next 4–8 weeks. Fever may or may not be present. Most patients report loss of appetite and loss of energy. CSD lymphadenopathy rarely develops overnight, and it is unlikely to have been present for more than 3 months before presentation. Nodes tend to be large, with an average diameter of 6–7 cm, but they may get as large as 10–13 cm. All patients have intimate contact with cats, usually kittens. The patient should be asked about cat exposure and examined for evidence of cat scratches, even if cat contact is denied. Some patients have a papule within the line of a healing scratch; it will have been present for about 2 weeks before the onset of lymphadenopathy and probably will have a tiny scab. Patients usually report that they have scratched or squeezed the papule, but that no pus has been expressed. The papule is not inflamed or tender. Most patients do not complain about the papule or associate it with the lymphadenopathy, so the physician must look carefully for the papule and cat scratches.

4. What lymph nodes are most commonly involved in CSD?

The most commonly involved lymph nodes are the anterior cervical, axillary, inguinal, femoral, preauricular, supraclavicular, and epitrochlear nodes. However, any lymph node in the body may be affected if it is in the path of lymphatic drainage from a site where *B. henselae* has been inoculated by cat scratch or bite.

5. Is a cat scratch necessary for transmission of CSD?

No. About one-third of patients in one study had no clear history of a cat scratch; however, all patients have a history of intimate contact with a cat or kitten.

6. Is lymphadenopathy present in all patients with CSD?

No. A syndrome called hepatosplenic CSD has been described in children who present with extremely high fevers (103–104° F), malaise, and anorexia. Lymphadenopathy is present in only 50% of such cases. Abdominal ultrasound or computed tomography (CT) is remarkable for multiple hypoechoic, hypodense areas in the liver and/or spleen. These lesions resolve completely. The development of antibody testing for *B. henselae* has allowed investigators to discover that hepatosplenic CSD is a common cause of fever of unknown origin (FUO). Estrada et al. found that 7 of 10 confirmed cases of CSD in patients who were initially admitted to affiliated hospitals in New Orleans with a diagnosis of FUO had hypoechogenic or hypodense areas involving the liver; the spleen was also involved in 2 of these cases. Liver transaminases were normal in all cases, and the mean erythrocyte sedimentation rate was 96 mm/hr (range: 45–150 mm/hr). All cases resolved clinically, and two cases with follow-up studies showed complete resolution of the lesions. Dunn et al. also have reviewed hepatosplenic CSD, its diagnosis, and association with fever and abdominal pain.

7. What are the demographics of patients with CSD?

CSD affects an equal number of children and adults and occurs equally in males and females. It is more common in warm climates than cold climates.

8. What pathognomonic physical finding is diagnostic of CSD?

The verrucous, non-erythematous, non-tender CSD papule within the line of a healed known cat scratch is diagnostic of CSD. If a characteristic papule and healed known cat scratch are found distal to an enlarged regional lymph node, a diagnosis of CSD may be made with certainty.

9. What is the best diagnostic test for CSD?

The diagnostic test of choice is a serologic test for antibody to *B. henselae*. Demers et al. showed that serologic tests for *B. henselae* antibody by immunofluorescent antibody had a specificity and sensitivity of 100%. Serologic tests are commercially available and include other methods such as enzyme-linked immunosorbent assay (ELISA).

10. Is intradermal skin testing useful for the diagnosis of CSD?

No. Intradermal tests have not been standardized or studied in a controlled manner. They are outdated and should not be used.

11. What is the role of fine-needle aspiration and incisional or excisional biopsy?

These procedures are usually not needed. Demers et al. found that of 39 patients with serologically or culture-proven CSD, fine-needle aspiration was diagnostic in only 3 cases. Incisional drainage is helpful in nodes that have progressed to liquefaction and necrosis (about 10% of cases). If a liquefied node is surgically incised, it should be drained and packed so that it will remain open and heal by secondary intention. Complete excision is not necessary. Incised, liquefied nodes will heal completely and will not develop chronic, draining fistulae.

12. What is the best way to look for *B. henselae* in tissues?

The best stain to demonstrate *B. henselae* is the Warthin-Starry silver stain, which enlarges the size of the organisms and makes them easier to see under the microscope. *B. henselae* is a gram-negative bacillus, but it is tiny and takes up Gram stain poorly.

13. How is *B. henselae* cultured?

B. henselae is cultured by sterilely obtaining blood from infected kittens or cats and plating it directly on 5% sheep's blood or chocolate agar. The agar plates should be placed first in airtight plastic bags with an activated carbon dioxide ampule that produces about 7–10% CO_2 and then in a 35° C incubator. *B. henselae* is a fragile and slow-growing organism; therefore, the plates should not be checked for 14 days. *B. henselae* appears as tiny, grayish-white, opaque, adherent colonies. The plates should be held for a total of 60 days before they are called negative. Seropositive humans with CSD usually have culture-negative blood and tissue samples. The bacteria is not often recovered from blood or lymph nodes in humans with CSD, but it is easily recovered from the blood of cats and kittens who are associated with humans who have CSD.

14. What is the treatment of choice for CSD?

No controlled trials have established an effective antibiotic treatment for CSD. In 1988 English et al. published in vitro data showing that CSD bacilli were sensitive to cefoxitin, cefotaxime, gentamicin, amikacin, tobramycin, netilmicin, and mezlocillin. In 1992 Margileth published a retrospective, uncontrolled study of 268 patients with CSD who were treated with 18 different antimicrobials, of which 14 were judged to be of little or no efficacy. The three most effective oral drugs were rifampin, ciprofloxacin, and trimethoprim-sulfamethoxazole. Gentamicin was the most effective intravenous drug. A reasonable option is to use no antibiotics in immunocompetent patients with mild or moderate typical CSD (regional lymphadenopathy), because the disease is benign and self-limited and resolves spontaneously in 2–3 months. Recent in vitro data suggest that azithromycin may be effective. A placebo-controlled trial is underway at the author's institution; if this study establishes efficacy, azithromycin will become the treatment of choice for CSD.

15. Can CSD be fatal?
A few deaths have been reported in immunocompromised patients with disseminated CSD, but no deaths due to CSD have been reported in immunocompetent patients.

16. How long does immunity to CSD last?
Demers et al. showed titers remained elevated in 20 of 24 patients observed for more than 3 months; in 4 patients titers reverted to less than 1:64 within as little as 6 weeks. None of the 24 patients had recurrent disease over the next year despite further scratches from the same cat. The literature indicates that recurrent CSD is extremely rare.

17. What other unusual manifestations of CSD may be seen by clinicians?
CSD encephalopathy is the sudden onset of generalized seizures with progression to coma and rapid return to consciousness within a few days. Relatives of such patients should be interviewed carefully about the patient's exposure to cats or kittens. Patients should be inspected for cat scratches, papules, and lymphadenopathy. If the patient has a history of intimate cat contact and the physical exam shows healed scratches, papules, or lymphadenopathy, a clinical diagnosis of CSD may be made; the prognosis for full recovery is excellent. Another unusual manifestation is the oculoglandular syndrome of Perinaud, which consists of eye involvement with a granuloma on the palpebral conjunctiva, bulbar conjunctival suffusion, and parotid gland enlargement on the ipsilateral side. In this syndrome the organism has been inoculated in the eye, the granuloma is the CSD papule, and the preauricular node is the regionally enlarged lymph node.

18. What are the most common pitfalls in the diagnosis and management of CSD?
The most common pitfalls are not taking a thorough history for cat and kitten exposure, not doing a thorough physical examination for cat and kitten scratches and papules, and not informing the patient that recovery will be slow, even after antibiotics are started.

19. Do *B. henselae*-infected kittens and cats appear to be sick?
No. Infected kittens and cats appear to be happy, healthy, and frisky.

20. Is it necessary to treat *B. henselae*-infected cats and kittens with antibiotics?
No. Antibiotic treatment is not recommended. One study reported that the cats ran away, bit, or fought when attempts were made to give them antibiotics. One researcher anecdotally acquired CSD after being scratched while trying to administer antibiotics to an infected cat. Infected kittens and cats spontaneously clear the bacteremia over time.

BIBLIOGRAPHY

1. Bass JW, Vincent JM, Person DA: The expanding spectrum of *Bartonella* infections. I. Bartonellosis and trench fever. Pediatr Infect Dis J 16:2–10, 1997.
2. Bass JW, Vincent JM, Person DA: The expanding spectrum of *Bartonella* infections. II. Cat scratch disease. Pediatr Infect Dis J 16:163–179, 1997.
3. Demers DM, Bass JW, Vincent JM, et al: Cat scratch disease in Hawaii: Etiology and seroepidemiology. J Pediatr 126:23–26, 1995.
4. Dunn MW, Berkowitz FE, Miller JJ, et al: Hepatosplenic cat scratch disease and abdominal pain. Pediatr Infect Dis J 16:269–272, 1997.
5. English CJ, Wear DJ, Margileth AM, et al: Cat-scratch disease: Isolation and culture of the bacterial agent. JAMA 259:1347–1352, 1988.
6. Estrada B, Silio M, Begue RE et al: Unsuspected hepatosplenic involvement in patients hospitalized with cat-scratch disease. Pediatr Infect Dis J 15:720–721, 1996.
7. Koehler JE, Glaser CA, Tappero JW: *Rochalimaea henselae* infection: A new zoonosis with the domestic cat as reservoir. JAMA 271:531–535, 1994.
8. Margileth AM: Antibiotic therapy for cat-scratch disease: Clinical study of therapeutic outcome in 268 patients and a review of the literature. Pediatr Infect Dis J 11:474–478, 1992.

XXI. Other Topics of Interest

65. ADULT IMMUNIZATION

Edward J. Yang, M.D.

1. Define the terms vaccine, toxoid, antitoxin, immune globulin, specific immune globulin, active immunization, and passive immunization.

Vaccine: a suspension of attenuated or killed microorganisms or fractions thereof administered to induce immunity and thereby prevent infectious diseases.

Toxoid: a modified bacterial toxin that has been rendered nontoxic but retains the ability to stimulate the formation of antitoxin.

Antitoxin: a solution of antibodies derived from the serum of animals immunized with specific antigens (toxins) (e.g., diphtheria, tetanus) and used to achieve passive immunity to effect treatment.

Immune globulin: a sterile solution containing antibody obtained from large pools of human blood plasma.

Specific immune globulin: special preparations obtained from donor pools preselected for a high antibody content against a specific disease (e.g., hepatitis B immune globulin [HBIG]; varicella zoster immune globulin [VZIG]).

Active immunization: production of antibody by the patient through administration of a vaccine or toxoid.

Passive immunization: provision of temporary immunity by administration of preformed antibodies (e.g., immunoglobulins).

2. What are some of the constituents of immunobiologics?

The specific nature and content of immunobiologics differ. Active and inert ingredients may differ slightly if the vaccine is produced by different manufacturers for the same microorganisms.

• **Active immunizing antigen.** In some vaccines, the antigen is a highly defined, single constituent (e.g., pneumococcal polysaccharide); in others, it is complex or ill-defined (live virus).

• **Suspending fluid.** The fluid may be sterile water, saline, or a complex fluid containing small amount of proteins or medium or biologic system in which the vaccine is produced (e.g., serum protein, egg antigen, cell culture-derived antigen).

• **Preservatives, stabilizers, antibiotics.** Trace amounts of chemicals are often used to inhibit or prevent bacterial growth in viral cultures or in the final product (antibiotics, e.g., neomycin) or to stabilize the antigen (glycine). Allergic reactions may occur if the recipient is sensitive to one of the additives (e.g., thimerosal, phenol, albumin, glycine, neomycin).

• **Adjuvants.** To enhance immunogenicity, many antigens are mixed with various substances or adjuvants (e.g., aluminum phosphate or aluminum hydroxide). Vaccines containing aluminum adjuvant should be injected deeply in muscle masses to avoid local irritation, inflammation, granuloma formation, or necrosis (e.g., hepatitis B vaccine).

3. Can multiple vaccinations be simultaneously administered?

Yes. Many of the commonly used vaccines can be safely and effectively administered simultaneously on the same day, but not at the same anatomic site.

• **Killed vaccines.** Most of the widely used killed vaccinations can be administered simultaneously at separate sites. However, when vaccines commonly associated with local or systemic reactions (e.g., cholera, parenteral typhoid, plague) are administered at the same time, theoretically the reactions may be accentuated. When feasible, it is advisable to administer such vaccines on separate occasions.

• **Live vaccines.** A live and a killed vaccine can be administered simultaneously without an impaired antibody response with the exception of cholera and live yellow fever vaccines. At least 3 weeks should elapse between administration of yellow fever and cholera vaccines because of interference in antibody response. Simultaneous administration of most live virus vaccines has not resulted in an impaired antibody response or increased rates of adverse reactions. Because of the theoretical possibility of interference in the development of the immune response to live virus, it is advisable to allow an interval of approximately 4 weeks between doses of different live virus vaccinations. Concern has been raised that oral live attenuated typhoid (Ty2la) vaccine may interfere with the immune response to oral polio vaccine (OPV) when administered simultaneously or soon after live oral typhoid vaccine. However, no published data support this immune response interference. Simultaneous administration of immunoglobulins and live mumps-measles-rubella (MMR) vaccines should be avoided for at least 6 weeks to 3 months after administration of immunoglobulin (IG) because of poor antibody response to MMR. OPV and yellow fever vaccines can be administered at any time before, with, or after IG administration.

• **Live virus.** Vaccination with live virus may interfere with the delayed type hypersensitivity (tuberculin test) response. Tuberculin testing, if otherwise indicated, can be done either on the same day or 4–6 weeks after live virus immunizations.

4. What constituents of vaccine may cause hypersensitivity reactions?

True allergic reactions to vaccine components are rare. Most reactions associated with vaccinations are nonimmunologic local or systemic adverse effects, such as redness, soreness, swelling, and fever. Four types of hypersensitivity reactions are associated with vaccine constituents:

1. Allergic reactions to egg or egg-related antigens.
2. Mercury sensitivity in some recipients of IG or vaccines.
3. Antibiotic-induced allergic reactions (e.g. neomycin). No currently recommended vaccine contains penicillin or penicillin derivatives.
4. Hypersensitive reactions to vaccine antigens or stabilizers.

5. List the vaccines that are contraindicated in persons with anaphylactic hypersensitivity to egg.

• **Influenza and yellow fever vaccines.** Egg protein is found in preparations using embryonated chicken eggs.

• **MMR vaccine.** MMR vaccines are prepared in chicken embryo cell culture. Protocols have been developed for testing and vaccinating patients with MMR who manifest anaphylactic reactions to egg ingestion. The revised recommendations of the Association of American Physicians (AAP) acknowledge that the MMR vaccine can be safely administered to all patients with egg allergy.

6. What vaccinations are indicated for adults with HIV infection?

In general, HIV-infected adults should not receive live-virus or live bacteria vaccines with the exception of MMR. However, evaluation and testing for HIV infection in asymptomatic persons is not necessary before a decision to use live virus vaccinations.

• **Tetanus-diphtheria:** administer when indicated (a booster for every 10 years).

• **Inactivated poliovirus (IPV):** administer IPV if polio vaccine is indicated; OPV is contraindicated.

• **MMR:** limited studies of MMR vaccination among both symptomatic and asymptomatic HIV-infected patients have not documented serious complications; therefore, administer if indicated.

• **Pneumococcal:** indicated for all HIV-infected persons.

- **Influenza:** annual influenza vaccination is indicated.
- **Hepatitis B virus:** indicated.
- **Haemophilus b (Hiv):** Highly consider, even in adults. The incidence of Hib disease may be higher among HIV-infected adults than non-HIV infected adults, and the disease can be severe.

7. A 19-year-old male patient has received no childhood vaccines. What is the immunization schedule for persons over 18 years of age who were not vaccinated at the recommended time in early infancy?

Timing	Vaccine(s)	Comments
First visit	Tetanus-diptheria, MMR*, hepatitis B, polio†	Primary polio vaccination is not routinely recommended for person over 18 yr
Second visit (6–8 weeks after first visit)	Tetanus-diphtheria, MMR, hepatitis B, polio	
Third visit (6 months after second visit	Tetanus-diphtheria, hepatitis B, polio	
Additional visit	Tetanus-diphtheria	Repeat every 10 yr

* Persons born before 1957 can generally be considered immune to measles and mumps and need not be vaccinated. Rubella (or MMR) vaccine can be administered to persons of any age, particularly to nonpregnant women of childbearing age.

† For previously unvaccinated persons over 18 years of age, inactivated poliovirus (IPV) is preferred. Polio immunization is recommended for certain adults, including the following:
- Travelers to areas or countries where poliomyelitis is or may be epidemic or endemic.
- Members of communities or specific population groups experiencing disease caused by wild polioviruses.
- Laboratory workers who handle specimens that may contain polioviruses.
- Health care providers in close contact with a polio patient.

8. List the vaccinations that are recommended for asplenia (functional or anatomic), including patients with sickle cell disease, thalassemia, or splenectomy.

Persons who have anatomic or functional asplenia have an increased risk of fulminant bacteremia with polysaccharide encapsulated bacteria; fulminant bacteremia is associated with a high mortality rate.

- **Pneumococcal:** indicated; reimmunization should be considered 6 or more years after immunization if the person is asplenic, has chronic renal failure, or has undergone organ transplantation.
- **Meningococcal:** indicated.
- **Hib:** Consider, even in adults
- **Influenza:** recommended.

When elective splenectomy is planned, vaccination should precede surgery by at least 2 weeks, if possible.

9. What are the recommendations for using live virus vaccination in patients on chronic corticosteroid treatment?

The exact amount and duration of systemic corticosteroid administration that suppress the cellular immune system of a healthy person are not well defined. In general, steroid treatment does not contraindicate administration of live virus vaccines:

- With therapy of short duration (< 2 weeks).
- With long-term, alternative-day treatment with short-acting preparations.
- With maintenance physiologic doses (replacement therapy).
- With administration topically to skin or eyes, by aerosol for nasal or lung, by intraarticular, bursa, or by tendon injection.

Many clinicians believe that a dose equivalent to 2 mg/kg of prednisone is sufficiently immunosuppressive to raise concern about the safety of live virus vaccinations. Physicians should wait at least 3 months after discontinuation of treatment before live virus vaccinations in patients who have been on high-dose, systemic steroids for more than 2 weeks.

10. What are the recommendations for a pregnant woman who needs vaccination?

Vaccination of pregnant women is generally avoided because of unknown but theoretical risks to the fetus. The benefit of immunization among pregnant women usually outweighs the potential risk when the risk of disease exposure is high, the disease would cause a special risk to the mother, and the vaccine is unlikely to cause harm.

- **Killed vaccines.** Tetanus-diphtheria is the only vaccine routinely indicated for susceptible pregnant women for the prevention of neonatal tetanus. Previously vaccinated pregnant women who have not received a booster within the past 10 years should receive a booster dose. Hepatitis B, influenza, and pneumococcal vaccines are recommended for women at risk for infection and complications.
- **Live vaccines.** In general, live vaccines are contraindicated in pregnancy with the exceptions of poliomyelitis and yellow fever. OPV can be administered to pregnant women who are at substantial risk of imminent exposure to natural infection. Pregnant women who must travel to areas where the risk for yellow fever is high should receive yellow fever vaccine.
- **Passive immunization with immune globulin.** There is no known risk to the fetus with IG preparations.

11. Describe the guidelines for tetanus prophylaxis in routine wound management of adult patients.

Guidelines for Tetanus Prophylaxis in Routine Wound Management of Adult Patients

TYPE OF WOUND	HISTORY OF TETANUS IMMUNIZATION STATUS (DOSES)	
	THREE OF MORE DOSES	UNKNOWN OR < 3 DOSES
Clean, minor wounds		
Tetanus and diphtheria toxoids (TD) adult type	No*	Yes
Tetanus immune globulin (TIG)	No	No
All other wounds†		
Tetanus and diphtheria toxoids (TD) adult type	No*	Yes
Tetanus immune globulin (TIG)	No	Yes

* Yes, If > 10 years since last dose.
† Wounds contaminated with dirt, feces, soil, and saliva; puncture or missile wounds; avulsions; wounds from burns, frostbite, and crushing.

12. Can persons with a current or recent febrile illness receive vaccination?

All vaccines can be administered to persons with minor illness such as diarrhea, mild upper respiratory infection with low-grade fever, or other low-grade febrile illness. Most studies from developed and developing countries support the safety and efficacy of vaccination to persons with mild illness. Studies from pediatric immunizations suggest that failure to vaccinate pediatric patients with mild illness may seriously impede vaccination efforts. Persons with moderate or severe febrile illness should be vaccinated as soon as they have recovered from the acute illness. This precaution avoids superimposing adverse reactions of the vaccine on the underlying illness or mistakenly attributing a symptom of the underlying illness to vaccine.

13. Describe groups of people who should receive hepatitis B vaccination as adults.

- Persons with occupational risk of exposure to blood or body fluids (e.g., healthcare workers, emergency medical personnel, police officers)
- Hemodialysis patients
- Patients with bleeding disorders who receive certain blood products

- Sexually active homosexual or bisexual men
- Sexually active heterosexuals with a history of sexually transmitted disease or sex with more than 1 partner in the previous 6 months. (With the current effort to vaccinate all high school students who have not previously received the vaccine, a case can be made for vaccinating all sexually active adults.)
- Users of intravenous drugs
- International travelers who will live for more than 6 months in an area of high HBV endemicity and who otherwise will be at risk
- Inmates of long-term correctional facilities
- Residents and staff of institutions for developmentally disabled persons
- Adoptees from countries where HBV infection is endemic
- Household contacts and sexual partners of HBV carriers

14. Describe the general recommendations for adults who previously completed childhood immunizations and plan to travel to developing countries.

People who live in the United States or other developed nations are accustomed to an environment in which government and a high standard of living ensure the safety and quality of food and water. Animals are vaccinated against rabies, and mosquitoes and other disease-caring insects are controlled. When such persons travel to developing countries, they require consideration of additional vaccines to protect themselves. Vaccines such as yellow fever may be required for entry into certain countries, and immunization against typhoid fever, meningococcal meningitis, rabies, hepatitis A and B, or Japanese encephalitis may be recommended, depending on destination, planned activity, and length of stay. Travelers to some tropical and subtropical areas risk exposure to chloroquine-resistant malaria, dengue fever, and other viral diseases for which vaccines are not available. For travelers at risk, malaria chemoprophylaxis and insect precautions are important preventive behaviors.

Recommendations for Immunizations before Travel

IMMUNIZATIONS	BRIEF STAY (< 2 WK)	INTERMEDIATE (2 WK–3 MO)	LONG-TERM (> 3 MO)
Tetanus-diphtheria*	+	+	+
Polio[†]	+	+	+
Measles[‡]	±	+	+
Hepatitis A[§]	±	+	+
Hepatitis B	±	±	+
Yellow fever[//]	+	+	+
Typhoid fever[∞]	–	±	+
Meningococcal meningitis	±	±	±
Rabies[¶]	–	±	+
Japanese encephalitis	–	±	+

+ = recommended; ± = considered; – = not recommended.
* Yes when indicated (booster every 10 years).
[†] Travelers who have previously completed a primary series need an additional dose of the vaccine before traveling for the first time. OPV or IPV may be used.
[‡] A second dose should be given to travelers born after 1956 who travel to developing countries, have not previously received two doses of the vaccine, and otherwise do not have documented evidence of measles immunity.
[§] Active immunization for HAV should be completed 2 weeks before expected exposure. Otherwise IG is recommended.
[//] For endemic regions of Africa and South America.
[∞] Indicated for travelers who will consume food outside the international hotel circuit.
[¶] Indicated for travelers with high risk of wild animal exposure and for spelunkers.

An excellent source of comprehensive information is the annually revised publication *Health Information for International Travel*, published by the Centers for Disease Control and Prevention.

15. List groups of people who are at increased risk of contracting complicated _Streptococcus pneumoniae_ infection and who are recommended for pneumococcal vaccination.

S. pneumoniae is the principal cause of community-acquired pneumonia and second most common cause of bacterial meningitis in the United States. With an estimated 40,000 deaths/year, mortality from these diseases remains significant, especially in persons with debilitating medical conditions. Vaccination is recommended for the following groups:

- All adults aged 65 years and older
- Adults of all ages with chronic illnesses, including heart or lung diseases, diabetes, alcoholism, cirrhosis, or leak of cerebrospinal fluid
- Adults with immunosuppressive illness or conditions (e.g., HIV infection, organ transplantation, lymphoma), renal failure or asplenia (anatomic or functional, such as sickle cell disease)
- Persons living in special circumstances or settings with a high risk of getting pneumococcal disease, such as certain Native American Indian populations

Revaccination should be considered for persons who received the original pneumococcal vaccine (between 1977 and 1983) or who received the current vaccine (available since 1983) 6 or more years ago.

16. What are indications for use of immune globulin and hyperimmune globulin?

Immune globulin (human) is derived from the pooled plasma of adults. It consists primarily of the immunoglobulin fraction (at least 95% IgG and trace amounts of IgA and IgM), is sterile, and is not known to transmit hepatitis, HIV, or any infectious disease agents. Large numbers of donors, at least 1,000 per lot of final product, are used to ensure inclusion of a broad spectrum of antibodies. Indications for IG:

1. Hepatitis A prophylaxis. IG can prevent clinical disease resulting from hepatitis A virus in exposed susceptible individuals when given within 14 days of exposure. The usual dose is 0.02 ml/kg, given as soon as possible after exposure. For preexposure use for prolonged travel to counties where hepatis A is prevalent and active immunization for hepatitis A is unfeasible because of imminent departure, a high dose is warranted (< 3 months exposure, 0.02 ml/kg; for longer stays, 0.06 ml/kg every 5 mo).

2. Measles prophylaxis. IG administered to exposed, susceptible individuals will prevent or modify infection if given within 6 days of exposure. A single dose of 0.25 ml/kg (maximum =15 ml) is given as soon after exposure as possible.

Hyperimmune globulin or specific immune globulin differs from IG in the selection of donors and the number of donors whose plasma is included in the pool from which the product is prepared. Donors known to have high titers of the desired antibody, either naturally acquired or stimulated by immunization, are selected.

1. Hepatitis B immune globulin (HBIG). Recommended for prophylaxis of infants born to HBsAg positive mothers and susceptible persons with percutaneous, sexual, or mucosal exposure to HB virus.

2. Tetanus immune globulin (TIG). Recommended for people with serious wounds and < 3 doses of tetanus toxoid before the wound.

3. Rabies immune globulin (RIG). Recommended for postexposure prophylaxis of persons not previously vaccinated against rabies.

4. Varicella-zoster immune globulin (VZIG). Recommended for newborns of mothers who develop chickenpox within 5 days before and 48 hours after delivery, exposed newborns (over 28 weeks' gestation) of susceptible mothers, exposed preterm infants (< 28 weeks' gestation or < 1000 gm) and may be used for exposed, susceptible adults and pregnant women.

5. Cytomegalovirus immune globulin intravenous (CMV IGIV). Developed for prophylaxis of disease in seronegative transplant recipient patients.

17. True or false: Each year more children than adults die from vaccine-preventable diseases in the United States.

False. It has been estimated that about 1,000 children die each year, whereas at least 50,000–70,000 adults die from such diseases as pneumococcal infections, influenza, and hepatitis.

BIBLIOGRAPHY

1. Berkovich S, Starr S: Effects of live type 1 poliovirus vaccines and other viruses on the tuberculin test. N Engl J Med 274:67–72, 1966.
2. Brickman HF, Beaudry PH, Marks MI: The timing of tuberculin tests in relation to immunization with live viral vaccines. Pediatrics 55:392–396, 1975.
3. Centers for Disease Control and Prevention: General recommendations on immunization: Recommendations of the Advisory Committee on Immunization Practice (ACIP). MMWR 43(RR-1):1–38, 1994.
4. Centers for Disease Control and Prevention: Recommendations of the Advisory Committee on Immunization Practices (ACIP): Use of vaccines and immune globulins in persons with altered immunocompetence. MMWR 42(RR-4):1–18, 1993.
5. Committee on Infectious Diseases: 1997 Red Book, Report of the Committee on Infectious Diseases, 24th ed. Elk Grove Village, IL, 1997.
6. Fasano MB, Wood RA, Cooke SK, Sampson HA: Egg hypersensitivity and adverse reactions to MMR vaccine: J Pediatr 120:878–881, 1992.
7. Gardner P, Tiru CO: Adult Immunizations. Comprehen Ther 22:440–448, 1996.
8. Grabenstein JD: ImmunoFacts, Vaccines and Immunological Drugs. St. Louis, Wolters Kluwer, 1995.
9. Kaplan JE, Nelson DB, Schonberger LB, et al: The effect of immune globulin on the response to trivalent OPV and yellow fever vaccinations. Bull WHO 62:585–590, 1984.
10. Starr S, Berkovich S: The effects of measles, gamma globulin modified measles and vaccine measles on the tuberculin test. N Engl J Med 270:386–391, 1964.

66. INFECTIOUS CAUSES OF
NONINFECTIOUS DISEASES

Robert H. Gates, M.D.

1. What is essential mixed cryoglobulinemia?

Essential mixed cryoglobulinemia is a disorder caused by cold precipitable immunoglobulins consisting of polyclonal IgG and monoclonal IgM. Patients may develop purpura and skin necrosis in cold-exposed areas. Previously hepatitis B and other "occult" infections were believed to account for the presence of these immunoglobulins.

2. Current serologic and clinical response data point to what infection as the underlying cause of essential mixed cryoglobulinemia?

Hepatitis C virus (HCV). The serologic association of essential mixed cryoglobulinemia with chronic hepatitis C infection exceeds 80–90% by some reports. The positive response to alpha interferon provides further evidence for the cause-and-effect relationship. The suggestion has been made to change the name to hepatitis C-associated cryoglobulinemia.

The immune response to HCV also may include the development of rheumatoid factor, antinuclear antibodies, anticardiolipin, antithyroid, and anti-liver, kidney, and microsomal antibodies (anti-LKM) as well as HCV/anti-HCV immune complex formation and deposition. Although a cause-and-effect relationship remains to be proved, there are reports of HCV infection preceding or coincident with polyarthritis, rheumatoid arthritis, systemic lupus erythematosus, and polymyositis/dermatomyositis.

3. By definition a reactive arthritis follows an infection elsewhere in the body, often involving the genitourinary or gastrointestinal systems. Patients are frequently positive for the HLA-B27 histocompatibility antigen. What infections are commonly associated with a subsequent reactive arthritis?

Enteric infections	Genital Infections
Shigella spp.	*Chlamydia trachomatis*
Salmonella spp.	
Yersinia sp.	
Campylobacter/Helicobacter spp.	

4. *Bartonella henselae* is best known as the causative agent of cat scratch disease. Name two other conditions caused by infection with this organism.

Bacillary angiomatosis and peliosis hepatis.

5. What organism unquestionably plays a key role in the pathogenesis of peptic ulcer disease? With what other conditions has infection with this organism been associated?

Helicobacter pylori, which plays a key role in peptic ulcer disease, is also associated with chronic gastritis, maltomas (low-grade B-cell lymphomas of lymph tissues in gastric mucosa), and gastric carcinoma.

6. Of the inflammatory bowel disorders, Crohn's disease has long been suspected of having an infectious cause. Although cause and effect have not been established, what organism has been isolated occasionally from the small bowel of patients with Crohn's disease?

The use of polymerase chain reaction (PCR) has isolated *Mycobacterium paratuberculosis* with greater frequency, and directed therapy anecdotally is said to improve the clinical course of patients with Crohn's disease.

7. Infection with what bacterium may precede the development of Guillain-Barré syndrome?

Patients who develop Guillain-Barré syndrome after infection with *Campylobacter jejuni* tend to have a more severe clinical course and a more prolonged recovery time.

8. A well-known neurologic manifestation of Lyme disease (*Borrelia burgdorferi*) is acute seventh nerve paralysis (Bell's palsy). What viral infectious agent has now been highly associated with Bell's palsy?

Herpes simplex type 1 (HSV-1). PCR found HSV-1 in facial muscles innervated by the seventh nerve in patients with Bell's palsy but not in facial muscles of uninvolved patients.

9. Name the cause and best treatment for Whipple's disease.

Because of its protean presenting manifestations, Whipple's disease has been a perennial favorite for medicine board questions. It has long been considered a prime candidate for an underlying infectious etiology because of the finding of rodlike organisms with periodic acid-Schiff (PAS) stains in the macrophages obtained from jejunal biopsies of affected patients and clinical improvement with antibiotic therapy. In 1992 *Tropheryma whippelii*, an organism related to the actinomycetes, was discovered by PCR amplification of 16S ribosomal material obtained from involved tissue. A recent case series from France showed clinical improvement in 83% of cases treated with antibiotics. No relapse was observed after treatment with trimethoprim-sulfamethoxazole (TMP-SMX), alone or following a combination of penicillin and streptomycin. Diagnostic pitfalls noted included normal appearance of the jejunum by endoscopy early in the disease as well as a normal erythrocyte sedimentation rate. Because of the low risk of relapse and effectiveness against central nervous system disease, TMP-SMX is considered the drug of choice.

10. Epstein-Barr virus (EBV) has been implicated to a greater or lesser extent in the pathogenesis of what disorders?

Burkitt's lymphoma, nasopharyngeal carcinoma, B-cell lymphomas, and sarcoidosis.

11. Hemolytic uremic syndrome (HUS) may follow bloody diarrhea that most commonly is associated with the ingestion of undercooked hamburger. What is the most commonly associated infectious agent? What is the risk?

Escherichia coli O157:H7 causes about two-thirds of the cases of HUS occurring in about 10% of infected children under the age of 10. Recent attention has been drawn to vehicles other than undercooked hamburger, such as apple cider, that may transmit *E. coli* O157:H7.

12. Treatment of *E. coli* O157:H7-induced diarrhea with appropriate antibiotics lessens the risk of the subsequent development of HUS. True or false?

False. Patients treated with antibiotics have the same or increased risk for the development of HUS.

13. Match the following condition with the corresponding infectious agent.

1. Hepatocellular carcinoma	a. Human herpesvirus-8 (HHV-8)
2. Cervical carcinoma	b. Epstein-Barr virus
3. Gastric carcinoma	c. HTLV-1
4. Burkitt lymphoma	d. Human papilloma virus
5. Kaposi sarcoma	e. Hepatitis C and B viruses
6. Human T-cell lymphoma	f. *H. pylori*

Answers: 1e, 2d, 3f, 4b, 5a, 6c.

14. What agent has been suggested as playing a role in the development of juvenile-onset diabetes in the newborn by infection in utero?

Congenital rubella infection.

15. What agents have been implicated in the development of juvenile-onset diabetes in childhood?

Enteroviruses have been recovered from the pancreas of patients with recent onset of insulin-dependent diabetes, and serologic review has found IgM to enteroviruses in children with new-onset diabetes.

16. Which viral infection has been linked to polyarteritis nodosa?

Up to one-fourth of patients with polyarteritis nodosa have immune complexes containing hepatitis B antigen.

17. What are the spongiform encephalopathies?

The spongiform encephalopathies are neurodegenerative diseases typified by vacuoles in neurons and include those that affect animals, such as scrapie and bovine spongiform encephalopathy (the infamous mad cow disease), and those that affect humans, such as kuru and Creutzfeldt-Jacob disease.

18. What two agents have been implicated in the pathogenesis of spongiform encephalopathies?

Prions and *Spiroplasma* spp. Spiroplasma are bacteria that lack cell walls; they can cause spongiform encephalopathy under experimental conditions in rodents. Prions are proteinaceous infectious particles that contain no nucleic acids yet still manage to reproduce and spread spongiform encephalopathy.

CONTROVERSIES

19. Does *Mycobacterium tuberculosis* have a role in the pathogenesis of sarcoidosis?

Several investigators using PCR have found evidence of *M. tuberculosis* DNA in the tissues and bronchial alveolar washings from patients with sarcoidosis. Other investigators using the same techniques have failed to find *M. tuberculosis* DNA in such specimens. Although sarcoidosis long has been viewed as a disease with a possible infectious etiology, its pathogenesis remains to be elucidated.

20. Does *Chlamydia pneumoniae* have a role in the pathogenesis of atherosclerosis?

In 1996 evidence began to implicate *C. pneumoniae* in atherosclerosis and coronary artery disease (CAD). Elevated levels of IgG to *C. pneumoniae* were found in patients with atherosclerosis as well as in atheromas but not in the vessel walls of controls. These discoveries appeared to fit well with the observation of increased levels of C-reactive protein, a marker for inflammation, in patients with CAD and prior myocardial infarctions. Other infectious agents mentioned as possible sources of chronic inflammation contributing to atherosclerosis include herpesviruses, dental caries, cytomegalovirus, and *H. pylori*. According to most recent serologic data, seropositivity to *C. pneumoniae*, *H. pylori*, and cytomegalovirus is no different in patients with CAD and controls.

The role of *H. pylori* in the pathogenesis of peptic ulcer disease is well established. *C. pneumoniae* may be as important to CAD, but we must exercise caution lest we repeat the mistakes of the mid 1980s, which attributed chronic fatigue syndrome to Epstein-Barr virus infection on the basis of poorly controlled serologic data.

BIBLIOGRAPHY

1. Durand DV, Lecomte C, Cathebras P, et al: Whipple disease. Clinical review of 52 cases. The SNFMI Research Group on Whipple Disease. Societe Nationale Francaise de Medecine Interne. Medicine 76(3):170–184, 1997.
2. Lorber B: Are all diseases infectious? Ann Intern Med 125:844–851, 1996.
3. McMurray RW, Elbourne K: Hepatitis C virus infection and autoimmunity. Semin Arthritis Rheum 26:689–701, 1997.
4. Peeling RW; Brunham RC: Chlamydiae as pathogens: New species and new issues. Emerging Infect Dis 2:307–319, 1996.
5. Sharara AI: Chronic hepatitis C. South Med J 90:872–877, 1997.

67. FAMOUS PEOPLE WITH INFECTIOUS DISEASES

C. Kenneth McAllister, M.D.

In great deeds something abides.

J. L. Chamberlain, Brigadier General, Army of the Potomac, 1864

1. What National Football League championship lineman had recurrent abdominal infection with fistulae? What was the organism?

Jerry Kramer, Green Bay Packers. *Actinomyces israelii.*

2. What Civil War general spent more time with gastrointestinal infection than with strategy on July 3, 1863?

A.P. Hill, who suffered from amebic dysentery.

3. Name seven prominent figures who have died with HIV infection.

Rock Hudson, Liberace, Elizabeth Glaser, Perry Ellis, Amanda Blake, Ryan White, and Harry of "Harry and the Hendersons."

4. What U.S. Army post had the initial case of the "Spanish flu" in 1918–1919?

The cook at Ft. Riley, Kansas was the initial U.S. case of (H1N1) influenza during the worldwide pandemic.

5. Which army at El Alamein had more cases of dysentery?

The German Army under Rommel.

6. Match the following (each answer may be used more than once):

a. Walt Whitman	1. Died with Typhoid Pneumonia
b. Franklin D. Roosevelt	2. Syphilis
c. Peter the Great	3. Disseminated tuberculosis
d. Emily Bronte	4. Polio
e. Robert Louis Stevenson	5. Pulmonary tuberculosis
f. Jim Bowie	6. Wrote *The Wrong Box*

Answers: a–3; b–4; c–2; d–3; e–5, 6; f–1.

7. Who was the hero at Gettysburg of "Little Round Top"? With what major infections was he afflicted?

Lt. Col. Joshua Lawrence Chamberlain defended the Union Army's left wing at Little Round Top on July 2, 1865. He was said to be suffering from "heat stroke" and "malaria" during the battle. Later in his career he was afflicted with typhoid fever and chronic osteomyelitis.

8. Enrico Caruso, the renowned tenor, suffered from what pulmonary process?

Pneumococcal pneumonia with empyema.

9. Adolf Hitler had VDRLs performed on one or two occasions. What were the results? Who was his physician, and what therapy did he recommend for which primary diagnoses?

VDRLs were negative twice in the 1940s. Dr. Theodore Morrell recommended "anti-gas pills" that contained arsenical compounds after diagnosing the cause of Hitler's illness as "meteorism."

10. What illness perplexed King George of England around the time of the American Revolution?
Probably acute intermittent porphyria (vs. schizophrenia).

11. What killed Calamity Jane?
Aspiration pneumonia as a result of falling intoxicated into a watering trough.

12. Name three assassinated Presidents and their associated infections.
Abraham Lincoln—nosocomial CNS infection superimposed on gunshot wound to the brain.
James Garfield—intraabdominal sepsis following gunshot wound.
William McKinley—intraabdominal sepsis following gunshot wound.

13. Match the following (each disease may be used more than once):
a. Typhoid fever   1. Thomas J. Jackson
b. Hypertension   2. Joshua Chamberlain
c. Fatal pneumonia   3. Jonas Salk
d. Malarial fever   4. Franklin D. Roosevelt
e. Polio   5. Stephan Douglas
Answers: a–4, 5; b–4; c–1; d–2; e–4.

14. Who was the "Commerce Comet"? What maladies pained him?
Mickey Mantle suffered from musculoskeletal problems (chronic osteomyelitis) and chronic hepatitis and liver failure (he received a liver transplant in 1995).

15. What disease killed Alexander the Great at a young age?
"Fever"—a common cause of death in times of little or no medical diagnoses or records.

16. What creator of a famous children's program died of group A streptococcal bacteremia?
Jim Henson, creator of the Muppets.

17. Ludwig van Beethoven (1770–1827) had hearing loss attributed to Paget's disease of the bone. What other diagnosis was entertained?
Otitic syphilis.

18. What really killed Napoleon?
Probably intraabdominal sepsis, but other diagnoses are possible.

19. Who was Charles Hardin Holly? What caused his death? What is his greatest hit?
Buddy Holly, the innovative rock-'n'-roll artist from Lubbock, Texas, died in an airplane crash in Iowa in 1958. His greatest hit was probably "Peggy Sue/That'll Be the Day."

20. Which pulmonary infection was recently transmitted through "confined respiratory seating" on a international airline flight?
Pulmonary tuberculosis, according to a 1996 report in the *New England Journal of Medicine*.

21. What sexually transmitted disease afflicted the South's most renowned cavalry general?
James Euell Brown (JEB) Stuart of the Confederate Army developed gonococcal urethritis.

22. This noted physician is credited with the development of the modern medical training system with housestaff. His 1892 textbook of medicine remains a classic work. He suffered from a number of infections during his lifetime, including croup, osteomyelitis of the tibia, smallpox, cutaneous tuberculosis (acquired while performing autopsies), and recurrent pneumonias with terminal pneumonia yielding an empyema. The drainage of the empyema cavity caused a hemorrhage that killed him. Who was he?
Sir William Osler.

23. For trivia buffs, the following list reveals who had what when—just the thing for board games on long winter days.

1.	William the Conqueror	Intraabdominal sepsis	1080s
2.	Henry VIII Of England	Syphilis	1500s
3.	George Washington	Peritonsillar abscess	1700s
4.	Benjamin Franklin	Aspiration lung abscess	1700s
5.	Peter the Great	Syphilis (meningovascular)	1700s
6.	Frederick the Great	Gonorrheal urethritis with epididymitis	1700s
7.	John Paul Jones	Urinary tract infection with secondary pneumonia	1790s
8.	Jim Bowie	Typhoid pneumonia/pulmonary tuberculosis	1800s
9.	Napoleon	Syphilis, intraabdominal sepsis	1800s
10.	Lord Randolph Churchill	Neurosyphilis	1800s
11.	John Keats	Pulmonary tuberculosis	1800s
12.	Percy Bysshe Shelley	Pulmonary tuberculosis	1800s
13.	Lord Byron	Malaria	1800s
14.	Ludwig van Beethoven	Syphilis (otitic)	1800s
15.	Ivan I	Neurosyphilis	1600
16.	Cecil Rhodes	Pulmonary tuberculosis	1800s
17.	Emily and Charlotte Bronte	Pulmonary tuberculosis	1800s
18.	Henry David Thoreau	Pulmonary tuberculosis	1800s
19.	Walt Whitman	Pulmonary tuberculosis	1800s
20.	Robert Louis Stevenson	Pulmonary/miliary tuberculosis	1800s
21.	Calamity Jane	Aspiration pneumonia	1800s
22.	Jane Austen	Addison's disease, secondary tuberculosis	1817
23.	Charles Darwin	Chagas disease	1850s
24.	James Garfield	"Nosocomial" infection after assasination attempt	1850s
25.	Stephen Douglas	Typhoid fever	1850s
26.	Stonewall Jackson	Probable streptococcal pneumonia	1860s
27.	Stephen Crane	Pulmonary tuberculosis	1860s
28.	Elizabeth Barrett Browning	Pott's disease/lung abscess	1860s
29.	A.P. Hill	Amebic colitis	1860s
30.	J.E.B. Stuart	Gonorrheal urethritis with fistulas	1860s
31.	Franklin D. Roosevelt	Polio	1900s
32.	Oscar Wilde	Bacterial meningitis	1900s
33.	William McKinley	Intraabdominal sepsis after assasination	1900s
34.	Clarence Darrow	Mastoiditis	1900s
35.	Woodrow Wilson	Influenza/Economo's encephalitis	1919
36.	Rudolph Valentino	Intraabdominal sepsis	1920
37.	Enrico Caruso	Pneumococcal pneumonia with empyema	1920
38.	Adolf Hitler	Syphilis	1940s
39.	Eleanor Roosevelt	Miliary tuberculosis	1950s
40.	Mickey Mantle	Chronic staphylococcal osteomyelitis	1950s
41.	Red Shoendiest	Pulmonary tuberculosis	1950s
42.	John F. Kennedy	Addison's disease secondary to tuberculosis	1960s
43.	Jerry Kramer	Abdominal actinomycosis	1960s

BIBLIOGRAPHY

1. Berger SA, Edberg SC: Infectious diseases in persons of leadership. Rev Infect Dis 6:802, 1984.
2. Dale PM: Medical Biographies: The Ailments of Thirty-three Famous Persons. Norman, OK, University of Oklahoma Press,1952.
3. Fabricant N: Thirteen Famous Patients. Philadelphia, Chilton, 1960.
4. Panati C: Extraordinary Endings of Practically Everything and Everybody. New York, Harper and Row, 1989.
5. Park BE: The Impact of Illness on World Leaders. Philadelphia, University of Pennsylvania Press, 1986.
6. Sorsby A: Tenements of Clay. Friedman, 1974.

INDEX

Page numbers in **boldface type** indicate complete chapters.